HOW TO USE

This book is really two books in one. It can be used as a quick clinical reference for specific drugs or for more in-depth information about psychotropic drugs and drug classes.

Part One consists of 21 narrative chapters that provide an overview and basic discussion of the biologic bases of psychopharmacology as well as the uses of psychotropic drugs for specific psychiatric disorders across the lifespan.

Part Two contains a series of brief profiles for some of the most common psychotropic drugs, listed by generic name in alphabetic order, for quick reference in clinical situations. Clinical information and nursing considerations are provided in a consistent format for each drug.

A comprehensive index is located at the end of the book to speed your access to information.

Psychotropic Drugs

Psychotropic Drugs THIRD EDITION

Norman L. Keltner, RN, EdD
Professor
University of Alabama School of Nursing
University of Alabama at Birmingham
Birmingham, Alabama

David G. Folks, MD
Professor and Chairperson
Department of Psychiatry
University of Nebraska College of Medicine;
Professor of Psychiatry
Creighton University
Omaha, Nebraska

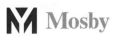

A Harcourt Health Sciences Company

St. Louis   London   Philadelphia   Sydney   Toronto

Mosby

A Harcourt Health Sciences Company

Vice President, Nursing Editorial Director: Sally Schrefer
Senior Editor: Terri Wood
Developmental Editor: Tom Stringer
Project Manager: Catherine Jackson
Project Specialist: Jeff Patterson
Book Designer: Judi Lang
Cover Design: Michael Warrell

THIRD EDITION

Mosby, Inc.
A Harcourt Health Sciences Company
11830 Westline Industrial Drive
St. Louis, Missouri 63146

Printed in the United States of America

Library of Congress Cataloging-in-Publication Data

Keltner, Norman L.
  Psychotropic drugs / Norman L. Keltner, David G. Folks.—3rd ed.
    p. ; cm.
  Includes bibliographical references and indexes.
  ISBN : 0-323-01003-2
  1. Mental illness—Chemotherapy. 2. Psychotropic drugs.
  3. Psychopharmacology. I. Folks, David G. II. Title.
    [DNLM: 1. Psychotropic Drugs—pharmacology. 2. Mental
  Disorders—drug therapy. 3. Psychopharmacology. QV 77.2 K29p
  2001]
  RC483.K45 2001
  616.89′18-dc21   00-045565

01 02 03 04 05 GW/FF 9 8 7 6 5 4 3 2

NOTICE

Pharmacology is an ever-changing field. Standard safety precautions must be followed, but as new research and clinical experience broaden our knowledge, changes in treatment and drug therapy may become necessary or appropriate. Readers are advised to check the most current product information provided by the manufacturer of each drug to be administered to verify the recommended dose, the method and duration of administration, and contraindications. It is the responsibility of the appropriately licensed health care provider, relying on experience and knowledge of the patient, to determine dosages and the best treatment for each individual patient. Neither the publisher nor the editor assumes any liability for any injury and/or damage to persons or property arising from this publication.

THE PUBLISHER

CONTRIBUTORS

Leland Allen, MD
Shelby Medical Center
Pelham, Alabama
Drugs of Abuse

Luis Bencomo, MD
Assistant Professor of Psychiatry
University of Nebraska College of Medicine
Omaha, Nebraska
Sexual Dysfunction

Teri Gabel, PharmD
Assistant Professor, College of Pharmacy
Assistant Professor, Department of Psychiatry
University of Nebraska College of Medicine
Omaha, Nebraska
Herbiceuticals in Psychiatry

Jonathan Leo, PhD
Assistant Professor of Anatomy
Western University of Health Sciences
Pomona, California
Neuropharmacology and Psychotropic Drugs

Lawrence Scahill, RN, PhD
Yale University School of Nursing
New Haven, Connecticut
Psychopharmacology for Children;
Psychopharmacology for Adolescents

Richard A. Sugerman, PhD
Western University of Health Sciences
Pomona, California
Functional Neuroanatomy;
Neuropharmacology and Psychtropic Drugs

Elizabeth Woodman Taylor, BSN
University of Alabama at Birmingham
Birmingham, Alabama
Drugs Used to Treat Extrapyramidal Side Effects

PREFACE

We developed the first edition of *Psychotropic Drugs* at the beginning of the 1990s, otherwise known as the *Decade of the Brain*. The beginning of the new millennium is an interesting time to look back and evaluate the significance of the *Decade*. Tremendous changes have occurred in psychopharmacologic interventions and, perhaps more importantly, in the approach to drug discovery. Dr. Sheldon Preskorn has described this shift as moving from a "chance discovery" approach to a "molecular targeting" approach.

The 1990s introduced unprecedented advances in the pharmacotherapy of depression and schizophrenia. Specifically, four selective serotonin reuptake inhibitors (SSRIs) were added to fluoxetine, and several newer and novel antidepressants (e.g., venlafaxine, nefazodone, mirtazapine) were marketed. As a result of receptor targeting refinement, some psychopharmacologists now divide antidepressants into seven or more categories based on distinct mechanisms of action. Antipsychotic therapy also evolved. Clozapine, an atypical antipsychotic drug, was introduced in that first year of the *Decade* and was followed by risperidone, olanzapine, quetiapine, and ziprasidone. Although it may be too early to assess the full impact of the *Decade*, it appears the call to focus on the biology of mental illness was taken seriously. Undoubtedly, significant advancements were made. We believe the *Decade of the Brain* will prove to be one of the most important periods in the history of psychiatric treatment.

Psychotropic Drugs, third edition, is divided into two parts, each uniquely contributing to an overall comprehensive discussion of chemical interventions in psychiatric care.

Part One, "Clinical Psychopharmacology," provides a narrative presentation in 21 chapters that will enable the reader to better integrate the wide-ranging nature of psychopharmacology into practice. Part One is further divided into four units, each organized around a significant conceptual theme.

Unit I, "Introduction to Psychotropic Drug Use," introduces the reader to psychotropic drug use and provides a brief historical perspective of these agents. In addition, chapters that review neuroanatomy and neurotransmitter mechanisms are so presented as to immerse those a bit "rusty" and challenge those who are more conversant with brain biology. This unit includes a new chapter on pharmacokinetics.

Unit II, "Drugs Used in the Treatment of Mental Disorders," focuses on the major categories of drugs used in psychiatric care. New chapters on dementia and amnestic delirium and sexual disorders have been added.

Unit III, "Drug Issues Related to Psychopharmacology," reviews electroconvulsive therapy, drugs of abuse, central nervous system stimulants, and drugs used to treat extrapyramidal side effects of psychotropic drugs. A new chapter on herbal medicines addresses the current needs of clinicians.

Unit IV, "Developmental Issues Related to Psychotropic Drugs," includes chapters on the psychopharmacologic treatment of children, adolescents, and the elderly.

Part Two, "Psychotropic Drug Profiles," features quick, handy profiles for 119 psychotropic drugs. This section has been streamlined in presentation but expanded in scope. It continues to provide important information in a handy format. Many drugs have been added, such as buprenorphine, citalopram, donepezil, mirtazapine, moclobemide, modafinil, olanzapine, quetiapine, rivastagmine, sildenafil, tiagabine, topiramate, vigabatrin, zaleplon, and ziprasidone. Each drug is profiled according to several selected categories such as classification, indications, contraindications, pharmacokinetics, and interactions. The combination of this feature with the extensive narrative explanation in Part One is unique among books on this topic.

Our goal at both the beginning and the end of the *Decade* is unchanged: To develop a readable, accurate, and current resource for clinicians and students. As with past editions, the third edition can be viewed as both a textbook and a reference. The reader can use the drug profiles for quick access to information and the text for in-depth study. This book is designed to meet the needs of both the on-duty clinician and the student of psychotropic drugs.

Acknowledgment

We would like to acknowledge our developmental editor, Mr. Jeff Downing. Jeff was tireless in his efforts to help us produce this edition. Jeff is young, bright, articulate, and hardworking. His skillful review of every word and his tactful but persistent approach in helping us remember that we were there to drain the swamp is appreciated. In other words, thanks, Jeff.

In addition, the authors wish to acknowledge and thank Ms. Elizabeth Woodman Taylor for her careful review of the Drug Profiles. We very much appreciate the scrutiny she gave this section. Finally, many thanks to Diana Dabney, Gina Howell, and Judy Evans for their efforts in manuscript preparation.

Norm Keltner and David Folks

Special thanks to my wife, Diane, and to Skyler and Connor who provided moral support for the project.

David Folks

CONTENTS

UNIT II

Drugs Used in the Treatment of Mental Disorders 77

UNIT III

UNIT IV

Developmental Issues Related to Psychotropic Drugs 467

PART TWO

PART ONE

CLINICAL PSYCHOPHARMACOLOGY

UNIT I

Introduction to Psychotropic Drug Use

CHAPTER 1

Psychiatric Care and Contemporary Treatment

Saugus, Massachusetts; December 24, 1840: ". . . thermometer below zero; drove to the poorhouse; was conducted to the master's family-room by himself; . . . thirteen pauper inmates; one insane man; one insane woman; one idiotic man; asked to see them; the two men were shortly led in; appeared decent and comfortable. . . . On the floor sat a woman, her limbs immovably contracted, so that the knees were brought upward to the chin; the face was concealed; the head rested on the folded arms; for clothing she appeared to have been furnished with fragments from many discharged garments; these were folded about her, yet they little benefited her, if one might judge by the constant shuddering which almost convulsed her poor crippled frame."
Dorothea Dix from her Massachusetts Memorial.[3]

The modern era of psychiatric care, including the discovery and use of psychotropic drugs, can be traced from events occurring near the end of the eighteenth century. The work of several individuals, including Philippe Pinel (1745-1826) in France, William Tuke (1732-1822) in England, and Dorothea Dix (1802-1887) in the United States, is particularly noteworthy because their efforts laid the foundation for compassionate and scientific treatment of people with mental illness. This era of treatment is referred to as *the period of enlightenment* and is considered the first of four significant benchmarks in the historical development of psychiatric care. Before this time, people with mental illness were often abused, neglected, or both.

Rosenblatt writes of the assistance, banishment, and confinement (the ABCs) of the preenlightenment era.[7] Assistance included efforts to help families cope with the problems of living with a mentally disordered family member. Banishment, or driving individuals with mental illness away from the "healthy," was a more common approach to mental illness and led to wandering bands of "lunatics," who frightened the public and stole or begged from them for survival. Just as often, however, these wandering bands were victimized by "sane" society. Confinement was the most calculated approach of the preenlightenment era. People with mental illness were often chained indiscriminately, the old to the young, men to women, the insane to the criminal or pauper, and by some accounts, the living to the dead. Confinement and the natural progression of this practice led to distorted and uninformed views of mental illness; for example, people with mental illness were thought to be immune from normal biologic stressors such as cold, heat, and hunger.[4] Whether such thinking was representative of the times or merely a rationalization for withholding resources is not documented. Nonetheless, people with mental illness suffered greatly. They were deprived of basic biologic needs, that is, shelter, clothing, and food, while their basic emotional needs also were not met. Confined mental patients, for example, were placed on display for the paying public and were forced to oblige their keepers in many vile and inhumane ways. This widespread abuse and neglect of individuals with mental illness ultimately stimulated a reaction among those who were enlightened—Pinel, Tuke, and Dix—that led to the first of the four significant benchmarks in psychiatric care.

BENCHMARKS IN PSYCHIATRIC CARE: THE ROAD FROM CONFINEMENT TO COMMUNITY

Benchmarks in psychiatric care are significant time periods during which converging forces led to a unique view of mental illness (Figure 1-1). The four benchmarks are the period of enlightenment, the period of scientific study, the period of psychotropic drugs, and the period of community mental health care. Each period represents a definite change in public perception of mental health and psychiatric problems; these changes in perception have led to new strategies and interventions to treat mental illness. A thorough investigation of these benchmarks is beyond the scope of this book. However, a brief description of the relationship between important events and the advent and use of psychotropic drugs follows.

Period of Enlightenment (Caring)

"One cannot ignore a striking analogy in nature's ways when one compares the attacks of intermittent insanity with the violent symptoms of an acute illness. It would in either case be a mistake to measure the gravity of the danger by the extent of trouble and derangement of the vital functions. In both cases a serious condition may forecast recovery, provided one practices prudent management."

Philippe Pinel, December 11, 1794[10]

The period of enlightenment is so named because reformers Pinel, Tuke, Dix, and others rejected the common reasoning of the day and initiated a humane approach to the care of people with mental illness. Affected individuals were no longer considered less than human but instead were to be treated as fellow humans deserving of adequate shelter, clothing, and food, which would be provided in a dignified manner. Pinel became superintendent of the French institutions Bicêtre (for men) and later Salpêtriére (for women). Dismayed by the living conditions at these institutions, he unchained the shackled, clothed the naked, fed the hungry, and disposed of whips and other instruments of cruel treatment. Pinel showed great understanding of his charges. His address to the Society for Natural History in Paris on December 11, 1794, readily demonstrates his vast insights into mental illness.[10] Tuke, on the other hand, developed a private institution to care for the psychiatric needs of his English Quaker brethren. In 1796, he established the York Retreat as "a place in which the unhappy might obtain refuge—a quiet haven in which the shattered bark might find a

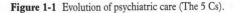

Confinement | Enlightenment | Caring → Curing → Chemicals → Community
Mid to late
1790s → 1800s → 1950s → 1960s →

Figure 1-1 Evolution of psychiatric care (The 5 Cs).

means of reparation or safety"[3] (quoted in Gollaher, 1995). Dix, an American reformer of intense religious conviction, visited the York Retreat and, upon returning to the United States, launched an effective campaign to change the treatment of people with mental illness. She played a direct role in the opening of 32 public mental hospitals.

The period of enlightenment was significant because the first evolutionary step toward a humane and scientific way of thinking was accepted, paving the way for the discovery of contemporary treatments, including psychotropic drugs. People with mental illness were now included in the human family, no longer to be chained and beaten but to be accorded dignity and access to humane treatment. This period set the stage for the period of scientific study.

Period of Scientific Study (Curing)

The second benchmark in the evolution of psychiatric care was the period of scientific study. Whereas the period of enlightenment represented a change in the way people perceived mentally ill individuals, during the period of scientific study, clinicians such as Kraepelin (1856-1926), Freud (1856-1939), and Bleuler (1857-1939) made significant contributions to the body of knowledge about mental illness. Not only were these individuals concerned with providing a humane atmosphere, but they also wanted to study mental illness and develop treatment strategies. The thrust of this period therefore was to move beyond caring to curing. Kraepelin, a gifted and thorough neurologist, carefully studied the course of serious mental illness. He laid the groundwork for those who study mental illness from a biologic perspective. Freud, through years of observation and treatment, developed an approach to working with patients—the psychoanalytic approach—which is still used and, more importantly, is the foundation for many other psychodynamic and psychotherapeutic approaches. Bleuler and others provided unique contributions to the understanding of mental illness, including descriptions of symptoms, course, etiology, prognosis, and treatment. In particular, Bleuler carefully described the symptoms of schizophrenia. Freud, Bleuler, and others laid the groundwork for those who study mental illness from a psychologic perspective.

The significance of the period of scientific study is the concerted effort of scientists during that period to identify causes and cures for emotional disturbances. The predominant approach that evolved from the work of Freud and his followers was a therapy based on dialog with patients, including psychoanalysis, individual therapy, and group therapy, which are still being used, studied, and refined today. The predominant approach that evolved from the work of Kraepelin and other neurologists was somatic, including the development of drug therapy, electroconvulsive therapy, and other nonpsychodynamic interventions.

Period of Psychotropic Drugs (Chemicals)

The milieu of theory development and scientific advances superimposed on a humane regard for people with mental illness further led to the discovery of psychotropic drugs (Box 1-1). In 1949, John Cade, an Australian physician, discovered that lithium was effective in treating bipolar illness. In the early 1950s, chlorpromazine (Thorazine) was developed and found to be effective in treating patients with schizophrenia and other psychoses. In the late 1950s, Ayd[1,2] and Kuhn[6] published the first articles on antidepressant therapy. Hence, within one decade, three major classes of psychotropic drugs—antimanic, antipsychotic, and

Box 1-1 Significant Points in the Evolution of Psychotropic Drugs

1930s	Benzodiazepines are first synthesized by Sternbach.
1948	Rapport, Green, and Page isolate "serotonin" from beef serum.
1949	John Cade, an Australian psychiatrist, reports on the efficacy of lithium in mania.
1949	The U.S. Food and Drug Administration bans lithium because of deaths in patients with cardiac disease.
1951	Chlorpromazine is developed as a nonsedating antihistamine. Laborit and others report diminished surgical anxiety in conscious patients.
1952	Delay and Deniker, two psychiatrists working with Laborit, administer chlorpromazine to a manic patient with successful results.
1952	Iproniazid, a derivative of the antituberculosis agent isoniazid, is identified as a monoamine oxidase inhibitor (MAOI).
1953	Bein isolates reserpine from rauwolfia. Reserpine, effective in treating psychosis, causes severe depression related to depletion of norepinephrine. Some suicides occur.
1954	Lehman publishes the first American article on chlorpromazine in the *Archives of Neurology and Psychiatry.*
1955	Researchers alter the molecular structure of chlorpromazine, developing new antipsychotic agents (e.g., haloperidol and fluphenazine).
1957	The first papers appear on MAOIs as antidepressants.
1957	Haloperidol (Haldol) is developed.
1958	Kuhn publishes the first article on tricyclic antidepressants in the *American Journal of Psychiatry.*
1960	Harris presents the first paper on the effectiveness of benzodiazepines in *The Journal of the American Medical Association.*
1970	The ban on lithium is lifted in the United States.
1980s	A new class of antidepressants is developed, the selective serotonin reuptake inhibitors (SSRIs).
1980s	The antiepileptic drugs carbamazepine and valproate are reported to have mood-stabilizing properties.
1990s	Atypical antipsychotic drugs that effectively treat negative symptoms are released in the United States. These new agents, sometimes referred to as *serotonin/dopamine antagonists,* include clozapine (Clozaril), risperidone (Risperdal), olanzapine (Zyprexa), and quetiapine (Seroquel).
1990s	Tacrine (Cognex) and donepezil (Aricept), drugs used to treat patients with Alzheimer's disease, are made available. Studies indicate that about 20% to 30% of cases improve. Newer drugs such as memantine and metrifonate may be available by the time this book is published.
2000	Rivastigmine (Exelon) is available for the treatment of Alzheimer's disease; ziprasidone (Zeldox) available for treatment of psychosis.

From References 2 and 6; and Rifkin A: Extrapyramidal side effects: a historical perspective, *J Clin Psychiatry* 48(9):3, 1987.

antidepressant—were discovered. These compounds significantly advanced the treatment of people with bipolar illness, psychosis, and depression, respectively.

The significance of this period was noted particularly as patients began to take psychotropic drugs consistently; the demand for observation, food and shelter, and ongoing treatment by a professional staff decreased. For example, in 1955, shortly after the introduction of chlorpromazine, state hospitals reached a peak census of 558,922 patients, but by 1997, that population had dropped to 70,000, representing a decrease of 85%.[9] Many mental health professionals believe the single most significant factor contributing to this decrease was the introduction of psychotropic drugs. The concept of the least restrictive alternative treatment milieu was a by-product of this period, and the fourth benchmark—the period of community mental health care—evolved.

Period of Community Mental Health Care (Community)

If the first three periods represent the evolution of psychiatric care, the period of community mental health care represents a revolution. A multitude of converging factors resulted in public demand for reforms in the mental health care system: films and books depicted an isolated, leaderless, and often cruel state hospital system that was perhaps contributing to the cause and perpetuation of mental illness; the promise of "talking" patients back to health was losing appeal as the public began to demand and expect faster results; and new emphasis on patient rights began to significantly affect the infrastructure of the public hospital, which previously had been immune to outside interference and criticism. However, the most influential factor contributing to the closing of many state hospital beds was the development of psychotropic drugs. As previously mentioned, patients were helped tremendously by these drugs insofar as patients were amenable to psychodynamic treatment and to other less restrictive treatment formats. Behaviors that necessitated inpatient care and locked units (e.g., agitation, withdrawal, delusions, hallucinations, suicidal ideations) were significantly relieved by the introduction or institution of psychotropic drugs. These agents enabled patients to respond more appropriately, to cooperate, and to comply with physicians, nurses, psychologists, and social workers. Because dialog with professionals occurred only a few times per week and because the aforementioned "problem" behaviors were better controlled by drugs, the economically attractive alternative of outpatient care was now possible.

Although the concept of community mental health care provides a multipronged approach to treatment modalities and levels of care, the outpatient dimension has been the approach most widely used. Today, many affected individuals, who only 40 years earlier would have been committed to a state hospital for treatment, are able to lead productive lives in or near their own homes because of the effectiveness of psychotropic drugs and community-based care.

The significance of the period of community mental health care has not yet been fully discovered. Neither the promise of psychotropic drugs nor the dream of community mental health care has been realized. The consequences of depopulating state hospitals, often referred to as *deinstitutionalization,* the subsequent rise in mental illness among an ever-growing homeless population, the overuse of emergency psychiatric services, and the flight of professionals from the community mental health arena remind us that much work remains to accomplish the objectives of the community approach. Because the promise of psychopharmacology is not yet realized, researchers continue to develop new drugs. This ongoing research and development of drugs remain critical elements in the goal to assist individuals with mental illness and psychiatric disturbances.

CONTEMPORARY ISSUES IN PSYCHOPHARMACOLOGY

Three questions seem appropriate for discussion in the concluding pages of this first chapter. The following are those three questions:

How should one study psychopharmacology?

How does one keep current in psychopharmacology?

What are the future directions of psychopharmacology?

The following material addresses these issues.

How to Study Psychopharmacology

As with students of any category of drugs, the serious student of psychotropic agents must master basic concepts to be fluent. Bypassing the basics leads to a practice based more on memorization than on understanding. Perhaps the two most important "basics" are pharmacokinetics and neuroreceptor functioning. For example, an important topic in psychopharmacology literature is the discussion of the cytochrome P-450 (CYP) isoenzymes. In fact, it is fair to say a clinician would be considered behind the times and perhaps unsafe if unable to appreciate the significance of, for instance, CYP inhibition by selective serotonin reuptake inhibitors (SSRIs). Without a grounding in pharmacokinetic principles, one would be hard pressed to grasp the full import of this system of drug breakdown.

Although most, if not all, psychotropic drugs affect neurotransmitter systems, it is becoming clear that effects on receptors may be the most significant aspect of drug therapy.[5] Stahl underscores this assertion when, in describing antidepressant efficacy, he suggests replacing the *monoamine hypothesis* of antidepressive activity with a *monoamine receptor hypothesis*.[8] Whereas all the chapters in Unit I support study of the specific drug categories found in Unit II, those chapters covering pharmacokinetics and receptor functioning may be the most critical chapters for the in-depth study of these medications.

Staying Current

Two approaches best anchor keeping abreast of developments in psychopharmacology. First, texts such as this one provide the latest information on drugs as well as foundational information for understanding basic drug paradigms. This book and similar works serve as excellent teaching and learning resources and reference entities. However, because the field is changing rapidly, additional sources of information are needed. Additional sources of information target new drugs and new conceptualizations of psychophysiology and drug mechanisms. Several newsletter-type subscriptions (with periodic updates), as well as online resources, ably serve this function. The underlying theme embedded in this section—with effort one can stay current—is heartening but requires perseverance.

Future Directions

Although no one has a crystal ball, it appears that several psychopharmacologic trends will continue, and thus those trends hold considerable promise for improved patient care.

1. *Greater drug specificity:* There will be a continued emphasis on developing agents with more specific activity. For instance, greater specificity for targeting brain receptors, neurotransmitters, second messenger systems, and/or "downstream" mechanisms will be a fundamental goal of research.

2. *Faster onset of action:* Because the delay in onset of action of psychotropic drugs is a major treatment concern, particularly with antidepressants, antipsychotics, and antimanic agents, a concerted effort to reduce lag time will be a major thrust of new drug development.

3. *Better understanding of the combined use of psychotropic drugs and psychotherapy:* Recent encouraging research supports the long-held belief of many professionals that the best treatment results occur when well-managed medications are bolstered by psychotherapy (and vice versa). It is anticipated that more attention will be focused on extrapolating the nuances of this synergy.

4. *Augmentation and combination strategies:* To provide the best possible psychopharmacologic response, more research will address chemical augmentation of agents or the development of new drug combinations.

Although the foregoing is not an exhaustive accounting of psychopharmacologic trends, these points capture four directions that, if realized, will enhance psychiatric care considerably.

REMARKS

The foregoing discussion is meant to serve as a historical foundation for the remainder of this book and to describe, albeit briefly, social and scientific factors associated with the development and use of psychotropic drugs. The four benchmarks in psychiatric care illustrate the steady movement by the psychiatric community to develop humane (benchmark one) and scientific treatments (benchmarks two and three) in the least restrictive environment (benchmark four). Those who have discovered and developed psychotropic drugs owe a conceptual debt to Pinel and Tuke for changing the world's view of people with mental illness and to Freud and the early scientists who studied mental illness and were determined to find a cure. However, the community mental health movement has demonstrated to the psychiatric community and to the lay public that drug therapy alone is not sufficient to help many psychiatrically disordered individuals. Continuing research is needed to identify more effective treatment approaches and to refine existing therapeutic interventions and techniques, including the research and development of new psychotropic agents.

REFERENCES

1. Ayd FJ Jr: A preliminary report on Marsilid, *Am J Psychiatry* 114:459, 1957.
2. Ayd FJ Jr: The early history of modern psychopharmacology, *Neuropsychopharmacology* 5(2):71, 1991.
3. Gollaher D: *Voice for the mad: the life of Dorothea Dix,* New York, 1995, The Free Press.
4. Foucault M: *Madness and civilization,* New York, 1973, Vintage.
5. Keltner NL: Neuroreceptor function and psychopharmacologic response. *Issues in Mental Health Nursing* 21:31, 2000.
6. Kuhn R: The treatment of depressive states with G 22355 (imipramine hydrochloride), *Am J Psychiatry* 115:459, 1958.
7. Rosenblatt A: Concepts of the asylum in the care of the mentally ill, *Hosp Community Psychiatry* 35:685, 1984.
8. Stahl SM: Basic psychopharmacology of antidepressants. Part I. Antidepressants have seven distinct mechanisms of action, *J Clin Psychiatry* 59(suppl 4):5, 1998.
9. Torrey EF: The release of the mentally ill from institutions: a well-intentioned disaster, *Chronicles of Higher Education* 43(40):B4, 1997.
10. Weiner DB: Philippe Pinel's "Memoir on Madness" of December 11, 1794: a fundamental text of modern psychiatry, *Am J Psychiatry* 149(6):725, 1992.

CHAPTER 2

Functional Neuroanatomy

In this chapter, the nervous system is viewed from a functional perspective. This chapter identifies many of the areas, which comprise the nervous system; briefly reviews their anatomic and physiologic relationships; and discusses one or more of their functions. It also attempts to demonstrate that, in general, the nervous system (1) contains multiple overlapping systems, (2) has highly interrelated structures, and (3) features some areas that function together more like a "committee" in producing movements and evoking emotions rather than any one specific area acting alone in controlling movements or emotions. This chapter starts by presenting the nervous system from the level of the cerebral cortex and then works its way down to the spinal cord. In this section, basic anatomic relationships are emphasized, including the organization of the spinal cord. The next section describes the peripheral nervous system, including the autonomic nervous system. Following that, the two major motor systems, the *corticospinal tract* and *basal ganglia*, are compared and contrasted. The corticospinal tract interconnects many neural structures between the cerebral cortex and the spinal cord. The discussion on the basal ganglia emphasizes its relationship with the corticospinal tract and the neurotransmitters involved in basal ganglia pathways and diseases. Olfaction, emotions, and memory are discussed in the section on the limbic structures. The last topic is a summary listing of chemical pathways and their distribution. This summary should make the reader aware of some of the large number of neurotransmitters within the nervous system and that these neurotransmitters overlap in many areas. This chapter serves as the basic reference for the other chapters in this book in terms of neuroanatomic structures and functions.*

The nervous system is artificially divided into the *central nervous system* (CNS) and *the peripheral nervous system* (PNS) (Figure 2-1). The CNS is made up of the brain, which fills the cranial vault, and the spinal cord, which lies within the vertebral canal. The CNS is often presented as if the brain and spinal cord are separate entities; however, they are logically viewed as one functional unit. For example, motor information is transmitted from the cerebral cortex down the spinal cord and ultimately to the body musculature; sensory information from the body, including skeletal muscles, ascends the spinal cord to higher levels. Integration of information takes place in association neurons (interneurons) throughout the nervous system. Integration of information means that association neurons in many areas "talk" to each other and determine how people perceive and react to stimuli, move their body parts, and think about their lives.

---

*For more information about any one of the topics covered, please refer to the references section of this chapter.

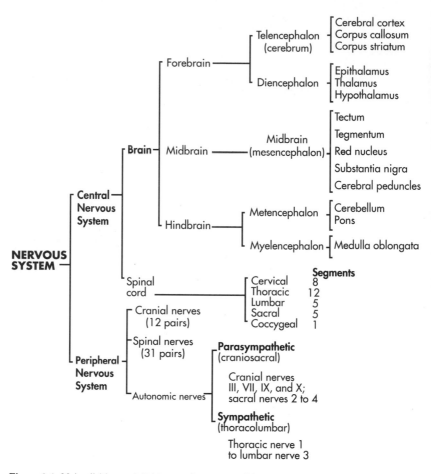

Figure 2-1 Major divisions, subdivisions, and structures of the nervous system. One can quickly determine from this figure the subdivisions of the nervous system and which structures are found in those subdivisions.

CENTRAL NERVOUS SYSTEM

The brain may be divided into three sections based on embryologic development: the forebrain (prosencephalon), the midbrain (mesencephalon), and the hindbrain (rhombencephalon). The forebrain is further separated into the *telencephalon* (cerebrum) and the *diencephalon* ("through" brain).

Telencephalon (Cerebrum)

The telencephalon forms the thick outer coverings of the two cerebral hemispheres and constitutes the bulk of the nervous system. These cerebral hemispheres are made up of the *cerebral cortex*, certain *limbic structures*, the *corpus striatum*, and a multitude of nervous system pathways that interconnect the cerebral lobes and descend into the spinal cord. The cerebral cortex (Figures 2-2 and 2-3) is divided by various authors into up to six lobes: frontal, temporal, parietal, occipital, insular (Figure 2-4), and

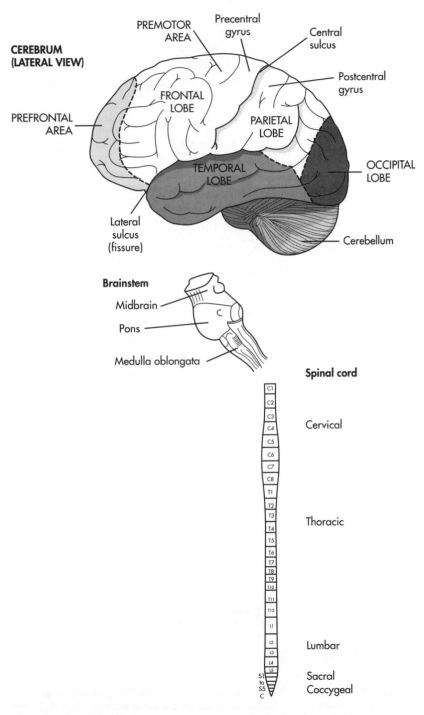

Figure 2-2 Expanded view of the central nervous system showing its major components. (From McCance KL, Heuther SE: *Pathophysiology: the biologic basis for disease in adults and children*, ed 3, St Louis, 1998, Mosby.)

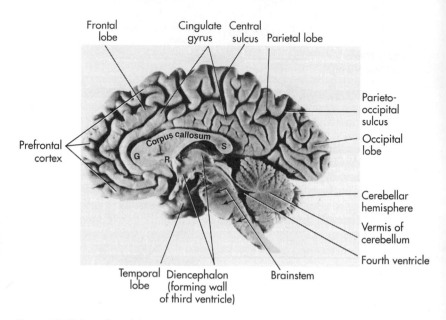

Figure 2-3 Major regions of the cerebrum, cerebellum, and brainstem as seen in the sagittal plane of this right hemisphere. (From Nolte J: *The human brain*, ed 4, St Louis, 1999, Mosby.)

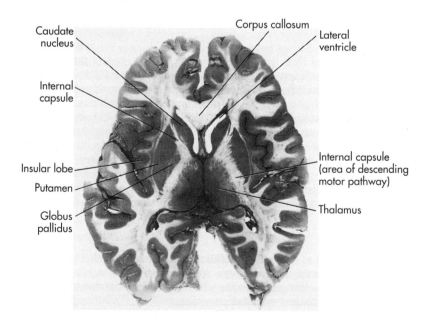

Figure 2-4 Basal ganglia and surrounding structures as seen in an approximately horizontal section. (From Nolte J: *The human brain*, ed 4, St Louis, 1999, Mosby.)

limbic (Figure 2-5). All anatomists accept the first four as cerebral lobes. The last two lobes are more controversial. The insular cortex (Island of Reil) is buried deep within the depth of the *lateral sulcus* (fissure) and is involved in visceral functions such as pain and taste. The *limbic lobe* (see Figure 2-5) consists primarily of the *septal area, cingulate gyrus, isthmus,* and *parahippocampal gyrus* of the temporal lobe, and it is involved in behavioral and memory functions. Deep in the core of the cerebrum is the corpus striatum, which is involved in motor functions and dysfunctions (e.g., Parkinson's disease), and it is described in detail later in this chapter. Neurons in the gray matter of the cerebral cortex interconnect through long and short pathways with many other CNS areas and create functional systems. These systems are involved in functions such as seeing, hearing, movement, and feelings. When huge numbers of cortical neuron axons come together, they can form some very large pathways. The corpus callosum (see Figures 2-3 and 2-4), which interconnects the two cerebral hemispheres, is a massive structure that is found inferior to the cingulate gyrus and superior to the lateral ventricles. The corona radiata and internal capsules (see Figure 2-4) are areas of white matter containing specific pathways that carry motor and sensory information, as well as other information, to and from the cerebral cortex (Box 2-1).

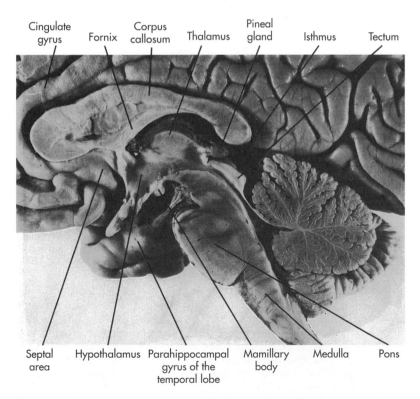

Figure 2-5 Major features of the diencephalon, brainstem, and cerebellum as seen in the sagittal plane. The limbic system, which is composed of the septal area, cingulate gyrus, isthmus, and parahippocampal gyrus, is identified. (From Nolte J: *The human brain,* ed 4, St Louis, 1999, Mosby.)

Box 2-1 Clinical Correlations

1. Surgical lesioning (destruction) of the corpus callosum to stop epileptic foci from crossing through the corpus callosum from one cerebral hemisphere to the other cerebral hemisphere results in people who have "split-brains." Split-brain studies have taught us a great deal about left- and right-brain functions.[6]
2. Classically, it is accepted that language processing is normally found in the left cerebral hemisphere and involves areas and pathways in the frontal, parietal, and temporal lobes, which include Broca's and Wernicke's areas. Recently, researchers using magnetic resonance imaging technology have identified additional areas, including an extensive area in the left prefrontal area.[3]

Diencephalon

The diencephalon (see Figures 2-3, 2-4, and 2-5) is approximately the size of a thumb from its distal tip to the first joint. The thalamus makes up most of the diencephalon. The *thalamus* (see Figures 2-3, 2-4, and 2-5) functions as the major sensory relay nuclear area to and from the cerebral cortex. People are normally conscious of sensory information that synapses in the cerebral cortex. The cerebral cortex is the site of consciousness. Part of the thalamus has input from all the sensory modalities except for olfaction. The other part of the thalamus functions with the basal ganglia in regulating gross motor movements. The *epithalamus* includes the pineal gland (see Figure 2-5), which is an endocrine gland that secretes melatonin and is involved in diurnal rhythms. The hypothalamus forms the lateral walls of the third ventricle and resides between the thalamus and the pituitary gland. The *hypothalamus* is considered the highest level of the autonomic nervous system and has both sympathetic and parasympathetic function. The hypothalamus maintains homeostasis by controlling and influencing such bodily functions as temperature regulation, food and water intake, gastrointestinal activity, and cardiovascular and endocrine activity. The hypothalamus is influenced by neural pathways from other nervous system areas and has cells that act as chemoreceptors by "sampling" cerebrospinal fluid and blood. One reason the hypothalamus can sample blood is because the blood-brain barrier is not complete in this area.

Hypothalamus-pituitary-portal system. The hypothalamus affects the pituitary gland in two ways (Figure 2-6). The first mode is by hypothalamic neurons producing either releasing or inhibiting hormones. These neurons project to the base of the hypothalamus (median eminence) and release their hormones into blood vessels that are part of the pituitary portal system. The portal system consists of capillary beds in the hypothalamus and pituitary gland, which are interconnected by a *portal vessel*. These hormones are thus transmitted to the cells in the *anterior pituitary*, where they cause either the release or inhibition of anterior pituitary hormones into the blood. The second mode is by the direct projection of hypothalamic neurons onto the capillaries in the *posterior pituitary*, and these neurons release their hormones directly into the pituitary blood supply (Box 2-2). In both cases, the hormones affect specific cells throughout the body.

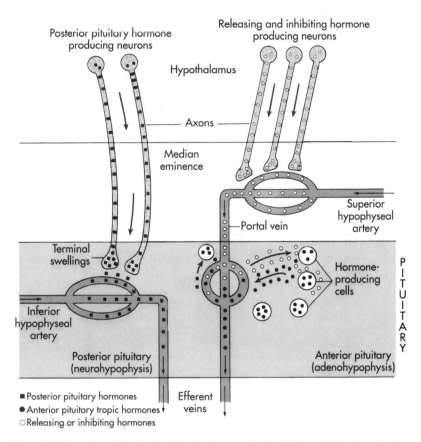

Figure 2-6 Anatomic and functional relationship between the hypothalamus, the pituitary gland, and its blood supply. *Arrows* indicate the direction and movement of hormone molecules. Note that the anterior pituitary gland receives blood from the median eminence, which contains hypothalamic releasing and inhibiting hormones. (From Berne RM, Levy MN: *Physiology,* ed 4, St Louis, 1998, Mosby.)

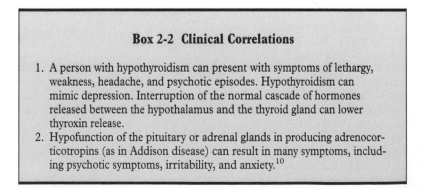

Box 2-2 Clinical Correlations

1. A person with hypothyroidism can present with symptoms of lethargy, weakness, headache, and psychotic episodes. Hypothyroidism can mimic depression. Interruption of the normal cascade of hormones released between the hypothalamus and the thyroid gland can lower thyroxin release.
2. Hypofunction of the pituitary or adrenal glands in producing adrenocorticotropins (as in Addison disease) can result in many symptoms, including psychotic symptoms, irritability, and anxiety.[10]

Lower Central Nervous System

The midbrain (which is the highest level of the brainstem), hindbrain, cerebellum (a component of the hindbrain), reticular formation, and spinal cord reside below the forebrain. The *brainstem* (see Figure 2-2) is a collective term for the midbrain, pons, and medulla oblongata. The cerebellum is an expansive area attached to the posterior surface of the pons and resembles its Latin name, "little brain." The most caudal portion of the CNS is the spinal cord.

Midbrain. The midbrain (Figure 2-7) is the caudal (inferior) continuation of the CNS below the forebrain. It is about 1.5 cm long and is significantly narrower than the forebrain. The midbrain consists of the *tectum* ("roof"), the *tegmentum* ("cover") (which includes the *red nucleus* and the *substantia nigra*), and the *cerebral peduncles.* The tegmentum forms the central portion of the midbrain. The *ventral tegmental area* (VTA) is the portion of the tegmentum between the red nucleus and the substantia nigra. As is set forth in subsequent chapters, dopaminergic tracts arising out of the VTA are important in the understanding of schizophrenia and substance abuse. The red nucleus and substantia nigra are large structures in the midbrain that are easily identified with the naked eye. The red nuclei may be seen on freshly cut brains as large, vaguely reddish, round circles and are involved in the ascending pathway from the cerebellum to the thalamus. The substantia nigra, as its name implies, is black. The black coloration is caused by melanin pigment found in neurons within the substantia nigra. This is the site of dopaminergic neurons. The substantia nigra is discussed again in the section on motor systems. The cerebral peduncles are basically a continuation of axons from motor neurons that project from the cerebral cortex through the corona radiata and internal capsule. The cerebral peduncles form prominent bulges on the anterior (ventral) surface of the midbrain.

Hindbrain. The hindbrain (see Figures 2-2, 2-3, and 2-5) consists of the pons, medulla oblongata, and cerebellum. The pons is an expansive area approximately 2.5 cm long that lies between the midbrain and the medulla oblongata. Some of the fibers in the cerebral peduncles continue into the pons near the ventral surface of the brainstem, where many of them synapse in large nuclei in the pons. These *pontine nuclei,* in turn, project their axons to the contralateral (opposite) cerebellar

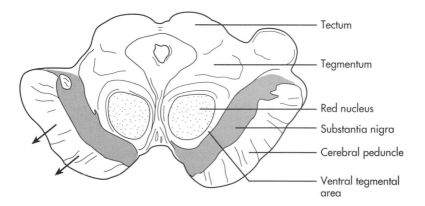

Figure 2-7 Cross section through tectum of the midbrain. The substantia nigra loses dopamine neurons, which results in Parkinson's disease. Corticospinal pathway *(arrows)* descends through the cerebral peduncle on its way to the spinal cord. The ventral tegmental area projects dopamine neurons to the nucleus accumbens (not shown). All are bilateral structures.

hemisphere. Each cerebellar hemisphere has its control over the ipsilateral (same) side of the body, while the cerebral cortex controls the contralateral side of the body.

The medulla oblongata is about 3 cm long and narrows until it is continuous with the cervical spinal cord at the level of the foramen magnum. The motor fibers from the cerebral cortex continue on the anterior surface of the medulla oblongata. These fibers are known collectively as the *pyramids* because they form two pyramidal bulges. The *decussation of the pyramids,* that is, the crossing of the motor pathways contralaterally, takes place at the lower level of the medulla oblongata and results in the cerebral cortex having contralateral control of the body. The pons and the medulla oblongata contain the central nuclei associated with the last 8 of the 12 cranial nerves and also contain autonomic control centers.

Cerebellum. The cerebellum (see Figure 2-2) consists of two hemispheres separated by a central portion called the *vermis* (see Figure 2-3). The cerebellar hemispheres and most of the vermis simultaneously receive (through complex ascending pathways from the spinal cord) sensory input from muscles and joints. They also receive motor signals from the cerebral cortex that indicate how the muscle is being directed. The various areas of the cerebellum then communicate with the cerebral cortex to coordinate the final motor activity. These cerebellar areas function to coordinate muscle synergy and activity, but they do not initiate movements. The cerebellum also functions to maintain equilibrium. The central processing of balance information occurs in a small part of the vermis and each cerebellar hemisphere (Box 2-3).

Reticular formation. The reticular formation resides within the brainstem. It comprises a discontinuous series of large nuclei located within the midbrain that extends inferiorly through the pons and the medulla oblongata, as well as through many multisynaptic ascending and descending neural pathways. The reticular formation may be conceived of as a primitive brain buried deep within the brainstem. Input from most sensory pathways synapse in the reticular formation, where it is integrated and then projected to the thalamus or the hypothalamus, or both. There are also minor motor pathways from the reticular formation descending to the spinal cord. The reticular formation is a polysynaptic integration area that affects motor, sensory, and visceral functions. The reticular formation, part of which constitutes the reticular activating system, is important to understanding the anatomy of behavior. This system and where it projects is further discussed in Chapter 3.

Spinal cord. The spinal cord (Figures 2-2 and 2-8) is approximately 42 to 45 cm long and 1 cm wide. In the normal adult, the spinal cord ends between lumbar

---

Box 2-3 Clinical Correlation

Lesions in the cerebellum can cause loss of coordinated motor movements on the same side of the body as the lesion occurs. This results in the person having difficulty maintaining balance while walking. In rare cases, dementia and psychosis have been diagnosed in patients with cerebellar diseases. The cerebellum has been shown to be involved in modulating higher functions.[10,11] The issue of whether dementia and psychoses are caused by cerebellar lesions is a controversial topic.

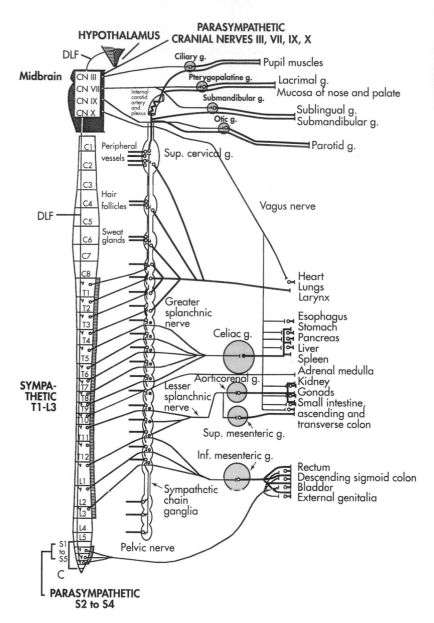

Figure 2-8 Diagram of the entire autonomic nervous system. Sympathetic portions of the central nervous system are shown as horizontally lined areas; the parasympathetic portions are shown as stippled areas. Preganglionic neurons are represented as solid lines, and postganglionic neurons are represented as dashed lines. The dorsal longitudinal fasciculus *(DLF)* interconnects the hypothalamus with the spinal cord autonomic areas. *G*, Ganglion.

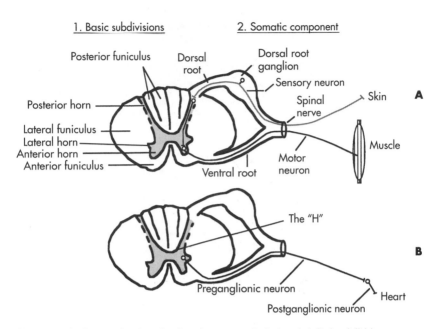

Figure 2-9 **A,** Cross section through a thoracic segment of spinal cord. *1,* Basic subdivisions of horns (gray matter) and funiculi columns (white matter areas composed of ascending and descending pathways). *2,* Somatic components of a spinal nerve illustrate a sensory neuron entering the spinal cord through the dorsal root, a motor neuron leaving the spinal cord through the ventral root, and an interneuron connecting these two neurons. The sensory and motor neurons run together in spinal nerves in the PNS. **B,** Cross section through a thoracic segment of spinal cord. Sympathetic (visceral) motor pathways are made up of preganglionic and postganglionic neurons that synapse on visceral organs.

vertebrae L1 and L2. That is why lumbar punctures are performed below L2. Internally, the spinal cord (Figure 2-9, *A, 1*) is divided into gray and white matter, cell bodies, and cell processes, respectively. The gray matter is shaped like an H and fills the central portion of the cord. The posterior (dorsal) part of the H (the posterior [dorsal] horn) is concerned with sensory information; the anterior (ventral) part of the H (the anterior [ventral] horn) is related to somatic (skeletal muscle); and the lateral part of the H is involved in visceral motor actions. The white matter is divided into posterior, lateral, and anterior areas (funiculi). In general, the posterior area contains ascending sensory pathways; the lateral and anterior areas transmit both ascending sensory and descending motor pathways. According to classical theories on pain pathways, pain information ascends in both the anterior and lateral areas.

The spinal cord is organized in segments. There are 8 cervical, 12 thoracic, 5 lumbar, and 5 sacral segments, and 1 coccygeal segment. This arrangement is reflected in the *dermatomes* of the body (Figure 2-10). For example, sensory nerves from the fourth and twelfth thoracic vertebrae (T4 and T12) subserve a narrow band from skin at the level of the nipples to the umbilicus, respectively (Box 2-4).

PERIPHERAL NERVOUS SYSTEM

The peripheral nervous system is made up of 31 pairs of spinal nerves and 12 pairs of cranial nerves. The peripheral nervous system can be divided into a *somatic* (body in

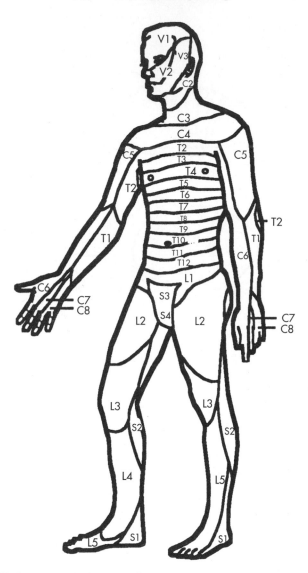

Figure 2-10 Dermatomes. Cutaneous distribution of spinal nerves for sensory input from the skin. *C,* Cervical nerves; *L,* lumbar nerves; *S,* sacral nerves; *T,* thoracic nerves; *V,* trigeminal nerve. (Courtesy Richard Sugerman.)

general) nervous system and an autonomic nervous system. The spinal nerve is considered a prototype for the entire peripheral nervous system. The spinal nerve (see Figure 2-9, *A, 2*) contains motor and sensory neurons. The motor axons originate from neurons in the anterior (ventral) and lateral horns (see Figure 2-9, *A* and *B*), pass through the ventral root into the *spinal nerve,* and terminate in skeletal (somatic) muscle, cardiac muscle, smooth (visceral) muscle, or glands. Visceral motor neurons have two neurons leading to visceral organs, whereas somatic motor neurons have only one neuron going to skeletal muscle. The spinal cord receives

Box 2-4 Clinical Correlations

1. New information concerning pain information indicates that pain information can be found in the posterior columns. Surgeons have cut the posterior columns to relieve pain in patients.[12]
2. A transection of the spinal cord at the fourth cervical vertebra (C4) results in quadriplegia, a total loss of motor and sensory functions from the level of the superior surface of the shoulders and below. A transection at this level does not interfere with the ability of males to perform sexually because the autonomic nuclei in the spinal cord below the transection are able to function without input from the brain. Tactile information from the genital area in men does not cross the transection; therefore no conscious sensations are felt.[9]

sensory information from sensory neurons. At the distal ends of many sensory neurons are specialized "transducers" that change sensory modalities like pressure into action potentials. For example, a free nerve ending when excited by a needle prick (e.g., injection) changes the tissue damage from the prick into an action potential, which is interpreted as pain by the nervous system. This information travels from neurons through the spinal nerve and dorsal root before synapsing in the posterior (dorsal) horn of the cord. As stated earlier, sensory modalities are consciously perceived if they travel through the thalamus and continue on to the cerebral cortex. The cranial nerves may be considered modified spinal nerves. Some cranial nerves are primarily motor, others are mainly sensory, and still others are a mixture of somatic and visceral, motor and sensory.

Autonomic Nervous System

The autonomic nervous system (see Figure 2-8) receives visceral input and transmits visceral motor output. The autonomic nervous system is further divided into the parasympathetic (craniosacral) and the sympathetic (thoracolumbar) nervous systems. The parasympathetic nervous system is divided into cranial and sacral portions. The cranial part has neuronal components within the oculomotor (CN III), facial (CN VII), glossopharyngeal (CN IX), and vagus (CN X) nerves, whereas the sacral part is composed of neuronal elements located in the second through fourth sacral nerves. The sympathetic nervous system is associated with the spinal nerves in a continuous column from the first thoracic nerve to the third lumbar nerve. Although sympathetic neurons originate within the thoracic portion and part of the lumbar portion of the spinal cord, they innervate visceral *effector organs* (glands, cardiac and smooth muscle) throughout the body. The anatomy of the visceral motor portion of the autonomic nerves differs from that of the somatic motor nerves. Each somatic motor neuron projects its axon out of the spinal cord and innervates a skeletal muscle. Each somatic neuron has its cell body in the anterior (ventral) horn of the spinal cord. The visceral nerve is made up of two neurons that are referred to as the *preganglionic* and *postganglionic neurons* (see Figure 2-9, *B*). The preganglionic neurons of the autonomic nervous system have their cell bodies in the lateral horns of the spinal cord or the brainstem. In the spinal cord, the myelinated axons of the preganglionic neurons join with the axons of the somatic

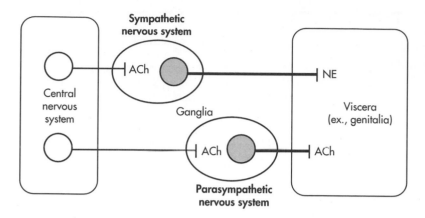

Figure 2-11 Major differences between the sympathetic and parasympathetic systems. The axons of preganglionic sympathetic neurons end in ganglia near the spinal cord, whereas those of preganglionic parasympathetic neurons travel a longer distance and reach ganglia near the innervated organ. The preganglionic neurons of both systems use acetylcholine *(ACh)* as their neurotransmitter, but at the synapses of postganglionic neurons, the parasympathetic system uses ACh, and the sympathetic system uses norepinephrine *(NE)*. (From Nolte J: *The human brain,* ed 3, St Louis, 1993, Mosby.)

motor neurons in the ventral root and leave in the spinal nerve. Many of the preganglionic axons then leave the spinal nerve to enter the *sympathetic chain ganglia.* These preganglionic axons synapse on the dendrites or cell body of the postganglionic neuron either in the sympathetic chain ganglia, other ganglia, or *plexuses.* The cell bodies of the postganglionic neurons are organized into either ganglia or plexuses. When many neuronal cell bodies are in a connective tissue capsule outside the CNS, they are called a *ganglion.* If the cell bodies are spread out, as in the wall of the gut, they are called a *plexus.* The sympathetic chain ganglia, the largest of the autonomic structures, run parallel to the vertebral column and extend from the base of the skull to the end of the coccyx. Generally, sympathetic preganglionic neurons have short axons, and postganglionic neurons have to travel some distance to their effector organs, whereas parasympathetic preganglionic neurons have long axons and postganglionic neurons are found near their effector organs.

Preganglionic neurons use *acetylcholine* as their neurotransmitter (Figure 2-11). The postganglionic neurons send their unmyelinated axons to their visceral effector organs. In general, the parasympathetic postganglionic neurons use acetylcholine as their neurotransmitter, and the sympathetic postganglionic neurons use *norepinephrine* as their neurotransmitter.

In general, both the sympathetic and parasympathetic systems innervate the same visceral organs. Sympathetic responses cause the heart to beat faster and push more blood, whereas the parasympathetic system slows the heart rate down and maintains its activity at its "normal," or relaxed, state. The rise in activity of one of these systems is balanced by the decrease in activity of the other system. Both sympathetic and parasympathetic systems function to some degree at the same time.

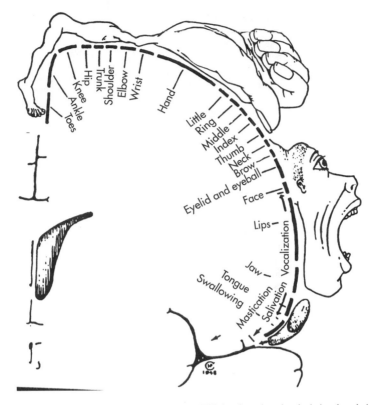

Figure 2-12 Homunculus of the precentral gyrus. This is a frontal section depicting the relative amount of cortex subserved in controlling the motor functions of various body areas. (From Penfield W, Rasmussen T: *The cerebral cortex of man*, New York, 1950, Macmillan.)

SUPRASPINAL MOTOR PATHWAYS

The term *supraspinal* motor pathway refers to pathways concerned with motor activity that involve cortical and subcortical (including brainstem nuclei) structures. The two major motor systems that are traditionally included are the *corticospinal tracts* (pyramidal system) and the *basal ganglia system* (extrapyramidal system). These systems function as an integrative whole in accomplishing motor activity.

Corticospinal Tracts

The corticospinal tract originates from the *precentral gyrus*, the most caudal *gyrus* ("hill") of the frontal lobe, with significant contributions from adjacent cortical areas. The motor strip located within the precentral gyrus is often called the *primary motor cortex* and has an inverted body pattern in the form of a *homunculus* ("little man") (Figure 2-12). The foot and leg muscles are represented on the medial surface of the precentral gyrus, and in order descending over the lateral surface of the gyrus, are the buttock, thorax, arm, hand, and facial muscles. This homunculus

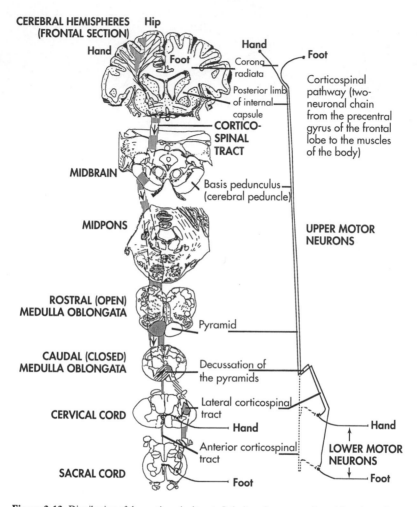

Figure 2-13 Distribution of the corticospinal tract. *Left,* Actual representation; *right,* schematic. Upper and lower motor lesions are clinical terms. Upper motor lesions (damaging the *upper motor neurons*) can result in permanent paresis, whereas lower motor neurons (damaging the *lower motor neurons*) can result in short- or long-term paralysis.

(somatotopic) organization is maintained throughout the CNS. Motor and sensory information are both organized in specific patterns throughout the nervous system.

The cortical neurons (Figure 2-13) project from the precentral gyri ipsilaterally (same side) through the corona radiata, the internal capsule, the cerebral peduncles, and the basal pons and form the pyramids at medulla oblongata levels. In the inferior medulla oblongata, about 70% to 85% of the pyramidal fibers decussate (cross) contralaterally, forming the *lateral corticospinal tract,* which ultimately synapses either directly or indirectly on alpha motor neurons in the spinal cord. Therefore the right cerebral cortex gives rise to the left lateral corticospinal tract and vice versa. This pathway controls voluntary, precise motor movements (Box 2-5). ·

Box 2-5 Clinical Correlation

A left cerebral hemisphere stroke, which involves the precentral gyrus and the premotor cortex, including the lower portion of the frontal lobe (Broca's area), results in right-side paralysis and difficulty with speech as well as possible global confusion and lethargy.[10]

Box 2-6 Clinical Correlations

1. The loss of caudate GABA neurons due to degeneration is believed to be responsible for causing Huntington's chorea.[1]
2. The degenerative loss of a significant number of dopaminergic neurons in the substantia nigra, which gives rise to the nigrostriatal pathway, results in Parkinson's disease.[8]
3. Children with attention-deficit hyperactivity disorder have been found to have significantly smaller right prefrontal cortices, right caudate nuclei, and right globus pallidi than normal children.[2]
4. A general lesion of the subthalamic nucleus can result in hemiballismus, whereas a specific surgical lesion can reduce the effects of Parkinson's disease.[1]

Basal Ganglia (System)

The basal ganglia (formerly, *extrapyramidal system*) form a group of subcortical nuclei that receives somatosensory information from the body and cerebellum and motor information from the cerebral cortex and integrates that information in a complex feedback system that modulates and stabilizes somatic motor activity.

Sensory: Body/cerebellum → Basal ganglia ← Cerebral motor information

Lesions of the basal ganglia result in abnormal motor movements such as those seen in Parkinson's disease, Huntington's chorea, and hemiballismus (Box 2-6).

The basal ganglia can be defined in several ways. A strict anatomic definition of the basal ganglia includes the following structures: *corpus striatum* (consisting of both the *caudate* and *lentiform nuclei*), claustrum, and *amygdala*. For our purposes, the claustrum and amygdala are not discussed as part of the basal ganglia motor system.*

A simplified illustration of many of the interrelationships of the nuclei and tracts of the basal ganglia is presented in Figure 2-14. The pathways, shown in the form of neurons projecting to anatomic areas, describe only general basal ganglia

---

*Because several terms are used to identify basal ganglia, this textual interruption is used to reduce potential confusion. *Basal ganglia* is roughly synonymous with *corpus striatum*.
Corpus striatum = caudate nucleus + lentiform nucleus (putamen + globus pallidus [internal pallidum + external pallidum])
Striatum = caudate nucleus and putamen

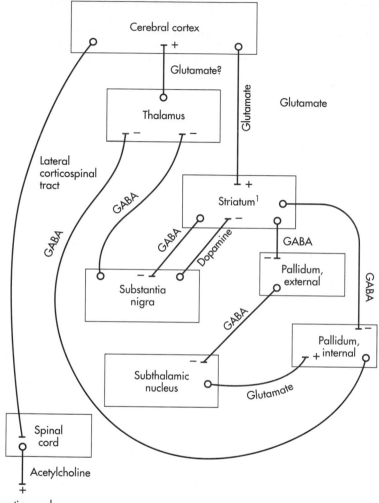

Figure 2-14 Simplified diagram of the basal ganglia and their major interconnections. The lateral corticospinal tract is the major pathway for motor movement and is modulated by the basal ganglia. [1]Striatum = putamen and caudate nuclei. The striatum also contains peptides and acetylcholine. *GABA,* Gamma aminobutyric acid; +, excitatory synapse; –, inhibitory synapse. Globus pallidus includes the external and internal pallidum.

relationships and do not attempt to represent all of the many direct and indirect basal ganglia pathways. Neurotransmitters for these connections are indicated in Figure 2-14, if they have been identified.

Neurons located in the frontal and parietal lobes, especially neurons in or near the precentral and postcentral gyri, project their axons to the *striatum* (which includes the *caudate and putamen nuclei*). These axons carry motor information, which descends through the corona radiata and the internal capsule and synapse in the striatum. The caudate nucleus integrates this motor information before projecting it to the putamen. The putamen integrates cortical and basal nuclei information before sending that information on to the globus pallidus. The globus pallidus is subdivided into an *internal pallidum* and an *external pallidum*. Most neurons within the putamen secrete gamma-aminobutyric acid (GABA) as their primary neurotransmitter and are referred to as *GABA (gabanergic) neurons*. GABA is an inhibitory neurotransmitter. The *striatonigral pathway*, which transmits GABA as its neurotransmitter, has its origins in the putamen and its insertion in the substantia nigra. The putamen also receives projections from *dopamine-secreting neurons* located within the substantia nigra via the *nigrostriatal tract*. The globus pallidus sends a significant number of gabanergic axons to the *subthalamic nucleus*, the substantia nigra (the tract is not shown in Figure 2-14), and three specific nuclei of the thalamus. The subthalamic nucleus projects *glutaminergic* neurons (excitatory neurons) to the internal pallidum and to the putamen (the tract is not illustrated).

Information from the basal ganglia passes to the thalamus and then, by way of *thalamocortical fibers*, ascends through the internal capsule and corona radiata, to terminate in the frontal lobe, especially the *premotor cortex*, which lies immediately anterior to the precentral gyrus. These cerebral motor cortical areas integrate and then help direct motor movements through the lateral corticospinal tract.

The following are the three major feedback loops within the basal ganglia:

1. Cerebral cortex ⇒ Caudate nucleus ⇒ Putamen ⇒ Globus pallidum ⇒ Thalamus ⇒ Cerebral cortex
2. Globus pallidus ⇔ Subthalamic nucleus
3. Putamen ⇔ Substantia nigra

The basal ganglia provide examples of chemical pathways that affect the stability of movement. In Parkinson's disease and Huntington's chorea, these pathways are complicated but usually one neurotransmitter is primarily involved. In the next section, the pathways and structures are involved in higher-level psychologic functions and appear to be even more complicated than the basal ganglia pathways.

LIMBIC STRUCTURES—"LIMBIC SYSTEM"

The term *limbic structures* (*limbus* means border) refers to all the structures involved in feeding, defense, reproduction, and emotional responses, as well as areas involved in the consolidation of memory. The term *limbic system* is commonly used to describe these structures as an interrelated system. However, it is not possible to describe a precise limbic system because there are many interdependent systems. Therefore the term *limbic system* has lost favor with many people in the field.[4] Limbic structures include the limbic lobe (see Figure 2-5) and associated structures. The limbic lobe, as stated earlier, consists of the septal area, cingulate gyrus, isthmus, parahippocampal gyrus, and the hippocampus. The limbic lobe is not a separate anatomic division within the CNS but comprises structures that are border areas of the frontal, parietal, and temporal lobes. The other associated limbic structures include the amygdala, hippocampus, hypothalamus (including the *mamillary bodies*), thalamus (anterior/medial nuclei), cerebral cortex, olfactory cortex, reticular formation, and striatum.

It is difficult to discuss fully in this chapter all the limbic structures and their interconnections. This chapter presents the olfactory and memory portions of the limbic structures, because they are central to the understanding of the limbic structures. For further discussions of limbic structures, refer to the neuroscience texts in the reference and additional reading sections of this chapter.

How do odors get into the brain, and where does odor information first go?

We are conscious of an odor if that information is "picked up" by olfactory receptors in our nose and that information is sent by way of the olfactory tract to the primary olfactory area (parahippocampal gyrus and part of the amygdala). The parahippocampal gyrus is located medially on the temporal lobe, and the amygdala is a large nucleus deep within the parahippocampal gyrus. Olfactory information travels from the primary olfactory area to many limbic structures.

Where does olfactory information travel to cause salivation and nausea? The amygdala sends two tracts (stria terminalis and diagonal band) to the septal area of the frontal lobe. The septal area connects caudally to the hypothalamus through the *medial forebrain bundle.* The medial forebrain bundle also sends projections to the reticular formation and *salivatory nuclei* (nuclei that evoke salivation). The hypothalamus also connects to the autonomic nuclei in the brainstem through the dorsal longitudinal fasciculus (see Figure 2-8). Following these pathways, pleasant information (e.g., food), descends from the nose to nuclei that can cause a person to salivate. Unpleasant odors descend further into the brainstem and the spinal cord and can evoke vomiting reflexes. The amygdala, hypothalamus, septal area, other limbic structures, and even cerebral cortex are all involved in interpreting what the odor is, reviewing previous experience with that odor, and formulating what visceral reactions a person will have to that odor. All of these areas are considered olfactory areas and are involved when people smell odors (Box 2-7).

Where is the memory consolidation circuit in the CNS? The *Papez circuit* forms the largest group of structures of the limbic structures. It is interconnected with many other limbic structures and the cerebral cortex of the frontal lobe. The Papez circuit forms a feedback loop within the CNS and helps in the consolidation of long-term memories and bringing rational thinking and visceral feelings together.

Hippocampus $\xrightarrow{\text{Fornix}}$ Mamillary body → Thalamus ↔ Frontal lobes
$\uparrow$ Parahippocampal gyrus ← Cingulate gyrus

It is now known that bilateral lesions of Papez's circuit, particularly those involving the fornix, result in profound loss of recent memory.[8] It is well documented that the removal of tumors from the third ventricle, which interrupts the fornix bilaterally, results in a patient who is no longer able to lay down new or recent memory. Patients

---

Box 2-7 Clinical Correlations

1. Electrical stimulation of the amygdala and hypothalamus in humans and animals can cause fear and defensive and aggressive behaviors.[7]
2. Epileptic seizure discharges (often originating from the temporal lobe) and electrical stimulation to the amygdala have been reported to evoke hallucinations or memories. Olfactory memories, such as memories associated with the smell of bread, have been reported.
3. Potentiating neuron receptors (increasing the number of receptors) makes neurons more sensitive to a transmitter. Benzodiazepine (Valium) potentiates the GABA receptors in the amygdala. When GABA is released, the inhibitory action of GABA is enhanced, resulting in the reduction of anxiety in patients.[5]
4. Electrical stimulation of the septal area in humans can evoke sexual arousal.[7]

with these kinds of injuries to the structures of the Papez circuit may have intact long-term memory, but their ability to make new memories is often severely impaired. Therefore it is thought that the integrity of Papez's circuit is vital for the ability to learn.

The amygdala and Papez's circuit appear to have reciprocal connections with the cerebral cortex, especially the frontal lobe. These pathways probably allow for the evaluation of "visceral feeling" from the limbic areas with the "cold" logic of the frontal lobe. The frontal lobes evaluate the consequences of acting on these feelings. It is likely that the violent behavior sometimes demonstrated by Alzheimer's patients may take place because the cortex in general, and the frontal lobes in particular, are atrophied as a result of neuronal death and the modulating effect of the cerebral cortex's "cold" logic is reduced or absent. All of the other limbic structures and their interconnections are not reviewed here. We hope that this brief summary of the limbic structures is sufficient to illustrate the complexity and diversity of the emotional parts of the CNS.

CHEMICAL PATHWAYS IN THE CNS

A list of the connections between CNS structures has been compiled in this section (Figure 2-15). The pathways have been grouped by the predominant neurotransmitter secreted by the neurons. This list should be used as a reference for discussions in the following text concerning drugs and their sites of action. Included with each neurotransmitter is a general statement as to whether it is excitatory or inhibitory. Please be aware that neurotransmitters can be inhibitory at one synapse and excitatory at another. Many areas in the CNS receive more than one of the eight neurotransmitters listed. Some of these pathways were presented in the discussion of the basal ganglia and limbic structures. Many of these neurotransmitters are involved in schizophrenia and depression. An oversecretion or undersecretion of a number of neurotransmitters or hormones could cause nearly identical signs or symptoms. That is why a single drug or combination of drugs might balance the system of one patient but not be as effective in another patient.

Proposed Anatomic Basis for Addiction and How We Can Use Neurochemical Pathway Information

An exciting new area concerning the anatomic and chemical basis for addiction has opened up in recent years. The *mesolimbic dopamine pathway* (often referred to as a *system*) has been shown to be very important in the understanding of addiction. The central portion of this pathway has dopamine neurons projecting from the ventral tegmental area (VTA) (see Figure 2-7) to the *nucleus accumbens* in the basal forebrain (just inferior to the caudate nucleus in Figure 2-4). This pathway can be thought of as the "anatomic bases of positive reinforcement."[5] Substances of abuse, as well as some other addictive chemicals, affect the nucleus accumbens. It has been reported that opioids in the brain remove the inhibiting pathways that modulate the VTA. The VTA then increases its release of dopamine into the nucleus accumbens, which then enhances the reward aspects of opioids. The nucleus accumbens also appears to be involved in drug cravings and withdrawal symptoms. Glutamate, GABA, serotonin, acetylcholine, and neuropeptides appear to be involved in the mesolimbic pathway. Glutamate neurons project from the frontal cortex, thalamus, amygdala, and hippocampus to the nucleus accumbens, and GABA neurons project from the nucleus accumbens back to the VTA (Figure 2-16). How all the chemicals and areas interact in this pathway has yet to be fully ascertained. This story is still unfolding,

Text continued on p. 36

I. Dopamine Projections: Inhibitory

A. MIDBRAIN:

1. Mesolimbic pathway
   Ventral tegmental
   area → Nucleus accumbens, amygdala, lateral septal nuclei, striatum

2. Mesocortical pathway
   Ventral tegmental
   area → Prefrontal cortex, anterior cingulate gyrus, entorhinal cortex (limbic area)

3. Nigrostriatal pathway
   Substantia nigra → Putamen and caudate nuclei

B. HYPOTHALAMUS:
(Tuberoinfundibular pathway)

Hypothalamus →
- Median eminence of hypothalamus; intermediate pituitary
- Dorsal and rostral hypothalamus
- Lateral septal area
- Spinal cord
- Thalamus

II. Norepinephrine Projections: Inhibitory

Locus ceruleus
(midbrain)

Dorsal bundle → Entire neocortex; amygdala; olfactory tubercle; hippocampus; spinal cord

Ventral bundle → Midbrain; entire hypothalamus; preoptic area; nucleus stria terminalis

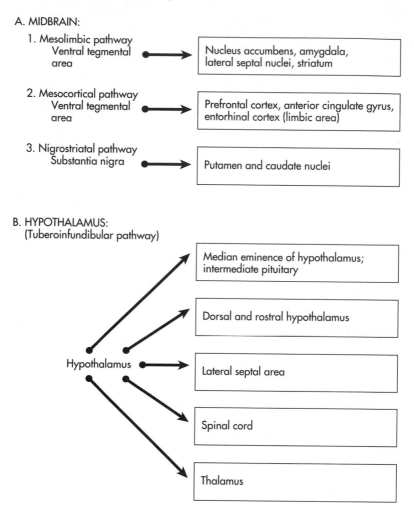

Figure 2-15 A diagram of major neurotransmitter pathways.
Continued

III. Serotonin Projections: Excitatory

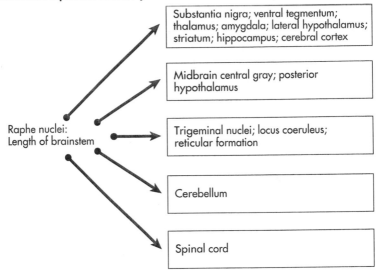

Raphe nuclei:
Length of brainstem

- Substantia nigra; ventral tegmentum; thalamus; amygdala; lateral hypothalamus; striatum; hippocampus; cerebral cortex
- Midbrain central gray; posterior hypothalamus
- Trigeminal nuclei; locus coeruleus; reticular formation
- Cerebellum
- Spinal cord

IV. Acetylcholine Projections: Excitatory

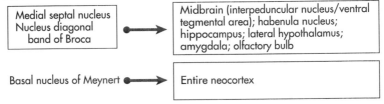

Basal forebrain:

| Medial septal nucleus
Nucleus diagonal band of Broca | → | Midbrain (interpeduncular nucleus/ventral tegmental area); habenula nucleus; hippocampus; lateral hypothalamus; amygdala; olfactory bulb |

Basal nucleus of Meynert ⟶ Entire neocortex

V. Gamma-Aminobutyric Acid (GABA) Projections: Inhibitory

1. Local projections:

   Many of the GABA neurons affect other neurons locally. In the central nervous system, 30% of the synapses in nuclei and gray matter secrete GABA.

2. Long projections:

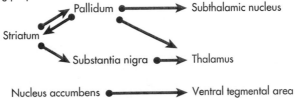

Pallidum ⟷ Subthalamic nucleus
Striatum
Substantia nigra ⟶ Thalamus
Nucleus accumbens ⟶ Ventral tegmental area

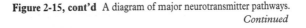

Figure 2-15, cont'd A diagram of major neurotransmitter pathways.
Continued

VI. Glutamate Projections: Excitatory

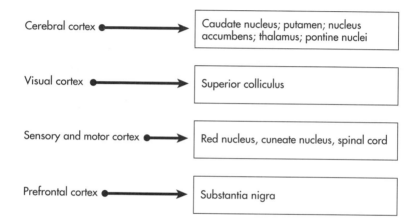

Cerebral cortex ⟶ Caudate nucleus; putamen; nucleus accumbens; thalamus; pontine nuclei

Visual cortex ⟶ Superior colliculus

Sensory and motor cortex ⟶ Red nucleus, cuneate nucleus, spinal cord

Prefrontal cortex ⟶ Substantia nigra

VII. Aspartate Projections: Excitatory

Widely distributed throughout the central nervous system

⟶

VIII. Glycine Projections: Inhibitory/excitatory

Many of the glycine neurons affect other neurons locally

Figure 2-15, cont'd A diagram of major neurotransmitter pathways.

Mesolimbic System

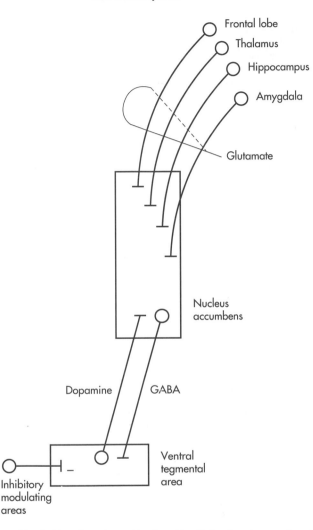

Figure 2-16 Mesolimbic pathway (system) has been identified as the primary pathway involved in substance abuse. The ventral tegmental area projects dopamine neurons to the nucleus accumbens. Opioids inhibit the modulating areas that affect the VTA and allow increased amounts of dopamine to be released into the nucleus accumbens, enhancing the reward aspects of the opioids. Glutamate neurons from the prefrontal cortex, thalamus, and hippocampus project to the nucleus accumbens. There is also a GABA pathway from the nucleus accumbens to the ventral tegmental area. This is a more complicated system than this diagram indicates.

and it is hoped that future findings will produce new methods of treatment for substance abuse patients.

REFERENCES

1. Adams RD, Victor M, Ropper AH: *Principles of neurology,* ed 6, New York, 1997, McGraw-Hill.
2. Barkley RA: Attention-deficit hyperactivity disorder, *Sci Am* 279:66, 1998.
3. Binder JR, and others: Human brain language areas identified by functional magnetic resonance imaging, *J Neuroscience* 17(1):353, 1997.
4. Brodal P: *The central nervous system,* ed 2, Oxford, 1998, Oxford University Press.
5. Charney DS, Nestler EJ, Bunney BS: *Neurobiology of mental illness,* New York, 1999, Oxford University Press.
6. Ganzzaniga MS: The split brain revisited, *Sci Am* 279:50, 1998.
7. Isaacson RL: *The limbic system,* New York, 1982, Plenum.
8. Kiernan JA: *Barr's the human nervous system: an anatomical viewpoint,* ed 7, Philadelphia, 1998, JB Lippincott.
9. Rampin O, Bernabe J, Giulinao F: Spinal control of penile erection, *World J Urol* 15:2, 1997.
10. Rowland LP: *Merritt's textbook of neurology,* ed 7, Philadelphia, 1983, Lea & Febiger.
11. Schmahmann JD, Sherman JC: The cerebellar cognitive affective syndrome, *Brain* 121:561, 1998.
12. Willis WD, and others: A visceral pain pathway in the dorsal column of the spinal cord, *Proc Natl Acad Sci USA* 96:7675, 1999.

ADDITIONAL READING

Berne RM, Levy MN: *Physiology,* ed 3, St Louis, 1993, Mosby.

Crill WE: The milieu of the central nervous system. In HD Patton, and others, editors: *Textbook of physiology,* vol 1, Philadelphia, 1989, WB Saunders.

Doane BK, Livingston KF, editors: *The limbic system: functional organization and clinical disorders,* New York, 1983, Raven.

Franck JAE, and others: The limbic system. In HD Patton, and others, editors: *Textbook of physiology,* vol 1, Philadelphia, 1989, WB Saunders.

Khan AU: *Neurochemistry of schizophrenia & depression,* Clover, 1998, AJ Publisher.

Lindsley DF, Holmes JE: *Basic human neurophysiology,* New York, 1984, Elsevier.

McCance KL, Heuther SE: *Pathophysiology: the biologic basis for disease in adults and children.* St Louis, 1998, Mosby.

McGinty JF, editor: Advancing from the ventral striatum to the extended amygdala: implications for neuropsychiatry and drug abuse, *Ann New York Acad Sci* vol 877, 1998.

Narabayashi H: Stereotaxic vim thalamotomy for treatment of tremor, *Eur Neurol* 29:29, 1989.

Neuwelt EA, editor: Implications of the blood-brain barrier and its manipulation, vol 2, *Clinical aspects,* New York, 1989, Plenum.

Nolte J: *The human brain: an introduction to its fundamental anatomy,* ed 3, St Louis, 1993, Mosby.

Papez JW: A proposed mechanism of emotion, *Arch Neurol Psychiatry* 38:725, 1937.

Pritchard TC, Alloway KD: *Medical neuroscience,* Madison, 1999, Fence Creek Publishers.

Rowland LP: Blood-brain barrier, cerebrospinal fluid, brain edema, and hydrocephalus. In Kandel ER, Schwartz JH, editors: *Principles of neural science,* New York, 1985, Elsevier.

Siegel GJ, and others, editors: *Basic neurochemistry,* ed 6, Philadelphia, 1999, Lippincott-Raven.

Squire LR: Mechanisms of memory, *Science* 232:1612, 1986.

CHAPTER 3

The Pharmacokinetic Basis
of Therapeutics

The primary objectives of drug therapy are to prevent and cure disease. Often, these goals are not achievable, and the secondary objectives are to use drugs to mitigate the progressive, devastating, or disabling aspects of disease. The nature of the disease determines the amount of drug or drugs to be given and the duration of therapy. This chapter discusses the fate of drugs and the absorption, distribution, binding, biotransformation, and excretion of drugs and their metabolites in the body. This chapter also focuses on drug interactions, with particular emphasis on cytochrome P-450 isoenzymes and their induction or inhibition, which leads to interference with drug metabolism. In addition, age-related issues pertinent to the geriatric patient are discussed briefly. For further discussion of psychopharmacology for geriatric patients, see Chapter 21.

Appropriate drug therapy can improve the quality of life, whereas injudicious drug therapy may be harmful. Medications are given for a variety of diagnostic, prophylactic, and therapeutic purposes. Prescribed medications bring about desired effects in most patients, but they may also prove to be inert and ineffective in some cases. They may even evoke totally unexpected responses and precipitate serious reactions.

The use of drugs in the treatment of disease is termed *pharmacotherapeutics*. However, the use of drugs is not always necessary in managing a disease. A drug may be used substitutively, supportively, prophylactically, symptomatically, diagnostically, or correctively. Drugs may eliminate or reduce the symptoms of a disease without influencing the actual pathologic condition. A drug may be used to diagnose a disease. In most cases, drugs do not cure diseases, but rather, they ease or eliminate the associated symptoms. In alleviating symptoms, drugs may also induce adverse effects, which may or may not be acceptable to a patient.

PHARMACOKINETIC PRINCIPLES

Pharmacokinetic principles address the absorption, distribution, biotransformation (metabolism), and excretion (elimination) of drugs and their metabolites (Figure 3-1).

Absorption

Absorption is defined as the movement of the drug from its administrative site to the bloodstream. The *oral* absorption of drugs entails multiple physical and chemical factors that influence the rate and extent to which drugs are absorbed. Drug particle size may compromise the rate of dissolution of a drug that increases significantly as the size of the drug particle decreases. The more soluble drugs are absorbed faster and more completely than are relatively insoluble ones. The oral bioavailability of numerous drugs has been increased by a reduction in particle size.

Sites of administration of drugs

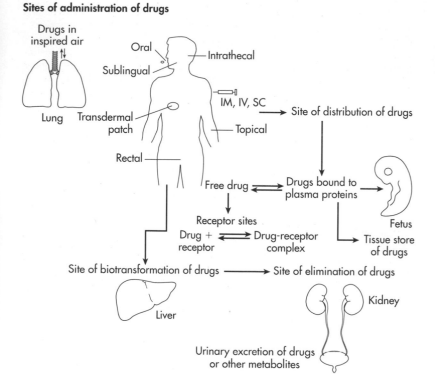

Figure 3-1 Pharmacokinetic basis of therapeutics. *IM,* Intramuscular; *IV,* intravenous; *SC,* subcutaneous. (Adapted from Ebadi M: *Pharmacology, an illustrative review with questions and answers,* ed 3, Philadelphia, 1996, Lippincott-Raven Press.)

Buccal and *sublingual* absorption compared with other routes of administration offer advantages that include the following:
1. Being noninvasive
2. Producing a rapid onset of action
3. Providing high blood levels
4. Preventing first-pass effects
5. Circumventing the exposure of drugs to the acidic and digestive fluid of the stomach

In addition, drugs may be easily applied, sufficiently localized, and if necessary readily retrieved.

The *intranasal* route of administration is best for drugs that either undergo extensive degradation or are poorly absorbed after oral administration. Drugs that are routinely administered intranasally include peptides, such as vasopressin, and more recently, nicotine.

The *oral* administration of drugs, which is the route of choice, is sometimes impractical or impossible to use under certain circumstances such as conditions in which an individual has severe nausea and vomiting, in patients with convulsions, just before surgery, and in uncooperative patients. The *rectal* route is desirable in some of these cases.

Ionization. Ionization is the degree of disassociation of drugs and the pH of the internal medium, which play an important role in the transfer of drugs across biologic membranes. Most drugs are either weak acids or bases. Therefore, in solution, they exist in nonionized and ionized forms. The nonionized forms of various compounds are more lipid-soluble and can penetrate the cellular membranes. The rate of passage of many drugs across various membranes becomes a function of the dissociation constant (pKa) of the drug and the pH of the internal medium. For example, phenytoin, an acid with a pKa of 8.3, is insoluble at the pH of gastric juice (i.e., 2.0) and is absorbed from the upper part of the intestinal tract.

Surface area. Because both ionized and nonionized drugs are absorbed from subcutaneous and intramuscular sites of injection, ionization does not appear to play as important a role in the passage of drugs across the capillary wall. Although drugs such as acetylsalicylic acid are best absorbed from an acidic medium such as that in the stomach, most of the aspirin is nevertheless absorbed in the upper small intestine, which has a considerably greater absorptive surface area. Similarly, the perfusion rate of the intestine is considerably greater than that of the stomach. In fact, most drugs, whether ionized or not, and whether acidic, basic, or neutral, are absorbed mostly from the small intestine. Consistent with this is the observation that buffered acetylsalicylic acid preparations are dissolved faster and are absorbed better in the intestine. Similarly, patients with achlorhydria (absence of hydrochloric acid in the stomach) or those who have undergone gastrectomy have little difficulty with the absorption of orally ingested drugs.

Blood flow. The absorption of drugs in solution from intramuscular and subcutaneous sites of injection is limited by the perfusion rate. Increasing the blood flow enhances the absorption of drugs, whereas decreasing the blood flow reduces absorption. Massaging the site where a drug has been administered therefore increases the rate of absorption. Placing an ice pack on the site retards it. One may take advantage of this concept and deliberately retard the absorption of drugs by reducing the peripheral circulation. For instance, local anesthetics are often combined with epinephrine, a vasoconstricting substance, and injected as a mixture. The vasoconstriction causes a bloodless field of operation. Epinephrine prevents the rapid absorption of local anesthetics and thus both enhances their duration of action and prevents systemic toxicity.

Gastric emptying time. Because drugs are mostly absorbed from the upper part of the small intestine, the rate of gastric emptying time plays a crucial role in drug absorption. If absorption is desired, drugs should be taken on an empty stomach. Meals, especially those with a high fat content, retard absorption. The desire for rapid absorption of drugs necessitates that the interactions between food and drugs be monitored carefully.

Hepatic first-pass effect. Several mechanisms account for the development of an inadequate plasma concentration of a drug and its active metabolites following oral administration. By far, the most important reason for an inadequate plasma concentration after the oral administration of a drug is the first-pass effect, which is the loss of a drug as it passes through the liver for the first time. For example, nitroglycerine, which is used in the management of patients with angina pectoris, is given sublingually. Taken orally, nitroglycerine is rapidly inactivated in the liver, and the resulting concentration is inadequate to be of immediate value to the patient.

Sublingually administered nitroglycerine bypasses the liver and enters the superior vena cava, whereupon it profuses the coronary circulation.

Distribution

Distribution is defined as movement of the drug from the blood to the rest of the body. Important distribution issues include blood flow and protein binding (which affects the drug leaving the bloodstream). Other significant functions discussed here are the site of action, potency and efficacy, affinity and intrinsic activity, and physiologic and pharmacologic antagonism of drugs.

Blood flow. For a drug to have an effect, it must reach the site in question. Typically, this is done via the circulatory system. Most tissue has adequate blood supply, and because no cell is more than two cells away from a capillary, a drug molecule is always close to the intended site of action. However, drug molecules may not be free to enter the extracellular space due to protein binding.

Binding of various drugs to plasma proteins. In an ideal therapeutic regimen, a sufficient amount of the drugs should reach the locus of action (receptor site) to bring about the desired effect, but not so much as to produce toxicity. Furthermore, the drugs should not disappear too rapidly from the locus of action, or their therapeutic effects will be transient and hence of limited value. The binding of drugs to plasma proteins and various subcellular components tends to accomplish these objectives. Human plasma contains more than 60 different proteins. The most abundant one is albumin.

The percentage of protein-binding drugs at therapeutic levels varies dramatically. Some drugs, such as allopurinol, heparin, and isoniazid, do not become bound. Other drugs, such as theophylline, become bound to the extent of only 4% to 15%. Some drugs, such as dicumarol and diazepam, are bound extensively to plasma proteins at levels of 97% or more. The binding sites of proteins are not unlimited and are subject to saturation. When this occurs, toxicity may develop following further drug administration because the latter portion of the drug remains free. Consistent with this view is the observation that toxic manifestations of drugs are quite common and considerably higher in individuals who have hypoalbuminemia or altered plasma and tissue protein concentrations, or both. The intensity of the effect of a displaced drug on a patient will simply depend on the blood level of a free drug and its nature. At times, the effect may be highly undesirable and even fatal. For example, displacement of a highly bound drug, such as dicumarol, an oral anticoagulant, which has great affinity for binding sites, can cause serious hemorrhage. Because only 3% of the anticoagulant is free, an additional displacement of 3% increases its effects by 100%.

The site of action of drugs. Most drugs exert their potent and specific effects by forming a bond, generally reversible, with a cellular component called a *receptor site*, which should be differentiated from acceptor or silent sites where drugs are stored. Drugs that interact with a receptor and elicit a response are called *agonists*. Drugs that interact with receptors and prevent the action of agonists are termed *antagonists*. For example, acetylcholine, which causes bradycardia, is an agonist; atropine, which blocks the action of acetylcholine and prevents bradycardia, is an antagonist.

Potency and efficacy. The relative effects of drugs are often judged in terms of their potency (a measure of the dosage required to bring about a response) and their efficacy (a measure of their inherent ability to exert an effect). When the pharmacologic properties of two compounds are compared, one may prove to be more potent and efficacious than the other. For example, morphine is more efficacious than aspirin. On the other hand, two compounds may be equally efficacious, but one could be more potent. Haloperidol and chlorpromazine are both efficacious neuroleptics in the management of schizophrenia, but haloperidol is more potent.

Affinity and intrinsic activity. A drug's affinity and intrinsic activity also need to be differentiated. *Intrinsic activity* refers to a drug's ability to bind to the receptor, which results in pharmacologic actions. Affinity is a measure of the degree to which a drug binds to the receptor whether it exerts a pharmacologic action (as an agonist) or simply blocks the receptor (as an antagonist).

Pharmacologic and physiologic antagonism. If two drugs, one an agonist and the other an antagonist, bind to an identical receptor site, either producing or preventing an effect, this association is called *pharmacologic antagonism.* Naloxone, atropine, and diphenhydramine are pharmacologic and specific antagonists of morphine, acetylcholine, and histamine at their respective receptor sites. In *physiologic antagonism,* the drugs do not bind to the same receptor sites but produce functionally opposite results. For example, histamine produces vasodilation, whereas epinephrine produces vasoconstriction; however, they interact with two separate receptor sites. Physiologic antagonism is used extensively in medicine, especially in overcoming the toxicity of pharmacologic agents. For instance, diazepam (Valium) may be used to overcome the central nervous system (CNS) excitation produced by physostigmine, an acetylcholinesterase inhibitor, which results in an increased acetylcholine concentration. Diazepam overcomes the acetylcholine-mediated CNS excitation by enhancing the activity of GABA, an inhibitory neurotransmitter.

Biotransformation (Metabolism)

Biotransformation may be defined as the enzyme-catalyzed alteration of drugs by the living organism. Although few drugs are eliminated unchanged, urinary excretion is a negligible means of terminating the action of most drugs or poisons in the body. As a matter of fact, the urinary excretion of a highly lipid-soluble substance, such as pentobarbital, would be so slow that it would take the body a century to rid itself of a single dose of the agent. Therefore mammalian animals have developed systems that allow the conversion of most lipid-soluble substances to water-soluble ones so that they may be easily excreted by the kidney.

Factors that modify the metabolism of drugs. Many environmental factors and pathophysiologic conditions inhibit or stimulate the activity of drug-metabolizing enzymes and hence may alter the outcome of a therapeutic regimen. Pharmacogenetics, the immaturity of drug-metabolizing enzyme systems, and the drug-drug interactions are a few of the factors that have been shown to alter drug metabolism.

Pharmacogenetics represents the study of the hereditary variation of the handling of drugs. Pharmacogenetic abnormalities may be entirely innocuous until the affected individual is challenged with particular drugs.

The liver is the principle metabolic organ, and hepatic disease or dysfunction may impair drug elimination. Any alteration in the serum albumin or bilirubin levels indicates impaired liver function. Similarly, skin bruising and bleeding tendency indicate decreased production of clotting factors by the liver.

The influence of age. Drug metabolism is qualitatively and quantitatively deficient in newborns. For example, chloramphenicol toxicity may occur in a newborn who fails to conjugate chloramphenicol with glucuronic acid because of inadequate activity of hepatic glucuronyl transferase. Thus a newborn should receive lower-than-usual dosages of chloramphenicol (i.e., 25 to 50 mg/kg of body weight). The elderly are also prone to toxicity from numerous drugs, including cardiac glycosides. A dose of digitoxin, which may be totally therapeutic and innocuous for a patient at age 60, may produce severe toxicity and even death in the same patient at age 70. In short, the ability of the liver to metabolize drugs and of the kidney to excrete metabolites declines with age.

Enzyme induction and inhibition. The activities of microsomal drug-metabolizing enzymes in humans can be enhanced by altering the levels of endogenous hormones, such as androgens, estrogens, progestational steroids, glucocorticoids, anabolic steroids, norepinephrine, insulin, and thyroxine. This effect can also be elicited by the administration of exogenous substances such as drugs, food, preservatives, coloring agents, insecticides, volatile oils, urea herbicides, and polycyclic aromatic hydrocarbons.

Patients are often given several drugs at the same time. The possibility that one drug may accelerate or inhibit the metabolism of another should always be kept in mind. When this phenomenon occurs (multiple drug use), the removal of an enzyme inducer could be hazardous. In some cases, a drug may induce its own metabolism, which results in a lower plasma level of the drug, which may affect its relative effects or side effects. For example, long-term treatment with drugs such as chlorpromazine or phenobarbital, which stimulate their own metabolism, should be expected to result in decreased effectiveness and decreased toxicity over time.

Excretion (Elimination)

Excretion is defined as removal of the drug from the body.

Renal excretion of drugs. An orally administered drug will gradually begin to be absorbed. As the amount of drug in the body increases by 50%, the amount of the drug at the absorption site should decrease by the same amount. The absorbed drug will gradually be metabolized or excreted, mostly by the kidneys.

Besides the renal elimination, drugs and their metabolites are eliminated in bile, breast milk, and perspiration, as well as by the lungs. The excretion of drugs into breast milk may be a significant concern during lactation, and the excretion of drugs, especially gaseous anesthetics from the lungs, also becomes important in specialized circumstances.

The amount of the drug and/or its metabolites that appear in the urine depends on the amount of drug undergoing glomerular filtration, tubular secretion, and tubular resorption. Metabolism plays a major role in drug excretion because the metabolic process causes drugs to be more water-soluble substances and thus more readily excreted. Drugs are excreted when they are in free form, but plasma protein-bound drugs and tissue-stored drugs are not excreted. The excretion of drugs from the kidneys, like the absorption of drugs from the gastrointestinal tract, depends on lipid solubility, the degree of ionization of drugs, and the pH of the urine. Nonionized lipid-soluble drugs are resorbed and not eliminated. Generally, drugs that are bases are excreted when the urine is acidic, whereas acidic compounds are excreted in greater quantities if the urine is alkaline. For example, in phenobarbital (weak acid and a pKa of 7.3) poisoning, alkalinization of the urine with sodium bicarbonate is helpful in eliminating the phenobarbital. In amphetamine toxicity, acidification of the urine with ammonium chloride is useful.

Significance of blood flow on drug clearance. In general, the rate of extraction of a drug from the blood and the rate of clearance by the kidney depend on blood flow and the ability of the kidney to extract the drug (the extraction ratio). If all of the drug is removed as it traverses the kidneys, the extraction ratio is 1. The higher the blood flow, the higher the rate of excretion of the drug, and the clearance is said to be profusion-rate limited. For example, the extraction ratio of digoxin—one of the cardiac glycosides—is low, and toxicity is likely to occur in those with renal failure. Similarly, the hepatic extraction of digitoxin is low, and toxicity is likely to occur in those with hepatic failure. Consequently, cardiologists have long recognized that digitoxin and digoxin should be avoided in patients who have liver and renal failure, respectively.

Half-life of a drug. The half-life of a drug, or its elimination half-life, is the time required for its concentration in the blood to be reduced by one half. Both the intravenously and orally administered identical drugs have the same half-lives once they reach the general circulation. When given at regular intervals, a drug or its metabolite reaches a plateau concentration after approximately 4 to 5 half-lives. This plateau changes only if the dose, frequency of administration, or both are altered.

PHARMACODYNAMIC PRINCIPLES

Pharmacodynamics may be defined as the study of the actions and effects of drugs on organ tissue cellular and subcellular levels. Therefore pharmacodynamics provides information about how drugs bring about their beneficial effects and how they cause their side effects. By understanding and applying the knowledge gained in studying pharmacodynamics, clinicians are able to provide effective and safe therapeutic care to their patients (Figure 3-2). Pharmacodynamics considers the sites, modes, and mechanisms of actions of drugs. For example, if a patient with multiple fractures receives a subcutaneous injection of 10 to 15 mg of morphine, analgesia, sedation, respiratory depression, emesis, myosis, suppression of the gastrointestinal tract, and oliguria may ensue. These diversified effects occur at multiple peripheral and central sites and through the influence of numerous modes and mechanisms of action.

Site of Action

The receptor site, where a drug acts to initiate a group of functions, is that drug's site of action. For example, the central site of action of morphine includes the cerebral cortex, hypothalamus, and medullary center.

Mode of Action

The character of an effect produced by the drug is called the *mode of action* of that drug. Morphine, by depressing the function in the cerebral cortex, hypothalamus, and medullary center, is responsible for decreasing pain perception (analgesia), inducing narcosis (heavy sedation), depressing the cough center (antitussive effect), initially stimulating and then depressing the vomiting center, and depressing respiration.

Kinetic (what body does to drug)

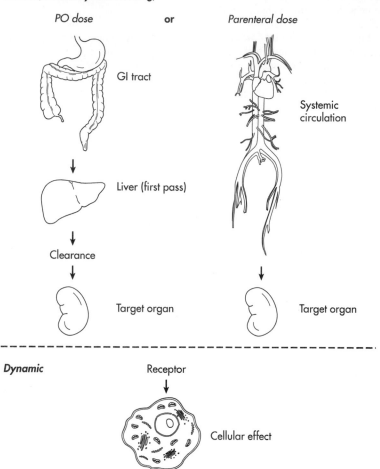

Figure 3-2 Relationship of pharmacokinetics to pharmacodynamics.

Mechanism of action. The identification of the molecular and biochemical events leading to an effect is called the *mechanism of action* of that drug. For instance, morphine causes respiratory depression by depressing the responsiveness of the respiratory center to carbon dioxide.

Cellular sites of actions of drugs. Because drugs are very reactive, many elicit their effects or side effects, or both, by interacting with coenzymes, enzymes, or nucleic acids, as well as other macromolecules in physiologic processes such as transport mechanisms. A full discussion of this topic is beyond the scope of this chapter.

ADVERSE REACTIONS AND DRUG INTERACTIONS

Patients may be prescribed as many as 10 to 15 drugs concomitantly. Many drug combinations, when used inappropriately and injudiciously, have the inherent potential to interact adversely, leading to side effects and potentially death. Occasionally, drug interactions are beneficial and actually enhance the therapeutic effectiveness of another drug (augmentation effect) or cause diminution of toxic reactions (antidote effect). Whether drugs are given individually or in combination, some side effects or adverse reactions are inevitable. Nevertheless, many adverse reactions of drugs or drug-drug interactions are avoidable or may be substantially minimized. The varied and complex mechanisms involved can be broadly classified as *pharmacokinetic interactions* or *pharmacodynamic interactions.* In pharmacokinetic interactions, drugs interfere with and/or alter the absorption, distribution, biotransformation, or excretion of other drugs. In pharmacodynamic interactions, drugs modify the intended and expected actions of other drugs.

Iatrogenic Reactions

Iatrogenic reactions include any adverse reaction produced unintentionally by the clinician or the patient. For example, side effects of many histaminic preparations may result in heavy sedation. Although sedation may be desirable for some patients, it may interfere with daytime activities.

Allergic Reactions

Drug allergy refers to those drug reactions occurring in a patient who has previously been exposed to the drug or sensitized to another drug, developing antibodies to that drug. The immunologic mechanisms involved may be varied and complex, involving anaphylactoid immediate reactions, cytotoxic reactions, or delayed allergic reactions. A careful history before the administration of drugs, in conjunction with a watchful monitoring of patients, may decrease the incidence of drug-induced allergic reactions.

Idiosyncratic reactions. *Idiosyncrasy* refers to abnormal, unexpected, or peculiar reactions seen in only certain patients. For example, succinylcholine may cause prolonged apnea in patients with pseudocholinesterase deficiency, and hemolytic anemia may be seen after the administration of a number of drugs in individuals with glucose-6-phosphate dehydrogenase deficiency. Although these reactions are unavoidable when they occur unexpectedly for the first time, they may be circumvented in patients who have previously shown such abnormal reactions.

OTHER PHARMACOKINETIC AND PHARMACODYNAMIC CONSIDERATIONS
Tolerance and Tachyphylaxis

Tolerance refers to the decreased responses following the long-term administration of drugs. Although it is generally accepted that tolerance may occur following the use of many depressant drugs such as benzodiazepines and barbiturates, it may also occur following the use of other agents such as carbamazepine, an anticonvulsant and mood stabilizer, or chlorpromazine, a neuroleptic. *Tachyphylaxis* refers to a quickly developing tolerance brought about by the rapid and repeated administration of a drug. Although tachyphylaxis is innocuous and is not regarded as a major clinical problem, not appreciating tolerance as an entity may have devastating consequences. For example, respiratory depression is not seen in a morphine-tolerant patient, and a dosage that far exceeds the normal therapeutic level is required to induce an analgesic effect. However, tolerance is lost or lessened following the discontinued administration of morphine. Therefore, in a once tolerant patient, administering a dose of morphine that was innocuous before (i.e., when the patient was tolerant) may prove fatal by causing severe respiratory depression.

Supersensitivity

Supersensitivity refers to the increased responsiveness to a drug that results either from denervation or following administration of a drug (a receptor antagonist) for a prolonged period. For example, the blocking of dopamine receptors by haloperidol may cause supersensitivity, upregulating dopamine receptors (e.g., supersensitivity of nigrostriatal dopamine receptors is associated with tardive dyskinesia).

Volume of Distribution

The pharmacokinetic parameter that describes how widely a drug is distributed in the body is *volume of distribution* (Vd). Volume of distribution is only an apparent volume, not the volume of any specific anatomic entity. The volume of distribution is determined by the characteristics of both the drug in question and the patient. Highly lipophilic drugs have large volumes of distribution primarily because of the extensive penetration into peripheral adipose tissue. Patients with more adipose tissue will therefore have higher volumes of distribution for lipophilic drugs than patients with higher percentages of lean body mass. It is important to note that elderly patients will tend to have higher volumes of distribution for many lipophilic psychotropic drugs than younger individuals, even if they retain normal body weight, because their proportion of adipose tissue to total body weight increases while the fraction of lean body mass correspondingly decreases.[1] In contrast, children generally have less adipose tissue than adults and thus might be expected to have smaller volumes of distribution.[3]

Another characteristic of a drug that will strongly influence its pharmacokinetic volume of distribution is the extent to which it binds plasma proteins. Many psychotropic medications bind to albumin and other plasma proteins, leaving only the unbound, or free, portion of the drug to diffuse to central receptors and produce a behavioral response. Most psychotropic drugs are highly protein bound, and any condition, for example renal failure, that reduces plasma protein binding can alter the interpretation of total plasma drug concentrations.[10]

Elimination of Drugs

Drug elimination is perhaps the single most important pharmacokinetic concept applied to the process of clearance. It is the best independent variable for describing the capacity of a given individual to remove a particular drug. Clearance is unique for each drug and each individual. Clearance is usually accomplished by a clearing organ or organs, and for most psychoactive drugs, with the exception of lithium, this organ is the liver. Clearance cannot exceed the rate at which blood is delivered to the clearing organ. Clearance is determined by the properties of the drug in question and the characteristics of the individual. The clearance of a drug may vary widely in populations and is generally given in milliliters per minute. For example, in a healthy adult, the clearance of a 10-mg oral dose of diazepam may vary as much as 15 ml/min to well over 50 ml/min. Clearance and volume of distribution act together to determine the pharmacokinetic parameter referred to as *elimination half-life* (t½). Elimination half-life is the time required for the plasma concentration of a drug to decline by 50%, assuming that the distribution process has reached equilibrium (steady state). The relationship between elimination half-life and clearance is intuitively obvious. If clearance is decreased, elimination half-life is increased. A larger volume of distribution is also associated with a longer elimination half-life. The mathematic relation among volume of distribution, elimination half-life, and clearance is shown as follows: t½ = 0.693 times volume of distribution over clearance.[10] For highly lipophilic drugs acting on the CNS, the volume of distribution can be a major determinant of the duration of drug action, particularly after single intravenous doses. The larger the volume of distribution, the more rapidly the drug will disappear from the plasma and the shorter its duration of action. Again, most psychotropic drugs are cleared by the liver, and many of the metabolites formed in this process may also have considerable biologic activity. For example, desmethyldiazepam is formed by the hepatic demethylization of the benzodiazepine diazepam and has pharmacologic activity similar to that of the parent drug.

Steady State

Most psychoactive drugs are administered chronically in the effort to achieve a long-term therapeutic effect. The pharmacokinetic parameter that is most important in achieving this aim is the steady-state plasma concentration of the medication in question, as well as concentrations of any active metabolites that may be present. If the patient's clinical response is at all related to the plasma concentration of the medication, this concentration becomes a critically important variable. Steady state means that the overall average total concentration of the drug and any metabolites will not change as long as the daily dose is not altered or other factors do not change clearance. For many psychotropic drugs, behavioral response is directly related to steady-state plasma concentration, which is determined by the relationship between dosing rate and clearance. The clinician chooses the dosing rate, which may then be modified by patient compliance. Then, as previously noted, the characteristics of the drug and the physiology of the patient determine clearance. Factors that may alter clearance include old age and disease states, as well as certain drug-drug interactions. Any factor that reduces clearance will increase steady-state plasma concentrations of a drug if the dosing rate remains the same. Conversely, as clearance increases, higher rates of infusion or larger or more frequent oral doses are necessary to produce a steady-state plasma concentration.

Half-life. Half-life is another important variable that must be considered at steady state. It determines both the time required to achieve steady-state plasma concentrations after treatment has started, as well as the time required to wash out a drug if treatment is stopped after steady state has been achieved. The importance of half-life in determining the time required to achieve steady state is illustrated in Figure 3-3. Four half-lives are required to reach within 10% of the steady-state condition. Although elimination half-life may vary from drug to drug, this value of 4 half-lives to achieve within 10% of steady state is constant for all medications. Thus, for drugs with long half-lives (the dash line in Figure 3-3), the approach to steady state is slow. Half-life also determines the time required to wash out a drug. In fact, washout is the mirror image approach to steady state (Figure 3-4). Four half-lives are

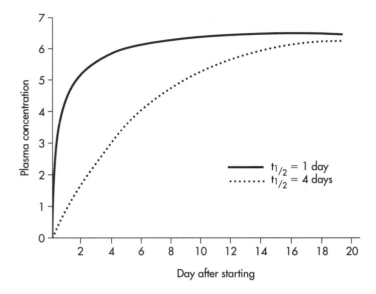

* For a drug with a $t_{1/2}$ of 1 day (solid line), the time required is about 5 days. For a drug with a $t_{1/2}$ of 4 days, the time required is about 20 days.

Figure 3-3 Effect of elimination half-life ($t^{1/2}$) on time required to reach steady state. (From Reference 9.)

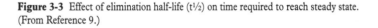

required to achieve more than 90% elimination of a drug from the body. The longer the half-life of a given drug, the longer this period will be. The speed with which a drug is washed out has substantial clinical importance. Toxicity can be resolved for drugs with short elimination half-lives, but rebound and withdrawal phenomenon tend to be less problematic for medications with longer elimination half-lives because their concentrations decrease more gradually when dosing is stopped.

Induction and Inhibition of Enzymes

Because most psychotropic drugs are cleared via biotransformation in the liver, a process that involves the activity of hepatic enzymes, any condition or event that alters this activity can markedly alter drug clearance and thus steady-state plasma concentrations. Clinically important changes in plasma concentrations of psychotropic medications can result from drugs that either induce or inhibit hepatic enzymes. Similarly, psychotropic drugs that inhibit or induce hepatic enzymes may also alter drug metabolism accordingly. Many drug-metabolizing enzymes are located in the endoplasmic reticulum of the liver; compounds that increase their synthesis or activity are referred to as *inducers*. Barbiturates are among the best known inducers of hepatic enzymes. When coadministered with a number of other psychotropic drugs, barbiturates increase their clearance and thus reduce steady-state plasma levels. Carbamazepine also has enzyme-inducing properties. One of the most potent inducers is the antituberculous agent rifampin.

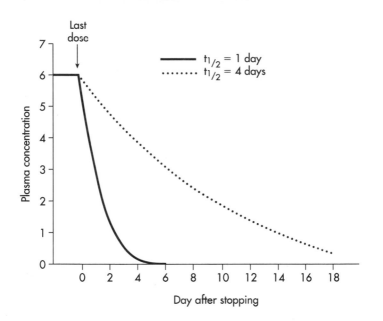

* For a drug with a $t_{1/2}$ of 1 day (solid line), the time required is about 5 days. For a drug with a $t_{1/2}$ of 4 days, the time required is about 20 days.

Figure 3-4 Effect of elimination half-life ($t^{1/2}$) on time required to wash out a given drug. (From Reference 9.)

Drug Interactions and Cytochrome P-450 Enzymes

Recent advances in pharmacogenetics and molecular biology have led to an increased understanding of drug metabolism and the potential for drug interactions when more than one drug is prescribed. Multiple drugs may be prescribed for existing illnesses, used in the context of augmentation for treatment-resistant illness, or simply used as an antidote to control adverse effects caused by another drug.[4] Cytochrome P-450 isoenzymes are significantly involved in the biotransformation of 80% to 90% of drugs as they are converted from lipid-soluble to water-soluble compounds. The enzymes are classified by family, subfamily, and specific gene and are designated by a number, a letter, then a number sequence. The key cytochrome P-450 enzymes involved in the metabolism of psychotropic drugs include 2D6, 1A2, 3A3/4, and 2C9/10/19 (Table 3-1). These are among some 34 cytochrome P-450 isoenzymes that have been identified in humans.[7]

The genetic ability to produce P-450 isoenzymes will vary by race or ethnic group. Genetic polymorphism describes the genetic makeup of an individual that codes for the inherent production of a specific hepatic enzyme. Individuals may be extensive metabolizers or poor metabolizers of certain drugs because of their genetic inability to produce, or produce in sufficient quantity, a given enzyme. Individuals who are poor metabolizers make up approximately 30% of the population. These individuals may manifest their characteristic poor metabolism through heightened sensitivity to even the lowest dosages of a particular drug.

Table 3-1 Key Cytochrome P-450 Enzymes: Partial Listing of Possible Inhibitors and Probable Substrates

Substrates of 2D6

Antidepressants: secondary TCAs, venlafaxine, fluoxetine, paroxetine, trazodone, mirtazapine

Antipsychotics: thioridazine, risperidone, perphenazine, haloperidol, clozapine

Antiarrhythmics: type IC (encainide, flecainide, mexiletine, propafenone)

β-*Blockers:* propranolol, metoprolol, timolol

Analgesics: oxycodone, dextromethorphan

Other: sparteine, brofaromine, mianserin, maprotiline, debrisoquin, remoxipride, chlorpheniramine

2D6 Inducers

No known inducers

2D6 Inhibitors

Paroxetine, fluoxetine, fluphenazine, sertraline (>100 mg), quinidine, haloperidol, cimetidine, thioridazine, amitriptyline, oral contraceptives, clomipramine, desipramine, norfluoxetine, levopromazine, noriluoxetine

Substrates of 1A2

Acetaminophen, caffeine, theophylline, amitriptyline, imipramine, clomipramine, clozapine, fluvoxamine, haloperidol, phenacetin, verapamil, antipyrine, tacrine, R-warfarin, estrogen, mirtazapine, olanzapine, phenothiazines

1A2 Inducers

Cigarette smoking, omeprazole, charcoal-broiled foods, some cruciferous vegetables, cabbage

1A2 Inhibitors

Fluvoxamine, enoxacin, fluoroquinolines, β-estradiol, furafylline, ciprofloxacin (fluoxetine and paroxetine at high dosages), erythromycin

Substrates of 3A3/4

Antidepressants: amitriptyline, imipramine, clomipramine, sertraline, mirtazapine, nefazodone, fluoxetine (minor), bupropion

Benzodiazepines: midazolam, alprazolam, diazepam, triazolam

Antiarrhythmics: lidocaine, quinidine, calcium channel blockers, propafenone, amiodarone, disopyramide

Antibiotics: erythromycin

Antihistamines: terfenadine, astemizole

Anticonvulsants: carbamazepine, valproate, lamotrigine, ethosuximide

Other: cyclosporine, dexamethasone, codeine, pimozide, zolpidem, cisapride, prednisone, tirilazad, alfentanil, vinblastine, lovastatin, pravastatin, fluvastatin, atorvastatin, dapsone, oral contraceptives, testosterone, diltiazem, dextromethorphan, codeine

3A3/4 Inducers

Steroids, rifampin, carbamazepine, phenobarbital, phenytoin

3A3/4 Inhibitors

Nefazodone, fluvoxamine, sertraline (>100 mg), cimetidine, diltiazem, verapamil, ketoconazole, erythromycin, fluoxetine, progestogens, gestodene, grapefruit juice, troleandomycin, paroxetine

Substrates of 2C9/10/19

Hexobarbital, propranolol, nirvanol, ibuprofen, tolbutamide, tertiary TCAs, S-warfarin, mephobarbital, phenytoin, omeprazole, proguanil, moclobemide, diazepam, citalopram, mephenytoin, piroxicam, naproxen

2C Inducers

Rifampin, isoniazid

2C Inhibitors

Paroxetine, fluoxetine, fluvoxamine, progestogens (2C19), omeprazole, moclobemide, ketoconazole, sertraline, fluconazole, sulfaphenazole

TCAs, Tricyclic antidepressants.

In addition to genetic polymorphism, cytochrome P-450 enzymes may be induced or inhibited by drugs and other ingested chemicals, by some food substances, and by cigarette smoking.[2] Induction may occur as a drug stimulates an increase in a hepatic enzyme that metabolizes either another administered drug or the drug itself—a phenomenon known as *autoinduction*.[6] A drug that is metabolized through a specific enzyme is referred to as a *substrate* of that enzyme. Increased enzyme activity results in faster metabolism and a shorter-than-expected half-life with potential loss of pharmacologic effect over time. In contrast, enzyme inhibition may occur, resulting in a significant increase in circulating plasma concentrations of a drug being metabolized by that particular enzyme. Consequently, the potential for increased adverse effect or toxicity may occur at standard dosing regimens.

Enzyme inhibition and induction alike may alter the process of achieving steady-state dosing. Enzyme inhibition may result in a significant rise in drug plasma levels, whereas induction occurs at a slower rate because enzyme production is not accelerated immediately but takes place over several days or weeks. These processes have implications, especially for patients with comorbid psychiatric and general medical conditions, and for those who smoke cigarettes and use over-the-counter agents. Awareness of cytochrome P-450 enzymes and their metabolic activity can facilitate patient safety and medication efficacy for those who are taking more than one medication. Some drug-drug interactions may allow lower dosing of a secondary agent, thereby reducing cause or side effects accordingly. Other combinations may allow maximum symptom relief through augmentation. However, patients may be at greater risk for significant and potentially harmful drug reactions when drugs inhibit the activity of enzymes necessary for metabolism of other drugs being coprescribed. An excellent review of the nursing considerations pertinent to cytochrome P-450 isoenzymes may be found in Applegate.[2]

PHARMACOKINETICS AND AGING
Interactions

Intercurrent medical illness and "obligatory polypharmacy" is encountered when prescribing psychotropic drugs in the elderly.[5] Thus the consideration of drug-drug interactions in this population is especially important. Whereas rigorous systematic drug-drug interaction studies are lacking in the elderly, the fund of knowledge currently available is sufficient to make some common decisions when prescribing. The importance of the P-450 enzyme system has been noted. This system is responsible for metabolizing many drugs (see Table 3-1). Thus, if one knows the specific P-450 enzymes that metabolize a particular drug that is to be coprescribed, then potential adverse drug-drug interactions can be predicted. Certainly, age-associated decreases in metabolism and elimination of drugs are sufficient to require special consideration before prescribing drugs in the elderly, particularly if multiple drugs are being prescribed. If one considers carefully the concomitant drugs that may inhibit P-450–mediated metabolism of other more toxic drugs, genetic deficiency of P-450 enzymes (e.g., 2D6), and medical illnesses (e.g., liver and renal failure) that will lead to further elevation of drug levels and delay in drug clearance, the likelihood of adverse events when multiple drugs are used in the elderly becomes truly amazing. In consideration of the pharmacokinetic and pharmacodynamic principles discussed, when prescribing drugs in the elderly, one might add to the often heard recommendation, "start low and go slow," another admonition, "keep it as simple as possible."[5]

Table 3-2 Pharmacokinetic Changes with Aging

Absorption	Metabolism
↑ Gastric pH	↓ Hepatic mass
↓ (Delayed) gastric emptying	↓ Hepatic blood flow
↓ Splanchnic blood flow	↓ Phase I metabolism
↓ Intestinal motility	= (Unchanged) phase II metabolism
Distribution	**Elimination**
↑ Body fat	↓ Creatinine clearance
↓ Total body water	↓ Glomerular filtration rate
↓ Albumin	↓ Tubular secretion
↑ α_1-acid glycoprotein	↓ Creatinine production

Absorption

The time to maximum concentration (T_{max}) following oral drug dose generally is not delayed despite age-related decrements in gastrointestinal functioning. The maximum concentration (C_{max}) of drug in plasma following an oral dose generally is unaffected by age as well.

Distribution

Table 3-2 shows the age-related changes that affect distribution, including increased body fat, decreased total body water, decreased albumin, and increased α_1-acid glycoprotein. All four of these effects can influence the way drugs distribute in tissues and bind with plasma proteins.[5] As a result of increased body fat, lipid-soluble drugs, which are used extensively as psychotropics, a larger volume of distribution occurs in older patients. Thus drugs with larger volumes of distribution in adipose tissue will make efforts to decrease toxic levels by hemodialysis relatively ineffective. By contrast, hydrophilic drugs will have smaller volumes of distribution in the elderly because of the decrease in total body water.

With respect to protein binding, drugs that are highly bound to albumin, such as carbamazepine, may show increased fractions of free drug because binding sites may become saturated more quickly in the elderly. It is the free, unbound drug that exerts pharmacodynamic actions, whether they are desirable or adverse. The free fraction, however, is also subject to metabolism and elimination. Thus a drug highly bound to albumin may or may not be more prone to cause toxicity, depending on the capacity for such protein binding and the presence of other albumin-bound drugs that may displace potentially toxic drugs from their binding sites. Finally, levels of α_1-acid glycoprotein become elevated with increasing age, which may affect distribution of a variety of psychotropic drugs, including tricyclic antidepressants, thioridazine, and methadone. The clinical consequences of increased α_1-acid glycoprotein have not been systematically studied in older adults.

Metabolism

Aging results in decreased liver size and blood flow and possibly decreased activity of hepatic microsomal enzymes, at least in terms of early phase metabolism.

Elimination

From age 40, a linear decline in the glomerular filtration rate occurs, and by age 60, the decline becomes exponential. Thus a drug such as lithium that depends on renal excretion for its elimination is likely to accumulate to potentially toxic levels unless the dosage is adjusted downward. In addition to the age-related decline in renal function, clearance by the kidney may be further impaired by nonsteroidal antiinflammatory drugs, resulting in a greater risk of lithium toxicity in older patients.

PHARMACOKINETICS AND CULTURE

Ethnicity and culture exert powerful influences on the effects of a wide array of medications, including most psychotropics. Also, patients' divergent beliefs, expectations, dietary practices, and genetic constitutions must be taken into consideration in psychopharmacotherapy. Because of immigration and increased ease and flexibility of movements around the globe, societies within a given country have become more heterogenous, requiring clinicians to understand not only how illness may present differently across ethnicities or cultures, but how treatment modalities and side effects may also be different. Many psychotropic agents have been reported to have disparate effects in cross-national and cross-cultural studies of dosing and side effect profiles. Most of these reports involve ethnic differences in Caucasians contrasted with non-Caucasians, particularly Asians, African-Americans, and Hispanics, with virtually no attention given to Native Americans.[12]

Drug Metabolism and Action

As previously discussed, numerous factors are involved in determining how an individual responds to a particular medication. Mechanisms responsible for cross-ethnic differences in drug response are similar to those that determine interindividual variability in the dosage range and side effect profiles and can be classified as pharmacokinetic, pharmacodynamic, and social-cultural factors. Of these various factors, metabolism has been identified as most likely to contribute to interindividual and cross-ethnic variation.[13] In recent years, a large number of drug-metabolizing enzymes, as well as the genes responsible for encoding these enzymes, have been characterized. Many of these enzymes and their genes are present in two or more distinct forms within a given population, a condition known as *polymorphism*. Substantial ethnic variations exist in the frequency of these gene mutations (genotypes) and the enzyme activity (phenotypes) of many of these polymorphic drug-metabolizing enzymes. Because the enzymes responsible for the metabolism of many medications vary in their activity, significant differences result in the pharmacokinetics of the drug, in turn, resulting in variations in therapeutic dosage ranges and side effect profiles. The activities of many of these enzymes show substantial cross-ethnic differences. Among these, the cytochrome P-450 enzyme system has received the most attention, particularly because this system clearly relates to clinical issues in the use of psychotropic medications. With the exception of lithium, most psychotropic medications are highly lipophilic; consequently, for these medications to be excreted from the body, they must undergo biotransformation to make them less fat soluble and more water soluble (as previously discussed). Thus the cytochrome P-450 isoenzymes, as discussed, manifest distinct interindividual and cross-ethnic variations.

Such cross-cultural diversity is most clearly seen in the P-450 isoenzymes CYP 2D6 and CYP 2C19. In any given population, these isoenzymes have been found to be bimodally distributed. A certain proportion of people, deficient in the activity of

Table 3-3 Ethnicity and Genetic Polymorphism (Pms) of CYP 2D6 and CYP 2C19

	CYP 2D6 (% Pms)	CYP 2C19 (% Pms)
African-Americans	1.9%	18.5%
African blacks	0%-8.1%	—
American Indians	0%-5.2%	0%
Asian Indians	—	20.8%
Caucasians	3%-8.9%	2.5%-6.7%
East Asians	0%-2.4%	17.4%-22%
Hispanics	1%-4.5%	4.8%
Sans bushmen	19%	—

these enzymes, are classified as poor metabolizers. In contrast, those without such deficiencies are classified as extensive metabolizers. The substantial cross-ethnic differences in the frequency of the poor metabolizer is summarized in Table 3-3, which shows the frequency of poor metabolizers in both enzymes and studies involving different populations. An example of the wide variation is the CYP 2D6 poor metabolizer rate ranging from less than 1% in some studies of Asians to as high as 19% among Sans bushmen. Other examples are shown in the table. A significant proportion of psychotropics, including most neuroleptics and antidepressants, are metabolized by CYP 2D6. In contrast to these two enzymes, there is no clear evidence of genetic polymorphism with regard to CYP 3A4 and CYP 1A2, two other cytochrome P-450 isoenzymes that are important for the metabolism of some of the psychotropic agents, particularly those used to treat anxiety disorders (e.g., several benzodiazepines, tricyclic antidepressants, and selective serotonin reuptake inhibitors).[7] However, some evidence of ethnic differences in the activity of these enzymes do exist; for example, the calcium channel blocker nifedipine, a substrate for CYP 3A4, is reported to be metabolized more slowly in South and East Asians and Hispanics.[12]

Other pharmacokinetic factors that have ethnic differences include variations in protein binding. Because plasma proteins are genetically determined, polymorphism may also result in ethnic differences. Some studies have suggested this possibility, but specific contributions of plasma protein binding to different responses across ethnic groups remains to be determined. The fat content of the body may differ across ethnic groups, leading to differences in the volume of distribution and thus the pharmacokinetics of lipophilic drugs. This, in fact, has been identified as one of the reasons for the greater effect of benzodiazepines in Asians as compared with Caucasians.[12]

Regarding ethnicity and pharmacodynamics, much less work has been done to show substantial interindividual and cross-ethnic differences. In addition, studies are under way to demonstrate differences in psychotropic response in different ethnic groups. Certainly, there have been frequent reports of ethnic differences in psychotropic response, but these have mostly been based on clinical impressions and survey.[14]

REFERENCES

1. Abernathy DR, Greenblatt DJ: Drug disposition in obese humans: an update, *Clin Pharmacokinet* 11:199, 1986.
2. Applegate M: Cytochrome P450 isoenzymes: nursing considerations, *J Am Psychiatr Nurses Assoc* 5:15, 1999.

3. Bartlett HL, and others: Fat-free mass in relation to stature: ratios of fat-free mass to height in children, adults, and elderly subjects, *Am J Clin Nutr* 53:1112, 1991.

4. Carson SW: Pharmacokinetic and pharmacodynamic drug interactions with polypharmacotherapy of treatment-resistant affective and obsessive-compulsive disorders, *Psychopharmacol Bull* 32:555, 1996.

5. Catterson ML, Preskorn SH, Martin, RL: Pharmacodynamic and pharmacokinetic considerations in geriatric psychopharmacology, *Psychiatric Clin North Am* 20(1):205, 1997.

6. DeVane CL: Pharmacogenetics and drug metabolism of newer antidepressant agents, *J Clin Psychiatry* 55(suppl 12):38, 1994.

7. DeVane CL: Pharmacokinetics of the newer antidepressants: clinical relevance. *Am J Med* 97(6A):13S, 1994.

8. DuPont RL: The pharmacology and drug interactions of the newer antidepressants, *Essential Psychopharmacol* 2(1):33, 1997.

9. Greenblatt DJ: Effect of elimination half-life ($t_{1/2}$) on time required to reach steady state, *J Clin Psychiatry* 54(9 Suppl):8, 1993.

10. Greenblatt DJ, Sellers EM, Koch-Weser J: Importance of protein binding for the interpretation of serum or plasma drug concentration, *J Clin Pharmacol* 22:259, 1982.

11. Lesser IM, Lin KM, Poland RE: Ethnic differences in the response to psychotropic drugs. In Friedman S, editor: *Anxiety disorders in African Americans,* New York, 1995, Raven Press.

12. Lesser IM, Smith M, Poland RE, Lin KM: Psychopharmacology and ethnicity. In Friedman S, editor: *Cultural issues in the treatment of anxiety,* New York, 1997, The Guilford Press.

13. Lin KM, Poland RE: Ethnicity, culture, and psychopharmacology. In Bloom FE, Kupfer DI, editors: *Psychopharmacology: the fourth generation of progress,* New York, 1995, Raven Press.

14. Lin KM, Poland RD, Nakasaki G: *Psychopharmacology and psychobiology of ethnicity,* Washington, DC, 1993, American Psychiatric Press.

CHAPTER 4

Neuropharmacology and Psychotropic Drugs

JONATHAN LEO AND RICHARD A. SUGERMAN

The discovery that drugs affect the nervous system has had a profound influence on human culture. Since it was first found that smoking or ingesting substances could have effects on consciousness, sensorium, and moods, scientists have searched for the mechanisms of action of these drugs. Early neuropharmacologic studies involved the purification of plant alkaloids such as morphine, cocaine, and reserpine. Following the serendipitous discovery of lithium salts in 1949, psychotropic drugs have been used extensively to treat psychiatric disorders. In fact, 20% of all prescriptions written are for psychotropic drugs. Antihistamines, sympathomimetics, and various other over-the-counter agents are also used to affect the nervous system.

Eighty percent of the U.S. population uses psychoactive drugs for nonmedicinal purposes.[13] Alcohol and tobacco account for most recreational drug use; however, 20% of the population abuses illegal substances such as cocaine, opiates, stimulants, hallucinogenics, or marijuana. These drugs significantly affect society and the lives of many individuals and their families.

Any drug acting on the central nervous system (CNS) will encounter the blood-brain barrier. The blood-brain barrier plays an important role in normal physiology by protecting neurons from harmful substances found in the bloodstream. There are tight junctions in the capillaries of the brain that are not found in other organs, such as the liver or spleen, that will prevent certain drugs from getting into the brain. Thus the blood-brain barrier controls fluctuations of ions such as K^+ and Ca^{2+}. Transporters facilitate transfer of substances such as glucose and amino acids across the blood-brain barrier. Lipophilic compounds also cross the blood-brain barrier quite readily. Alcohol is an example of one drug that readily crosses the blood-brain barrier. A classic example of a drug delivery dilemma and a solution to the problem involves Parkinson's patients who have a shortage of dopamine. Dopamine will not cross the blood-brain barrier, so these patients are given L-dopa, a precursor of dopamine, that readily crosses the blood-brain barrier. Overall, the complexity of the brain makes treating neuropsychiatric disorders challenging. The basic processes, as such, are described in this chapter.

Neurons are the basic subunit of the nervous system. They transmit information by sending action potentials (waves of electrical depolarization) down their processes and on to other neurons. Most action potentials travel from one neuron to another by sending a chemical called a *neurotransmitter* across a minute space (a synapse) that separates these cells, to evoke the next action potential. It is in or around these synapses that many drugs act on the nervous system.

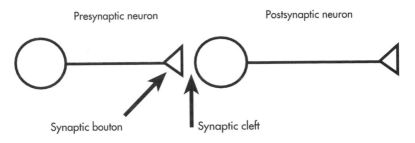

Presynaptic neuron   Postsynaptic neuron

Synaptic bouton   Synaptic cleft

Figure 4-1 Two-neuron chain showing the presynaptic and postsynaptic neurons interconnected by a synapse. The synapse is composed of a synaptic bouton *(triangle)*, which is on the presynaptic membrane, the synaptic cleft, and the postsynaptic membrane, which in this instance is the dendrite or cell body *(circle)* of the postsynaptic neuron.

SYNAPTIC TRANSMISSION

Figure 4-1 depicts two neurons. The first neuron is the presynaptic neuron, and its axon is going to a dendrite of the second neuron, or postsynaptic neuron. The presynaptic membrane often has on its surface synaptic boutons, button-shaped or bulb-shaped projections on the end of the axon, which are directly opposite the postsynaptic membrane. Synaptic boutons are about 1 μm wide and contain synaptic vesicles carrying neurotransmitters. An action potential arriving at a synaptic bouton (Figure 4-2) causes a change in the membrane potential of the bouton by opening calcium channels and allowing extracellular calcium (Ca^{2+}) to enter the bouton. The increased intracellular calcium in the bouton triggers the vesicles to fuse with the bouton's cellular membrane and release the transmitter into the synaptic cleft, a 20-nm space between the cells. The neurotransmitter then diffuses across the synaptic cleft to the postsynaptic membrane of the next neuron, where it binds only to specific receptors. For example, the neurotransmitter acetylcholine (ACh) binds only with the ACh receptors on the postsynaptic membrane of the next neuron. This binding allows sodium ions into and potassium ions out of opened channels. If enough ACh diffuses to the postsynaptic membrane (receptors), an action potential can be generated by the postsynaptic neuron. Most neurotransmitters, after binding to the receptors, are quickly and actively "reuptaken" by the presynaptic boutons or surrounding glial cells. ACh is an exception to this general principle. It is broken down in the synaptic space by the enzyme acetylcholinesterase. The rapid degradation of ACh allows only a short burst of activity at the postsynaptic membrane.

Types of Synapses

At one time, neuroscientists were aware of only a few types of synapses. The classic axon synapsed on the dendrites, somas (cell body), and axons—the axodendritic, axosomatic, and axoaxonic synapses, respectively. With the advent of the electron microscope, scientists found somatosomatic synapses. In addition, electron micrography has allowed scientists to find reciprocal synapses between two neurons, for example, dendrodendritic synapses.[21] These reciprocal synapses probably form minuscule local positive or negative feedback loops. Furthermore, many neurons receive input from more than 1500 other neurons. Thus the true complexity of the neuronal milieu begins to be apparent.

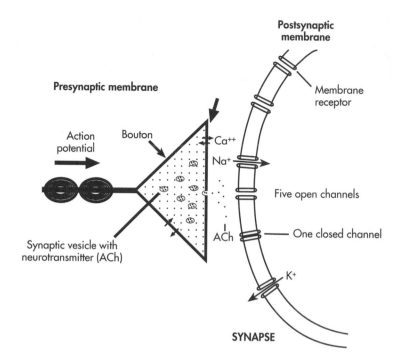

Figure 4-2 An action potential opens calcium ion channels and allows Ca^{2+} to enter the presynaptic membrane *(bouton)*. The Ca^{2+} triggers the vesicles to fuse with the membrane and release the neurotransmitter acetylcholine *(ACh)* into the synaptic cleft. Two molecules of ACh then bind with an ACh receptor on the postsynaptic membrane of the target cell, which allows sodium (Na^{2+}) influx and potassium (K^+) efflux through opened channels in the target cell membrane. The channels are normally closed, except when activated by the ACh-receptor complex.

MEMBRANE RECEPTORS

Receptors are cell membrane proteins that are stimulated by specific neurotransmitters. The "fluid mosaic model" of the cell membrane depicts the receptors as floating within the lipid bilayer. Both the mobility and the number of receptors are important parameters that determine how the cell will respond to a stimulus. Conditions that change these parameters will affect the biologic characteristics of the cell. The number of receptors on a cell is constantly changing based on the surrounding physiologic conditions. Cells will tend to upregulate receptors in response to low neurotransmitter levels or to downregulate receptors when a neurotransmitter is plentiful. The ability of the cell to change the numbers of receptors on the cell membrane has important implications for theories of psychotropic drug activity. The mobility of receptors will also affect the physiology of the cell. For instance, alcohol is thought to change the mobility of the receptors within the membrane.

These receptors, or proteins, are depicted as hollow tubes that extend their openings between the extracellular and intracellular spaces. These openings are referred to as *pores* or *channels*. When a neurotransmitter binds with its specific receptor, a conformational change takes place that opens or closes the channel to the flow of specific ions, for example, sodium, potassium, and chloride. The ACh receptor molecule is a glycoprotein with a molecular weight of 268,000 and five separate polypeptides that extend into the extracellular space.[10] The exposed polypeptides help in providing the specificity for the receptors. Classically, pharmacologists working with ACh have operationally defined ACh receptors as either nicotinic or muscarinic, depending on which alkaloid, either nicotine or muscarine, has an excitatory (agonistic) effect at the synapse. For example, ACh receptors that are stimulated by nicotine are nicotinic, and ACh receptors that are stimulated by muscarine are muscarinic. ACh receptors at the neuromuscular junction of skeletal muscle and in autonomic ganglia are nicotinic, whereas ACh receptors found on effector organs such as glands, smooth muscle, and cardiac muscle are muscarinic. In the brain, the muscarinic receptors outnumber the nicotinic receptors by 10-fold to 100-fold. Therefore ACh has more than one type of receptor. In addition, the excitatory effects of ACh at the receptors can be blocked selectively by different agents or antagonists. For example, nicotinic receptors on skeletal muscle are selectively blocked by curare, whereas muscarinic receptors are blocked by atropine. Scopolamine results in sedation and amnesia by blockade of the central muscarinic receptors, whereas cigarette smoking and coffee activate the nicotinic receptors, which leads to alertness. Thus the presence of specific agonists and antagonists for the membrane receptors has enabled scientists to classify receptors for ACh and other neurotransmitters into more than one type. Scientists now know that there are many different types of receptors that are specific for individual neurotransmitters.

Mechanisms of Receptor Action

When a neurotransmitter binds with a receptor, ion channels are opened or closed, allowing specific ions to start or stop moving across the postsynaptic membrane and evoking local changes in the membrane potential. In neuron excitation, when a sufficient amount of neurotransmitter binds with a threshold-level number of receptors, an action potential takes place and travels along the entire length of the neuron. When the neurotransmitter-receptor complex results in direct change of the membrane potential, it is referred to as *first messenger transmission*. First messenger transmission requires only a few milliseconds to initiate its changes to the cell membrane. First messenger transmission also can initiate a series of intracellular reactions by triggering secondary messenger transmission, which causes not only delayed ion channel opening or closing but also the regulation of many cell functions. These secondary messengers are cell membrane proteins that relay the message from the neurotransmitter-receptor complex to a chain of chemical reactions in the neuroplasm of the cell.[19]

One common second messenger is cyclic adenosine $3',5'$-monophosphate (cAMP), or simply cyclic AMP. When a neurotransmitter, such as epinephrine, binds to its receptor, there is an allosteric change (conformational change in the protein) in the receptor, which causes a G-protein to associate with the enzyme adenylate cyclase, which is found in the membrane. Adenylate cyclase then synthesizes cAMP, which activates protein kinase A and, in turn, leads to phosphorylation (addition of a phosphate to an organic compound) of intracellular proteins. The phosphorylation of the proteins can now have numerous effects on cellular processes (Figure 4-3).

Another extensively studied second messenger is the Ca^{2+}-calmodulin complex (see Figure 4-3). When a neurotransmitter binds to a receptor, calcium channels

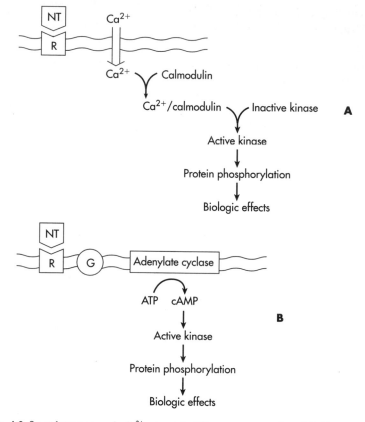

Figure 4-3 Second messengers. **A,** Ca^{2+}-calmodulin. When a neurotransmitter *(NT)* binds to the receptor, this allows an influx of calcium into the cell, which binds to calmodulin to form a complex, which in turn activates a kinase. The activated kinase now leads to protein phosphorylation, which leads to biologic effects. **B,** Cyclic AMP. When neurotransmitter binds to the receptor, this causes the related G-protein to bind to adenylate cyclase, which produces cAMP from adenosine triphosphate (ATP). This in turn activates a kinase, phosphorylates proteins, and leads to biologic effects.

open and intracellular calcium levels increase. The calcium binds with calmodulin, an intracellular molecule, and the resulting Ca^{2+}-calmodulin complex activates a protein kinase that leads to phosphorylation of intracellular proteins and subsequent biologic effects such as protein synthesis. In the past decade, it has also been shown that calcium will activate nitric oxide synthase (NOS) to produce the gaseous messenger nitric oxide (NO). Because NO is a free radical that will react with numerous molecules, it has been implicated in many normal physiologic processes such as vasodilation, peristalsis, learning and memory, and erection, to name just a few. Thus hormones and neurotransmitters can activate intracellular mechanisms to initiate such processes as cell division and protein synthesis. Whereas first messenger transmission can be viewed as evoking rapid, direct membrane changes, the second messengers tend to have more complex and longer-term effects on cellular physiology.

NEUROTRANSMISSION
Neuron Excitation and Inhibition

Neuron excitation of the postsynaptic membrane is caused by the stimulation of the receptor by the neurotransmitter. Neurons, like most cells, have a resting membrane potential, but neurons are excitable and have the ability to rapidly alter their membrane potential in response to a stimulus. The stimulus, typically a neurotransmitter, can cause a depolarization or a hyperpolarization of the membrane. An excitatory transmitter, such as glutamate, will cause an influx of sodium ions into the neuron, resulting in depolarization of the postsynaptic membrane. Inhibition, or hyperpolarization, is caused by an efflux of potassium ions or an influx of chloride ions. Neurotransmitters are sometimes classified as excitatory or inhibitory, but the mechanism of action actually depends on the postsynaptic receptor. For instance, dopamine can be either excitatory or inhibitory, depending on the receptor that it activates.

Defining Neurotransmitters

The following specific criteria are used to define a chemical as a neurotransmitter:

1. The chemical must be found in the presynaptic boutons and must be released when the neuron is stimulated.
2. The chemical must somehow be inactivated after it is released. Two mechanisms of inactivation have been found. The most common is reuptake of the chemical by the presynaptic membrane, and the second is the degradation of the chemical by an extracellular enzyme.
3. If the chemical is applied exogenously at the postsynaptic membrane, the effect will be the same as when the presynaptic neuron is stimulated. The quantity of chemical applied must be in a sufficient concentration.
4. The chemical applied to the synapse must be affected in a manner similar to that of the normally occurring chemical (e.g., enzymatic degradation).

ACTION AND SYNTHESIS OF NEUROTRANSMITTERS

Neurotransmitters have been divided into four major groups or systems: cholinergics, monoamines, neuropeptides, and amino acids (Table 4-1). In this section, neurotransmitters are classified by major group or system, and their sites of action, their modes of synthesis, and their mechanisms of action are discussed. Neurotransmitters occur in neurons and tracts in too many locations to discuss in detail; therefore only significant anatomic locations are mentioned.

Cholinergic System

The neurotransmitter in the cholinergic system is ACh.[16,23] ACh is found in the peripheral nervous system (PNS) at the myoneural junction of skeletal muscle, in autonomic ganglia, at parasympathetic postganglionic-effector synapses, and in the CNS within the spinal cord, basal ganglia, and cerebral cortex. The molecular weight of ACh is 136, whereas the typical ion is in the range of 20 to 30. Several pathways in the brain have been identified as ACh tracts. The basal nucleus of Meynert projects fibers to the cerebral cortex and has been implicated as a site of lesion in Alzheimer's disease. The septal area, an area rostral to the hypothalamus, sends ACh fibers to the hippocampus. ACh is synthesized by the union of acetylcoenzyme A

Table 4-1 Classification of Neurotransmitters and Pathways

Neurotransmitter	Chemical transmitter	Location found	Major pathways
Cholinergic systems	ACh	Myoneural junctions, postganglionic neurons, autonomic ganglia, parasympathetic postganglionic neurons	Basal nucleus of Meynert to cerebral cortex, septal area (rostral to hypothalamus) to hippocampus
Monoamine systems	Dopamine	Substantia nigra, ventral tegmental area	Nigrostriatal, mesolimbic, tuberoinfundibular mesocortical
	Norepinephrine	Locus ceruleus	Locus ceruleus (in pons) to thalamus, cerebral cortex, cerebellum, and spinal cord; lateral midbrain to hypothalamus and basal forebrain
	Epinephrine	Red nucleus	Central tegmental tract
	Serotonin	Raphe nuclei	Central brainstem nuclei up to forebrain and down to spinal cord
Neuropeptides	Enkephalins	Spinal cord, hypothalamus, midbrain, and the like	
	Endorphins	Spinal cord, hypothalamus, midbrain, and the like	
	Substance P	Spinal cord, hypothalamus, and many other places	
Amino acids	GABA	Most common transmitter in brain	Purkinje cells to deep cerebellar nuclei; striatal nigro
	Glycine	Spinal cord, brainstem, and many other CNS areas	
	Glutamate	Widely distributed in the CNS	
	Asparate	Hippocampus, dorsal root ganglion	

ACh, Acetylcholine; *ACTH,* adrenocorticotropic hormone; *CCK,* cholecystokinin; *CNS,* central nervous system; *GABA,* gamma-aminobutyric acid; *VIP,* vasoactive intestinal polypeptide.

(acetyl-CoA) and choline in the axonal boutons and is stored in synaptic vesicles (Figure 4-4, *A*).

As stated earlier, ACh is released from the presynaptic membrane, crosses the synaptic cleft, and attaches to its receptor. Acetylcholinesterase in the synaptic cleft breaks down the ACh into its component molecules (Figure 4-4, *B*). Much of the choline in the bouton is obtained by reuptake from the synaptic cleft and is used subsequently for ACh synthesis. It was also stated earlier that ACh has two major categories of membrane receptors: nicotinic and muscarinic. Both nicotinic and muscarinic receptors can be further divided into subtypes, which are beyond the scope of this review. The nicotinic receptors are found at the postsynaptic membrane at the myoneural junction and the autonomic ganglia. The nicotinic receptor is a ligand gated ion channel that allows sodium to enter the cell. The muscarinic receptors are located on parasympathetic effector organs and in the CNS, but they are coupled to G-proteins that use second messengers. Thus acetylcholine is a fast transmitter when it binds to the nicotinic receptor but a slow transmitter when it binds to the muscarinic receptor.

Both the nicotinic receptor and muscarinic receptors are composed of five polypeptide subunits. They both have two alpha subunits that bind to Ach, but they differ in the remaining three units. This is thought to be the basis for the functional differences between the two receptors. There is an important physiological connection between the dopamine D_2 receptor and the ACh receptors in the striatum. In the normally functioning brain, the dopamine released from the substantia nigra projections to the striatum binds to the D_2 receptor. One of the actions of the D_2 receptor is to decrease the release of ACh within the striatum. In Parkinson's patients, there is extensive degeneration of the substantia nigra, resulting in less dopamine released into the striatum and thus less inhibition of the cholinergic interneurons within the striatum. The fact that there is less inhibition of the cholinergics results in an excess of ACh in the striatum of Parkinson's patients. A common drug therapy for Parkinson's patients is to give a cholinergic muscarinic blocker such as benztropine to decrease the striatal levels of ACh to normal and thus restore movement to normal. It is interesting that there are essentially three transmitter systems involved in the basal ganglia loop, which is implicated in Parkinson's disease: dopamine, acetylcholine, and GABA. Pharmacologic efforts to treat the disease have been most successful with attempts to alter the activity of the dopaminergic and cholinergic systems. Attempts to develop drugs that act on the GABA-ergic system have not been as successful, most likely because the GABA-ergic receptors are so ubiquitous within the CNS.

Monoamine Systems

Neurotransmitters containing one amine group are called *monoamines*.[16,24] These include the catecholamines (dopamine, norepinephrine, and epinephrine), serotonin, and histamine. The term *adrenergic* refers to neurons activated by catecholamines, which are adrenalin-like substances also derived from the adrenal gland. The catecholamines are common neurotransmitters that are widely dispersed in the CNS and PNS. Dopamine neurons project from the substantia nigra to the putamen via the nigrostriatal pathway, a major pathway affected in Parkinson's disease. Additional dopamine synthesizing sites are located in the caudate nucleus, amygdala, and temporal lobe. Dopamine is also produced in the ventral tegmental area (VTA). Dopaminergic fibers from the VTA project to various areas of the limbic system, including the nucleus accumbens, olfactory tubercle, septum, amygdala, and cortical areas. Many antipsychotic drugs, as well as cocaine and amphetamines, are thought

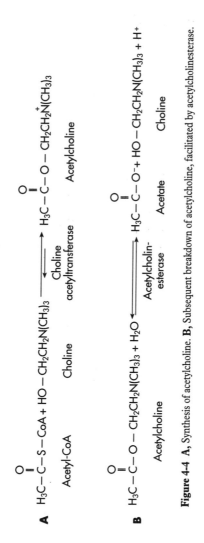

Figure 4-4 **A,** Synthesis of acetylcholine. **B,** Subsequent breakdown of acetylcholine, facilitated by acetylcholinesterase.

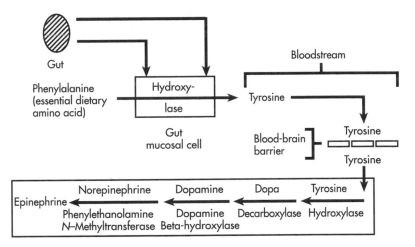

Figure 4-5 Normal synthesis of the catecholamines.

to act on the dopaminergic pathways in these areas. High concentrations of dopamine appear to be involved in schizophrenia. Norepinephrine cells in the locus ceruleus (in the pons) send their processes to the thalamus, cerebral cortex, cerebellum, and spinal cord. Norepinephrine is also the neurotransmitter of the sympathetic postganglionic neurons. Epinephrine (adrenalin) is found in neurons that run from the red nucleus to the medulla oblongata in the central tegmental tract. Serotonin is found in central midbrain nuclei (raphe nuclei) and in neuronal processes up to the forebrain and down to the spinal cord. The catecholamines are all derived from tyrosine (Figure 4-5).

Catecholamines. Tyrosine is found in the neurons, where it is converted to levodopa (L-dopa) and then to dopamine. Dopamine is then taken up into storage vesicles and converted to norepinephrine within the vesicles in some cells. There are several classes of catecholamine receptors (five dopaminergic receptors and four adrenergic receptors), and these receptors appear to influence ion channels by secondary messenger mechanisms. The dopamine receptors, D_1 and D_2, are clinically significant because of their role in numerous psychiatric conditions. When dopamine binds to the D_1 receptor, there is an upregulation of cAMP, whereas activation of the D_2 receptor results in downregulation of cAMP. As mentioned earlier, the D_2 receptor also inhibits ACh release from the striatum, and disruption of this pathway has been implicated in Parkinson's disease. The administration of L-dopa, the precursor for dopamine, thus restores the ability of the nigrostriatal tract to inhibit the striatum. Information concerning the D_3, D_4, and D_5 receptors continues to evolve, and their role in psychosis is discussed in Chapter 5.

Serotonin. Serotonin, or 5-hydroxytryptamine (5HT), is derived from tryptophan within the CNS. Serotonin receptors function via both first and second messenger systems. In the brain, the major site of serotonin is found in the raphe nuclei. The raphe nuclei are found in the brainstem and project widely to the forebrain, cerebellum, and spinal cord. Serotonin has a significant effect on sensory perception, arousal, and emotions. Lysergic acid diethylamide (LSD), which in the 1950s was found to cause hallucinations, has been shown to exert its effect by depressing serotonin-containing neurons. There are several subdivisions of the serotonin receptors. The $5HT_3$ receptor, which has been implicated in schizophrenia and depression, is a ligand gated receptor, and has been found in the entorhinal cortex and in the PNS. The $5HT_1$ receptor, which has several subtypes, is inhibitory and is coupled to a G-protein that inhibits cAMP. The $5HT_2$ receptor is excitatory and causes depolarization of neurons in the cerebral cortex. Serotonin is involved in the spinal pain pathway, in facilitating motor activity, and possibly in modulating human behavior. Both norepinephrine and serotonin have been implicated in depression. $5HT_3$ is also widely distributed in the stomach and probably accounts for the gastrointestinal upset commonly found when taking antidepressants.

Histamine. Histamine is found in low quantities in the brain. Its precursor is histidine, which is the chemical that crosses the blood-brain barrier. Histamine neurons are located primarily in the hypothalamus, and their processes extend to many CNS areas. The receptors for histamine initiate secondary messenger transmission. Histamine is believed to be involved in body functions such as the regulation of biorhythms and thermoregulation and in neuroendocrine functions.

The monoamines can be excitatory or inhibitory transmitters, depending on the action mediated by their receptors. These receptors primarily give rise to secondary messenger transmission that can be slow acting initially but have an extended duration of action. Therefore, for a full understanding of the action of neurotransmitters, one needs to understand the action of the specific receptors.

Neuropeptides

Neuropeptides are proteins that act as neurotransmitters or hormones. These are highly diverse proteins that have a common ability to excite or inhibit the activity of cell membranes. This discussion is limited to the neuropeptides that act as neurotransmitters in the CNS. Some of these proteins are released from their neurons in a manner similar to that of other transmitters. However, these neurotransmitters may enter either synaptic clefts or the bloodstream (pituitary hormones). Receptors on the postsynaptic membrane initiate secondary messenger transmission. Neuropeptides have been found to be released in conjunction with other neurotransmitters. For example, ACh and vasoactive intestinal polypeptide (VIP) have been shown to be released from cortical neurons at the same boutons.[4] Therefore the principle that one neuron releases one neurotransmitter (Dale's principle) does not reflect current information. Theoretically, then, one might expect to find multiple transmitters from the same neuron working synergistically or antagonistically on the postsynaptic receptors. Hence the quantity and distribution of the receptors are important in forming neural circuits.

The synthesis of neuropeptides is hypothesized to be performed in one of two ways: by messenger ribonucleic acid (mRNA) or by enzymatic action. Large neuropeptides are proteins that originate from the interaction of mRNA with polyribosomes on the endoplasmic reticulum in the cell body. Because these proteins will be involved in secretory processes, they are transported to the Golgi apparatus as prohormones, where they are packed in membranes and shipped by axonal transport to the cell processes for storage, degradation to the active molecule, and release.[11,20] Small neuropeptides can be synthesized by means of enzymatic action through glycolysis, the citric acid cycle, and related mechanisms.

Opioids. In 1975, Hughes and others discovered that the brain contains its own opioid system and that the system appears to be involved in pain and pleasure.[12] The receptors of this system are stimulated by endogenous, opioid-like chemicals and morphine and can be blocked by naloxone, a narcotic antagonist. The chemicals are called *endorphins* and are defined as endogenous molecules of the body that have an opioid-like action. The term *endorphin* encompasses a large group of diverse neuropeptides. In this section beta-endorphin and a smaller group of endorphins called enkephalins are discussed. These chemicals are widely distributed throughout the CNS.

Beta-endorphin. Beta-endorphin, which contains 31 amino acids, is an excellent representative of the endorphin group. It has been found to be 48 times as potent as morphine. Beta-endorphin has been localized to the hypothalamus, with projecting processes to the midbrain and other CNS locations. It is synthesized from the prohormone proopiomelanocortin, which is broken down in vesicles into adrenocorticotropin, or adrenocorticotropic hormone (ACTH), beta-lipotropin, and a number of other active neuropeptides. Beta-lipotropin is further processed into beta-endorphin and another peptide. Under stress, beta-endorphin and ACTH are released simultaneously into the blood, which helps demonstrate the common prohormone origins.[14]

Enkephalins. Enkephalins are specific endorphins. They are all pentapeptides. Enkephalins are widely distributed throughout the CNS, primarily in small neurons that are locally active. The prohormones for enkephalins are proenkephalin and prodynorphin. The synthesis is similar to that of endorphin formation in that a number of neuropeptides are formed when the cell dismantles the prohormones. The enkephalins have been implicated in physiologic areas such as pain perception, taste and olfaction, arousal, emotional behavior, vision and hearing, neurohormone secretion, motor coordination, and water balance.[5,11,15,22]

Substance P. Substance P was discovered in 1931 from the precipitate of horse brain. It is made up of a chain of 11 amino acids. The activity of substance P was shown at that time to be similar to that of ACh, but it was not blocked, as ACh is, by atropine. Substance P is found in great quantities in the dorsal horn of the spinal cord and is widely distributed throughout the CNS. In the spinal cord, it appears to be the neurotransmitter of the small-diameter, peripheral pain neurons.[5]

Somatostatin. Somatostatin is produced inside the brain and in D cells of the pancreas. It is made up of a chain of 14 amino acids. One fourth of the brain somatostatin has been localized to the hypothalamus, and it is also found in the small-diameter, peripheral pain neurons with substance P. Somatostatin is both a hormone and a neurotransmitter. Somatostatin affects the postsynaptic membrane by hyperpolarizing (inhibiting) the membrane.[5,6]

Other neuropeptides that are beyond the scope of this review include vasoactive intestinal polypeptide, cholecystokinin, adrenocorticotropic hormone, neurotensin, and angiotensin II.

Amino Acid Transmitters

The amino acid transmitters are a special group of amino acids that are normally found in cells. They are formed, like many other amino acids, as products during the normal cellular processes of glycolysis and the citric acid cycle (Figure 4-6).[16] These chemicals include gamma-aminobutyric acid (GABA), glycine, glutamate, and aspartate. GABA and glycine are well-known inhibitory transmitters; glutamate and aspartate are excitatory transmitters. These amino acid transmitters are widely distributed throughout the nervous system.

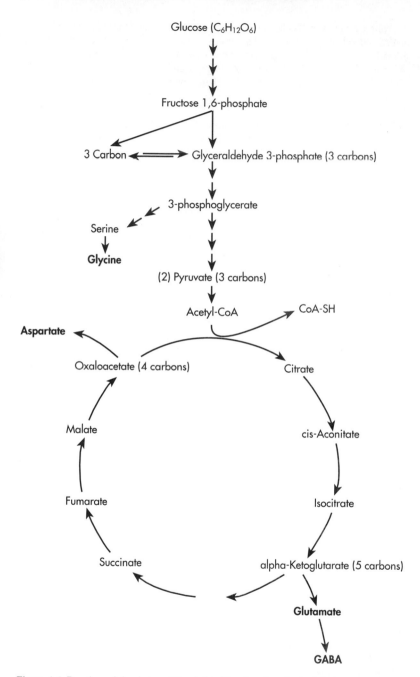

Figure 4-6 Reactions of glycolysis and the citric acid cycle and synthesis of glycine, aspartate, glutamate, and gamma-aminobutyric acid *(GABA)*.

GABA. GABA receptors have been localized on all neurons that have been investigated, which indicates a ubiquitous distribution in the nervous system.[4] GABA receptors are designated A and B.[8] Type A receptors function by first messenger transmission, whereas type B receptors use the indirect secondary messenger transmissions. Both receptors, when activated, result in an influx of chloride ions into the neuron, which causes hyperpolarization of the membrane potential (inhibition). Glial cells, which form a dense network around neurons, have an affinity for GABA, and by removing it from the synaptic cleft, they prevent GABA buildup.[2,8] GABA is synthesized by the decarboxylation of glutamate (see Figure 4-6) via alpha-ketoglutaric acid from the citric acid cycle.

Glycine. Glycine has been localized in the cerebellum, brainstem, and spinal cord. Both glycine and GABA have been isolated from the two types of Renshaw cells, from interneurons, and in the spinal cord. The receptor for glycine uses the fast-acting first messenger transmission. The storage mechanism within the neuron for both glycine and GABA has not yet been determined. The mechanism for inhibition is the same as that described for GABA. Glycine is synthesized directly from serine, which is derived from glycolysis (see Figure 4-6).[4,18]

Glutamate. Glutamate is the primary excitatory neurotransmitter in the mammalian nervous system. The most extensively studied glutamate receptor subtype is the *N*-methyl-D-aspartate (NMDA) receptor. The non-NMDA receptor is also referred to as the *aminomethylisoxazole propionate* (AMPA) *receptor.*[3]

NMDA receptor. The NMDA receptor has certain properties that set it apart from classical receptors. Namely, it is both ligand and voltage gated. When glutamate is released into the synaptic cleft, it binds to the NMDA receptor; however, this alone will not activate the receptor. At membrane potentials less than −50 mV, the concentration of Mg^{2+} in the extracellular fluid will block the ion flow through the receptor (Mg-block).[17] To activate the receptor, the Mg-block must be released, an event that occurs when the membrane is depolarized by glutamate binding to the AMPA receptors (also referred to as the *non-NMDA receptors*). Unlike the non-NMDA receptors, the activation of the NMDA receptor allows calcium to flow into the cell. It has been known for some time that the increase in intracellular calcium following NMDA receptor activation will lead to increases in NO levels by activating the enzyme NOS. The brain is a good source of NOS. Before the discovery of NOS in the brain, several investigators had shown that in several regions of the brain, excitatory amino acids produced elevated levels of cyclic guanosine monophosphate (cGMP). In 1988, it was shown that stimulation of NMDA receptors induced a calcium-dependent increase in NO, which in turn led to increased levels of cGMP in the presynaptic cell (Figure 4-7).[7] NO is extensively investigated in numerous pathologic states such as Parkinson's disease, Huntington's disease, and Alzheimer's disease. In summary, glutamate binds to the NMDA receptor, which leads to an influx of calcium into the cell. The increase in intracellular calcium activates NOS, which produces NO, and the NO in turn binds to guanylate cyclase in the presynaptic cell, which produces cGMP. Under normal physiologic conditions, the NMDA-NO pathway is important in many biologic functions, but overstimulation of this pathway has been implicated in numerous diseases.

Aspartate. Aspartate is found in the hippocampus and the dorsal root ganglion. Its activity is similar to that of glutamate. Aspartate is synthesized (see Figure 4-6) directly from oxaloacetic acid, again a primary chemical in the citric acid cycle. It is

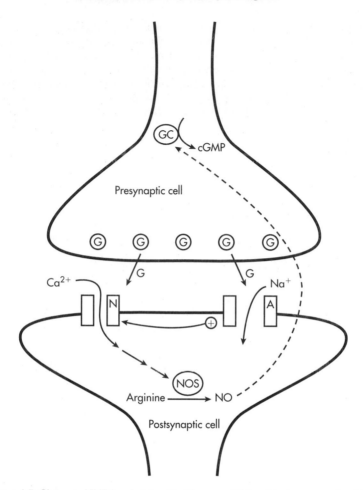

Figure 4-7 Glutamate-NMDA and nitric oxide. Glutamate *(G)* found in the presynaptic cell is released and binds to the AMPA receptor *(A)* on the postsynaptic cell, which allows an influx of Na^{2+}. The increased Na^{2+} leads to a membrane depolarization, which along with binding of glutamate to the NMDA receptor (N) allows an influx of Ca^{2+} into the cell. The increased intracellular calcium activates nitric oxide synthase *(NOS)*, which produces nitric oxide *(NO)*. NO is a gas that diffuses back to the presynaptic cell to activate guanylate cyclase *(GC)* and produces cyclic guanosine monophosphate *(cGMP)*, which leads to functional changes in the presynaptic cell. This pathway has been implicated in normal learning and memory and also in several pathologic conditions.

difficult to distinguish between glutamate and aspartate by means of current technology.

NEUROTRANSMITTERS AND NEUROCHEMISTRY OF BEHAVIOR

It is important to recognize that all neurotransmitters and pathways have multiple functions. Only a few are discussed in this review. Furthermore, more than one neurotransmitter may be released at any synapse. When this occurs, the synergistic effect or a differential effect may take place. Finally, receptors select which transmitter will activate or inhibit the neuron. The following section discusses some of these neurotransmitters with respect to the neurochemistry of behavior. In addition, the functional neuroanatomic pathways rising from the reticular formation (see Chapter 2) are known to be involved in the integration, modulation, and regulation of several neurotransmitter systems such as the acetylcholine, norepinephrine, serotonin, and dopamine systems. A basic understanding of these systems is useful when considering the actions and effects of pharmacologic agents. Moreover, current neurophysiologic studies, postmortem studies, and molecular genetics studies are seeking to further clarify the role of these systems in the behavioral neurobiology of pharmacologic agents.

In this chapter, neurochemical systems have already been characterized with respect to their neurochemical transmission and communication between presynaptic and postsynaptic receptors. In addition, the potential for transmission at the postsynaptic receptor sites through ion channels and the influence of second messenger systems have been discussed. Also, projections arising from the reticular formation, including the locus ceruleus, dopaminergic tracts arising from the VTA and substantia nigra, and serotonergic tracts arising from the raphe nuclei, have been presented in Table 4-1 and are important to understanding the proposed effects of psychotropic drugs.

The neurochemistry of many behaviors and mechanisms of several classes of psychotropic agents may best be understood through an appreciation of the interaction among the neuroanatomic structures and the interplay of the neurochemical systems, especially in the case of certain pharmacologic compounds that have been discovered or developed along these conceptual frameworks. For example, the initial observations leading to the neurochemical explanations of many behaviors were stimulated in the 1950s by Laborit, a French anesthesiologist, who was trying to invent a cocktail to relieve anxiety and stress associated with surgical procedures. In Laborit's work with a chemist to invent a new antihistamine, chlorpromazine was identified as the active ingredient of his cocktail. The cocktail was then given to schizophrenic and psychotic patients in a French asylum and shown not only to calm the patients but also to reduce other symptoms such as hallucinosis, paranoia, and agitation. This experiment resulted in the dramatic changes in psychiatric care and treatment, as discussed in Chapter 1, and in many historical advances; in addition, it led to the neurochemical studies of chlorpromazine and other chemicals, which were believed to be useful in clinical practice.

Chlorpromazine, from the phenothiazine class, or family, was found to be similar in structure to dopamine, especially in its ring structure and tailed nitrogen. The molecule was found to fit, or interact, with the dopamine receptor and to act as a dopamine antagonist, preventing transmission of dopamine impulses believed to be responsible for schizophrenic and other psychotic symptoms. It was observed that a concentration of approximately 600 mg/day was necessary for the desired clinical effect, probably because of its relatively low affinity for the dopamine receptors. Other drugs in the phenothiazine family found later include triflupromazine, trifluoperazine, fluphenazine, and others that are much more potent, have a higher affinity for the receptor and are much more likely to be clinically effective at lower dosages. Two potent nonphenothiazine drugs are haloperidol and thiothixene. These agents are discussed in Chapter 5.

Further study of the phenothiazine family of agents resulted in additional delineation of the dopaminergic tracts. The mesolimbic and mesocortical tracts were identified as the main ones responsible for schizophrenic behavior. The nigrostriatal tract is involved in symptoms that are associated with Parkinson's disease. Thus, when chlorpromazine is administered to a patient, it interacts with dopamine receptors in the terminal portion of the striatum and can result in extrapyramidal symptoms that mimic Parkinson's disease. These symptoms are referred to as *pseudoparkinsonian symptoms* and include dyskinetic movement, dystonia, and other frank parkinsonian symptoms. The development of tardive dyskinesia, which is discussed in detail in Chapter 5, as well as other undesired effects, results from the *upregulating* of dopamine receptors, particularly D_2 receptors.

In the past decade, there has also been research progress in the biologic and neuropharmacologic basis of drug abuse and the so-called reward pathway. The reward pathway consists of the limbic system, the nucleus accumbens, and the globus pallidus and involves several neurotransmitters such as serotonin, dopamine, and epinephrine. These systems are thought to be important in rewarding certain behaviors, and when the system is disrupted, the individual feels a variety of negative emotions such as anxiety, anger, and a craving for a substance that can alleviate these negative emotions. This chemical imbalance ultimately leads to a variety of behavioral disorders. The most extensively investigated aspect of this system is the D_2 receptor. Specifically, it is thought that in chronic alcoholics there is a possible reduction in the D_2 receptors in certain areas of the limbic system. Furthermore, genetic studies suggest that there is a relationship between the A1 allele for the D_2 receptor and severe chronic alcoholism. These findings have also been replicated with cocaine users and even polysubstance users. The fact that the D_2 receptor has been implicated as the basis for abuse of several different drugs has given rise to the model of dopamine being instrumental in *the final common pathway.* [1]

As with the discovery of antipsychotic agents, the antidepressant drugs were discovered serendipitously. After the success of treating patients with tuberculosis using isonicotinic acid was established, pharmaceutical companies began seeking to create similar compounds. This research resulted in the development of iproniazid, which underwent clinical trials. The moods of tuberculous patients who had been taking this drug for 3 to 4 months improved significantly, although the tuberculosis did not. Iproniazid, which acts as a monoamine oxidase (MAO) enzyme inhibitor, has many effects on neurotransmitters, including the potentiation of norepinephrine and serotonin, neurotransmitters thought to play a key role in depression. Because it took 3 to 4 months to see these effects, these drugs did not have significant abuse potential and this class of drug (MAO inhibitors) was later developed as a conventional antidepressant (see Chapter 6). Another pharmaceutical company attempted to develop alternative forms of chlorpromazine and developed a compound called *imipramine.* When scientists tested this drug, they found that it is also successful in treating depression. This compound was the predecessor to the tricyclic antidepressants and was later noted to block the reuptake of various biogenic amines.

The discovery of the MAO inhibitors and tricyclic antidepressants resulted in further consideration of depression as an illness in which both mood and behavior were affected and induced by neurochemical changes. The biogenic amine theory of depression resulted from this thinking. Subsequent hypotheses included the serotonin hypothesis. Because the vast majority of serotonin is produced in the CNS by the raphe nuclei that supply the limbic system and frontal cortical system, this distribution made serotonin a likely suspect in the cause of depressive illness. Tricyclic antidepressants prevented the reuptake of this neurochemical from the synapse by the presynaptic terminal, which in turn increased the relative amount of serotonin in the synapse and corrected the relative deficiency. The initial result was a greater-than-normal response because of the supersensitivity of the serotonin receptor site. In short, these receptor sites were hungry for serotonin and these pharmacologic agents, the MAO inhibitors and the tricyclic antidepressants, enabled those receptors to have an increased supply.

Subsequently, the norepinephrine hypothesis of depression was developed. The major nuclei of the norepinephrine production are found within the locus ceruleus. This structure, the virtual command and control center of norepinephrine, sends projections to the limbic system and cortex in a manner similar to that of serotonin. Norepinephrine was also deemed to be important in certain depressive syndromes, particularly when a decrement of norepinephrine production was occurring. It was proposed that certain agents, in particular, tricyclic antidepressants, acted with norepinephrine as they did with serotonin. That is, they blocked the reuptake of norepinephrine at the presynaptic terminal and supersensitized the postsynaptic membrane. Thus a greater synaptic supply of norepinephrine was available.

The action of the tricyclic antidepressants showed a lag time of approximately 2 to 5 weeks before any effects of treatment were seen. Furthermore, the amount of neurotransmitter in the synapse increased immediately because of the block of the reuptake by the presynaptic terminal. However, the changes in the sensitivity of the postsynaptic receptors occurred over time. This seems to be the critical step in how this class of agents has its clinical effect. In addition, effects at differential receptor sites are now thought to be critical to the clinical efficacy of these and other antidepressant compounds, including novel agents such as bupropion and newer agents such as the selective serotonin reuptake inhibitors.

Many other agents that affect neurotransmitter systems outlined in this chapter are discussed in chapters specific to disorders. For example, generalized anxiety disorder that occurs in patients with persistent, severe, and disabling anxiety may involve the GABA-benzodiazepine chloride system. Psychostimulants such as amphetamines and methylphenidate (Ritalin) may cause brief periods of euphoria but are more commonly used to treat attention deficit hyperactivity disorder (ADHD).

Glutamate and the NMDA receptor have received considerable attention in the past decade because of their roles in both development and neuronal cell death. The term *activity-dependent learning* was first used in 1949 by Hebb[9] to refer to the fact that the nervous system needs to be active for it to learn and that learning must be due to functional changes at the synaptic level. The glutamate-NMDA-NO pathway has been strongly implicated as the biochemical and molecular basis for activity-dependent learning. The functional changes at the synaptic level following activation of the NMDA receptor are an example of the brain's plasticity. The term *plasticity* refers to the brain's ability to adapt and change in response to activity or to the environment.

When the NMDA receptors and the non-NMDA receptors on the postsynaptic cell are occupied by glutamate, the NMDA channels open and allow calcium into the cell. The increased calcium then activates NOS to produce NO that leads to functional changes in the presynaptic cell and ultimately leads to a strengthening of the synapse between the presynaptic and postsynaptic cell. The downside of this intricate and finely tuned system is that it is very susceptible to damage. It had been known since the 1970s that following a stroke there was increased levels of glutamate in the region of damage. It has now been shown that much of the neuronal damage results from the excess glutamate overstimulating the NMDA receptors, leading to increased calcium and higher-than-normal levels of NO. Alterations in the glutamate-NMDA receptor pathway have also been implicated in schizophrenia, Alzheimer's disease, Parkinson's disease, drug reinforcement, AIDS dementia, and several other neurologic conditions.

Other connections between neurotransmitter systems and identified psychiatric disorders include the role of ACh and other cholinergic systems in memory processes. The degeneration of cholinergic neurons of the basal nucleus of Meynert into the hippocampus is one of the many features found in Alzheimer's disease. Endorphins and enkephalins are known to be important in pain perception. Cholecystokinin and neurotensin may also be important in schizophrenia. A deficiency in somatostatin may be found to occur in individuals with Alzheimer's disease. These neurochemical systems, as they are being explored, have certainly furthered the understanding of the biology of behavior, including the cause and course of many significant neuropsychiatric syndromes.

The introduction of computed tomography, magnetic resonance imaging, and other imaging techniques, including single photon emission computed tomography and positron emission spectroscopy, may also be useful in elucidating the biologic basis of psychiatric syndromes. These technologies have also been useful, through the use of radioisotopes, in the study of the influence of pharmacologic agents on certain receptor sites and structures. These technologies allow us to view the inside of the brain, including the ventricular system, receptor sites, and brain tissues. Positron emission spectroscopy scanning with the use of radioisotopes, which are taken up readily into the cells, may also further enhance our understanding of the relative value of pharmacologic agents.

Molecular genetics, through which certain disorders based on specific chromosomal defects can be identified, may allow the discovery and development of novel drugs and targeted actions. This could certainly open up further development of chemical treatments for psychiatric disorders. However, it must be kept in mind that complex human traits are caused by interactions between numerous genes and the environment. The human brain and especially psychiatric disorders are so complex that it would be a mistake to succumb to the notion that these disorders are simply due to a single faulty gene. The challenge for neuroscience in the next century is to determine the relative contributions of genes and the environment to these psychiatric disorders and to wisely use this information in the treatment of patients. This is indeed an interesting time to study the neurochemistry of behavior.

REFERENCES

1. Blum K, Cull JG, Braverman ER, Comings DE: Reward deficiency syndrome, *Am Sci* 84: 132, 1996.
2. Crill WE: The milieu of the central nervous system. In Patton HD and others, editors: *Textbook of physiology,* vol 1, Philadelphia, 1989, WB Saunders.
3. Davies J: NMDA receptors in synaptic pathways. In Wilkins JC and others, editors: *The NMDA receptor,* Oxford, 1989, Oxford University Press.
4. Detwiller PB, Crill WE: Synaptic transmission. In Patton HD and others, editors: *Textbook of physiology,* vol 1, Philadelphia, 1989, WB Saunders.
5. Dorsa DM: Neuropeptides as neurotransmitters. In Patton HD and others, editors: *Textbook of physiology,* vol 2, Philadelphia, 1989, WB Saunders.
6. Erulkar SD: Chemically mediated synaptic transmission: an overview. In Siegel GJ and others, editors: *Basic neurochemistry,* New York, 1989, Raven.
7. Garthwaite G: Glutamate, nitric oxide, and cell signaling in the nervous system. *Trends Neuroscience* 14:60, 1991.
8. Gottlieb DI: GABAergic neurons, *Sci Am* 258:82, 1988.
9. Hebb DH: *The organization of behavior,* New York, 1949, John Wiley.
10. Hille B: Neuromuscular transmission. In Patton HD and others, editors: *Textbook of physiology,* vol 1, Philadelphia, 1989, WB Saunders.
11. Holaday JW: *Endogenous opioids and their receptors: current concepts,* Kalamazoo, Mich, 1985, Upjohn.
12. Hughes H and others: Identification of two related pentapeptides from the brain with potent opiate agonist activity, *Nature* 258:577, 1975.

13. Hyman SE, Nestler EJ: *The molecular foundations of psychiatry,* Washington, DC, 1993, American Psychiatric Press.
14. Kelly DD: Central representation of pain and analgesia. In Kandel ER, Schwartz JH, editors: *Principles of neural science,* New York, 1985, Elsevier.
15. Kutchai HC: Cellular physiology. In Berne RM, Levy MN, editors: *Physiology,* ed 3, St Louis, 1993, Mosby.
16. Mathews CK, Van Holde KE: *Biochemistry,* Redwood City, Calif, 1990, Benjamin Cummings.
17. Mayer ML, Westbrook GL, Guthrie PB: Voltage dependent block by Mg^{2+} of NMDA responses in spinal cord, *Nature* 308:261, 1984.
18. McGeer PL, McGeer EG: Amino acid neurotransmitters. In Siegel GJ and others, editors: *Basic neurochemistry,* New York, 1989, Raven.
19. Patton HD: The autonomic nervous system. In Patton HD and others, editors: *Textbook of physiology,* vol 1, Philadelphia, 1989, WB Saunders.
20. Schwartz JH: Chemical messengers: small molecules and peptides. In Kandel ER, Schwartz JH, editors: *Principles of neural science,* New York, 1985, Elsevier.
21. Shepard GM: *Neurobiology,* New York, 1983, Oxford University.
22. Simon EJ, Miller JB: Opioid peptides and opioid receptors. In Siegel GJ and others, editors: *Basic neurochemistry,* New York, 1989, Raven.
23. Taylor P, Brown JH: Acetylcholine. In Siegel GJ and others, editors: *Basic neurochemistry,* New York, 1989, Raven.
24. Weiner N, Molinoff PB: Catecholamines. In Siegel GJ and others, editors: *Basic neurochemistry,* New York, 1989, Raven.

UNIT II

Drugs Used in the Treatment
of Mental Disorders

CHAPTER 5

Schizophrenia and Other Psychoses

*"To live with schizophrenia is to live with uncertainty, to always have
the threat of regression as a reality. After four years out of the hospital
and feeling myself impervious, in 1996 I relapsed. I felt totally
defeated, having all but forgotten that I had a chronic psychotic illness.
It was nothing short of heartbreak."*

Patricia J. Ruocchio, 1999

HISTORICAL CONSIDERATIONS
Description

Psychosis is a disruptive mental state in which an individual struggles to distinguish the external world from his or her internally generated perceptions. Common symptoms of psychosis include hallucinations, delusions, and difficulty with thought organization. Psychosis can be present in the following disorders:

- Schizophrenia
- Acute mania
- Depression
- Drug intoxication
- Dementia
- Delirium

Schizophrenia is one of the most common and important forms of psychosis and will be used as the prototype disorder for this discussion. Schizophrenia is a serious and for most a lifelong psychotic illness. *The Diagnostic and Statistical Manual of Mental Disorders,* Fourth Edition (DSM-IV), describes schizophrenia as a psychiatric disorder characterized by social withdrawal and disturbances in thought, motor behavior, and interpersonal functioning.[4] These criteria are depicted in Box 5-1. Individuals with schizophrenia may appear dull and colorless, dependent and apathetic, emotionally isolative, or agitated and threatening. These and other characteristic symptoms determine which subtype is assigned, that is, paranoid, catatonic, disorganized, undifferentiated, or residual (Box 5-2, p. 80).

Prevalence and Cost

The cost in human suffering is incalculable (see Box 5-3, p. 81, for a review of statistical realities of schizophrenia). At any given time, about 1% of the adult population meets conventional criteria for schizophrenia, with a lifetime prevalence between 1% and 2%.[127,129] Economic costs, both direct and indirect, are estimated in the tens of billions of dollars each year. Direct health care costs are 2.5% of total health care expenditures (including such expenditures as treatment, medications, hospitalization, institutionalization, board and care, and day treatment). Examples of indirect costs include lost productivity of patients and families and wages lost related to suicide.[52,130]

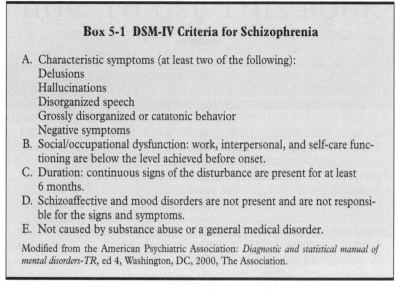

Box 5-1 DSM-IV Criteria for Schizophrenia

A. Characteristic symptoms (at least two of the following):
   Delusions
   Hallucinations
   Disorganized speech
   Grossly disorganized or catatonic behavior
   Negative symptoms
B. Social/occupational dysfunction: work, interpersonal, and self-care functioning are below the level achieved before onset.
C. Duration: continuous signs of the disturbance are present for at least 6 months.
D. Schizoaffective and mood disorders are not present and are not responsible for the signs and symptoms.
E. Not caused by substance abuse or a general medical disorder.

Modified from the American Psychiatric Association: *Diagnostic and statistical manual of mental disorders-TR,* ed 4, Washington, DC, 2000, The Association.

Age of Onset

Typically, schizophrenia is first diagnosed in late adolescence or early adulthood. The earlier the onset, the poorer the long-term prognosis and the greater the neuroleptic resistance.[117] Men develop schizophrenia earlier in life than do women. Box 5-4 (p. 81) lists the variables associated with a more favorable outcome.

Gender Issues Related to Schizophrenia

Box 5-5 (p. 82) captures some of the gender issues related to schizophrenia. Although there is near equal incidence of schizophrenia for men and women, several gender-based differences have been documented. For example, women have a later onset of schizophrenia by about 5 years and have a documentable bimodal distribution for age of onset. That is, a small (about 10%) but distinct cohort of women are initially diagnosed with schizophrenia after menopause.[130] The early delay in symptoms compared with men and the significant number of postmenopausal diagnoses of this disorder are thought to be related to the protective function of estrogen. It is believed the dopamine-antagonizing effects of estrogen "protect" women during times of high estrogen and that protection subsides as estrogen levels decrease. Women also have less severe courses of this illness, exhibit less aggression and better social relationships, have more positive symptoms, have fewer structural abnormalities, and have less cerebral lateralization.

THE EVOLUTION OF DIAGNOSTIC CONSIDERATIONS IN UNDERSTANDING SCHIZOPHRENIA

Science attempts to classify, categorize, and subordinate. Morel was the first to assign a name to the psychiatric symptoms we now refer to as *schizophrenia*. In 1856, while treating an adolescent boy, he used the phrase *démence précoce* (precocious dementia) to describe the group of observed symptoms. Over the next several years, Kahlbaum, Hecker, and Kraepelin contributed the diagnostic terms *catatonia, hebephrenia,* and

---

Box 5-2 DSM-IV Criteria for Schizophrenia Subtypes

Paranoid:
A. Preoccupation with one or more delusions or frequent auditory hallucinations
B. None of the following is prominent: disorganized speech, disorganized behavior, flat or inappropriate affect, catatonic behavior

Disorganized:
A. All of the following are prominent: disorganized speech, disorganized behavior, flat or inappropriate affect
B. Does not meet criteria of catatonic type

Catatonic:
At least two of the following are present:
A. Motoric immobility, waxy flexibility, or stupor
B. Excessive motor activity (purposeless)
C. Extreme negativism or mutism
D. Peculiar movements, stereotypy of movements, prominent mannerisms, or prominent grimacing
E. Echolalia or echopraxia

Undifferentiated:
Characteristic symptoms are present, but criteria for paranoid, catatonic, or disorganized subtypes are not met.

Residual:
A. Characteristic symptoms (criterion A [see Box 5-1]) are no longer present; criteria are unmet for paranoid, catatonic, or disorganized subtypes
B. There is continuing evidence of disturbance, such as the presence of negative symptoms or criterion A symptoms, in an attenuated form (e.g., odd beliefs, unusual perceptual experiences)

Modified from the American Psychiatric Association: *Diagnostic and statistical manual of mental disorders-TR*, ed 4, Washington, DC, 2000, The Association.

---

paranoia, respectively. Kraepelin, the best scientist of the group, engaged in a rigorous study of a variety of disorders now recognized as schizophrenia. He noted the symptomatic commonalties among catatonia, hebephrenia, and paranoia, and in 1896, he used Morel's term to group them under the label *dementia praecox.* Kraepelin believed schizophrenia resulted from neuropathologic disturbance and attempted to distinguish florid symptoms from those characterized by persistent losses or deficits.[96] Kraepelin envisioned a progressive deteriorating course for patients suffering from the latter. These individuals, he recognized, experienced a disabling trajectory of impairment and had little hope of recovery.[8] Kraepelin described the fundamental deficit in schizophrenia as "annihilation of the will."[102]

The term *schizophrenia* was not developed until the 1900s when Bleuler used it in his book subtitled *The Group of Schizophrenias.* Bleuler argued against the use of the term *dementia praecox* because he observed that schizophrenia did not always follow a

Box 5-3 Statistical Realities of Schizophrenia

1. About 1% of the population suffers from schizophrenia.
2. Prevalence is roughly the same for men as for women.
3. Peak onset for men is 18 to 25 years of age.
4. Peak onset for women in 24 to early 30s.
5. For 95% of sufferers, the disease lasts a lifetime.
6. Approximately 75% of taxpayer mental health expenditures are for schizophrenia.
7. Individuals with schizophrenia occupy 25% of inpatient hospital beds.
8. Approximately 15% of individuals with schizophrenia do not respond to traditional antipsychotic medications, and 70% are only partial responders.
9. Half of the patients experience serious side effects to the medication.
10. Unemployment reaches 70% to 90%, and individuals with schizophrenia constitute 10% of all people classified as permanently disabled.
11. Direct health care costs are 2.5% of total health care expenditures.
12. Indirect costs are estimated at $46 billion.
13. From 20% to 50% of these individuals attempt suicide, and 10% are successful in fatally injuring themselves.
14. Individuals with schizophrenia have a 20% shorter life span.

Adapted from News in mental health nursing. *J Psychosoc Nurs* 35(2):6, 1997; American Psychiatric Association: *Am J Psychiatry* 154(suppl 4):1, 1997; and Richards SS, Musser WS, Gershon S: *Maintenance pharmacotherapies for neuropsychiatric disorders*, Philadelphia, 1999, Brunner/Mazel.

Box 5-4 Prognositc Variables Associated with Better Long-Term Outcomes

Older age at onset
Female gender
Family history of affective disorder
No family history of schizophrenia
Good premorbid functioning
Higher IQ
Married
Acute onset with a precipitation stressor
Fewer prior episodes (both number and length)
Advancing age
Minimal comorbidity
Paranoid subtype
Predominantly positive symptoms (delusions, hallucinations)
Not disorganized
Not negative (flat affect, alogia, avolition)

Adapted from American Psychiatric Association: *Am J Psychiatry* 154:(suppl 1)4, 1997.

Box 5-5 Gender Based Issues Related to Schizophrenia

1. Women have later onset of schizophrenia.
2. Women have a less severe course of illness.
3. Women are prescribed 60% of all antipsychotic drugs.
4. Thirty percent of all antipsychotics are prescribed to women during childbearing years (ages 20 to 50).
5. Dopamine receptor decline is slower in women.
6. Women have less cerebral lateralization (may confer greater brain resilience).
7. Women tend to have more positive symptoms and fewer negative symptoms.
8. Estrogen modulates dopaminergic functions and seems to play a protective role for women.
9. At times when estrogen is high (e.g., pregnancy), symptoms may improve in women with schizophrenia.
10. At times when estrogen is low (e.g., premenstruation, postpartum, post-menopausal), symptoms may worsen in women with schizophrenia.
11. Women have fewer structural brain abnormalities.
12. Women have a better response to lower dosages of conventional antipsychotic drugs.

Adapted from Promedica Research Center: *Women and schizophrenia*, Tucker, Ga, 1997; The Promedica Research Center, Lilly Center for Women's Health: *Sex based differences in antipsychotic therapy*, Chicago, 1997, The Center; and Richards SS, Musser WS, Gershon S: *Maintenance pharmacotherapies for neuropsychiatric disorders*, Philadelphia, 1999, Brunner/Mazel.

---

deteriorative course, nor did it always develop at an early age.[27] Bleuler's contribution broadened Kraepelin's concept by focusing on symptoms rather than strictly clinical outcomes. Kraepelin's paradigm of schizophrenia did not anticipate recovery. Because of Bleuler's wider grouping, pessimism eased and some clinicians began to record improvements in their patients. Bleuler himself estimated that 25% of his patients fully recovered.[78] Influenced by Freud and other psychodynamic theorists, Bleuler explored psychologic explanations for schizophrenia, yet he never abandoned the biologic theories of Kraepelin. Nonetheless, his psychodynamic views held sway and greatly influenced the conceptualization of schizophrenia as presented in the *Diagnostic and Statistical Manuals I and II.*

In 1980, the third edition of the *Diagnostic and Statistical Manual* was printed.[3] Wilson, noting the transforming nature of this document, stated, "DSM-III is commonly declared to be the most significant factor in promoting what has been called the 'remedicalization' of American psychiatry."[170] During the last half of the twentieth century, this remedicalization of psychiatry has resulted in biologic paradigms and a renewed respect for Kraepelin's work. In fact, it is not uncommon to find the terms *Kraepelinian* and *non-Kraepelinian* used to differentiate individuals in terms of severity and prognosis.[88,95] In contrast, the introduction of the DSM-III resulted in the view that Bleuler's contributions, albeit significant, had softened the diagnostic criteria and obscured the deteriorating course of the illness.

DSM-IV and Clinical Subtyping

Early efforts to categorize schizophrenia yielded the subtypes catatonic, hebephrenic, paranoid, and simple schizophrenia. Paranoid and catatonic subtypes are still reflected in the current official (DSM-IV) diagnostic classification system given in Box 5-2.

The most clinically useful subtyping approach, in our view, is derived from Kraepelin's work. As noted earlier, Kraepelin differentiated between florid symptoms (positive symptoms) and those characterized by loss and deficit (negative symptoms). Biologically oriented diagnosticians, such as Strauss, Carpenter, and Bartko; Crow, Andreasen, and Olsen; and Andreasen and others, have developed two subtypes, positive and negative schizophrenia.[7,8,45,150] This dichotomy is based on well-designed research. Positive (type I) schizophrenia presents a different constellation of symptoms than does negative (type II) schizophrenia. In 1997, the American Psychiatric Association (APA) Guidelines recognized an expansion of this dichotomy to include a *disorganized* category.[5] Disorganized symptoms include disorganized speech, disorganized behavior, and poor attention. Box 5-6 contrasts type I and type II.

Type I is positive in the sense that symptoms are an embellishment of normal cognition and perception. The symptoms are "additional," for example, hallucinations, delusions, thought disorders, or bizarre or agitated behaviors. Positive symptoms are believed to be caused by a hyperdopaminergic process affecting mesolimbic areas. Type II is labeled negative because symptoms are essentially an absence of what should be, for example, lack of affect, lack of energy, and so forth. Type II is thought to be related to a hypodopaminergic phenomenon in the prefrontal cortex or even a nondopaminergic process (e.g., glutamatergic system dysfunction).[50,117] According to biologic theory, traditional antipsychotic drugs (drugs that primarily antagonize dopamine D_2 receptors) are likely to be more beneficial in individuals with positive schizophrenia. Because negative schizophrenia is not specifically related to hyperdopaminergic function, the use of dopamine D_2 antagonists or traditional antipsychotics is less effective and their continuous administration more controversial.[77] In addition to neurotransmission abnormalities, several well-documented structural and functional changes, primarily associated with negative schizophrenia, have been identified.

BIOLOGIC EXPLANATIONS OF SCHIZOPHRENIA

Kraepelin's tireless work encouraged others to search for postmortem findings that would indicate evidence of neuropathology in the brains of individuals with schizophrenia. Although efforts to find neuropathologic markers for schizophrenia have been attempted for many years, early attempts proved so futile that schizophrenia was oftentimes referred to as the *graveyard of neuropathologists*.[166] The work was so inconclusive that biologically oriented clinicians lost credibility and the psychodynamic approach prevailed for some time. As the science of understanding schizophrenia grew and as technology allowed, supporters of a biologic view became more influential. As noted previously, the publication of the DSM-III proved to be a major turning point in psychiatry.

Ventricular Enlargement

Johnstone and her colleagues were the first to definitely report enlarged ventricles among some individuals with schizophrenia.[79] Although several brain disorders are characterized by increased ventricular size, the increased ventricular brain ratios

Box 5-6 Positive and Negative Symptoms of Schizophrenia

Positive (Type I)

Prognosis: good
Precipitating factors: yes
Onset: acute
Sensorium: dreamlike quality
Intellectual impairment: none
Pathophysiology: D_2 hyperactivity

Pathoanatomy: VBRs normal
Response to typical neuroleptics: good
Effect of levodopa; increases symptoms

Negative (Type II)

Prognosis: poor
Onset: chronic
Family history: more than type I
Sensorium: clear
Intellectual impairment: yes
Pathophysiology: possibly hypodopaminergic, decreased CBF

Pathoanatomy: increased VBRs, other changes (see text)
Response to typical neuroleptics: varies
Response to atypical neuroleptics: good
Effect of levodopa: minimal

Positive symptoms
Abnormal thought form
Agitation, tension
Associational disturbances
Bizarre behavior
Conceptual disorganization
Delusions
Excitement
Feelings of persecution
Grandiosity
Hallucinations
Hostility
Ideas of reference
Illusions
Insomnia
Suspiciousness

Negative symptoms
Alogia
Anergia
Anhedonia
Asocial behavior
Attention deficits
Avolition
Blunted affect
Communication difficulties
Difficulty with abstractions
Passive social withdrawal
Poor grooming and hygiene
Poor rapport
Poverty of speech

(VBRs) found in schizophrenia are considered to be neurodevelopmental as opposed to the neurodegenerative processes identified in other disorders (e.g., Alzheimer's disease).* The assertion that schizophrenia is not neurodegenerative is supported by the absence of gliosis, the telltale sign of ongoing cellular breakdown. Imaging technology (magnetic resonance imaging [MRI] and computed tomography [CT]) makes it appealing to study ventricular size in these patients; however, MRI and CT diagnostic capabilities are limited. Roughly 50% of individuals with schizophrenia fall within the range of normal subjects when their VBRs are compared with those of controls.[37] This is not to imply that there is no loss of periventricular gray matter but rather to recognize the need for better control subjects. As with other research efforts, monozygotic twin studies have been helpful in establishing the overall significance of ventricular enlargement in individuals with schizophrenia. Whereas an individual case might "hide" when contrasted to the general population, monozygotic comparisons have yielded significant findings for ventricular size in the affected twin.[133,167]

Temporal Lobe Reduction

Temporal lobe reductions are evident in schizophrenia.[54,69,163,169] Reversed asymmetry has also been observed in some studies.[163] That is, normally the left temporal lobe is larger than the right, but this asymmetry is reversed in schizophrenia. The planum temporale, which composes the superior aspect of the temporal lobe, is involved in the generation and understanding of language. Reversed asymmetry in this region has been hypothesized to account for difficulties in understanding language, interpreting tone and emotional quality of language, inability to organize internal thoughts (thought disorder), and/or dyslexic (difficulty with written language) difficulties associated with schizophrenia.[163]

Hippocampal and Entorhinal Cortex Reductions

Although neuronal loss is not reported consistently in the literature, there is accumulating evidence that neuronal loss occurs in both the hippocampus and its immediate extension, the entorhinal cortex.† Decreased synaptic density is reported as well. Both the hippocampus and the entorhinal cortex are involved in memory and learning. Disruptions in these areas decrease the ability to learn and impair memory function. Roberts and colleagues state hippocampal neuron loss may reach 20%, and Torrey believes this loss, probably caused by viral infection, may be the major cause of schizophrenia.[159]

Cortical Atrophy

Scientists have observed for at least 100 years the diminished size of brain cortices in individuals with schizophrenia. Overall, a 5% reduction in brain weight and a 7% decrease in cortical thickness have been reported.[133,144] Negative symptoms such as cognitive slowing, alogia, avolition, anergia, apathy, withdrawal, and inappropriate or flattened affect could logically be connected to these prefrontal changes. Particularly associated with declines found in this population is an underdeveloped dorsolateral prefrontal cortex (DLPFC).[166]

*References 6, 30, 38, 54, 61, 109.
†References 11, 13, 29, 34, 109, 135, 153, 167.

Decreased Cerebral Blood Flow

A hypometabolic state occurs in schizophrenia (most often type II) and seems to be particularly apparent in the DLPFC and in the prefrontal poles (i.e., hypofrontality). This decrease in cerebral blood flow (CBF) is thought to contribute to diminishing the effectiveness of higher tasks performed by these brain areas (i.e., cognition, inhibition, goal setting, abstraction, spontaneity, and recent memory).[19,72]

ANTIPSYCHOTIC DRUGS

Antipsychotic drugs, as implied, are used primarily in the treatment of psychoses and are particularly important in prevention of relapse. Unfortunately, noncompliance is high. Table 5-1 presents a comparative description of these drugs. Specifically some or all antipsychotic drugs are approved for the treatment of the following conditions[22]:

- Acute and chronic psychoses (schizophrenia, manic phase of bipolar disorder, delusional disorder)
- Prophylaxis of schizophrenia
- Prophylaxis of bipolar disorder
- Agitated aggressive behavior in dementia (loxapine, risperidone, clozapine)
- Gilles de la Tourette's syndrome (primarily haloperidol, risperidone, pimozide)
- Antiemetic uses (chlorpromazine)

Unapproved indications include the following[22]:

- Antimanic and antidepressive mood stabilization
- Delusional depressive disorder
- Psychosis associated with Parkinson's disease
- Agitation in major depression
- Huntington's disease
- Impulsivity
- Augmentation of refractory obsessive-compulsive disorder
- Porphyria
- Refractory hiccups
- Itching

For other uses of antipsychotic drugs, see Table 5-2.

History of Antipsychotics

Phenothiazines (without antipsychotic properties) were first synthesized in the late 1800s. In 1950, Charpontier, a French scientist, synthesized chlorpromazine (Thorazine) from another phenothiazine, promethazine (Phenergan), while attempting to develop a better antihistamine.[14] This new medication caused mild antihistaminic effects but was highly sedating. Laborit, a physician, used the drug to calm anxious surgery patients. He observed, "There is not any loss of consciousness . . . [but] a state of tranquility or ataraxia."[14] Not long after, two other French physicians, J. Delay and P. Deniker, administered chlorpromazine to 38 acutely psychotic patients. They reported, "manic excitation and more generally psychotic agitation, aggressiveness and delusive conditions of schizophrenia improved, but deficiency symptoms did not change markedly."[14] From this serendipitous beginning, we see both the promise and the frustration associated with these drugs. Chlorpromazine and the many chlorpromazine-like drugs eventually developed were from the very beginning much more effective in treating the positive symptoms of schizophrenia than the negative symptoms, or as Delay and Deniker called them, the *deficiency symptoms*. This admission in the first report helped identify

Table 5-1 Major Traditional and Atypical Antipsychotic Drugs

Drug	Dosage range (mg/day)	D_2 receptor occupancy	5HT2* receptor occupancy	Half-life (hr)	Rate of EPSEs	Rate of anticholinergic effects	Rate of orthostasis	Rate of sedation	Rate of weight gain	Cost per tablet (mg/$)
Traditional agents										
High-potency drugs										
Fluphenazine (Prolixin)	0.5-20	xxxxx	xxx	13-56	High	Low	Low	Low	Low	1/0.45
Haloperidol (Haldol)	1-15	xxxxx	xxx	12-36	High	Low	Low	Low	Low	0.5/0.19
Thiothixene (Navane)	8-30	xxxx	xxx	34	High	Low	Low	Moderate	Moderate	1/0.21
Trifluoperazine (Stelazine)	20-80	xxxx	xx	13	High	Low	Moderate	Low	Low	1/0.50
Moderate-potency drugs										
Loxapine (Loxitane)	20-250	xxxx	xxxx	8-30	High	Moderate	Moderate	High	Low	5/0.53
Molindone (Moban)	5-255	xxxx	x	6.5	High	Moderate	Low	High	Low	5/0.66
Perphenazine (Taractan)	12-64	xxxx	xxxx	9-21	High	Low	Low	Moderate	None to low	2/0.45
Low-potency drugs										
Chlorpromazine (Thorazine)	30-800	xxx	xxxx	16-30	Moderate	High	High	High	High	200/0.18
Thioridazine (Mellaril)	150-800	xxxxx	xxx	9-30	Low	High	High	High	High	20/0.49
Atypical agents										
Clozapine (Clozaril)	300-900	xx	xxxx	4-12	Low	High	High	High	High	100/3.52
Olanzapine (Zyprexa)	5-20	xx	xxxx	21-54	Low	Moderate	Low	High	Moderate	5/4.51
Quetiapine (Seroquel)	300-400	xxx	xxxx	4-10	Low	Low	Moderate	Moderate	Moderate	100/1.89
Risperidone (Risperdal)	4-16	xxxxx	xxxxx	20-24	Low†	Low	High	High	Moderate	2/3.10
Ziprasidone (Zeldox)	80-160	xx	xxxxxx	5-10	Low	Low	Low	Low	Low	n/a

Adapted from References 19, 103, and 130.

x, Very low; xx, low; xx, moderate; xxxx, high; xxxxx, very high.

*Assumes normal dosage and normal plasma concentrations.

†Risperidone can cause significant levels of EPSEs at higher dosage levels.

Table 5-2   Other Uses of Antipsychotic Drugs (Not FDA Approved)

General uses
Agitation in major depression
  Porphyria
  Hiccups
  Adjunctive to anesthesia
  Relief of itching

Specific agents
Clozapine: antimanic, antidepressant, mood-stabilizing properties; delusional major
  depression, psychosis associated with Parkinson's disease
Risperidone: antimanic, antidepressant, mood-stabilizing properties; delusional major
  depression, augmentation of refractory obsessive-compulsive disorder
Pimozide: augmentation of refractory obsessive-compulsive disorder

Adapted from Reference 22.

the first of two overarching goals of antipsychotic therapy: the search for *greater efficacy*. The second goal was soon apparent as reports of serious and debilitating side effects trickled in: the need for *greater tolerability*. For the past five decades, the two goals, efficacy and tolerability, have dominated antipsychotic research.

Chlorpromazine was introduced in public hospitals in about 1954. Before the use of antipsychotic drugs in these facilities, hundreds of thousands of patients with severe psychiatric disturbances were hospitalized, sometimes under poor conditions. Social isolation, physical restraint, and occasional treatment with aggressive measures (e.g., psychosurgery or lobotomy) were used. These treatments rarely restored the patient to a state that enabled productive social or occupational functioning, and affected individuals often were unable to interact rationally with others.

Although some of the hopes and expectations for antipsychotic drugs have not been realized, these drugs have had a dramatic impact on psychiatric care and therapeutic outlook. Their use has resulted in earlier and more effective treatments, abandonment of ineffective or restrictive treatments, and a decline in public hospital patients. The latter is particularly noteworthy. In 1955, before the widespread use of these agents, more than 558,000 patients were in state hospitals. By 1997, that number had dropped by 85% to approximately 70,000.[159] In short, many patients who previously would have been hospitalized are now living and functioning well in the community, largely because of the efficacy of antipsychotic drug treatment. On the other hand, the restrictive admission policies created by the community mental health movement legislation have made it difficult to hospitalize some individuals needing the structure and care available in hospital settings. Furthermore, funding mandates embedded in these legislative acts made it financially attractive to treat in the community (typically at federal expense) rather than in public state hospitals (at state expense). Sadly, many individuals with serious mental illnesses have not done well and are not doing well in the community. Although a range of community services are available, a significant number of these individuals are referred to as *recidivistic* because they revolve in and out of the state hospital system or are found among the large homeless population. These realities indicate more than psychopharmacologic treatment is needed to bring about the best outcomes for people with schizophrenia.

Three Approaches to Classifying Antipsychotic Drugs

1. Chemical classification system based on molecular structure: *Traditional drugs*
2. High versus low potency based on D_2 receptor antagonism: *Traditional drugs*
3. Traditional versus atypical antipsychotics; *Atypical drugs*

Classification based on molecular structure (traditional drugs). Antipsychotic drugs can be generally classified in three overlapping ways. The first and most accurate system is based on *chemical classification*. These drugs have diverse chemical properties, but all of those available before 1990 (the traditional drugs) are considered equieffective. Anecdotal reports suggest switching chemical classifications (e.g., from a phenothiazine to a thioxanthene) when treatment failure occurs. Theoretically, this utilizes inherent chemical differences; however, research supporting this strategy is not conclusive.

Overarching chemical classes of antipsychotics
- Benzisothiazolyl (atypical) (e.g., ziprasidone)
- Benzisoxazole (atypical) (e.g., risperidone)
- Butyrophenones (traditional) (e.g., haloperidol)
- Dibenzodiazepine (atypical) (e.g., clozapine)
- Dibenzothiazepine (atypical) (e.g., quetiapine)
- Dibenzoxazepine (traditional) (e.g., loxapine)
- Dihydroindolone (traditional) (e.g., molindone)
- Diphenylbutylpiperdine (traditional) (e.g., pimozide)
- Phenothiazines (traditional) (e.g., chlorpromazine, fluphenazine, thioridazine)
- Thienobenzodiazepine (atypical) (e.g., olanzapine)
- Thioxanthenes (traditional) (e.g., chlorprothixene, thiothixene)

Classification based on potency or D_2 receptor occupancy (traditional drugs). A second means of classifying antipsychotic drugs is based on *potency* or the ability to antagonize or occupy dopamine D_2 receptors. Clinical effectiveness occurs when 60% to 75% of these receptors are blocked. These drugs (drugs that block D_2) have been the principal means of treating psychosis for more than 40 years yet have not been very effective in ameliorating negative and cognitive symptoms.[161] Although less precise than chemical classification, the potency-based approach has proven more clinically useful. Essentially, some drugs are required in much larger doses to achieve clinical results similar to those of other drugs. For example, about 100 mg of chlorpromazine is required to achieve the same clinical effect as 2 mg of haloperidol (Haldol). Drugs that are one to four times as potent as chlorpromazine are designated as low potency, and those 20 or more times as potent are designated high potency.[62] Accordingly, chlorpromazine is referred to as a *low-potency antipsychotic drug* and haloperidol as a *high-potency* one. Prescriptive preferences are mainly related to a drug's potential for producing adverse effects, and those effects can be reliably predicted based on potency. That is, low-potency drugs tend to produce more significant autonomic (anticholinergic and antiadrenergic) side effects, whereas high-potency agents tend to cause more severe extrapyramidal side effects (EPSEs). Low-potency agents are also thought to be more sedating. As noted, this approach to classification is less precise. Several drugs do not neatly fit the high or low category (e.g., loxapine, molindone, and perphenazine) and are placed in a "moderate potency" category. Many individuals tolerate these drugs well. Interestingly, anticholinergic agents are used to treat EPSEs, and antipsychotic drugs with more potent anticholinergic effects are known to produce fewer EPSEs. In other words, low-potency agents seem to have a "built-in" treatment for extrapyramidal side effects. Box 5-7 identifies the putative effects of receptor blockade of selected neurotransmitters.

Box 5-7   Effects of Antipsychotic Drugs on Selected Neurotransmitter Receptors

Receptor: Effects of receptor blockade

D_1, D_5: ? antipsychotic effect

D_2: *mesolimbic tract,* antipsychotic effect (all antipsychotic drugs antagonize this receptor); *nigrostriatal tract,* extrapyramidal side effects (EPSEs); *tuberoinfundibular tract,* prolactin elevation and associated effects; *mesocortical tract,* ? secondary negative symptoms

D_3: ? antipsychotic effect on negative symptoms

D_4: ? antipsychotic effect on positive symptoms

$5HT_1$: ? mood, cognitive symptoms

$5HT_{2A}$: ? antipsychotic effect on negative symptoms; ? reduction in EPSEs

$5HT_{2C}$: weight gain

$5HT_3$: ? nausea

M: can restore acetylcholine/dopamine balance and relieve EPSEs; anticholinergic side effect

H_1: sedation, orthostasis, weight gain

Alpha-1: orthostasis, dizziness, sedation, ? antipsychotic effect

Alpha-2: sexual dysfunction

GABA: lowers seizure threshold

Adapted from References 22, 76, 91, and 103.
M, Muscarinic.

Atypical drugs. Antipsychotic drugs available in the United States between 1950 and 1990 have been referred to as *traditional* or *typical antipsychotics.* All of the antipsychotic agents developed and released since 1990 are the putative *atypical antipsychotics.* The third approach to classifying antipsychotics contrasts traditional or typical antipsychotics with newer or atypical antipsychotics. The first atypical antipsychotic marketed in the United States was clozapine in 1990. Since then, several more atypical agents have been developed, including risperidone, olanzapine, quetiapine, sertindole (not marketed in the United States), and ziprasidone (Food and Drug Administration [FDA] approval pending). As mentioned, all traditional drugs (drugs developed before 1990) have similar efficacy. Clozapine and the other atypical antipsychotics have greater efficacy for treatment resistant patients and appear more effective in treating negative symptoms, particularly risperidone and olanzapine.[152] Whereas typical antipsychotic drugs block dopamine D_2 receptors in the limbic system and striatum, accounting for both their effect on positive symptoms and their extrapyramidal effects, atypical agents produce less D_2 receptor blockade yet effectively antagonize other dopamine (principally D_1 and D_4) and the serotonin $5HT_2$ receptor subtypes.[50,110,136] Atypical agents have been defined as antipsychotic drugs with the following characteristics[31,50,55,93,136]:

- Reduced or no risk for EPSEs (reduced D_2 antagonism in nigrostriatal tract)
- Increased effectiveness for negative and/or cognitive symptoms
- No elevation in prolactin (reduced D_2 antagonism in tuberoinfundibular tract)
- Antagonization of $5HT_2$
- Minimal risk for tardive dyskinesia

Box 5-8 Areas of Concentration for Dopamine Receptor Subtypes

D_1: Found in motor neurons in the basal ganglia and may be the principal dopamine-stimulating receptor for motor function.
- It has no direct role in controlling psychotic symptoms.
- It does influence D_2 receptor function.

D_2: Located in neurons of both the limbic and motor centers. Dopamine stimulation of D_2 receptors activate psychomotor pathways.
- Overactivation is thought to be the cause of positive symptoms.
- D_2 receptors are modulated when the D_1 receptor is blocked, but this does not occur in schizophrenia.

D_3 and D_4: Found primarily in limbic centers. Dopamine stimulation of D_3 may suppress behavior; overstimulation of D_3 may be associated with negative symptoms. D_4 receptors are located on neurons that influence thought processes and may be related to positive symptoms.

D_5: Found only in the limbic regions, including hippocampal gyrus and nucleus accumbens. May be an important dopamine-stimulating receptor for behavior.

From Seeman P: Dopamine receptors as new targets for novel drugs, *Curr Approach Psychoses* 4:8, 1995.

Neurochemical Views of Schizophrenia

The dopamine hypothesis. A neurochemical approach affords the best explanation for the effectiveness of antipsychotic agents.[156] The most important of these views is the dopamine hypothesis. Yaryura-Tobias, Diamond, and Merlis observed that L-dopa worsened the symptoms of schizophrenia, and coupling this observation with the fact that the dopamine antagonist chlorpromazine was an effective antipsychotic, Matthysse conceptualized the so-called dopamine hypothesis of schizophrenia.[111,175] This hypothesis states that the symptoms of schizophrenia (e.g., hallucinations and delusions) are caused by increased levels of dopamine in the brain. This original hypothesis proved to be too broad, however. Although there are five types of dopamine receptors, with a total of more than 20 subvariants, the dopamine hypothesis embraces only the dopamine D_2 receptor.[142] The atypical antipsychotics, through their more novel mechanisms of action, prompted researchers to move beyond this traditional view of schizophrenia as a purely hyperdopaminergic disorder and led them to recognize and distinguish the separate functions of major dopaminergic pathways (Box 5-8).[128] More recent investigations explore other neurochemical processes as well, including roles for serotonin, glutamate, glycine, gamma-aminobutyric acid (GABA), acetylcholine (ACh), norepinephrine, and very importantly, a hypodopaminergic theory.[80,84,130]

The importance of $5HT_2$ antagonism. The notion of a serotonergic role in schizophrenia was first postulated by Woolley and Shaw in 1954 but was overshadowed by the more conceptually pleasing dopamine hypothesis.[173] Today, there is an appreciation for the role of serotonin in schizophrenia and atypical agents, by definition, antagonize the serotonin $5HT_2$ receptor.[26] This theorized role for serotonin in schizophrenia helps clarify the clinical and neurochemical puzzlement: Why do atypical antipsychotic drugs help patients refractory to treatment and patients with negative symptoms more than the traditional antipsychotics do? To answer this question it is important to review the assumptions that link the more difficult to treat symptoms with the atypical agents. First, negative symptoms are thought to be related to a hypodopaminergic process. Second, serotonin inhibits dopamine. Third, drugs that antagonize $5HT_2$ receptors in the cortex are presumed to block the inhibiting nature of serotonin neurons on dopamine, thus increasing frontal lobe dopamine levels. Fourth, this liberation of dopamine helps "normalize" frontal lobe function.

As discussed earlier, positive schizophrenia is associated with a hyperdopaminergic disorder of the limbic region, and negative schizophrenia may be associated with a hypodopaminergic process of the frontal cortex. Hence drugs that block dopamine in limbic areas will modify positive symptoms, and drugs that block serotonin $5HT_2$ in cortical areas will liberate dopamine. Stated another way, typical antipsychotics antagonize dopamine receptors limbically, whereas atypical antipsychotics antagonize serotonin $5HT_2$ receptors cortically. As is noted in the section discussing specific agents, several of the traditional drugs also antagonize serotonin $5HT_2$ and risperidone elevates prolactin, confounding supposed differences between traditional and atypical antipsychotics. Figure 5-1 briefly describes the dopamine antagonizing effects of antipsychotic agents on four major dopaminergic tracts.

Glutamate and glycine contributions to schizophrenia. Glutamate is a product of the Kreb's cycle and has been implicated in schizophrenia.[44,160] Glutamate is an excitatory neurotransmitter, and with related excitatory amino acids (e.g., aspartate), it mediates fast excitatory neurotransmission in the central nervous system (CNS).[161] Glycine, an inhibitory neurotransmitter, is synthesized directly from serine, which is derived from glycolysis.[112] Research suggests a decrease in glutamate exists in individuals with schizophrenia and is associated with both positive and negative symptoms.[94,146,160] Both glutamate and glycine contribute to N-methyl-D-aspartate (NMDA) receptor regulation, which is essential for smooth cognitive processes. Overstimulation of NMDA receptors is associated with neurotoxicity (excitotoxicity). Interest in the link between NMDA receptors and psychosis grew out of observations about the abuse of phencyclidine (PCP). PCP is a noncompetitive antagonist of the NMDA system and this antagonism can result in the manifestation of psychosis, including positive, negative, and cognitive symptoms.[44,160] Thus far, efforts to normalize these neurotransmitter systems have failed to produce encouraging results.

A role for gamma-aminobutyric acid? GABA is an important inhibitory neurotransmitter, and evidence suggests that individuals with schizophrenia have unusually low levels of this amino acid. Furthermore, the enzyme that catalyzes the synthesis of GABA is thought also to be deficient in individuals with schizophrenia. Inadequate inhibition in the frontal cortex related to decreased levels of GABA may account for the loss of filtering/selective attention (inability to ignore inconsequential stimulation such as background noise) so often found among individuals who have schizophrenia. Most cortical GABA dysfunction occurs in a layer of neurons still developing at birth, and defects in this layer may be the result of the types of perinatal insult mentioned previously.

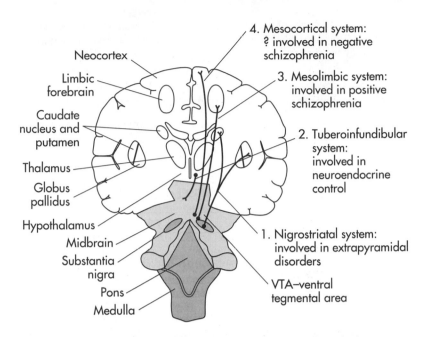

Neocortex

Limbic
forebrain

Caudate
nucleus and
putamen

Thalamus

Globus
pallidus

Hypothalamus

Midbrain

Substantia
nigra

Pons

Medulla

4. Mesocortical system:
? involved in negative
schizophrenia

3. Mesolimbic system:
involved in positive
schizophrenia

2. Tuberoinfundibular
system:
involved in
neuroendocrine
control

1. Nigrostriatal system:
involved in extrapyramidal
disorders

VTA–ventral
tegmental area

Figure 5-1 Four dopaminergic tracts important for understanding the actions of antipsychotic drugs. *1*, Nigrostriatal system: when antipsychotic drugs antagonize this system, a pseudoparkinsonism or extrapyramidal effect occurs. *2*, Tuberoinfundibular system: when antipsychotic drugs antagonize this system, the dopamine inhibition of the hypothalamic hormone prolactin is lifted and can lead to gynecomastia and galactorrhea. *3*, Mesolimbic system: when antipsychotic drugs antagonize this system, a decrease in the symptoms of schizophrenia occurs (primarily positive symptoms). This is the effect that makes these drugs antipsychotic. *4*, Mesocortical system: when antipsychotic drugs antagonize this system, it is thought the disorder can be worsened in some patients and cause "secondary" negative symptoms. Atypical antipsychotics, on the other hand, antagonize serotonin $5HT_2$ in the cortex, which is thought to liberate dopamine. That is, it is suspected a mesocortical hypodopaminergic state contributes to negative symptoms. Atypical drugs are thought to enhance dopaminergic function in the frontal cortex. Much remains to be understood about the role of the mesocortical dopaminergic tract in schizophrenia.[133]

Pharmacologic Effects (Therapeutic Effects)

Chlorpromazine and the other traditional antipsychotic drugs are used primarily to treat schizophrenia and other psychotic states. Well-designed clinical research has produced impressive evidence for their effectiveness.[47] Not all patients improve, but approximately 75% of the patients with positive symptoms respond to antipsychotics. Of those refractory to traditional agents, about 30% respond to clozapine. A positive response related to these drugs is usually noted in 1 to 2 weeks, with improvement continuing for up to 6 to 8 weeks once appropriate dosage is established.[130]

Central nervous system effects. CNS effects include emotional quieting, sedation, and psychomotor slowing; thus at one time these drugs were generally referred to as *major tranquilizers*. The emotional quieting enables the patient to take advantage of other forms of therapeutic intervention, for example, psychoeducation programs, therapeutic relationships, and therapeutic milieu. Sedative effects are welcomed by the many patients who have chemically and psychologically induced insomnia.

Psychiatric Symptoms Modified by Antipsychotic Drugs

As previously discussed, traditional antipsychotic drugs are effective in treating the positive symptoms of schizophrenia (see Box 5-6). Negative symptoms are more responsive to the newer atypical drugs. Unfortunately, neuroleptics can cause negative symptoms, so differentiating drug-induced negative symptoms from negative schizophrenia can be difficult. Psychotic symptoms associated with other disorders, for example, mania, depression, organic mental syndromes, or disorders of cognitive impairment, may also respond to antipsychotic drugs.

Perceptual disturbances. In general, the more bizarre the behavior associated with psychosis, the more likely that an antipsychotic drug will be found beneficial. Hallucinations and illusions usually diminish or remit with the use of these drugs. Even when symptoms are not fully eradicated, antipsychotic drugs may enable the individual to understand that hallucinations and illusions are, indeed, not real or can be tolerated without influencing behavior.

Thought disturbances. The use of antipsychotic drugs may also improve reasoning and decrease ambivalence and delusions or suspiciousness. Because disturbed reasoning, ambivalence, and delusional thinking may produce frustration and behavioral consequences, an antipsychotic agent can free the patient from these symptoms while improving the ability to communicate and cooperate with others.

Motor disturbances. Individuals with schizophrenia and other psychotic disorders are often found to be hyperactive or agitated because of internal turmoil and perhaps because of the disturbed neurochemistry. Antipsychotic drugs may slow or normalize psychomotor activity. Some drugs, such as chlorpromazine, trifluoperazine, thioridazine, clozapine, molindone, risperidone, and olanzapine, are inherently sedating, and this effect may be particularly useful for agitated and combative persons.

Altered consciousness. Mental confusion found among psychotic and schizophrenic patients may be caused by the anxiety and disturbed processing of thought associated with psychosis. Some mental health professionals believe these symptoms are among the most disabling. Antipsychotic drugs can be effective in decreasing disturbances of thought and in clearing mental confusion.

Interpersonal disturbances. Schizophrenic patients often have a history of asocial behavior and social withdrawal and may have few if any close personal relationships. Inconsistent relationships with family members are common as well. Individuals with schizophrenia may invest little energy in their appearance and may be oblivious to behaviors that offend others. When combined with introspective, self-focused speech and the resultant ineffective communication patterns, isolation is reinforced. Antipsychotic drugs, together with other forms of therapy, may enable patients to become less self-focused and to divert their attention from themselves to others.

Affective disturbance. Depression is common in schizophrenia and occurs most often after symptom improvement (i.e., postpsychotic depression) and during times of remission. Depression and negative schizophrenia share some symptoms, such as flat affect, apathy, anhedonia, and/or avolition, and it may be difficult to distinguish one from the other. Depression should be treated with antidepressants and psychotic symptoms with antipsychotics. It is thought that ziprasidone (Zeldox), which blocks the reuptake of both serotonin and norepinephrine, may be effective in treating comorbid schizophrenia and depression.

Pharmacokinetics

Absorption after oral intake of antipsychotics is variable. Peak plasma levels are usually seen within 1 to 6 hours.[121] A tranquilizing effect from many of these drugs occurs within an hour or so after oral ingestion. Antipsychotic effects usually occur within 1 to 2 weeks, with improvement continuing in most patients for up to 6 to 8 weeks.[130] Antipsychotics tend to be highly lipophilic and accumulate in fatty tissue, from which they are released slowly. Traces of metabolites are found in the urine months after therapy has stopped, which may explain why some patients who abruptly stop their medication continue to experience an antipsychotic effect for a time. This slow release from fatty stores may also account for noncompliance because the patient who stops taking his or her medication does not experience an immediate return of symptoms.

Antipsychotics are highly bound to plasma proteins (91% to 99%) and appear to have an increased effect in older individuals who have decreased protein-binding capabilities, although other explanations are plausible as well. Antipsychotics are metabolized in the liver by the cytochrome P-450 (CYP-450) system and have half-lives on average of 10 to 30 hours, with some exceptions (see Table 5-1). Impaired hepatic function and interactions with drugs that inhibit the CYP-450 system can extend half-lives and therefore can extend effect. Antipsychotic substrates of specific P-450 isoenzymes include the following:

- *IID6:* thioridazine, risperidone, perphenazine, haloperidol, clozapine; most antipsychotics are metabolized by IID6[130]
- *IA2:* clozapine, haloperidol, olanzapine, phenothiazine
- *IIIA3/4:* pimozide, ziprasidone, quetiapine

Interestingly, the IA2 isoenzyme is induced by cigarette smoking, and that behavior may be linked to inconsistent effects on antipsychotic substrates.[9]

Antipsychotic Administrative Forms

Oral antipsychotics. Many antipsychotic drugs are available in oral and parenteral forms. Oral administration is the favored route for many reasons, not the least of which is patient preference. When a patient is not responding to an antipsychotic drug, reassessment is necessary. Two questions guide assessment of the patient's response and raise the possibility of a change of drug. These questions are as follows:

1. Is the patient taking the drug as prescribed (compliance)?
2. Has the drug been given a fair trial (3 to 6 weeks)?

If the answer to the first question is "no," then drug forms such as depot injections that effectively circumvent patient noncompliance tendencies may be needed.

Noncompliance. Oral drugs are easily "cheeked"; that is, an inpatient under the watchful eye of a nurse can tuck the pill or tablet in the side of the mouth and only pretend to swallow. Among those individuals managing their own medication, many simply do not take the drug as it was prescribed. Blair estimates that 46% of patients take less of their medication than prescribed.[23] Ongoing psychoeducation programs for patients and their families and development of a therapeutic alliance are considered effective approaches to diminishing noncompliance. Noncompliance is the leading cause of relapse.

Relapse. Review of the literature concerning the level of relapse provides various views as to the extent of this problem. Johnson suggests that about one third of all patients with schizophrenia will relapse within 2 years.[77] Hogarty and Ulrich indicate that 40% of patients taking medication will relapse within a year after hospitalization, and rates of 65% and 80% have been demonstrated for "off-drug" individuals at 1 year and 2 years, respectively.[66] Their research also indicates that relapse rates can be halved if psychosocial treatment is available. The risk of relapse is increased by a factor of five when antipsychotic therapy is discontinued.[134] Taking a long-term perspective, relapse rates as high as 90% have been found in patients 15 years after their first episodes.[120] Of course, the other implication in this study is that some maintenance programs are effective. To reduce relapse, first-episode patients should be treated with antipsychotics for 2 years and multiepisode patients should be treated for 5 years or more.[55]

Parenteral and depot forms. Another form of administration of antipsychotic drugs is the parenteral route (Box 5-9). Parenteral drugs are usually used to treat acutely disturbed patients or those who represent significant compliance risks. Both haloperidol and fluphenazine are available in long-acting or depot-injectable forms that require injection as seldom as every 2 to 3 weeks with fluphenazine decanoate (half-life of 14 days), to once per month with haloperidol decanoate (half-life of 21 days). These depot compounds are particularly beneficial in community outpatient clinics and have several advantages and disadvantages.[15]

The following are advantages of depot compounds:
1. Overcoming noncompliance
2. Circumvention of reduced bioavailability and metabolism associated with oral antipsychotic drugs
3. Achievement of stable plasma levels

The disadvantages of depot injections include the following:
1. Inability to withdraw drugs rapidly should problems develop
2. Lengthy process to adjust dosage related to extended half-lives

---

Box 5-9 Antipsychotic Drugs Available for Injection

Chlorpromazine (Thorazine)	Haloperidol decanoate (Haldol LA)
Chlorprothixene (Taractan)	Loxapine (Loxitane)
Fluphenazine (Prolixin)	Mesoridazine (Serentil)
Fluphenazine decanoate	Perphenazine (Trilafon)
(Prolixin Decanoate, Modecate)	Thiothixene (Navane)
Haloperidol (Haldol)	Trifluoperazine (Stelazine)

The following depot drugs are available in the United States:
1. Fluphenazine decanoate:
   - Usual dose range: 12.5 to 50 mg
   - Usual duration: 2 to 3 weeks
2. Haloperidol decanoate:
   - Usual dose range: 50 to 300 mg
   - Usual duration: 3 to 4 weeks

Oral dosage is typically stabilized before long-acting forms are initiated related to the disadvantage noted first above. Once an oral regimen has reached steady state and symptoms are stabilized, the process of switching from oral to depot preparations can commence. Because long-acting agents take months to arrive at steady state, a considerable period of time exists in which both oral and depot forms must be given. The oral forms are gradually tapered downward.

Side Effects

The antipsychotic drugs produce numerous side effects because of their PNS and CNS actions (Boxes 5-10A and 5-10B). Side effects caused by PNS autonomic blocking (anticholinergic and antiadrenergic blockade) are more likely to be caused by low-potency forms such as chlorpromazine.[131] EPSEs are more likely caused by high-potency drugs such as haloperidol.

Peripheral nervous system effects
Anticholinergic effects. Anticholinergic PNS effects are related to the blockade of parasympathetic functions of several cranial (Table 5-3, p. 101) and other parasympathetic nerves. Dry mouth (cranial nerves [CN] VII and IX), blurred vision and photophobia (CN III), and decreased lacrimation (CN VII) are common but are often managed with nondrug interventions. Mydriasis (CN III) can increase intraocular pressure, which can aggravate glaucoma. Other relatively common anticholinergic effects are constipation and urinary hesitance (CN X). Although sweating is controlled by the sympathetic system, its postsynaptic neurotransmitter is ACh and hence is decreased with anticholinergics. Patients with a history of glaucoma or prostatic hypertrophy are not ordinarily placed on regimens of these drugs. Patients with cardiovascular disease should be evaluated carefully before these drugs are prescribed because of tachycardia caused by blockade of CN X. Sudden death related to arrhythmias and decreased cardiac output has been reported, with thioridazine (Mellaril) implicated most often.[114]

Antiadrenergic effects. Hypotension caused by antagonism of noradrenergic alpha-1 receptors is the major antiadrenergic effect of antipsychotic drugs. Hypotension often occurs when the individual stands or changes position suddenly (orthostatic hypotension). Elderly persons are particularly prone to orthostasis; thus precautions against falls must be instituted.[62] In addition, hypotensive episodes can trigger reflex tachycardia in an already tachycardia-prone heart (e.g., CN X blockade), which can lead to general cardiovascular inefficiency. Thus low-potency antipsychotic drugs are usually not prescribed for individuals with severe hypotension, heart failure, or a history of arrhythmias.

Central nervous system extrapyramidal side effects.
EPSEs develop in up to 60% to 90% of patients receiving antipsychotic medications, and up to 50% of readmissions are related to these side effects.[5,25] EPSEs can be roughly grouped into acute and chronic categories. Acute EPSEs occur early on in treatment (in the first

Box 5-10A Side Effects of Antipsychotic Drugs and Appropriate Clinical Interventions

Peripheral nervous system effects

Constipation

Encourage high dietary fiber and increased water intake; give laxatives as
    ordered.

Dry mouth

Advise patient to take sips of water frequently; provide sugarless hard
    candies, sugarless gum, and mouth rinses.

Nasal congestion

Give over-the-counter nasal decongestant if appropriate.

Blurred vision

Advise patient to avoid potentially dangerous tasks. Reassure patient that
    normal vision typically returns in a few weeks, when tolerance to this
    side effect develops. Pilocarpine eye drops can be used on a short-term
    basis.

Mydriasis

Advise patient to report eye pain immediately.

Photophobia

Advise patient to wear sunglasses outdoors.

Hypotension or orthostatic hypotension

Ask patient to get out of bed or chair slowly. He or she should sit on the side
    of the bed for 1 full minute while dangling feet, then slowly rise. If hypo-
    tension is a problem, measure blood pressure before each dose is given.
    Observe to see whether changing to another antipsychotic agent is
    indicated.

Tachycardia

Tachycardia is usually a reflex response to hypotension. When intervention
    for hypotension (previously described) is effective, reflex tachycardia
    usually decreases. With clozapine, hold the dose if pulse rate is greater
    than 140 pulsations per minute.*

Urinary retention

Encourage frequent voiding and voiding whenever the urge is present.
    Catheterize for residual fluids. Ask patient to monitor urine output
    and report output to nurse. Older men with benign prostatic hypertrophy
    are particularly susceptible to urinary retention.

Urinary hesitation

Provide privacy, run water in the sink, or run warm water over the
    perineum.

Sedation

Help patient get up early and get the day started.

Weight gain

Help patient understand an appropriate diet; diet pills should not be taken.

Box 5-10A   Side Effects of Antipsychotic Drugs and Appropriate Clinical Interventions—cont'd

Agranulocytosis

A high incidence of agranulocytosis is associated with clozapine. White blood cell (WBC) count should be performed weekly for 6 months and then, if there are no apparent problems, every 2 weeks from then on. When baseline WBC count is less than 3500 cells/mm^3, treatment should not be initiated. After treatment begins, a WBC count of less than 3000 cells/mm^3 and a granulocyte count of less than 1500 cells/mm^3 indicate treatment interruption to monitor for infection. If no signs of infection are present, treatment can resume. If the WBC count is less than 2000 cells/mm^3 and the granulocyte count is less than 1000 cells/mm^3, stop therapy and do not rechallenge the patient. If infection develops, antibiotics should be prescribed.

Central nervous system effects
Akathisia

Be patient and reassure the patient who is "jittery" that you understand the need to move and that appropriate drug interventions can help. Akathisia is the chief cause of noncompliance with antipsychotic regimens. Treatment options include switching to a different antipsychotic drug, starting an antiparkinson drug, reducing the dosage of the current drug, or waiting for tolerance to develop (in some cases).

Dystonias

If a severe dystonic reaction occurs, give antiparkinson or antihistamine drugs immediately, as needed, and offer reassurance. Intramuscular route is typically indicated in this situation.

Drug-induced parkinsonism

Assess for the three major parkinsonism symptoms—tremors, rigidity, and bradykinesia. Antiparkinson drugs are usually indicated.

Tardive dyskinesia

Assess for signs by using the Abnormal Inventory Movement Scale (AIMS). Because antipsychotic drugs mask tardive dyskinesia, withdrawal dyskinesia is not uncommon. Anticholinergic agents worsen tardive dyskinesia, which is one reason these drugs are not always prescribed for prophylactic use. However, young men taking large doses of high-potency antipsychotic drugs may warrant prophylactic antiparkinson drugs.†

Neuroleptic malignant syndrome

Be alert for this potentially fatal side effect by assessing for fever, rigidity, and tremor. Encourage adequate water intake for all individuals taking antipsychotic drugs.

Seizures

Seizures occur in approximately 1% of patients receiving antipsychotic drug treatment. Clozapine causes an even higher rate, up to 5% of patients taking 600 to 900 mg/day. For dosages of clozapine greater than 600 mg/day, an electroencephalogram should be performed. If a seizure occurs, it may be necessary to discontinue clozapine.

*From Jaretz N, Flowers E, Millsap L: *Perspect Psychiatr Care* 28:19, 1992.
†From American Psychiatric Association Task Force on Tardive Dyskinesia: *Am J Psychiatry* 137:1163, 1980.

Box 5-10B Major Adverse Responses to Antipsychotic Drugs in Summary

Neuroleptic malignant syndrome (NMS)

Caused by: a hypodopaminergic state

Offending agents: high-potency antipsychotics primarily

Signs and symptoms:
- Agitation
- Altered levels of consciousness
- Autonomic hyperactivity
- Electrolyte imbalance
  - Hyperkalemia
  - Hyponatremia
  - Metabolic acidosis
- Hyperreflexia
- Hyperthermia*
- Diaphoresis
- Tachypnea
- Impaired breathing
- Muscular rigidity*
- Muteness
- Pallor
- Rhabdomyolysis-acute myoglobinuric renal failure

*Cardinal symptoms

Anticholinergic side effects

Caused by: blockade of cholinergic receptors (muscarinic receptors)

Offending agents: anticholinergic drugs such as the low-potency antipsychotics and anticholinergic antiparkinson drugs.

Signs and symptoms:
- Anhidrosis
- Blurred vision
- Constipation
- Diminished lacrimation
- Dry mouth
- Mydriasis
- Tachycardia
- Urinary hesitancy

Extrapyramidal side effects (EPSEs)

Hypokinetic types

Caused by: hypodopaminergic state

Offending agents: typically high-potency antipsychotics

EPSEs:
- Akathisia
- Akinesia
- Dystonia
- Drug-induced parkinsonism

Hyperkinetic type

Caused by: nigrostriatal receptor supersensitivity

Offending agents: typically high-potency antipsychotics

EPSE: tardive dyskinesia

---

month of treatment), with chronic forms developing later. The likely order of development, definition, and incidence of each follows[130,162]:

1. *Dystonic reaction:* Spastic contraction of muscle groups; 10% of patients, most within the first 3 days.
2. *Akathisia:* Restlessness, an irresistible need to move manifested objectively and subjectively; 20% to 25% of patients usually within first 10 days.

Table 5-3 Anticholinergic Effect on Cranial Nerves with Parasympathetic Functions

Cranial nerve	Parasympathetic function	Anticholingeric effect
III	Constricts pupils	Mydriasis (dilates pupils)— blurred vision
	Alters shape of lens	Impairs accommodation
VII	Salivation	Dry mouth
	Lacrimation	Decreased tearing
	Nasal mucus secretion	Dry nasal passage
IX	Salivation	Dry mouth
	Nasal mucus secretion	Dry nasal passage
X	Slows heart rate	Tachycardia
	Promotes peristalsis	Slows peristalsis—constipation
	Constricts bronchi	Dilates bronchi

Mechanism of action: Blockade of the muscarinic receptors of these four cranial nerves.

3. *Akinesia:* Difficulty with movement; up to 33% of patients, with most cases developing by the third week of treatment.
4. *Parkinsonism:* Tremor, rigidity, bradykinesia; up to 20% of patients, usually developing after weeks to months.
5. *Tardive dyskinesia:* Abnormal, involuntary skeletal muscle movements of the face, tongue, trunk, and extremities; it occurs at an annual cumulative rate of 5% and eventually affects 20% to 35% of patients; usually developing after months of continuous use.[22,55]

Abnormal involuntary movement disorders develop because of a drug-induced imbalance between two major neurotransmitters: dopamine and ACh. As dopamine D_2 receptors are antagonized or occupied at levels between 60% and 75%, an optimal clinical effect occurs. At blockade levels not much higher (greater than 75% occupancy) EPSEs develop.[141,143] This imbalance is caused more readily by high-potency antipsychotic drugs; however, all antipsychotics can cause EPSEs.

Dystonias. Dystonic reactions occur very early in treatment and are characterized by involuntary contractions of voluntary muscles controlling posture, gait, or ocular movement. Positions become frozen and, although frightening, are not typically dangerous. Dystonias occur early in treatment, often appear suddenly, and can recur. Risk factors include young age, male gender, use of high-potency agents, regimen using high dosages, and drugs being given via the intramuscular route. About 10% of patients starting antipsychotic therapy develop dystonias. The following three specific dystonic reactions bear special mention:

1. *Oculogyric crisis* is a dystonic reaction in which the eyes roll upward. This is a terrifying experience for the patient.
2. *Torticollis* is a contracted state of the cervical muscle that produces torsion on the neck.
3. *Laryngeal-pharyngeal dystonia* is associated with gagging, cyanosis, respiratory distress, and asphyxia (particularly in young men). *It is life-threatening and requires immediate intervention.*

All dystonic conditions respond to intramuscular anticholinergic drugs (see Chapter 17).

Akathisia. Akathisia manifests as subjective and objective restlessness.[46] It is a common EPSE, usually occurs within the first 10 days of treatment, is less responsive to treatment than dystonia and parkinsonism, and probably accounts for more noncompliant behavior than do other EPSEs. Akathisia was first described in 1911, long before antipsychotic drugs were available, suggesting other variables contribute to its occurrence (e.g., iron deficiency). Subjectively, the patient often feels jittery or uneasy. He or she may report a lot of "nervous energy." Objectively, the patient is restless and literally cannot sit still. Planasky and Johnston discovered that 79% of suicidal schizophrenic patients had akathisia.[126]

Unfortunately, restlessness and verbal reflections of subjective anguish can be misinterpreted as a worsening of psychosis. Because akathisia can present as agitation, the clinician should not mistake the two; they have different treatment protocols.[56] If additional antipsychotic medication is given, akathisia will worsen. Akathisia may respond to anticholinergic drugs such as trihexyphenidyl (Artane) or benztropine (Cogentin) but can also be resistant to this intervention. Benzodiazepines (e.g., lorazepam) may also be useful. However, Keepers and Casey suggest other approaches may work, including waiting for tolerance to develop or decreasing the dosage of the antipsychotic agent.[89]

Akinesia. *Akinesia* refers to an absence of or an impairment of movement. More often, a state of bradykinesia, a slowing of movement, exists. Akinesia is experienced by about 33% of patients taking antipsychotic drugs.[162] Movement is difficult to initiate and difficult to maintain. The patient lacks spontaneity in movement and speech. Paradoxically, these same symptoms (for different reasons) are common in schizophrenia. If a manifestation of schizophrenia is occurring, more medication may be indicated; if it is akinesia, more medication will worsen the symptoms.

Parkinsonism. Parkinsonism occurs in approximately 20% of patients taking antipsychotics and develops within weeks to months. Symptoms mimic those of Parkinson's disease, that is, tremors, rigidity, and bradykinesia. As would be expected, antipsychotic drugs intensify the symptoms of Parkinson's disease and should be avoided if possible for persons with this condition. Parkinsonian symptoms must be differentiated from the negative symptoms of schizophrenia because treatment approaches are different. Anticholinergic agents are effective and are most often used for drug-induced parkinsonism. Use of dopaminergic drugs such as levodopa is not indicated because of their inherent potential to increase psychotic symptoms. Amantadine (Symmetrel), possessing both anticholinergic and dopaminergic properties, is the exception and is ordered in the treatment of drug-induced parkinsonism for some individuals.

Tardive dyskinesia. Tardive dyskinesia (TD) manifests as abnormal, involuntary movements of the face, tongue, trunk, and extremities. It is the most dreaded EPSE and was once thought to be irreversible. The term *tardive* means "late appearing," and TD typically appears after months of continuous use. Traditional antipsychotic drugs are the major culprits, but all antipsychotics, perhaps with the exception of clozapine, can cause TD. Although the other EPSEs are hypokinetic disorders caused by dopamine deficiency, TD is a hyperdopaminergic disorder related to dopamine receptor hypersensitivity. Because striatal dopaminergic receptors can become supersensitive, TD also develops when antipsychotic dosage reductions or withdrawal is instituted. Cholinergic deficits are also suspected. Although anticholinergic antiparkinsonism drugs are beneficial for most other EPSEs, they can exacerbate TD, no doubt related to cholinergic irregularities. Tardive dyskinesia has an annual prevalence rate of 5%, and a mean prevalence of 20% to 35% of continuous users develop it.[18] Most will have mild symptoms, but about 10% will develop a debilitating form of TD.[5] Sometimes, TD appears when psychotropic agents are being withdrawn or reduced in dosage. This phenomenon, referred to as *withdrawal dyskinesia*, may be reversible and subsides with time.

TD usually affects the muscles of the mouth and face and can also occur in the trunk and extremities. Signs of TD include lip smacking, grinding of the teeth, rolling or protrusion of the tongue, tics, and diaphragmatic movements, which may impair breathing. These involuntary movements fluctuate in severity and disappear during sleep. They can be controlled with great effort, but most individuals cannot sustain the effort for long. TD is most severe in young men and most common in women older than 70.[10] High dosages of antipsychotics and concurrent EPSEs increase the risk of TD.[164]

TD can be irreversible; however, if caught during the early stages, symptoms can be reversed or decreased in severity. Early detection and gradual dosage reductions (to 50%) have proven capable of mitigating the impact of TD.[5] Patient and family education should emphasize early detection by careful monitoring. The Abnormal Involuntary Movement Scale (AIMS) provides a mechanism for assessing TD. The dopamine agonist bromocriptine (Parlodel) has been used to treat this side effect, as has clonazepam (Klonopin) and vitamin E (which apparently works by neutralizing free radicals). Another approach involves the use of clozapine.[18,39,51,151] Numerous clinical trials have substantiated the efficacy of low dosages of clozapine in the treatment of TD.

Neuroleptic malignant syndrome. Neuroleptic malignant syndrome (NMS) is a potentially lethal hypodopaminergic side effect of antipsychotic drugs. Traditionally, a morbidity rate of 1% with a mortality rate of up to 30% was widely reported in the literature.[92] Increased vigilance by physicians, nurses, and others has significantly reduced both the morbidity and mortality of the syndrome.[24,68,86,145] Current thinking indicates an incidence of less than 1%. Before 1984, apparently 25% of patients developing NMS died, and since 1984, that percentage has declined to less than 12%.[145] The American Psychiatric Associations estimates that 5% to 20% of untreated cases (some as a result of misdiagnosis) result in death.[5] Risk factors for NMS include being male; being younger; having a diagnosis of mood disorder, dementia, or delerium; having dehydration; having a dosage rapidly titrated; and using concomitant psychotropics.[5,103] However, NMS is not related to toxic drug levels and may occur after only a few doses.[101] Onset can occur within minutes or can occur months after drug initiation but most often occur within the first 2 weeks of treatment.

Important symptoms associated with NMS include hyperthermia, Parkinson-like symptoms of muscular rigidity and tremors, altered consciousness, increase in some laboratory values, and autonomic disturbances. Perhaps the two cardinal symptoms are elevated body temperature (up to 108° F with temperatures of 101° to 103° F more likely) and rigidity. Rigidity can range from muscle hypertonicity to severe lead pipe rigidity.[124] Altered consciousness includes confusion and even unresponsiveness. The muteness found in some patients may also be related to state of consciousness. Patients with NMS typically show a spike in creatinine phosphokinase (CPK) levels and an increase in white blood cell (WBC) count. CPK levels may reach 100,000 U/L while WBC counts range to 40,000/mm^3.[124] The increase in CPK is caused by muscle rigidity and the subsequent rhabdomyolysis. Autonomic dysfunction includes hypotension, tachycardia, sialorrhea, sweating, and urinary incontinence.

As noted, fever, rigidity, tremors, altered consciousness, and autonomic disturbances are associated with NMS. Because many patients do not associate these symptoms with their antipsychotic medication, emergency room personnel and primary care providers may be contacted first. These health care professionals should always rule out NMS in their patients taking antipsychotics who develop high temperatures. Other risk factors include prolonged use of restraints; coadministration of lithium; poorly controlled EPSEs; withdrawal from anticholinergic medications; diagnosis of alcoholism, organic brain syndrome, or previous brain injury; extrapyramidal disorder (e.g., Parkinson's disease); iron deficiency; and catatonia.[124] Pharmacologic treatment has included bromocriptine (Parlodel), a dopamine agonist; dantrolene (Dantrium), a skeletal muscle relaxant via suppression of calcium release; and amantadine (Symmetrel), another dopaminergic agent (see Chapter 17). Dursun and others found vitamins E and B_6 effective for a 74-year-old woman thought to be a poor candidate for the more conventional medications just mentioned.[48]

Prophylactic treatment of EPSEs. Prophylactic use of anticholinergic agents has been debated because these drugs have their own set of side effects and a potential for abuse. Nonetheless, Tesar finds prophylactic administration particularly effective in preventing dystonic reactions.[155] In his study, only 13% of patients receiving prophylactic anticholinergic drugs experienced dystonias, compared with 46% not taking anticholinergics. Because 90% of dystonic reactions occur within the first 3 days of treatment, anticholinergics can be discontinued fairly soon for most patients. Typical anticholinergics used for EPSEs are trihexyphenidyl 2 to 5 mg or benztropine 2 mg by mouth or intramuscularly for patients beginning high-potency antipsychotic treatment (see Chapter 17).

Other side effects. Other side effects that may occur in association with antipsychotic drugs include the following[22]:

- *Other CNS effects:* weight gain (up to 40% of patients) with low-potency and most atypical agents, sedation (most common side effect), insomnia, anxiety, dysphagia, dose-related lowering of seizure threshold (about 1% for most antipsychotics; about 5% with clozapine at dosages greater than 600 mg/day), memory loss related to anticholinergic blockade of cholinergic memory pathways, and heat dysregulation mediated by antagonism of hypothalamic D_2 receptors
- *GI effects:* anorexia, sialorrhea (about 30% of patients taking clozapine)
- *Sexual dysfunction:* resulting from altered D_2 activity, ACh blockade, alpha-2 blockade; impaired ejaculation, decreased libido, erectile dysfunction (23% to 54%), retrograde ejaculation reported with thioridazine and risperidone
- *Endocrine effects:* elevated prolactin levels (i.e., galactorrhea [risperidone can cause incidence of 1% to 5%], gynecomastia in men and women), lactation, weight gain, hypoglycemia or hyperglycemia, polydipsia, polyurea; chronic prolactin elevation leads to sexual dysfunction and osteoporosis
- *Skin:* blue-gray skin rash, sun-sensitive skin (primarily with low-potency phenothiazines)
- *Hepatic effects:* jaundice (typically occurs in first month), elevation of liver enzymes
- *Ocular effects:* pigmentary retinopathy (particularly with thioridazine [maximum dose of 800 mg/day] and chlorpromazine)
- *Hematologic effects:* leukopenia (up to 10% with chlorpromazine), agranulocytosis (see the following discussion)

Agranulocytosis Another major life-threatening side effect of potentially most, if not all, antipsychotics is agranulocytosis. *Agranulocytosis* is clinically defined as a granulocyte count less than 500 cells/mm³. Patients who develop agranulocytosis have initial symptoms of sore throat, malaise, fever, or bleeding and eventually become as sick as those undergoing chemotherapy.[59] Fatalities are typically caused by overwhelming infection as the body loses its ability to fight. Although theoretically this is a concern for all antipsychotics, the relative risk is greatly increased with the atypical drug clozapine. Clozapine is a drug that has been around for more than 40 years but was first marketed in the United States only in the past decade. This reluctance by the FDA to approve clozapine was based on the high incidence of agranulocytosis associated with this drug. Most specifically, a report out of Finland for the months of June and July 1975 revealed a clozapine-caused tragedy. During those 2 months, 9 of 18 patients who developed clozapine-related agranulocytosis died.[74] FDA approval for marketing in 1990 was contingent on an intense monitoring system developed by the manufacturer, Sandoz, Inc. From their introduction of clozapine (Clozaril) in 1990 to June of 1996, 728 cases of leukopenia (defined as a WBC count between 2000 and 3000 cells/mm^3 or a granulocyte count of 1000 to 1500 cells/mm^3) and 464 cases of agranulocytosis were reported.[53] During that same period, 13 deaths occurred.[140] Currently, it is thought that the incidence of agranulocytosis is about 0.8% after 1 year and 0.9% after 18 months.[2] This compares with a morbidity of less than 1 per 1000 for most other antipsychotics. The rigid protocols established by the manufacturer and close monitoring by concerned clinicians account for this reduction in incidence.

Feldman proposes the following three possible mechanisms for the pathogenesis of agranulocytosis[53]:

1. The clozapine metabolite desmethylclozapine may have a direct cytotoxic effect on marrow cells.
2. The release of the granulocyte-stimulating factor may be suppressed by clozapine, resulting in hematologic imbalance.
3. Clozapine may induce antibody formations that are toxic to peripheral neutrophils and their committed precursors.

Treatment with clozapine should not be initiated if the WBC count is less than 3500 cells/mm^3. Once treatment commences, weekly monitoring of WBCs is required for 6 months and, if no concerns develop, then biweekly. After termination of clozapine therapy, weekly blood counts should continue for 4 weeks. Patients whose WBC counts drop below 3500 cells/mm^3 but remain above 3000 cells/mm^3 should be followed carefully (with twice-weekly differential counts until the WBC count is greater than 3500) while clozapine is continued. Therapy must be interrupted if the count drops below 3000 cells/mm^3 and/or the granulocyte count is below 1500 cells/mm^3. At these levels, infection can easily develop. However, if no sign of infection is noted, therapy can resume. If the WBC count is below 2000 cells/mm^3 and the granulocyte count is below 1000 cells/mm^3, clozapine must be discontinued. If agranulocytosis is diagnosed and infection develops, antibiotic therapy and reverse isolation are indicated. Development of infection significantly increases the risk of dying. Reversal of agranulocytosis has been achieved with granulocyte-colony stimulating factor.[59,64]

Treatment Implications

Individual profiles for each antipsychotic can be found in Part 2 of this book.

Therapeutic versus toxic levels. Antipsychotic drugs have a wide therapeutic index, and although overdoses are seldom fatal for any of these drugs, they are even less likely with high-potency agents. Symptoms of overdose are an extension of adverse effects previously mentioned and include CNS depression (somnolence to coma), hypotension, and EPSEs. Restlessness or agitation, convulsions (antipsychotic drugs lower the seizure threshold), hyperthermia, increased anticholinergic symptoms, and arrhythmias also indicate an overdose. Treatment is mostly supportive, with gastric lavage to empty the stomach. Antiparkinson drugs for severe EPSEs and vasoconstrictors (e.g., norepinephrine) can be used for severe hypotension. *Epinephrine* aggravates hypotension and should not be used to treat this hypotension.

Use in pregnancy. Although the risks to the fetus are statistically low, exposure to antipsychotic drugs during the first trimester should still be avoided. Richards and colleagues state that weeks 4 through 10 are particularly dangerous times to give pregnant women antipsychotics.[130] During the remainder of the pregnancy, the lowest possible dosage is desirable. If possible, antipsychotic drugs should be discontinued to reduce the risk of transient neonatal toxicity.[42] Neonatal EPSEs, withdrawal symptoms, and evidence of antipsychotics in breast milk are all complications of continuing antipsychotic drug use during pregnancy.

Use in the elderly. The elderly have decreased hepatic metabolism capability, and their age-related nigrostriatal and cholinergic degeneration make them pharmacodynamically more susceptible to the effects of antipsychotic drugs. They seem particularly susceptible to TD. Current studies reveal prevalency rates ranging from 29% in neuroleptic naive patients to 60% in chronically institutionalized populations.[36,75,172] Hence, as with most medications prescribed for the elderly, the clinician should start low and go slow. Although more sensitive to the effects of both low-potency (anticholinergic and antiadrenergic) and high-potency (EPSEs) drugs, most clinicians prescribe higher-potency agents to avoid the multiple consequences of cholinergic blockade and orthostasis. A dosage equivalent of 0.5 to 2 mg of haloperidol is typically adequate.

Withdrawal. Withdrawal symptoms include various gastrointestinal problems, autonomic symptoms (e.g., tachycardia, tremors, sweating), and insomnia. Effects of abrupt withdrawal may be delayed because of the large volume of distribution of these agents. As noted earlier, phenomena related to dopamine receptor supersensitivity can emerge as these agents are withdrawn, namely, TD or psychosis.

Patient education. Patient education is important when caring for people who are taking antipsychotic drugs. The clinician should use discretion in selecting the content of education sessions though, because patients may become anxious about potential side effects. The focus should be on symptoms that can be seen or felt. Some patient education issues have been discussed throughout this chapter. Recommendations not previously mentioned include the following:

- Avoid hot tubs, hot showers, and hot tub baths because hypotension is potentiated and may cause falls.
- Avoid abrupt drug withdrawal, thereby reducing the risk of EPSEs, particularly TD, and antipsychotic withdrawal psychosis (supersensitivity psychosis [parallel to withdrawal dyskinesia]).
- Use sunscreen to prevent sunburn.
- Adhere to the drug regimen as prescribed. Noncompliance is the primary cause of symptom exacerbation.
- Pay attention to and communicate symptoms of sore throat, malaise, fever, or bleeding. Such signs and symptoms may indicate the emergence of agranulocytosis.
- Adopt appropriate dress in hot weather and increase fluid intake to prevent heat stroke. Because of drug-mediated hypothalamic changes and anhidrosis, individuals using antipsychotics are vulnerable to hyperthermia.

**Box 5-11 Instructions to Provide to Individuals
Prescribed Antipsychotic Drugs**

Take medications only as prescribed.

Take the correct dosage.

Do not give your medications to another person.

If you forget to take your medication on time, wait until your next scheduled dose and get back on schedule (there may be exceptions to this guideline, e.g., once-per-day dosing).

Do not take street drugs or alcohol when taking your prescribed medication.

Tell your doctor or your nurse practitioner about all the drugs prescribed for you.

Before taking over-the-counter drugs, check with your doctor or nurse practitioner.

Do not stop your medication just because you start to feel better.

These drugs tend to be stored in body fat, so even after you stop taking them they are still working to make you feel better. Sometimes, patients confuse this with not needing the medication any longer.

Box 5-11 presents patient education guidelines for taking these medications.

Interactions

Antipsychotic drugs inhibit and are inhibited by many other drugs.[9,165] Because these drug-drug interactions can be serious, it is important first to know potential offending agents and second to advise the family and patient accordingly. As noted in the pharmacokinetic discussion, most antipsychotics are metabolized by the CYP-450 IID6 isoenzyme. Drugs that inhibit this system will increase serum levels of most antipsychotics, and because most antipsychotics are themselves IID6 inhibitors, the serum levels of many other drugs can be increased as well. The following is a partial list of CYP-450 system inhibitors and inducers:

- *IID6 inhibitors (will* elevate *serum levels of most antipsychotics):* paroxetine, fluoxetine, sertraline (more than 100 mg), quinidine, haloperidol, cimetidine, thioridazine, amitriptyline, oral contraceptives, clomipramine, desipramine, norfluoxetine, levopromazine
- *IA2 inhibitors (will* elevate *serum levels of clozapine, haloperidol, olanzapine, all phenothiazines):* fluvoxamine, enoxacin, fluoroquinolones, beta-estradiol, furafylline, ciprofloxacin, (fluoxetine and paroxetine at high dosages), erythromycin
- *IA2 inducers (will* decrease *the serum levels of clozapine, haloperidol, olanzapine, all phenothiazines):* cigarette smoking, omeprazole, charcoal-broiled foods, some cruciferous vegetables, cabbage[9]

Agents such as alcohol, antihistamines, antianxiety drugs, antidepressants, barbiturates, meperidine, and morphine have additive effects that can cause profound CNS depression. The clinician should check prescriptions for the possible inadvertent combination of these and antipsychotic drugs and should advise the patient to avoid both alcohol and certain over-the-counter medications, for example,

Box 5-12 Adverse Interactions of Antipsychotics with Other Drugs

Amphetamines: decrease in antipsychotic effect; antipsychotics reverse amphetamine toxicity and psychosis

Antacids: impairment of absorption of chlorpromazine and perhaps other antipsychotics

Antiarrhythmics: impaired conduction with thioridazine, chlorpromazine, and pimozide

Anticholinergic antiparkinsonism drugs: increase in anticholinergic effect, delay in the onset of the effects of oral doses of antipsychotics, and the potential to increase the risk of hyperthermia

Antihistamines: potentiation of the QT interval with astemizole (Hismanal) and terfenadine (Seldane) (both off the American market), particularly with thioridazine and pimozide

Antihypertensives
    Methyldopa, enalapril: additive hypotension
    Guanethidine: decreased control of hypertension

Anticonvulsants
    Carbamazepine: increases in plasma levels of carbamazepine and decrease in neuroleptic serum levels
    Phenytoin: possible increase in phenytoin toxicity; decreased antipsychotic blood serum levels
    Valproic acid: decreased clearance of valproic acid, leading to neuro-toxicity, sedation, and so on

Barbiturates: respiratory depression and increased sedation; all decrease antipsychotic serum levels, hypotension

Benzodiazepines: increased sedation and impairment of psychomotor function

Beta-adrenergic blocking agents (propranolol): increased effect of either chlorpromazine or propranolol

Cimetidine: decreased chlorpromazine absorption; increased sedation with chlorpromazine; decreased metabolism of clozapine, olanzapine, and thiothixene

Diazoxide: possible severe hyperglycemia

Ethanol: impairment of psychomotor skills (e.g., driving); may worsen EPSEs

Insulin, oral hypoglycemics: weakened control of diabetes

L-dopa: decreased antiparkinsonism effect of L-dopa; L-dopa not effective for drug-induced parkinsonism; may exacerbate psychosis

Lithium: decreased antipsychotic effect; possible neurotoxicity when combined with haloperidol; lithium toxicity may be masked by antiemetic effect of antipsychotic drugs; increased EPSEs

Some information from Reference 22 and Ciraulo DA, Shader RI, Greenblatt DJ, Creelman W: *Drug interactions in psychiatry*, Baltimore, 1989, Williams & Wilkins.

**Box 5-12 Adverse Interactions
of Antipsychotics with Other Drugs—cont'd**

Narcotics: hypotension with chlorpromazine and meperidine; increased
sedation; hypotension augmented; respiratory depression augmented
Smoking: decreased serum levels of antipsychotics (smoking induces
cytochrome P-450 isoenzyme IA2)
SSRIs: increased antipsychotic serum levels; increased EPSEs
Trazodone: additive hypotension with phenothiazines
Tricyclics: possible ventricular arrhythmias with thioridazine; increased
blood serum levels of both antipsychotic and tricyclic; hypotension;
sedation; anticholinergic effect; increased risk of seizures.

---

cold medications and sleep aids. Box 5-12 provides a reference for specific
interactions between and among antipsychotics and other drugs.

TRADITIONAL ANTIPSYCHOTIC DRUGS BY CHEMICAL CLASSIFICATION

Following are brief summaries for traditional antipsychotic drugs organized by
chemical classification. For these agents, true therapeutic differences have not been
substantiated. Differences among individual drugs are primarily related to propensity
for certain side effects (see Table 5-1).[9,22]

Phenothiazines

The phenothiazines are divided into three subclasses: aliphatics, piperidines, and
piperazines.

Aliphatics: chlorpromazine, promazine, and triflupromazine. Chlorpromazine (Thorazine) was the first antipsychotic agent developed and remains an
important drug. Promazine (Sparine) and triflupromazine (Vesprin) are seldom
prescribed. Chlorpromazine is highly sedating and causes significant orthostasis. It
has moderate capability of causing EPSEs. It has the potential for causing significant
weight gain. It has a half-life of 16 to 30 hours. See Table 5-1 for more specific
information.

Piperidines: thioridazine and mesoridazine. Thioridazine is a tricyclic and is
almost as old as chlorpromazine. Until the release of the atypical agents, it was the
largest-selling antipsychotic in the United States.[174] It continues to enjoy favor
among many clinicians, and patients may respond to it when they do not respond to
newer agents. Thioridazine is sometimes prescribed for the short-term treatment of
depression accompanied by anxiety in adult patients and for agitation, anxiety,
depressed mood, tension, sleep disturbances, fears, and other symptoms in geriatric
patients. In children with severe behavioral problems marked by combativeness,
thioridazine has been beneficial. Thioridazine has a lower risk of EPSEs, but
important concerns about eye toxicity exist. For example, in prescribing thioridazine,

the maximum daily dose is 800 mg. At higher dosages, there is a risk of pigmentary retinopathy, which decreases visual acuity, impairs night vision, and is characterized by pigment deposits on the fundus. Thioridazine is also associated with weight gain, higher rates of falls regardless of age, retrograde ejaculation and other sexual dysfunction, and has been linked to fatal arrhythmias.[105] It is an inhibitor of CYP-450 IID6 and can interfere with the metabolism of other drugs. Conversely, thioridazine is metabolized by this same system and its serum levels are elevated if coadministered with other inhibitors of IID6. It has a half-life of 9 to 30 hours. Mesoridazine is not prescribed as often as thioridazine but has the advantage of being available as an injectable and is more easily metabolized. Mesoridazine is sometimes preferred in alcohol abusers or other persons with liver disease. Elderly persons are highly sensitive to mesoridazine-induced hypotension.

Piperazines: fluphenazine, trifluoperazine, and perphenazine. Piperazines are mildly sedating and seldom cause orthostatic hypotension. These drugs cause significant levels of EPSEs. The two most prescribed piperazines are fluphenazine (Prolixin) and trifluoperazine (Stelazine). Fluphenazine, a high-potency antipsychotic, is available in a long-acting or depot form, fluphenazine decanoate. In this form, fluphenazine benefits patients who do not comply with a daily oral medication regimen. An injection can be given every 2 to 3 weeks. Fluphenazine hydrochloride has a "regular" duration and is available in tablet and concentrate forms. Fluphenazine inhibits the CYP IID6 isoenzyme system and has a half-life of 13 to 56 hours.

Trifluoperazine is prescribed relatively often. It is available in tablet, concentrate (unpleasant taste), and parenteral forms. It is indicated for excessive anxiety, tension, agitation, and psychotic manifestations. Side effects include severe EPSEs but milder levels of orthostasis, sedation, and anticholinergic reactions. It has a half-life of approximately 13 hours.

Perphenazine is often used with antidepressants for patients who are both psychotic and depressed. It is metabolized and inhibits the IID6 isoenzyme. Its serum levels are elevated by drugs that inhibit this system. Perphenazine has a half-life of 9 to 21 hours. It can be given by itself or is available in a fixed-dose combination with amitriptyline (Elavil). The fixed-dose combination of perphenazine/amitriptyline is named Triavil.

Butyrophenones: Haloperidol and Droperidol

Haloperidol (Haldol) is a high-potency drug and tends to cause EPSEs but has fewer anticholinergic, sedating, and hypotensive side effects than do the low-potency agents. Haloperidol is commonly prescribed and is used extensively in older adults (because of fewer anticholinergic and hypotensive effects) and in pediatric psychiatry. Haloperidol is also used for Gilles de la Tourette's syndrome (see Chapters 20 and 21). It has a half-life of 12 to 36 hours. Haloperidol is metabolized by the CYP IID6 and IA2 isoenzymes. It is an inhibitor of IID6. There is a "window" of dosage with this drug to obtain a therapeutic effect. Dosages above or below this window (serum levels between 4 and 22 ng/ml) are not as effective.[20,132] In other words, both undermedicating and overmedicating decrease the therapeutic value of haloperidol.

Haloperidol decanoate (Haldol LA) is a long-acting depot form and can be given every 3 to 4 weeks (or with longer intervals). This preparation is particularly beneficial for patients with compliance difficulties.

Droperidol is used as an antiemetic and in the management of delirium.

Thioxanthenes: Chlorprothixene and Thiothixene

Chlorprothixene (Taractan) and thiothixene (Navane) have different potencies. Chlorprothixene is similar to chlorpromazine and is a low-potency drug. It exhibits moderate extrapyramidal, anticholinergic, and hypotensive effects. It causes moderate to significant sedation as a result of its heavy blockade of histamine H_1 receptors. It is also a potent antagonist of $5HT_2$, which duplicates some of the sought after properties of the more expensive atypical drugs. It has a half-life of 8 to 12 hours. Thiothixene is 20 times as potent as chlorpromazine, more like the piperazine phenothiazines. Thiothixene is prescribed relatively often. Thiothixene causes relatively powerful EPSEs but significantly milder anticholinergic, orthostatic, and sedative effects. It has a half-life of about 34 hours.

Dibenzoxazepine: Loxapine

Loxapine (Loxitane) is available in capsule, concentrate, and parenteral forms. The concentrate is unpleasant and should be diluted with orange juice shortly before administration. Specific EPSEs have been reported in more than 20% of patients, particularly during the first few days of treatment. As with other agents, reduction of the loxapine dosage and administration of an antiparkinson drug usually control these side effects. It is associated with moderate to severe sedation, moderate orthostasis, and mild to moderate anticholinergic symptoms. Loxapine differs from other traditional antipsychotics because of its antagonism of a significant proportion of $5HT_2$ receptors.[83] It also demonstrates prominent blockade of dopamine D_4 receptors with an affinity for that receptor type comparable to clozapine. This receptor-blocking pattern is associated with less intense EPSEs and better outcomes for refractory and negative type schizophrenia.[83] The half-life of this drug is 8 to 30 hours.

Dihydroindolone: Molindone

Molindone (Moban) is about 10 times as potent as chlorpromazine. Side effects include significant levels of EPSEs but mild orthostasis, frequent but mild to moderate sedation, and a mild to moderate anticholinergic response. Available only for oral administration, molindone has several unique properties; for example, it provokes heavy menstruation in previously amenorrheal women and contains calcium ions that can interfere with the absorption of tetracycline antibiotics or phenytoin (Dilantin). Although many antipsychotics, particularly the atypical agents, cause weight gain, molindone may actually cause weight loss.[58] It has a half-life of about 6.5 hours.

Diphenylbutylpiperidine: Pimozide

Pimozide (Orap) is used primarily in the treatment of Gilles de la Tourette's syndrome (see Chapters 20 and 21). It can also be prescribed for augmenting therapy for refractory cases of obsessive-compulsive disorder. It is metabolized by the CYP IID6 and IIIA/4 isoenzyme systems. It inhibits the IID6 isoenzyme. It has a half-life of 29 to 55 hours.

Atypical Antipsychotics

Between the time chlorpromazine was introduced and the emergence of the first atypical drug in 1990, psychiatric researchers continually sought to develop more effective and better-tolerated antipsychotic drugs. During that 40-year span, pharmaceutical manufacturers developed a multitude of traditional antipsychotics.[67,116] As previously stated, these drugs were basically the same or "typical." They were equieffective with unique side effect profiles. Beginning in 1990 and continuing to this day, new atypical drugs are being developed, studied, and made available for individuals who have schizophrenia and other psychoses. First, clozapine (Clozaril) was marketed in 1990, followed by risperidone (Risperdal) in 1994, olanzapine (Zyprexa) in 1996, and quetiapine (Seroquel) in 1997. The next drug to be released will be ziprasidone (Zeldox). All of these drugs are touted as being atypical because they do the following:

1. Cause fewer EPSEs (reduced D_2 antagonism in nigrostriatal tract)
2. Are effective for negative and/or cognitive symptoms
3. Do not elevate prolactin (reduced D_2 antagonism in tuberoinfundibular tract)
4. Antagonize $5HT_2$ (theoretically accounting for improvement in negative symptoms)
5. Reduced risk for tardive dyskinesia

Related to the last characteristic, these drugs are at times marketed as serotonin/dopamine antagonists or SDAs.

Dibenzodiazepine: Clozapine

Clozapine has been referred to as the gold standard in the management of refractory schizophrenia.[122] Although it was first introduced in 1960, clozapine (Clozaril) was not marketed in the United States for three more decades because of its potentially fatal side effect, agranulocytosis.[16,138] As noted previously, 50% of the individuals (9 of 18 in a report by Idanpaan-Heikkila and others[74]) developing agranulocytosis from clozapine therapy died. This terrible development delayed use of clozapine in the United States another 15 years and then was approved for use only under the aforementioned rigid protocols.

Clozapine is a dibenzodiazepine derivative, and its pharmacologic features were unique among antipsychotic drugs when it was introduced. Whereas traditional antipsychotic drugs block dopamine D_2 receptors, clozapine produces a weaker blockade of D_2 receptors (about 45% occupancy with normal dosage compared with haloperidol's 80% blockade) but has a more significant blockade of dopamine D_1 and D_4 receptors and of serotonin $5HT_2$ receptors (approximately 90%).[28,81,93] The low affinity for D_2 explains the relative lack of EPSEs and prolactin-associated side effects. Clozapine also has a significant antagonism of alpha-1, alpha-2, muscarinic, and histamine H_1 receptors, accounting for other side effects.

Clozapine's primary importance is that patients resistant to other antipsychotics have responded to it.[115] Thirty percent of individuals refractory to traditional agents respond to clozapine. Although clinicians agree that clozapine treatment succeeds where treatment with other antipsychotics fails, its efficacy for purely negative symptoms remains unknown.[138] Nonetheless, clozapine and the other atypical agents that followed have reaffirmed the biologic nature of schizophrenia.[100] Clozapine also appears to have mood-stabilizing properties and with other atypical agents may be effective in the treatment of delusional major depression and psychosis associated with Parkinson's disease.[22,57,151]

Until the advent of clozapine, all antipsychotic drugs were considered equally effective. Some drugs helped some people more than other drugs, but one could not say, for instance, that haloperidol was superior to chlorpromazine. Clozapine is the first drug for which an improved rate of response is suggested. However, because of the high risk of agranulocytosis and death, certain precautions in the form of weekly or biweekly monitoring of WBCs and platelets must be observed by the clinician and patient. When WBCs and platelets are monitored frequently, impending bone marrow failure can be detected early, thus greatly reducing the risk associated with infections. As noted in Table 5-1, clozapine remains the most expensive antipsychotic on the market. Part of that expense is created by the required monitoring system. The side effect profile for clozapine is good overall, but it is far from the perfect drug. Beyond the potentially life-threatening agranulocytosis, clozapine causes significant sedation, orthostasis, the spectrum of anticholinergic symptoms, and weight gain (one report showed an average gain of 23.5 pounds).[137] At dosages between 600 and 900 mg/day, there is a 5% risk of seizures (or five times the risk with most antipsychotic drugs). A unique side effect of clozapine is the high rate of sialorrhea found among these patients. Upwards of 30% of individuals taking clozapine report significant hypersalivation.[73] Numerous anecdotal reports indicate that some patients must carry "spit" cups to collect their excessive droolings. Gagging is also common. Other autonomic effects include dizziness, tachycardia (approximately 25%), and hypotension. Finally, a significant level of leukopenia is reported among these individuals. Just as importantly, clozapine is not associated with TD and in fact may be therapeutic in the treatment of this disabling disorder.[104]

Clozapine has a half-life of 4 to 12 hours and, with its metabolite, is metabolized by CYP-450 isoenzymes IID6, IIC19, IA2, and IIIA4.[9,97] Clozapine inhibits IID6.[9] Interactions are likely with substrates and inhibitors of these enzymes. The following is an actual case report. Nonmedicinal substances can affect clozapine levels; for example, cigarette smoking induces IA2, thus causing decreased serum levels of clozapine. Conversely, grapefruit juice inhibits IIIA4, leading to increased levels of substrates of this enzyme.

> Fred White is a 37-year-old man who has struggled with schizophrenia since late adolescence. Because his illness was not manageable at times, he experienced several short hospitalizations. He eventually was placed involuntarily in the state hospital and was living there in 1990 when clozapine became available. After 4 months of taking clozapine, Mr. White was discharged from the state hospital. Mr. White did well on the drug for almost 3 years. In late 1992, Mr. White's WBC count began to drop. He was withdrawn from clozapine and placed on large doses of haloperidol. He was hospitalized "locally" on several occasions and then as a "last ditch effort" was rechallenged with clozapine after approval was granted from the manufacturer. Mr. White made impressive gains again but several months later was hospitalized for a decreasing WBC count. Mr. White's presenting symptoms were sore throat (so much so that he gave up eating and had trouble speaking), malaise, and fever (103° F). He was withdrawn from clozapine never to be rechallenged. At this writing, he is back in the state hospital.

Benzisoxazole: Risperidone

The next atypical antipsychotic drug available was risperidone (Risperdal). It was made available in 1994 and today is the most prescribed antipsychotic.[82,90,107] It blocks dopamine D_2 receptors more than clozapine (less than 80% versus 40%, respectively) and potently blocks serotonin $5HT_2$ receptors (78% to 88%).[28,50] Risperidone has a high affinity for D_4 and alpha-1 receptors and a relatively high affinity for D_3, H_1, and alpha-2 receptors[28]; thus it has antidopaminergic, antiserotonergic, and antiadrenergic properties.[22] It does not efficiently block cholinergic receptors.[99] Risperidone's receptor blocking profile accounts for the lack of serious side effects associated with it. Traditionally, risperidone is said to cause few EPSEs; however, at higher dosages (greater than 6 mg/day) and in large multicenter trials, EPSEs have been more common.[55] It also causes few anticholinergic side effects.[99] Because of antiadrenergic effects, orthostasis can be significant at the beginning of treatment.[22]

It is theorized that risperidone's blocking of $5HT_2$ in cortical regions of the brain accounts for improvements in negative symptoms seen with its use.[26,40,41,119] Because of its effects on D_2 receptors in the mesolimbic tract, risperidone also effectively treats positive symptoms. It is thought that alpha-1 blockade may play a role in risperidone's antipsychotic effects as well.[148] Risperidone's therapeutic range is important for many patients—risperidone ameliorates positive symptoms (hallucinations, delusions, bizarre behavior, and thought disorders) like traditional antipsychotics and is effective in diminishing negative symptoms associated with cortical dopamine deficiencies (alogia, flattened affect, avolition, and anergia).* Gutierrez-Esteinou and Grebb analyzed reports from the first 3 years of risperidone use (12 million patient-months of risperidone use) and found evidence supporting risperidone's efficacy for treatment-resistant, first-episode, and negative schizophrenia.[65]

Risperidone significantly blocks histamine H_1 receptors, causing sedation and weight gain. There are moderate levels of sexual dysfunction associated with risperidone related to both its dopamine-blocking activity and its antiadrenergic effects. Risperidone does not appear to cause agranulocytosis, TD, or neuroleptic malignant syndrome.[31] Other side effects, including insomnia, agitation, headache, anxiety, and rhinitis, appear routinely among recipients of risperidone. Less commonly reported side effects include dizziness, constipation, nausea, and tachycardia.

Risperidone is rapidly absorbed from the gastrointestinal tract and reaches plasma levels in about 1 hour.[106] The half-life of risperidone and its active metabolite (9-hydroxyrisperidone) is about 20 to 24 hours; thus once-a-day dosing is permitted. The metabolite is equally as potent as the parent compound.[99] Risperidone is a substrate of CYP IID6 and also an inhibitor of that enzyme. Predictably, interactions can occur with other drugs that are metabolized or inhibit this system; however, as Lam points out, such proposed effects might be mitigated by the subsequent decrease in the active metabolite.[98] Risperidone is not a substrate of CYP IA2; thus cigarette smoking, a common behavior among patients with schizophrenia, should not diminish serum levels.

Thienobenzodiazepine: Olanzapine

Olanzapine (Zyprexa) was the next atypical antipsychotic drug made available. It was released in September 1996. It is similar to clozapine in receptor affinity and antagonizes dopamine D_1, serotonin $5HT_2$, muscarinic, histamine H_1, and alpha-1 receptors. It has three metabolic routes, including a phase 1 oxidation by CYP IA2, IID6, and IIC.[49] It provides low inhibition for CYP IA2, CYP IID6, and CYP 3A4 isoenzymes. It has a half-life of 21 to 54 hours. It is well absorbed from the gastrointestinal tract; food has no effect on absorption.[21]

As with other newer atypical agents, sufficient investigations have yet to be done to state conclusively the efficacy of olanzapine for patients with refractory schizophrenia. However, a number of studies indicate olanzapine to be an effective antipsychotic.[33,43] In a large study of nearly 2000 patients, Tollefson and colleagues found olanzapine (at 15 mg/day) to be superior to haloperidol (at 10 mg/day), to have broad affinity for several neurotransmitters, to modulate mesolimbic function without significant extrapyramidal system antagonism, to spare dopamine blockade within the tuberoinfundibular tract, and to have a normalizing effect on NMDA receptors.[158] In fact, olanzapine appears to affect the glutamate system and can prevent the schizophrenic-like symptoms caused by NMDA antagonists PCP or ketamine.[157]

*References 1, 13, 31, 35, 41, 108.

As do the other atypical agents that follow, olanzapine does not cause agranulocytosis. Olanzapine has few significant side effects because of its receptor-antagonizing profile. Because of specific receptor affinities, olanzapine produces few extrapyramidal or orthostatic symptoms, and only mild to moderate anticholinergic symptoms, but it does cause significant sedation.[171] Increases in prolactin levels are transient.[76] Headache, light-headedness, dizziness, insomnia, and agitation are also reported.[21] Anecdotally, reports of mania, NMS, TD, and priapism have been published. Of particular concern for many individuals taking olanzapine is weight gain (Ganguli reviewed reports of patients who had average weight gains of 4.8, 12, and 16 pounds).[58] Among the atypical agents, only clozapine causes the same level of weight gain.[171] Although olanzapine is about 10 times as expensive as the traditional drugs, it is still less expensive than clozapine (see Table 5-1). Olanzapine has few significant drug interactions. Typical dosage is 5 to 40 mg/day. An intramuscular formulation is anticipated.

Dibenzothiazepine: Quetiapine

Quetiapine (Seroquel), another atypical antipsychotic, became available in September 1997. It has a pharmacodynamic profile similar to clozapine but does not cause agranulocytosis.[63,70,125] Quetiapine has a somewhat greater affinity for $5HT_2$ receptors (58% to 72%) than for dopamine D_2 receptors (27% to 44%).[32,63,113,123,149] EPSEs are not prominent side effects of quetiapine, probably related to this relatively low dopamine D_2 occupancy (threshold occupancy levels for EPSEs are approximately 75%). After chronic administration, quetiapine effectively blocks the mesolimbic dopaminergic system but not the nigrostriatal pathways, indicating a preference for mesolimbic sites over striatal neurons.[113,139] It has a high affinity for alpha-1 and histamine receptors and low affinity for alpha-2, dopamine D_1, and muscarinic receptors; hence orthostasis, dizziness, sedation, and weight gain are most commonly reported, whereas sexual dysfunction and anticholinergic responses to not occur often. Plasma prolactin levels, after a brief increase, normalize. This is related to quetiapine's low affinity for D_2 receptors within the tuberoinfundibular tract. Galactorrhea, menstrual irregularities, and gynecomastia are rarely reported.

Quetiapine is rapidly absorbed by the body and is 83% protein bound. Peak serum levels are achieved in 1.5 hours. It is metabolized in the liver by CYP IIIA4 and has no active metabolites. Clearance decreases with age, in those with renal or hepatic impairment, and when administered with CYP IIIA4 inhibitors. Inducers of this isoenzyme hasten elimination. The elimination half-life of quetiapine is 4 to 10 hours. It is excreted both in the urine (73%) and in the feces (20%), with 5% excreted unchanged.

Quetiapine is started at 25 mg twice daily for 1 day, then increased to 300 mg/day by day 4.[12] Research supports the efficacy and tolerability of quetiapine for people with schizophrenia, as indicated by the following advantages[12,32,63,118,149]:

1. Effectiveness for both positive and negative symptoms
2. Few EPSEs
3. Normal levels of prolactin
4. Normal hematologic profile
5. A lack of significant interactions with other drugs

Benzisothiazolyl: Ziprasidone

Ziprasidone (Zeldox), approved in August 2000, is similar in action to other atypical antipsychotic drugs. It acts on several neurotransmitter systems and has been shown to be effective for both positive and negative symptoms of schizophrenia at divided doses of 80 and 160 mg/day.[28,87,154] Ziprasidone has a high affinity for $5HT_2$ receptors and a moderate affinity for dopamine D_2 and D_3 receptor.[76] It has relatively low affinity for dopamine D_1, alpha-1 adrenergic, histamine, muscarinic, and alpha-2 receptors.[76] Ziprasidone occupies about 98% of $5HT_2$ only 4 hours after administration, which is higher than either clozapine or olanzapine.[28,71] The serotonin/dopamine antagonism ratio is greater for ziprasidone than for clozapine, risperidone, or halperidol[60] and accounts for the reduced incidence of EPSEs with this drug. Ziprasidone produces a low incidence of orthostasis, sedation, and anticholinergic effects.[55] There has been no evidence of compromised hematologic function and prolactin levels are normal, although transient increases occur during early therapy. Weight gain, a problem with other atypical agents, appears to be insignificant with ziprasidone.[87] Common side effects include nausea, dyspepsia, abdominal pain, constipation, somnolence, coryzal symptoms, and insomnia. Transaminase levels have increased in some individuals but return to normal on discontinuance of the drug.

Ziprasidone is also an agonist for the $5HT_{1A}$ receptor, while moderately inhibiting the reuptake of both serotonin and norepinephrine. This particular constellation of receptor affinities suggests a drug with the potential for alleviating the mood and anxiety commonly associated with schizophrenia.[28,60,85,87] This may be of particular importance because approximately 10% of patients with schizophrenia commit suicide.[154]

Ziprasidone is about five times more potent than chlorpromazine. Peak plasma levels are reached within 4 hours. Bioavailability increases to 60% if ziprasidone is taken with food. Protein binding for this drug is approximately 99%. It is metabolized by the CYP IIIA4 isoenzyme to inactive metabolites. The half-life is 5 to 10 hours. Pharmacokinetic studies have suggested that it has low potential for drug-drug interactions and does not inhibit the CYP system. An intramuscular form is anticipated.

Other Atypical Antipsychotic Drugs: Sertindole and Zotepine

Sertindole and zotepine are two new atypical agents not on the market at this time. Sertindole is a potent blocker of D_2, alpha-1, and $5HT_2$ receptors.[55,147] It does not significantly antagonize histamine or muscarinic receptors. It has a half-life of about 3 hours.[55] Because of the potential for cardiovascular problems (prolonged QT interval) sertindole was pulled from the U.S. drug approval process. It is currently available in Europe. Zotepine is a dibenzothiepine and blocks serotonergic, dopaminergic, histaminergic, and adrenergic receptors. It also blocks reuptake of norepinephrine. The side effect profile for zotepine reflects the receptors antagonized. Its blockage of noradrenergic reuptake may explain its seeming efficacy in depression associated with schizophrenia.

REMARKS

The dopamine hypothesis states that schizophrenia is caused by excessive levels of dopamine in the brain. Traditional antipsychotic drugs blocked dopamine receptors, accounting for their therapeutic effect. However, many patients did not improve or, if so, did not improve for long, so a perpetual search for more efficacious and better-tolerated drugs began. Many new antipsychotic drugs were developed in this quest, but it was not until 1990, when clozapine was marketed, that new ground was broken. These new or atypical antipsychotics also worked at the receptor level but demonstrated a more exquisite receptor profile. Essentially, the newer drugs appear to be more efficient for treatment-resistant individuals and patients exhibiting negative symptoms, while producing fewer adverse side effects. A notable exception is clozapine, which can cause the potentially lethal blood dyscrasia, agranulocytosis. Extrapyramidal, anticholinergic, antiadrenergic, antihistaminic, and prolactin-related side effects are the major obstacles to patient compliance with these medications. Noncompliance remains a major cause of symptom reemergence among this population. Overdoses of antipsychotics are seldom fatal, but drug interactions with other CNS depressants such as alcohol can be serious.

REFERENCES

1. Addington DE and others: Reduction of hospital days in chronic schizophrenia patients treated with risperidone: a retrospective study, *Clin Ther* 15:917, 1993.
2. Alvir JM, Lieberman JA: Agranulocytosis: incidence and risk factors. *J Clin Psychiatry,* 55(suppl B):137, 1994.
3. American Psychiatric Association: *Diagnostic and statistical manual of mental disorders,* ed 3, Washington, DC, 1980, The Association.
4. American Psychiatric Association: *Diagnostic and statistical manual of mental disorders-TR,* ed 4, Washington, DC, 2000, The Association.
5. American Psychiatric Association: *Practice guidelines for the treatment of patients with schizophrenia.* Washington, DC, 1997, The Association.
6. Andreasen NC: Positive vs negative schizophrenia: a critical evaluation. *Schizophr Bull* 11:380, 1985.
7. Andreasen NC, Olsen S: Negative vs. positive schizophrenia, *Arch Gen Psychiatry* 39:789, 1982.
8. Andreasen NC and others: Positive and negative symptoms in schizophrenia: a critical reappraisal, *Arch Gen Psychiatry* 47:615, 1990.
9. Applegate M: Cytochrome P450 isoenzymes: nursing considerations. *JAPNA* 5(1):15, 1999.
10. Appleton WS: *Practical and clinical psychopharmacology,* Baltimore, 1988, Williams & Wilkins.
11. Arnold SE and others: Smaller neuron size in schizophrenia in hippocampal subfields that mediated cortical-hippocampal interactions. *Am J Psychiatry* 152(5):738, 1995.
12. Arvanitis LA, Miller BG, the Seroquel Trial 13 Study Group: Multiple fixed doses of "Seroquel" (quetiapine) in patients with acute exacerbation of schizophrenia: a comparison with haloperidol and placebo, *Biol Psychiatry* 42:233, 1997.
13. Awouters F and others: Functional interaction between serotonin-S2 and dopamine-D2 neurotransmission as revealed by selective antagonism of hyper-reactivity to tryptamine and apomorphine, *J Pharmacol Exp Ther* 254(3):945, 1990.
14. Ayd FJ: The early history of modern psychopharmacology, *Neuropsychopharmacology* 5(2): 71, 1991.
15. Barnes TR, Curson DA: Long-term depot antipsychotics: a risk-benefit assessment, *Drug Safety* 10(6):464, 1994.
16. Barrett N, Ormiston S, Molyneux V: Clozapine: a new drug for schizophrenia, *J Psychosoc Nurs Ment Health Serv* 28:24, 1990.
17. Bartzokis G and others: Reliability of in vivo volume measures of hippocampus and other brain structures using MRI, *Magn Reson Imaging* 11(7):993, 1993.
18. Bassitt DP, Louza Neto MR: Clozapine efficacy in tardive dyskinesia in schizophrenic patients, *Eur Arch Psychiatry Clin Neurosci* 248(4):209, 1998.
19. Berman KF, Weinberger DR, Shelton RC, Zec RF: A relationship between anatomical and physiological brain pathology in schizophrenia: lateral cerebral ventricular size predicts cortical blood flow, *Am J Psychiatry* 144(10):1269, 1987.
20. Bernardo M and others: Monitoring plasma level of haloperidol in schizophrenia, *Hosp Community Psychiatry* 44(2):115, 1993.
21. Bever KA, Perry PJ: Olanzapine: a serotonin-dopamine receptor antagonist for antipsychotic therapy, *Am J Health-Sys Phar* 55(10):1003, 1998.
22. Bezchlibnyk-Butler KZ, Jeffries JJ: *Clinical handbook of psychotropic drugs,* Seattle, 1997, Hogrefe and Huber.

23. Blair DT: Risk management for extrapyramidal symptoms, *Qual Rev Bull J Qual Assur* 17: 116, 1990.
24. Blair DT, Dauner A: Neuroleptic malignant syndrome: liability in nursing practice, *J Psychosoc Nurs Ment Health Serv* 31(2):5, 1993.
25. Blair DT, Dauner A: Nonneuroleptic etiologies of extrapyramidal symptoms, *Clin Nurs Spec* 7(4):225, 1993.
26. Bleich A and others: The role of serotonin in schizophrenia, *Schizophr Bull* 14(2):297, 1988.
27. Bleuler E: *Dementia praecox or the group of schizophrenias*, New York, 1950, International Universities Press (Translated by J Zinkin).
28. Blin O: A comparative review of new antipsychotics, *Can J Psychiatry* 44:235, 1999.
29. Bogerts B and others: Post-mortem volume measurements of limbic and basal ganglia structures in chronic schizophrenia, *Schizophr Res* 3(5-6):295, 1990.
30. Bogerts B and others: Hippocampus-amygdala volume and psychopathology in chronic schizophrenia, *Biol Psychiatry* 33(4):236, 1993.
31. Borison RL and others: Risperidone: clinical safety and efficacy in schizophrenia, *Psychopharmacol Bull* 28(2):213, 1992.
32. Borison RL and others: ICI 204,636, an atypical antipsychotic: efficacy and safety in a multicenter, placebo-controlled trial in patiens with schizophrenia, *J Clin Psychopharmacol* 16(2):158, 1996.
33. Breier A, Hamilton S: Comparative efficacy of olanzapine and haloperidol for patients treatment-resistant schizophrenia, *Biol Psychiatry* 45:403:1999.
34. Breier A and others: Brain morphology and schizophrenia: a magnetic resonance imaging study of limbic, prefrontal cortex, and caudate structures, *Arch Gen Psychiatry* 49(12): 921, 1992.
35. Brown K and others: Overdose of risperidone, *Ann Emerg Med* 22(12):1908, 1993.
36. Byne W and others: Tardive dyskinesia in a chronically institutionalized population of elderly schizophrenic patients: prevalence and association with cognitive impairment, *Int J Geriatr Psychiatry* 13(7):473, 1998.
37. Cannon TD, Marco E: Structural brain abnormalities as indicators of vulnerability to schizophrenia, *Schizophr Bull* 20(1):89, 1994.
38. Casanova MF and others: A topographical study of senile plaques and neurofibrillary tangles in the hippocampi of patients with Alzheimer's disease and cognitively impaired patients with schizophrenia, *Psychiatry Res* 49(1):41, 1993.
39. Casey DE: Effects of clozapine therapy in schizophrenic individuals at risk for tardive dyskinesia, *J Clin Psychiatry* 59(suppl 3):31, 1998.
40. Chouinard G, Arnott W: Clinical review of risperidone, *Can J Psychiatry* 38(3):S89, 1993.
41. Claus A and others: Risperidone versus haloperidol in the treatment of chronic schizophrenic inpatients: a multicenter double-blind comparative study, *Acta Psychiatr Scand* 85(4): 295, 1992.
42. Cohen LS: Psychopharmacology: psychotropic drug use in pregnancy, *Hosp Community Psychiatry* 40:566, 1989.
43. Conley R and others: Olanzapine compared with chlorpromazine in treatment-resistant schizophrenia, *Am J Psychiatry* 155:914, 1998.
44. Coyle JT: The glutamatergic dysfunction hypothesis for schizophrenia, *Harv Rev Psychiatry* 3(5):241, 1996.
45. Crow TJ: Molecular pathology of schizophrenia: more than one disease, *Br Med J* 280: 66, 1980.
46. Dauner A, Blair DT: Akathisia: when treatment creates a problem, *J Psychosoc Nurs Ment Health Serv* 28(10):13, 1990.
47. Davis JM, Andrivkactis S: The natural course of schizophrenia and effective maintenance drug treatment, *J Clin Psychopharmacol* 6:2S, 1986.
48. Dursun S, Oluboka OJ, Devarajan S, Kutcher SP: High-dose vitamin E plus vitamin B6 treatment of risperidone-related neuroleptic malignant syndrome, *J Psychopharmacol* 12: 220, 1998.

49. Ereshefsky L: Pharmacokinetics and drug interactions: update for newer antipsychotics, *J Clin Psychiatry* 57(suppl 11):12, 1996.

50. Ereshefsky L, Lacombe S: Pharmacological profile of risperidone, *Can J Psychiatry* 38(3): S80, 1993.

51. Factor SA, Friedman JH: The emerging role of clozapine in the treatment of movement disorders, *Mov Disord* 12(4):483, 1997.

52. *Federal Task Force on Homelessness and Severe Mental Illness: Outcasts on Main Street,* Washington, 1992, Interagency Council on the Homeless.

53. Feldman J: Clozapine and agranulocytosis, *Psychiatr Serv* 47(11):1177, 1996.

54. Flaum M and others: Effects of diagnosis, laterality, and gender on brain morphology in schizophrenia, *Am J Psychiatry* 12(5):704, 1995.

55. Fleischhacker WW, Hummer M: Drug treatment of schizophrenia in the 1990s: achievements and future possibilities in optimizing outcomes, *Drugs* 53(6):915, 1997.

56. Foley JJ: Considerations in the use of benzodiazepines and antipsychotics in the emergency department, *J Emer Nurs* 19(5):448, 1993.

57. Friedman J: Olanzapine in the treatment of dopaminomimetic psychosis in patients with Parkinson's disease, *Neurology* 47(4):1085, 1996.

58. Ganguli R: Newer antipsychotics versus older neuroleptics: is weight gain still a problem? *Ther Adv Psychoses* July 6, 1999.

59. Gerson SL: G-CSF and the management of clozapine-induced agranulocytosis, *J Clin Psychiatry* 55(suppl B):139, 1994.

60. Goff D and others: An exploratory haloperidol-controlled dose-finding study in hospitalized patients with schizophrenia and schizoaffective disorder, *J Clin Psychiatry* 18(4):296, 1998.

61. Goldstein M, Tsuang MT: Gender and schizophrenia: an introduction and synthesis of findings, *Schizophr Bull* 16(2):179, 1990.

62. Gomez GE, Gomez EA: The special concerns of neuroleptic use in the elderly, *J Psychosoc Nurs Ment Health Serv* 28:7, 1990.

63. Green B: Focus on quetiapine, *Curr Med Res Opin* 15(3):145, 1999.

64. Gullion G, Yeh HS: Treatment of clozapine-induced agranulocytosis with recombinant granulocyte colony-stimulating factor, *J Clin Psychiatry* 55:401, 1994.

65. Gutierrez-Esteinou R, Grebb JA: Risperidone: an analysis of the first three years in general use, *Int Clin Psychopharmacol* 12(suppl 4):S3, 1997.

66. Hogarty GE, Ulrich RF: The limitations of antipsychotic medication on schizophrenia relapse and adjustment and the contributions of psychosocial treatment, *J Psychiatr Res* 32(3-4): 243, 1998.

67. Hollister LE: New antipsychotic drugs, *J Clin Psychopharmacol* 14(1):50, 1994.

68. Hooper JF, Herren CK, Goldwasser H: Neuroleptic malignant syndrome, *J Psychosoc Nurs Ment Health Serv* 27:13, 1989.

69. Howard R and others: Magnetic resonance imaging volumetric measurements of the superior temporal gyrus, hippocampus, parahippocampal gyrus, frontal and temporal lobes in late paraphrenia, *Psychol Med* 25(3):495, 1995.

70. Hustey FM: Acute quetiapine poisoning, *J Emerg Med* 17(6):995, 1999.

71. Ischikawa J, Meltzer H: Relationship between dopaminergic and serotonergic neuronal activity in the frontal cortex and the action of typical and atypical antipsychotic drugs, *Eur Arch Psychiatry Clin Neurosci* 249(suppl 4):90, 1999.

72. Ingvar DH, Franzen G: Abnormalities of cerebral blood flow distribution in patients with chronic schizophrenia, *Acta Psychiatr Scand* 50:425, 1974.

73. Jaretz N, Flowers E, Millsap L: Clozapine: nursing care considerations, *Perspect Psychiatr Care* 28:19, 1992.

74. Idanpann-Heikkila J, Alhava E, Olkinuora M, Palva I: Clozapine and agranulocytosis (letter), *Lancet* 2:611, 1975.

75. Jeste DV and others: Conventional vs newer antipsychotics in elderly patients, *Am J Geriatr Psychiatry* 7(1):70, 1999.

76. Jibson MD, Tandon R: New atypical antipsychotic medications, *J Psychiatr Res* 32:215, 1998.

77. Johnson DAW: Pharmacological treatment of patients with schizophrenia: past and present problems and potential future therapy, *Drugs* 39(4):481, 1990.

78. Johnstone EC, Geddes J: How high is the relapse rate in schizophrenia? *Acta Psychiatr Scand Suppl* 382:6, 1994.

79. Johnstone EC and others: Cerebral ventricular size and cognitive impairment in chronic schizophrenia, *Lancet* 2(7992):924, 1976.

80. Joyce JN: The dopamine hypothesis of schizophrenia: limbic interactions with serotonin and norepinephrine, *Psychopharmacology* 112 (1 suppl):S16, 1993.

81. Kane J: Newer antipsychotic drugs: a review of their pharmacology and therapeutic potential, *Drugs* 46(4):585, 1993.

82. Kane J: Risperidone, *Am J Psychiatry* 151(6):802, 1994.

83. Kapur A and others: PET evidence that loxapine is an equipotent blocker of 5-HT2 and D2 receptors: implications for the therapeutics of schizophrenia, *Am J Psychiatry* 14(11):1525, 1997.

84. Karson CN, Casanova MF, Kleinman JE, Griffin WS: Choline acetyltransferase in schizophrenia, *Am J Psychiatry* 150(3):454, 1993.

85. Keck P, Strakowski S, McElroy S: The efficacy of atypical antipsychotics in the treatment of depressive symptoms, hostility, and suicidality in patients with schizophrenia, *J Clin Psychiatry* 61(suppl 3):4, 2000.

86. Keck PE and others: Risk factors for neuroleptic malignant syndrome, *Arch Gen Psychiatry* 46:914, 1989.

87. Keck PE and others: Ziprasidone 40 and 120 mg/day in the acute exacerbation of schizophrenia and schizoaffective disorder: a 4-week placebo-controlled trial, *Psychopharmacology* 140:173, 1998.

88. Keefe RSE and others: Characteristics of very poor outcome schizophrenia, *Am J Psychiatry* 144(7):889, 1987.

89. Keepers GA, Casey DE: Clinical management of acute neuroleptic-induced extrapyramidal symptoms. In Masserman JH, editor: *Current psychiatric therapies,* New York, 1986, Grune & Stratton.

90. Keltner NL: Risperidone: the search for a better antipsychotic, *Perspect Psychiatric Care* 31(1):30, 1995.

91. Keltner NL: Neuroreceptor function and psychopharmacological response, *Iss Mental Health Nurs* 21:31, 2000.

92. Keltner NL, McIntyre CW: Neuroleptic malignant syndrome, *J Neurosurg Nurs* 17:362, 1985.

93. Kerwin RW: The new atypical antipsychotics, *Br J Psychiatry* 164:141, 1994.

94. Kim JS and others: Low cerebrospinal fluid glutamate in schizophrenic patients and a new hypothesis on schizophrenia, *Neurosci Lett* 20:379, 1980.

95. Kopelowicz A, Bidder TG: Dementia praecox: inescapable fate or psychiatric oversight? *Hosp Community Psychiatry* 43(9):940, 1992.

96. Kraepelin E: *Dementia praecox and paraphrenia, with historical introduction (1919),* New York, 1971, RE Krieger (Translated by RM Barclay).

97. Lam WFL: Clozapine and fluvoxamine, *Psychopharmacol Update* 10(2):2, 1999.

98. Lam WFL: Drug interaction potential of risperidone, *Psychopharmacol Update* 10(5):2, 1999.

99. Land W, Salzman C: Risperidone: a novel antipsychotic medication, *Hosp Community Psychiatry* 45(5):434, 1994.

100. Lawson WB: Drugs versus other therapies, *Hosp Community Psychiatry* 43(1):84, 1992.

101. Lazarus A, Mann SC, Caroff SN: *The neuroleptic malignant syndrome and related conditions.* Washington, DC, 1989, American Psychiatric Press.

102. Lewine RRJ: A discriminate validity study of negative symptoms with a special focus on depression and antipsychotic medication, *Am J Psychiatry* 147:1463, 1990.

103. Lieberman JA, Tasman A: *Psychiatric drugs,* Philadelphia, 2000, WB Saunders.

104. Littrell K, Magill AM: The effect of clozapine on pre-existing tardive dyskinesia, *J Psychosoc Nurs Ment Health Serv* 31(9):14, 1993.

105. Liu YJ and others: Thioridazine dose-related effects on biomechanical force platform measures of sway in young and old men, *J Am Geriatr Soc* 46(4):431, 1998.

106. Mannens G and others: Absorption, metabolism, and excretion of risperidone in humans, *Drug Metab Dispos* 21(6):1134, 1993.

107. Marder SR: Risperidone (Risperdal), *The decade of the brain* 8(3):5, 1997.

108. Marder SR, Meibach RC: Risperidone in the treatment of schizophrenia, *Am J Psychiatry* 151(6):825, 1994.

109. Marsh L and others: Medial temporal lobe structure in schizophrenia: relationship of size to duration of illness, *Schizophr Bull* 11(3):225, 1994.

110. Matsubara S and others: Dopamine D-1, D-2, and serotonin-2 receptor occupation by typical and atypical antipsychotic drugs in vivo, *J Pharm Exp Ther* 265(2):498, 1993.

111. Matthysse SW: The role of dopamine in schizophrenia. In Usdin E, Hamburg DA, Barchas J, editors: *Neuroregulators and psychiatric disorders*, New York, 1977, Oxford University Press.

112. McGeer PL, McGeer EG: Amino acid neurotransmitters. In Siegal GJ and others, editors: *Basic neurochemistry*, New York, 1989, Raven Press.

113. McManus DQ and others: Quetiapine, a novel antipsychotic: experience in elderly patients with psychotic disorders, *J Clin Psychiatry* 60(5):292, 1999.

114. Mehtonen OP, Aranko K, Malkonen L, Vapaatalo H: A survey of sudden death associated with the use of antipsychotic or antidepressant drugs: 49 cases in Finland, *Acta Psychiatr Scand* 84(1):58, 1991.

115. Meltzer HY: Duration of a clozapine trial in neuroleptic-resistant schizophrenia, *Arch Gen Psychiatry* 46:672, 1989.

116. Meltzer HY: New drugs for the treatment of schizophrenia, *Psychiatr Clin North Am* 16(2):365, 1993.

117. Meltzer HY and others: Age at onset and gender of schizophrenic patients in relation to neuroleptic resistance, *Am J Psychiatry* 154(4):475, 1997.

118. Migler BM, Warawa EJ, Malick JB: Seroquel: behavioral effects in conventional and novel tests for atypical antipsychotic drugs, *Psychopharmacology* 112:229, 1993.

119. Mok H, Yatham LN: Response to clozapine as a predictor of risperidone response in schizophrenia (letter), *Am J Psychiatry* 151(9):1393, 1994.

120. Ohmori T, Ito K, Abekawa T, Koyama T: Psychotic relapse and maintenance therapy in paranoid schizophrenia: a 15 year follow up, *Eur Arch Psychiatry Clin Neurosci* 249(2): 73, 1999.

121. Olin BR: *Drugs facts and comparisons*, ed 49, St Louis, 1995, Wolters Kluwer.

122. Oyemumi LK: Does lithium have a role in the prevention and management of clozapine-induced granulocytopenia? *Pediatr Ann* 29(10):597, 1999.

123. Parsa MA, Bastani B: Quetiapine (Seroquel) in the treatment of psychosis in patients with Parkinson's disease, *J Neuropsychiatry Clin Neurosci* 10:216, 1998.

124. Pelonero AL, Levenson JL, Pandurangi AK: Neuroleptic malignant syndrome: a review, *Psychiatr Serv* 49(9):1163, 1998.

125. Peusken J, Link CGG: A comparison of quetiapine and chlorpromazine in the treatment of schizophrenia, *Acta Psychiatrica Scand* 96:265, 1997.

126. Planasky K, Johnston R: The occurrence and characteristics of suicidal preoccupation and acts in schizophrenia, *Acta Psychiatr Scand* 47:473, 1971.

127. Regier DA and others: The de facto U.S. mental and addictive disorders service system: epidemiologic catchment area prospective 1-year prevalence rates of disorders and services, *Arch Gen Psychiatry* 50(2):85, 1993.

128. Remington GJ: Clinical considerations in the use of risperidone, *Can J Psychiatry* 38(3): S96, 1993.

129. Rice DP, Kelman S, Miller LS: The economic burden of mental illness, *Hosp Community Psychiatry* 43(12):1227, 1992.

130. Richards SS, Musser WS, Gershon S: *Maintenance pharmacotherapies for neuropsychiatric disorders*, Philadelphia, 1999, Brunner/Mazel.

131. Richelson E: Neuroleptic affinities for human brain receptors and their use in predicting adverse effects, *J Clin Psychiatry* 45:331, 1984.

132. Rifkin A and others: Dosage of haloperidol for schizophrenia, *Arch Gen Psychiatry* 48(2): 166, 1991.

133. Roberts GW, Leigh PN, Weinberger DR: *Neuropsychiatric disorders,* London, 1993, Wolfe.

134. Robinson D and others: Predictors of relapse following response from a first episode of schizophrenia or schizoaffective disorder, *Arch Gen Psychiatry* 56(3):241, 1999.

135. Rossi A and others: Magnetic resonance imaging findings of amygdala-anterior hippocampus shrinkage in male patients with schizophrenia, *Psychiatry Res* 2(1):43, 1994.

136. Roth BL, Ciaranello RD, Meltzer HY: Binding of typical and atypical antipsychotic agents to transiently expressed 5-HT1C receptors, *J Pharmacol Exp Ther* 260(3):1361, 1992.

137. Sachs GS: "Sanity versus vanity"—balancing the problem of weight gain and the benefits of psychotropic drugs, *Ther Adv Psychoses* July 5, 1999.

138. Safferman A and others: Update on the clinical efficacy and side effects of clozapine, *Schizophr Bull* 17(2):247, 1991.

139. Saller CF, Salama AI: Seroquel: biochemical profile of a potential atypical antipsychotic, *Psychopharmacology* 112:285, 1993.

140. Sandoz, Inc.: *Oral communication,* July 10, 1995.

141. Sedvall G: PET studies on the neuroreceptor effects of antipsychotic drugs, *Curr Approach Psychosis* 4:1, 1995.

142. Seeman P and others: Human brain D1 and D2 dopamine receptors in schizophrenia, Alzheimer's, Parkinson's and Huntington's disease, *Neuropsychopharmacology* 1(1):5, 1987.

143. Seeman P, Van Tol HH: Dopamine receptor pharmacology, *Trends Pharmacol Sci* 15(7): 264, 1994.

144. Selemon LD, Rajkowski G, Goldman-Rakic PS: Abnormally high neuronal density in the schizophrenic cortex: a morphometric analysis of prefrontal area 9 and occipital area 17, *Arch Gen Psychiatry* 52:805, 1995.

145. Shalev A, Hermesh H, Munitz H: The role of external heat load in triggering the neuroleptic malignant syndrome, *Am J Psychiatry* 145:110, 1988.

146. Sherman AD and others: Evidence of glutamatergic deficiency in schizophrenia, *Neurosci Lett* 121(1-2):77, 1991.

147. Silber C: Sertindole (Serlect), *The decade of the brain* 8(3):11, 1997.

148. Sleight AJ, Koek W, Bigg DC: Binding of antipsychotic drugs at alpha 1A- and alpha 1B-adrenoceptors: risperidone is selective for the alpha 1B-adrenoceptors, *Eur J Pharmacol* 238(2-3):407, 1993.

149. Small JG and others: Quetiapine in patients with schizophrenia, *Arch Gen Psychiatry* 54: 549, 1997.

150. Strauss J, Carpenter WT, Bartko J: The diagnosis and understanding of schizophrenia. Part III: speculation on the processes that underlie schizophrenic symptoms and signs, *Schizophr Bull* 1:61, 1974.

151. Spivak B and others: Clozapine treatment for neuroleptic-induced tardive dyskinesia, parkinsonism, and chronic akathisia in schizophrenic patients, *J Clin Psychiatry* 58(7): 318, 1997.

152. Stahl SM: What makes an antipsychotic atypical? *J Clin Psychiatry* 59(8):403, 1998.

153. Syvalahti EK: Biological factors in schizophrenia: structural and functional aspects, *Br J Psychiatry Suppl* (23):9, 1994.

154. Tandon R: Ziprasidone (Zeldox), *The decade of the brain,* 8(3):13, 1997.

155. Tesar GE: The agitated patient. Part II: pharmacologic treatment, *Hosp Community Psychiatry* 44(7):627, 1993.

156. Thompson LW: The dopamine hypothesis of schizophrenia, *Perspect Psychiatric Care* 26(3): 18, 1990.

157. Tollefson GD: Olanzapine (Zyprexa). *Decade Brain* 8(3):7, 1997.

158. Tollefson GD and others: Olanzapine verus haloperidol in the treatment of schizophrenia and schizoaffective and schizophreniform disorders: results of an international collaborative trial, *Am J Psychiatry* 154:457, 1997.

159. Torrey EF: A viral-anatomical explanation of schizophrenia, *Schizophr Bull* 17(1):15, 1991.

160. Tsai G and others: Abnormal excitatory neurotransmitter metabolism in schizophrenic brains, *Arch Gen Psychiatry* 52(10):829, 1995.

161. Tsai G and others: D-serine added to antipsychotics for the treatment of schizophrenia, *Soc Biol Psychiatry* 44(11):1081, 1998.

162. Van Putten T, Marder SR: Behavioral toxicity of antipsychotic drugs, *J Clin Psychopharmacol* 7:243, 1987.

163. Vita A and others: A reconsideration of the relationship between cerebral structural abnormalities and family history of schizophrenia, *Psychiatry Res* 3(1):41, 1994.

164. Walters VL and others: New strategies for old problems: tardive dyskinesia (TD). Review and report on severe TD cases treated with clozapine, with 12, 8 and 5 years of video follow-up, *Schizophr Res* 28(23):231, 1997.

165. Watsky EJ, Salzman C: Psychotropic drug interactions, *Hosp Community Psychiatry* 42(3): 247, 1991.

166. Weinberger DR: Implications of normal brain development for the pathogenesis of schizophrenia, *Arch Gen Psychiatry* 44:660, 1987.

167. Weinberger DR and others: Evidence of dysfunction of a prefrontal-limbic network in schizophrenia: a magnetic resonance imaging and regional cerebral blood flow study of discordant monozygotic twins, *Am J Psychiatry* 149(7):890, 1992.

168. White E, Cheung P, Silverstone T: Depot antipsychotics in bipolar affective disorder, *Int Clin Psychopharmacol* 8(2):119, 1993.

169. Wibble CG and others: Prefrontal cortex and schizophrenia: a quantitative magnetic resonance imaging study, *Arch Gen Psychiatry* 52(4):279, 1995.

170. Wilson M: DSM-III and the transformation of American psychiatry: a history, *Am J Psychiatry* 150(3):399, 1993.

171. Wirshing DA and others: Novel antipsychotics: comparison of weight gain liabilities, *J Clin Psychiatry* 60(6):358, 1999.

172. Woerner MG and others: Prospective study of tardive dyskinesia in the elderly: rates and risk factors, *Am J Psychiatry* 155(11):1521, 1998.

173. Woolley D, Shaw E: A biochemical and pharmacological suggestion about certain mental disorders, *Proc Natl Acad Sci USA* 40:228, 1954.

174. Wysowski DK, Baum C: Antipsychotic drug use in the United States: 1976-1985, *Arch Gen Psychiatry* 46(10):929, 1989.

175. Yaryura-Tobias YA, Diamond BI, Merlis S: The actions of L-dopa on schizophrenic patients (a preliminary report), *Curr Ther Res* 12:528, 1970.

CHAPTER 6

Mood Disorders

MOOD OR AFFECTIVE DISTURBANCES
Historical Considerations

Descriptions of mood disorders have been noted since ancient times. The term *melancholia* is attributed to Hippocrates, who thought the malady resulted from the influence of black bile and phlegm on the brain, which darkened the spirit. Descriptions of bipolar disorder can be traced to early in the second century, when Aretaeus of Cappadocia recognized the association between melancholia and mania. It was not until the end of the 1800s that another major contribution to our understanding of mood disorders was developed. In 1896, Kraepelin separated the functional psychoses into two groups: dementia praecox and manic-depressive psychosis. Subsequently, patients with chronic depression were included in this classification.[64] In 1917, Freud published *Mourning and Melancholia*, which described his theories of depression.[24] He noted that depression and grief had in common the process of mourning, that is, the response to the loss of a love object. He further observed that although grief was a healthy response, it differed from melancholia in that the latter involved intense expression of ambivalent, hostile feelings formerly associated with the object.

The controversy concerning endogenous (biologic) versus reactive depressions (reactions to life events) undoubtedly arose as a result of the differing viewpoints of Kraepelinians and Freudians. A large part of the existing literature assumes that the two basic forms of depression do indeed exist. However, clinical observations in the past three decades indicate that primary mood disorders are more appropriately divided into bipolar and unipolar forms. Other mood or "affective" spectrum disorders have been identified and subclassified as minor forms of mood disturbances.[1]

Epidemiology and Risk Factors

Estimates of the prevalence of mood disturbances depend on the sample of the population studied and the definition of the illness. For major depression, lifetime prevalence rates as high as 18% have been reported. The prevalence of bipolar disorder has been investigated primarily through treatment cases because it occurs less frequently. Approximately 1% of the population is affected by bipolar disorder.

Women are at greater risk than men for major depression, and age at onset is usually the late twenties. No ethnic differences are found; however, differences among social classes and familial differences have been shown. Depression is most common in lower socioeconomic groups and is likely to emerge in individuals with a positive family history of depression. Negative life events are often precipitators of a depressive disorder.

The occurrence of bipolar disorder is equal among men and women and among ethnic groups. Age at onset is typically the early twenties. This disorder is most common in higher socioeconomic groups and in some specific communities, for example, Old Order Amish. Family history is important insofar as genetic contributors are present, and often a positive family history is found among affected individuals. The relative effect of life events on the onset of an episode of mania is currently unknown.

Primary mood disorders are the psychiatric problem for which patients are most commonly admitted to hospitals. The National Institute of Mental Health (NIMH) estimates that 18 million individuals in the United States have major depression or a bipolar mood disorder at any given time at an annual cost to society of $40 billion and $30 billion dollars, respectively. Mood disturbance is also a common reason for psychiatric consultation; secondary depression or mania is often found among elderly and medically ill individuals or among substance users who are referred for consultation.

Generally, the cause and effects of mood disorders can be conceptualized as follows: disease, disability, psychosocial stressors, and genetic factors culminate in a mood disturbance—that is, depression or mania. The mood disturbance, in turn, can result in significant consequences to the individual, his or her family, and society. These sequelae include suicide, dependence on anxiolytic or sedative-hypnotic drugs, alcoholism, cognitive impairment, disability, increased rates of medical symptoms and health care utilization, and increased rates of mortality. Generally, mood disturbance increases an individual's dysfunction, suffering, and disability while diminishing the quality of life. Thus the impact of recognition and appropriate diagnosis and treatment of these conditions is considerable.

Diagnostic Considerations

Diagnostic criteria for major depression and mania (bipolar disorder) are presented in Boxes 6-1 and 6-2.

Minor forms of depression include dysthymic disorder and adjustment disorder. Mania subtypes include hypomania, mixed, and rapid cycling. These syndromes and

---

Box 6-1 Diagnostic Criteria for Major Depression

1. Five or more of the following:
   - Depressed mood*
   - Lack of pleasure or loss of interest*
   - Appetite disturbance or weight loss/gain
   - Sleep disturbance
   - Motor agitation or retardation
   - Fatigue or loss of energy
   - Guilt or worthlessness
   - Concentration difficulties or indecisiveness
   - Suicidal ideation or thoughts of death
2. Distress or impairment in social, occupational, or other areas of functioning
3. Symptoms not caused by substances or general medical conditions, or normal grief and bereavement

Modified from American Psychiatric Association: *Diagnostic and statistical manual of mental disorders-TR*, ed 4, Washington, DC, 2000, The Association.
*Must have one of these symptoms to qualify.

Box 6-2   Diagnostic Criteria for Bipolar Disorder: Mania

1. Euphoric, expansive, or irritable mood associated with social or occupational impairment
2. Three or more of the following:
   - Grandiosity
   - Decreased need for sleep
   - Pressured or hyperverbal speech
   - Flight of ideas or racing thoughts
   - Distractibility
   - Motor agitation or increased activity
   - Excessive involvement in activities
3. Not caused by a primary psychotic disorder, substances, or a general medical condition

Modified from American Psychiatric Association: *Diagnostic and statistical manual of mental disorders-TR*, ed 4, Washington, DC, 2000, The Association.

---

subtypes of depression and mania are commonly treated with pharmacotherapy. Residual categories or subsyndromal mood disturbance may also be a focus of treatment. It is recognized that a mood disturbance may be related to psychologic events, may be a component of another major psychiatric disorder, or may be associated with a seasonal pattern.[1] Some individuals with depression may meet threshold criteria for melancholia, the most severe form of depression. Melancholia is characterized by agitation, somatic or nihilistic delusions, loss of pleasure in all or almost all activities, increased depression in the morning, early morning awakening, and excessive or inappropriate guilt.

Major depression. The chief complaint of patients with major depressive disorder is usually psychologic, that is, mood disturbances, feelings of worthlessness, despair, or ideas of self-harm. However, a significant portion of depressed individuals complain of somatic disturbances combined with dysphoric mood. They may also describe themselves as being irritable, fearful, worried, or discouraged. Patients who somatize have a tendency to minimize feelings of dysphoria and focus on insomnia and anorexia (i.e., vegetative disturbances). Agitation may be so overwhelming in depressed individuals that other symptoms of mood disturbance go unnoticed. In contrast, some patients may have prominent motor retardation to the point that they become mute or even catatonic. Psychotic symptoms (e.g., suspiciousness and perceptual disturbances) may complicate a depressive episode. Delusions, hallucinations, or both may or may not be congruent with the mood disturbance per se. Depressed patients may or may not be able to identify precipitating events that have contributed to the illness. In fact, some of the "precipitators" actually may have occurred after the onset of depressive symptoms. For instance, a failed marriage may be either the cause of or the result of depression.

A variety of biologic correlates are known concomitants of depression. Some examples include reduction in slow-wave sleep, decreased rapid eye movement (REM) latency, and increased REM density. Heart rate variability and neuroendocrine disturbances (e.g., alterations in the response to dexamethasone or thyrotropin-

Table 6-1 Comparison of Dementia and Depression

Feature	Dementia	Depression
Onset	Insidious, indeterminate	Rapid, abrupt
Symptom duration	Longer	Shorter
Mood	Variable	Depressed
Cognitive deficits	Consistent	Inconsistent
Mental status assessment	Wrong answer	Refuses to attempt answer
Neurologic deficit	Aphasia, apraxia, agnosia	None

releasing factor) may also be present, but a discussion of these parameters is beyond the scope of this book (See Keltner, Folks, Palmer, and Powers, *Psychobiological Foundations of Psychiatric Care,* 1998).

Bipolar disorder. The cardinal features of mania are euphoria, hyperactivity, and disturbances of thinking and speech, for example, flight of ideas and pressured speech (see Box 6-2). Many bipolar patients are primarily irritable. Manic patients may have a mixed subtype that is a mixture of manic and depressive symptoms. Psychotic symptoms, especially persecutory and grandiose delusions, hallucinations, or ideas of reference, also complicate mania.

Suicide and other risks. There is a clear association between mood disturbance and suicide; in fact, 50% to 70% of people who commit suicide are retrospectively found to have had symptoms characteristic of depression. Of those with major depression or bipolar disorder, approximately 15% eventually die by suicide. Disregarding suicide, patients with primary mood disturbance show an increased rate of mortality when compared by age and sex with members of the general population. Alcoholism and accidents resulting from poor judgment are other risks of primary mood disorders, especially among patients with mania. The postpartum period is significant for mood disturbance, especially in women with bipolar disorder, who are likely to have episodes of depression or mania during the postpartum period.

Diagnostic dilemmas. Depressed patients may show impairment in concentration and short-term but typically not long-term memory. Sometimes, the memory impairment associated with depression mimics dementia. This condition is referred to as the *dementia syndrome of depression* or *depressive pseudodementia* (Table 6-1). Distinguishing between primary mood disturbance and grief can also be difficult (Table 6-2). Other differential diagnostic concerns include anxiety disorders, hypochondriasis or other somatoform disorders, and other major psychiatric syndromes such as schizophrenia and delirium. Syndromes involving a mood disturbance may be secondarily induced as a side effect of drugs, an effect of abused substances, or as a complication of general medical problems. Personality disorders, especially borderline, histrionic, narcissistic, or antisocial, must be considered when the patient presents with dysphoria or an irritable mood. In other words, many cases of depression will coexist with a general medical condition, a substance use disorder, or a personality disorder. Pharmacotherapy and other forms of treatment are indicated for these cases, similar to those without comorbidity.

Table 6-2 Comparison of Grief and Depression

Grief	Depression
Guilt/self-reproach	Guilt/self-reproach
Somatic symptoms	Somatic symptoms
Duration of 6 months or less	Duration of more than 6 months
Remains functional	Becomes debilitated
Usually not suicidal	Possibly suicidal

Treatment Considerations

Depression. The management of depression ideally combines an indicated medication with other appropriate interventions. Psychotherapy, including cognitive-behavioral, interpersonal, dynamic, group, or marital therapy, may contribute significantly to a positive clinical outcome. Studies have repeatedly suggested psychotherapy is more efficacious than nontreatment and that the combination of psychotherapy and antidepressant medication is more efficacious than drug treatment alone. Unfortunately, some patients will not comply with a combined approach: some refuse drug treatment, some cannot tolerate antidepressants (because of side effects), and still others do not want to "bother" with psychotherapy.

The best approach to the management of major depressive disorder is drug treatment, electroconvulsive therapy (ECT), or a combination of both. Choosing the most suitable antidepressant medication for a patient remains more of an art than a science. It is not yet clear how antidepressant medication shortens depressive episodes, and ECT may still be the most effective treatment available for major depression (see Chapter 14).

Bipolar disorder. Mania may be treated effectively with antipsychotics, mood stabilizers or alternative agents, or ECT. Of these methods, ECT is the least effective. Lithium or valproate (valproic acid [Depakene]) are the drugs of choice, but antipsychotic or anxiolytic agents may be particularly useful in active or agitated manic patients. The clinical utility of lithium, valproate, or other alternative agents such as carbamazepine (Tegretol) may be limited to the treatment of acute mania. However, growing evidence suggests that these drugs reduce morbidity; that is, they may prevent depression as well as mania.[37]

Other mood disorders. The use of drugs to treat other mood disturbances depends largely on the "target" symptoms that are present. The identification of target symptoms and a rationale for treatment are considered carefully before therapy is instituted. Individuals with dysthymic disorder, adjustment disorder with depressed mood, cyclothymia, or other subsyndromal mood disturbances may benefit greatly from drug treatment. Substantial data to support this conventional wisdom now exist and remain the subject of further studies.

ANTIDEPRESSANTS

The introduction of pharmacologic agents with antidepressant action in the 1950s revolutionized our thinking about the causes, pathogenic mechanisms, and management of depressive illness. As a consequence, many patients with depressive illness were able to function normally and lead productive lives. ECT, developed in the 1930s, remains an effective and safe modality for treatment of depressions that fail to respond to pharmacotherapy and is discussed in Chapter 14.

Before the 1950s but after the initial development of ECT, amphetamines to treat psychomotor retardation and barbiturates to treat agitation were used in patients with depression. There is little reason to use these drugs in contemporary settings. Moreover, the use of amphetamines with severe depression may actually worsen any associated agitation or psychosis.

The antidepressant actions of the monoamine oxidase inhibitors (MAOIs) were discovered serendipitously in the 1950s; these drugs were the first to have a true mood-elevating effect. Clinical pharmacologists also began to observe and correlate changes in brain chemistry with changes in mood and behavior. This in turn led to theories about the mechanisms of action of these drugs and the biologic contributors to psychiatric illness. Subsequently, in the late 1950s, the tricyclic antidepressants (TCAs) were introduced to treat depression. The TCAs were "discovered" as an outgrowth of attempts to find more effective antipsychotic drugs chemically related to the phenothiazines. The TCAs remain a viable pharmacologic treatment of depressive illness, although newer agents have been developed and are now used as first-line agents. Depending on molecular configuration, some of these newer agents are more correctly identified as bicyclic or tetracyclic. To reduce repetition, an encompassing classification, "heterocyclic," has been developed to embrace bicyclic, tricyclic, and tetracyclic antidepressants. Although these categories are not identical, it is common for all to be referred to as *tricyclic antidepressants*, or *TCAs*, in the literature. Figures 6-1 through 6-4 depict the chemical structures of many currently available antidepressants. Table 6-3 (p. 134) shows the starting dose, dosages range, suggested plasma level, half-life, metabolizing enzyme, and CYP-450 (P-450) inhibition potential of each listed antidepressant. The relative effects resulting from cholinergic, histaminergic, alpha-adrenergic, and dopaminergic blockade and reuptake inhibition of neurotransmitters are shown in Table 6-4 (p. 136). The last major group of antidepressants—the selective serotonin reuptake inhibitors (SSRIs)—were established in 1987. This class of drugs holds great promise as five are marketed in the United States at this writing. SSRIs are considered first-line agents for treating depression.

All of the antidepressant agents depicted in Figures 6-1 through 6-4 are effective in alleviating the symptoms of depressive illness. In fact, despite many clinical trials, it has not been demonstrated that one class of antidepressants is more efficacious than the others. Melancholia, including sadness and hopelessness, as well as vegetative, somatic, and motor symptoms, is responsive to drug treatment. The ability to reengage in social, occupational, and relationship functioning and to recapture quality of life is among the many benefits that may be derived from antidepressant therapy. Patients generally experience an improvement in energy level, a decrease in fatigue and psychomotor symptoms, and the disappearance of suicidal thoughts.

Neurochemical Theory of Effectiveness

Although a number of theories concerning the cause of depression have been promulgated, the efficacy of antidepressants is best understood from a neurochemical and neurobiologic perspective.[36] The biogenic amine theory of depression essentially implies that an imbalance or a relative deficiency exists of certain neurotransmitters or biogenic amines, for example, serotonin (indolamine hypothesis) and norepinephrine (catecholamine hypothesis). Specifically, deficiencies of

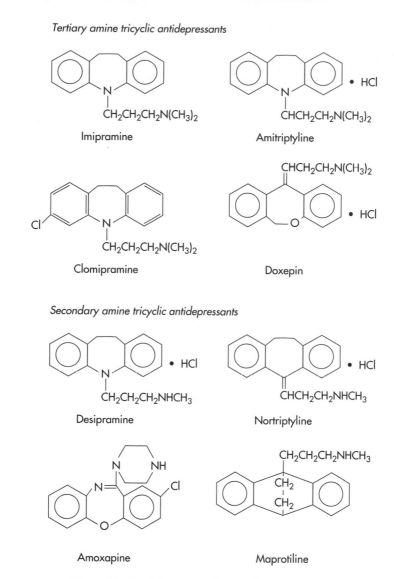

Figure 6-1 Chemical structures of heterocyclic antidepressants.

these substances result in a neurochemical imbalance. A related but slightly different view suggests alterations exist in the functioning of the receptor site or the secondary messenger systems that modulate the activity of the receptor site postsynaptically (hence the term *neuromodulator*). Neuromodulation via second messengers affects cellular enzymes, ion transport, and protein synthesis.

Psychopharmacologic treatment is based on the restoration of normality to neurotransmitter systems by doing the following:

1. Blocking neurotransmitter uptake in the presynaptic nerve ending
2. Inhibiting neurotransmitter breakdown
3. Stimulating the release of neurotransmitters

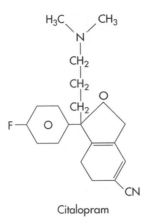

Citalopram

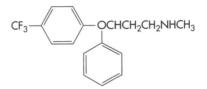

Fluoxetine

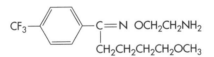

Fluvoxamine

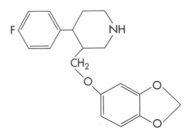

Paroxetine

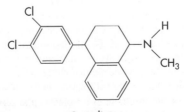

Sertraline

Figure 6-2 Chemical structures of selective serotonin reuptake inhibitor (SSRI) antidepressants.

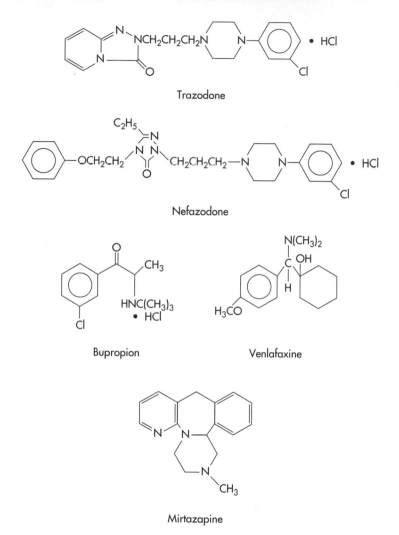

Figure 6-3 Chemical structures of atypical new-generation antidepressants.

4. Reducing stimulation at the site of the postsynaptic beta receptors (i.e., downregulation)

Point 4 merits further elaboration. The first three effects—increasing monoamine levels—occur fairly quickly, but the antidepressant effects take weeks to occur (about the same length of time for downregulation of beta receptors). Reduction of the beta-adrenergic receptor stimulation (4 in the preceding list) occurs through norepinephrine pathways or by normalizing/regulating receptor function and neurotransmission. Whether the amine-potentiating actions of antidepressants are either necessary or sufficient to account for the clinical actions of antidepressants remains uncertain. Thus considerable risk is taken when simply developing new antidepressants by screening for a chemical compound's ability to inhibit the uptake

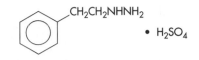

Phenelzine

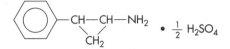

Tranylcypromine

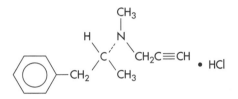

Selegiline

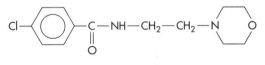

Moclobemide

Figure 6-4 Chemical structures of monoamine oxidase inhibitors.

of norepinephrine or serotonin or to otherwise alter neurochemical transmission. Nonetheless, this type of circular reasoning is tempting in view of the apparent association of these drugs' effects and the clinical response.[4]

Five new-generation agents, citalopram (Celexa), fluoxetine (Prozac), fluvoxamine (Luvox), paroxetine (Paxil), and sertraline (Zoloft), are classified as SSRIs and are widely prescribed for patients with depression, anxiety, and related disorders (e.g., bulimia, premenstrual dysphoria, and pain). Clomipramine (Anafranil), a TCA, possesses beneficial effects in the treatment of depressive as well as obsessive-compulsive disorder (OCD) by blocking the reuptake of both norepinephrine and serotonin. Other TCAs are primarily indicated for depression. A newer agent, venlafaxine (Effexor), also significantly inhibits both serotonin and norepinephrine reuptake (at higher dosages) and is indicated for depression and generalized anxiety. Furthermore, some effective antidepressants neither primarily block the uptake of monoamines nor inhibit monoamine oxidase but probably exert subtle influences on neuronal processes; nefazodone (Serzone) and mirtazapine (Remeron)

Text continued on p. 138

Table 6-3 Antidepressant Doses Half-Life and CYP-450 Effects and Metabolism

Drug dose	Starting (mg)	Therapeutic dose range (mg)	Comparable dose (mg)	Suggested plasma levels (ng/ml)	Elimination half-life (hr)	CYP-450 metabolizing enzymes (hr)	CYP-450 inhibition
SSRIs							
Citalopram (Celexa)	20	10-60	10		35 (mean)	3A4,2C19	1A2,2D6,2C19
Fluoxetine (Prozac)	20	10-80	10		48-216	2D6,3A4,2C	1A2,2D6,3A4,2C
Fluvoxamine (Luvox)	50	50-300	50		15-19	3A4	1A2,2D6,3A4,2C
Paroxetine (Paxil)	20	10-60	10		21 (mean)	2D6	1A2,2D6,3A4,2C
Sertraline (Zoloft)	50	50-200	25		26 (parent) 98 (metabolite)	2D6,3A4	1A2,2D6,3A4,2C
Atypical new generation							
Bupropion (Wellbutrin)	150	225-450	200	75-350	8-15 (parent) 20-27 (metabolites)	2D6,3A4	
Bupropion SR (Wellbutrin SR, Zyban)		150-300mg					
Venlafaxine (Effexor)	37.5	75-225	50		3-7 (parent) 9-11 (metabolite) 9-12 (absorption half-life)	2D6,3A4,2E 3A4	1A2,2D6 3A4,2C
Venlafaxine XR (Effexor XR)							

					2-4 (parent) 3-18 (metabolites)	2D5,3A4	1A2,2D6,3A4
Nefazodone (Serzone)	200	150-600	100				
Trazodone (Desyrel)	150	150-600	100		4-9	1A2, 2D6,3A4	2D6
Mirtazapine (Remeron)	15-45	7.5			35		None known
Nonselective cyclic agents							
Tricyclic							
Amitriptyline (Elavil)	25-50	75-300	50	250-285	31-46	1A2,2D6,3A4, 2C	2D6
Clomipramine (Anafranil)	25-50	75-300	50	300-1000	17-37	1A2,2D6,3A4, 2C	2D6
Desipramine (Norpramin)	25-50	75-300	50	400-1000	12-24	1A2,2D6[r]	2D6
Doxepin (Sinequan, Triadapin)	25-50	75-300	50	500-950	8-24	1A2	—
Imipramine (Tofranil)	25-50	75-300	50	500-800	11-25	1A2,2D6, 3A4,2C	2D6
Nortriptyline (Aventyl, Pamelor)	10-25	40-200	25	150-500	18-44	2D6	2D6,3A4,2C
Protriptyline (Triptil, Vivactil)	10-20	20-60	15	350-700	67-89	—	
Trimipramine (Surmontil)	25-50	75-300	50	500-800	7-30	1A2,2D6	

Table 6-4 Effects of Antidepressants on Neurotransmitters/Receptors*

	Amitriptyline	Clomipramine	Desipramine	Doxepin	Imipramine	Nortriptyline	Protriptyline	Trimipramine	Amoxapine	Maprotiline
NE uptake	++	++	++++	++	++	+++	++++	+	+++	+++
5HT reuptake	++	++++	+	++	++	++	++	+	++	+
DA reuptake	+	+	+	+	+	+	+	+	+	+
Blockade 5HT$_1$	++	+	+	++	+	+	+	+	++	+
Blockade 5HT$_2$	++	++	++	++	++	++	++	++	+++++	++
Blockade ACh	++	++	++	++	++	++	++	++	++	++
Blockade H$_1$	+++	++	++	++++	++	++	++	++++	++	+++
Blockade α_1	++	++	++	++	++	++	++	++	++	++
Blockade α_2	+	+	+	+	+	+	+	+	+	+
Blockade D$_2$	+	+		+	+	+	+	+	+	+
Selective	NE > 5HT	NE < 5HT	NE > 5HT	NE > 5HT	NE > 5HT	NE > 5HT	NE > 5HT	NE > 5HT	NE > 5HT	NE > 5HT

	Trazodone	Nefazodone	Bupropion	Venlafaxine	Citalopram	Fluoxetine	Fluvoxamine	Paroxetine	Sertraline	Mirtazapine
NE uptake	+	++	+	++	+	++	++	++	++	+
5HT reuptake	++	++	+−	+++	+++	+++	+++	++++	+++	+
DA reuptake	+−	+	++	+	+−	+	+	+	+−	−
Blockade $5HT_1$	+++	+++	+	+	+	+	+	+	+	−
Blockade $5HT_2$	+++	+++	+	+	+	++	+	+	+	+++
Blockade ACh	−	+	+	−	−	+	+	++	++	++
Blockade H_1	++	+−	+	−	+−	+	−	+−	+−	++++
Blockade α_2	+++	+++	+	−	+	+	+	+	++	+++
Blockade α_2	++	++	+−	+−	+−	+−	+	+	+	++
Blockade D_2	+	++	−	−	+−	+	+−	+−	+−	+
Selective	NE <5HT	NE <5HT	NE >5HT	NE <5HT	NE <5HT	NE <5HT	NE <5HT	NE <5HT	NE <5HT	−

Adapted from Seeman P: Receptor Tables vol 2: *Drug dissociation constants for neuroreceptors and transporters*, Toronto, 1993, SZ Research; and Richelson E: Synaptic effects of antidepressants, *J Clin Psychopharmacol* 16 (suppl 2)3: 1, 1996.

−, K_1 (nM) >100,000; +−, 10,000-100,000; +, 1000-10,000; ++, 100-1000; +++, 10-100; ++++, 1-10; +−, 0.1-1; >, $1/K_1$ (M) <0.001; +−, 0.001-0.01; +, 0.01-0.1; ++, 0.1-1; +++, 1-10; +++, 10-100; ++++, 100-1000.

NE, Norepinephrine; DA, dopamine; Ach, acetylcholine.

*The ratio of K_1 values (intrinsic dissociation constant) between various neurotransmitters/receptors determines the pharmacologic profile for any one drug.

are good examples of these drugs. Bupropion (Wellbutrin) is a novel agent that inhibits reuptake of dopamine and norepinephrine. Bupropion is also prescribed for smoking cessation (i.e., Zyban). Norepinephrine reuptake inhibitors (selective) are emerging as a new class of antidepressant and will likely be used for depression, anxiety, and attention deficit disorder. Thus it would seem that antidepressants with similar actions on neurotransmitters may be selectively beneficial for dissimilar disorders and that antidepressants with dissimilar actions on neurotransmitters may be selectively beneficial for similar disorders.

Although the influence of monoamines is the most studied neurochemical aspect of mood disorders, other important receptor interactions are useful in predicting clinical side effects and potential toxic effects (see Table 6-4). These effects account for nontherapeutic actions of antidepressants. Variable effects in blocking the reuptake of norepinephrine and serotonin and other effects undoubtedly account for some of the variability in side effect profiles as well as therapeutic effects.

TRICYCLIC AND HETEROCYCLIC ANTIDEPRESSANTS
Pharmacokinetics

The tricyclic and heterocyclic antidepressants are well absorbed from the gastrointestinal tract and are usually given orally. On average, their mean half-life is about 24 hours. Imipramine and amitriptyline are available in parenteral forms; clomipramine may be given intravenously. Antidepressant compounds are metabolized in the liver and some metabolites have active antidepressant effects and are marketed as such. For example, desipramine is a metabolite of imipramine; nortriptyline is a metabolite of amitriptyline.

Peak plasma concentrations of antidepressants are generally reached in 3 to 4 hours. These compounds are water soluble and are highly bound to plasma proteins (approximately 95%). Their effects are caused by a small fraction of free drug; thus even a small increase in free drug is potentially significant. Individuals with diminished liver function, decreased plasma proteins, and decreased total body water are particularly at risk for elevated serum levels. Antidepressant compounds are relatively lipophilic but are avidly bound to tissue and plasma proteins, making it virtually impossible to remove these agents by hemodialysis and thereby adding to the danger of acute overdoses.

The ratio of parent tertiary compound to the active secondary amine products varies markedly among patients by as much as fiftyfold.[4] The older TCAs, such as imipramine and amitriptyline, are tertiary amines and produce active metabolites, that is, the secondary amines desipramine and nortriptyline, respectively. Assays of antidepressant compounds may not be reliable, but such measurements do help confirm patient compliance with medication regimens and may be useful in evaluating unexpected or untoward clinical outcomes. Serum levels of imipramine, clomipramine, desipramine, and nortriptyline are reliable for determining therapeutic dosages.

Tolerance to many of the side effects of heterocyclic and other antidepressant compounds (e.g., sedation and the autonomic effects) is usual. Occasional symptoms suggestive of physical dependence have been reported, especially after a discontinuation of the drug, and a withdrawal or "discontinuation" syndrome consisting of malaise, chills, coryza, and muscle ache has been described. Therefore gradual withdrawal is considered a reasonable and standard practice. These compounds are eliminated in a manner similar to that of antipsychotic compounds.

The individual and structural characteristics and pharmacologic properties of the antidepressant medications are shown in Figures 6-1 through 6-4 and Tables 6-3 and 6-4.

Side Effects

Patients for whom TCAs are prescribed have both peripheral and central nervous system side effects.

Peripheral nervous system effects. Peripheral nervous system (PNS) side effects include anticholinergic effects on the peripheral autonomic nervous system, which often affect patient tolerance and may also affect compliance; anticholinergic effects include dry mouth and visual disturbances (e.g., blurred vision and photosensitivity resulting from mydriasis). These symptoms are more annoying than dangerous; however, the mydriatic action of the tricyclics can precipitate an acute attack of glaucoma. Moreover, TCAs should not be prescribed for individuals with narrow-angle glaucoma. Other anticholinergic side effects include slowing of the gastrointestinal tract, which can lead to constipation, and slowing of bladder function, which can bring about hesitancy or urinary retention. Elderly individuals are most susceptible to these side effects (see Chapter 21).

Anticholinergic effects on the cardiovascular system are common enough to warrant some consideration. Furthermore, inhibition of the sodium-potassium pump can affect cardiac conduction. Tachycardia, reflex tachycardia, and arrhythmias can lead to myocardial infarction, heart block, or both. Essentially, the potential reduction in cardiac conduction time is of greater concern than is the potential for inducing arrhythmias, except in patients who have a preexisting arrhythmia or bundle branch block. The TCAs possess a quinidine-like effect and may actually prove to be beneficial for patients with arrhythmia. In any event, patients with a history of cardiac problems should be evaluated carefully and closely monitored when receiving treatment with a TCA.

Patients with a corrected QT interval of 500 msec or more or a QRS complex 100 msec or greater are at more significant risk for adverse effects. The secondary amine TCA nortriptyline has gained some favor in the treatment of persons with cardiac conditions because of its ability to be monitored by means of serum level determinations and because of its relatively favorable profile with respect to the potential for causing orthostasis and other hemodynamic instabilities. Newer agents are much less likely to result in cardiovascular side effects. Alpha-adrenergic antagonism is responsible for orthostatic hypotension. Orthostasis can be very disabling and accounts for a significant percentage of noncompliance.

Central nervous system effects. A number of effects on the central nervous system (CNS) have been reported with the TCAs. Sedation (histamine blockade) is common but sometimes represents a "fringe therapeutic benefit," because insomnia often accompanies depression. Less pleasant CNS effects include confusion, disorientation, delusions, agitation, and hallucinations. These neuropsychiatric side effects are probably caused by CNS anticholinergic effects and may be found in as many as 5% to 15% of patients.[39] These CNS effects are more likely to occur when serum TCA levels are elevated. Other potential CNS effects include anxiety, insomnia, nightmares, ataxia, and tremors and are related to monoamine reuptake inhibition. Some patients report nightmares so terrifying that they avoid sleep even though they are sleep deprived. If TCAs are withdrawn abruptly, anticholinergic rebound can occur.

Treatment Implications

Therapeutic versus toxic levels. TCAs do not produce euphoria and are nonaddictive, so their potential for abuse is minimal. However, overdose of these agents is a real issue. When they were widely prescribed in the 1980s, TCA overdose accounted for 25% to 50% of all hospital admissions for psychotropic overdose.[29] Today they account for 7% of all deaths from intentional overdose.[71] The difference is slight between a therapeutic dose and a health-impairing or lethal dose; as little as a 1 week's supply can be fatal. TCA serum levels may be monitored, and acceptable therapeutic plasma values for some agents are shown in Table 6-5. Toxic blood levels may result in sedation, ataxia, agitation, stupor, coma, respiratory depression, convulsions, and exaggeration of the side effects previously mentioned. Cardiovascular events may occur suddenly and cause acute heart failure or sudden death. The onset of cardiotoxic effect may also be delayed; that is, it can occur after recovery from an acute overdose. For these reasons, all TCA overdoses should be considered serious; patients should be admitted to a hospital for monitoring.

TCAs (and possibly other antidepressants) have a paradoxic effect. Although they are effective antidepressants, they may energize suicidal patients. Apparently, as TCAs begin to exert their antidepressant effect, patients who otherwise might be too depressed to act on suicidal thoughts slowly begin to accrue the energy to act in self-destructive ways. Because of the potential lethality of TCAs, it is common for outpatients to be restricted to a 7-day supply when suicide is a risk. Inpatients should be watched for hoarding. Interventions for TCA overdose are given in the Drug Profiles section, under Amitriptyline.

Use in pregnancy. Depressive symptoms such as loss of appetite can interfere with fetal development by preventing adequate fetal weight gain. During pregnancy, TCAs with low anticholinergic effects, such as nortriptyline and desipramine, are preferred to those with high anticholinergic effects. The TCAs must be tapered off before delivery to prevent transient perinatal toxicity.[14] Although no data exist to suggest teratogenicity, TCAs are best avoided during pregnancy. A detailed discussion for antidepressant use in general is found later in this chapter.

Use in the elderly. There are numerous concerns when prescribing TCAs and heterocyclics for elderly patients. Because TCAs are primarily metabolized by the

---

Table 6-5 Tricyclic Antidepressant Blood Levels

Drug	Range (ng/ml)	Relationship
Imipramine and desipramine (combined levels)	150-250	Linear
Desipramine*	150-250	Linear; plateau above 250 ng/ml
	100-155	? Therapeutic window
Amitriptyline and nortriptyline* (combined levels)	100-250	Linear; ? therapeutic window
Nortriptyline*	50-140	Curvilinear; therapeutic window
Protriptyline	80-240	Linear; ? therapeutic window
Doxepin and desmethyldoxepin	120-250	Linear; ? therapeutic window
Maprotiline	150-250	Linear

*The only confirmed tricyclic antidepressants with a therapeutic window.

P-450 system and because this system is significantly reduced by aging, a greatly reduced dosage of these drugs is important. Furthermore, a general reduction in receptors can also cause a more intense reaction to TCAs. In particular, greater sensitivity to alpha-adrenergic blockade makes elderly individuals more likely to experience orthostasis and more prone to falls and fall-related injuries. In a like manner, older patients are more susceptible to anticholinergic effects and experience both PNS and CNS effects. A detailed discussion is provided in Chapter 21.

Side effect interventions. As noted previously, TCAs can cause both CNS and PNS side effects. Although some are simply annoying, others are significant, even dangerous, and warrant clinical attention. A common CNS effect is sedation. Sedation can be beneficial for a depressed patient with insomnia; for example, amitriptyline (Elavil) may be ordered to take advantage of its sedating properties. In other situations, when a patient must continue to work, sedation presents an array of problems, from dozing off at work to impairment of driving. This example underscores the need for individual consideration when prescribing TCAs.

Interactions. TCAs are primarily metabolized by the P-450 isoenzymes 2D6, 1A2, and 3A4. TCAs may compete for these isoenzymes, causing interactions in a couple of directions. Hence several serious drug interactions may occur with TCAs. These interactions can be categorized as CNS depression, cardiovascular and hypertensive interactions, and additive anticholinergic effects.

Central nervous system depression. When taken with drugs such as the antipsychotics, benzodiazepines, sedatives, antiepileptics, alcohol, and some antihypertensives (e.g., beta-blockers, clonidine, and reserpine), TCAs can increase CNS depression.

Cardiovascular and hypertensive effects. Cardiovascular arrhythmias or hypertension can occur when sympathomimetic drugs that increase norepinephrine levels in the synaptic cleft are given with TCAs. Interactants to avoid include norepinephrine, dopamine, ephedrine, and phenylpropanolamine. The latter is a major component of over-the-counter (OTC) weight-loss stimulants. MAOIs, another class of antidepressants, must also be avoided for similar reasons. The MAOI-TCA combination, although perhaps not as lethal as once thought, can cause a severe reaction, including high fever, seizures, and a fatal hypertensive crisis. Because MAOIs are not typically prescribed unless TCAs fail, care should be taken when switching the TCA-resistant patient to MAOIs. A minimum of 14 days should occur between the time TCAs are discontinued and the time MAOIs are given. TCAs block the release of several antihypertensives (e.g., clonidine) from presynaptic cells, thus contributing to the failure of some antihypertensives to control hypertension. TCAs, when combined with some SSRIs (discussed later in this chapter), may also become toxic as their metabolism is slowed through SSRI-mediated P-450 isoenzyme inhibition.

Additive anticholinergic effects. An "atropine-poisoning" effect can occur when TCAs are mixed with other anticholinergic drugs. Especially troublesome drugs include antipsychotic drugs, atropine, scopolamine, anticholinergic-antiparkinson drugs, and antihistamines. Elderly persons are at particular risk for this interaction, and all the central and peripheral anticholinergic effects mentioned in the side effects section can be intensified.

Patient education. In addition to discussion related to side effects, the following areas of education are worth discussing with the patient and his or her family:

- A "lag period" of 4 to 6 weeks occurs before full therapeutic effects are experienced.

- Certain interactants must be avoided, including OTC products (see the section on interactions).
- Patients susceptible to orthostatic hypotension should be asked to change positions slowly and to sit and dangle before arising from a reclined position.
- Abrupt discontinuation of TCAs can cause abdominal pain, anorexia, chills, sweating, diarrhea, fatigue, headache, malaise, myalgia, nausea, vomiting, weakness, and autonomic instability.
- Eye pain must be reported immediately.

SPECIFIC TRICYCLIC ANTIDEPRESSANTS
Tertiary Amines

Tricyclic antidepressants are usually divided into tertiary and secondary amine TCAs (based on their structure). The tertiary TCAs are older drugs and are relatively potent serotonin reuptake inhibitors.

Imipramine (Tofranil) is the oldest of the TCAs. Imipramine has relatively high anticholinergic and sedative effects; however, none of the newer antidepressant agents has proved to be more effective. Imipramine pamolate (Tofranil PM) is available in a single bedtime dose for adults. *Amitriptyline* (Elavil, Endep) preferentially potentiates serotonin and exerts the greatest anticholinergic and antianxiety effects among the tertiary amine TCAs. Amitriptyline is sedating and often prescribed to be taken at bedtime to enhance sleep. Amitriptyline is also available in a parenteral form and in a fixed-dose combination with the antipsychotic drug perphenazine (Triavil).

Clomipramine (Anafranil) is a TCA that has potent serotonic and norepinephrine reuptake inhibition. The parent compound preferentially potentiates serotonergic neurotransmission; this effect is the most potent among the TCAs and is comparable to the SSRIs. Therefore clomipramine is primarily indicated and used for OCD in the United States. The active metabolite of clomipramine is desmethylclomipramine, which preferentially potentiates noradrenergic neurotransmission. Thus clomipramine has a dual mechanism as a reuptake inhibitor of both norepinephrine and serotonin. Side effects of clomipramine are similar to those of other tertiary amine TCAs, especially imipramine. Sedation, anticholinergic effects, and orthostasis may limit its use. Serum levels are somewhat useful in achieving an optimal dose. Clomipramine is sometimes combined effectively with SSRIs, for example, sertraline for refractory OCD at one-fourth to one-third the usually effective dosages (see Tables 6-3 and 6-4).

Doxepin (Sinequan) is a TCA that potentiates serotonin preferentially. Doxepin is sedating, has significant anticholinergic activity, and is often touted as a drug that effectively enhances sleep and reduces anxiety. Doxepin has often been recognized as a compound well tolerated among cardiac patients; however, there is no substantial evidence to show that doxepin is superior to other tertiary (or secondary amine) TCAs.

Trimipramine (Surmontil) is a TCA that theoretically potentiates serotonin; however, this effect has not been clearly established. Trimipramine, like the other tertiary amine TCAs, is quite sedating and has moderate anticholinergic effects.

Secondary Amines

Secondary amine TCAs are represented by *desipramine* (Norpramin, Pertofrane), a TCA that potentiates norepinephrine preferentially. Desipramine is a naturally occurring metabolite of imipramine, and many clinicians have noted its utility in depressed elderly patients sensitive to anticholinergic effects and in elderly individuals with open-angle glaucoma or prostatic hypertrophy because of its lower incidence of anticholinergic effects. This drug is also considered less sedating than other tricyclics and therefore is sometimes referred to as an *activating* antidepressant agent.

Nortriptyline (Aventyl, Pamelor) is a TCA often preferred over tertiary amine compounds because it has a lower potential for sedation and anticholinergic effects. It is a natural metabolite of amitriptyline, and because of the reliability of its measured serum levels, it is often used in patients for whom toxicity or compliance is an issue.

Protriptyline (Vivactil) is different from other TCAs in that it is quite stimulating. Protriptyline may produce a greater incidence of tachycardia and cardiovascular problems than other tricyclics and certainly has a higher potential for anticholinergic side effects. Because some depressed patients have hypersomnia rather than insomnia, protriptyline enables these individuals to reduce their amount of sleepiness.

Heterocyclics

Maprotiline (Ludiomil) represents a tetracyclic antidepressant. It potentiates norepinephrine, has relatively mild potential for anticholinergic effects, and is sedating. Its neurochemical effects are similar to those of desipramine. Dosage increases are generally made more slowly than with the tertiary amine TCAs because this drug is almost twice as potent.

Amoxapine (Asendin), a secondary amine heterocyclic, is a novel compound not related to the TCAs. It is a metabolite of the antipsychotic drug loxapine and accordingly blocks dopamine receptors (D_1 and D_2). Amoxapine potentiates norepinephrine preferentially and, perhaps because of its neuroleptic effects, has a faster rate of onset of action than other antidepressants. However, extrapyramidal and other neuroleptic side effects, including tardive dyskinesia, have been reported with amoxapine related to the dopamine-blocking properties.

In addition to amoxapine and maprotiline, *trazodone* (Desyrel) represents the other heterocyclic that was introduced (in the 1980s) after the TCAs. Trazodone potentiates serotonin through $5HT_2$ receptor antagonism and is prescribed because of its virtual lack of anticholinergic effects and low potential for cardiac effects. Trazodone's absorption is increased by 20%—an unusual reaction—when it is taken with a meal. Another unique adverse reaction with trazodone is the potential for priapism (prolonged penile erection). This side effect tends to occur at higher dosages in younger men, but whether this is a dose-related response is not definitely known. Emergency or surgical intervention has been required in a small percentage of affected men. If priapism occurs, the patient should stop the medication and seek immediate medical advice.

SELECTIVE SEROTONIN REUPTAKE INHIBITORS

The SSRIs available in the United States are citalopram (Celexa), fluoxetine (Prozac), fluvoxamine (Luvox), paroxetine (Paxil), and sertraline (Zoloft). The SSRIs, as a class of antidepressants, have unique pharmacologic, therapeutic, and side effect profiles. The SSRIs are currently the first choice in antidepressant therapy with respect to market share. Generally, the SSRIs have a broad spectrum of application in depression, from the atypical to the more severely depressed. Other applications include the anxiety disorders, bipolar depression, eating disorders, and premenstrual dysphoria.[67] SSRIs are well tolerated for both long- and short-term therapy. Weight gain has been reported with paroxetine, but other SSRIs are relatively neutral with respect to weight effects. SSRIs carry a low risk of seizures and low lethality with overdose, with a relative risk of fatal overdose at one or two in a million.

Pharmacokinetics

The SSRIs differ in chemical structure, pharmacokinetics, and pharmacodynamics. They tend to be highly protein bound (80% to 98%) but have significant differences in half-lives, ranging from a few hours to 9 days or longer (when including fluoxetine's active metabolite). Steady state for fluoxetine can take up 6 to 8 weeks. These drugs are potent inhibitors of the P-450 isoenzyme system and can significantly affect the metabolism of other drugs. Fluvoxamine inhibits 1A2, 2C19, and 3A4 isoenzymes. Fluoxetine, paroxetine, fluvoxamine, and citalopram inhibit 2D6. Citalopram, fluoxetine, and paroxetine are substrates of the 2D6 isoenzymes.

Side Effects

The SSRIs lack cholinergic, histaminergic, and adrenergic adverse effects. More common side effects include gastrointestinal complaints, headache, dizziness, anxiety, agitation, insomnia, somnolence, and sexual dysfunction. Rarely, bradycardia or syndrome of inappropriate antidiuretic hormone (SIADH) may result as an idiosyncratic effect. The SSRIs differ in chemical structure, pharmacokinetics, and pharmacodynamics, resulting in subtle differences in side effects (see Figure 6-2 and Table 6-6). Patients who discontinue one SSRI because of side effects may be treated successfully with another.[9] Similarities among these agents' effects and side effects are greater than their individual differences. Less common side effects of the SSRIs include rash, lymphadenopathy, swollen joints, and other types of allergic phenomena. Dystonia and dyskinesias, including nocturnal myoclonus, have been reported. These effects usually require drug discontinuation. Serotonin syndrome, potentially fatal, can be a serious adverse effect of all SSRIs or of venlafaxine and clomipramine, especially if combined with an MAOI (including St. John's Wort). Tachycardia, confusion, malaise, and a maniclike state develop (Box 6-3). The final common pathway is very similar to neuroleptic malignant syndrome, with hyperthermia, profuse sweating, and cardiovascular collapse. This rare syndrome may develop so rapidly that patients may die before the clinician can intervene.

Sexual Dysfunction

Sexual dysfunction, that is, decreased libido, reduced sexual arousal, and impaired orgasmic function, may be associated with depression. However, the SSRIs (and venlafaxine) may interfere with sexual functioning to a greater extent than the TCAs or MAOIs. In up to one third of patients, SSRI antidepressants are estimated to either reduce libido, arousal, or orgasmic function or result in ejaculatory delay. As shown in Box 6-4, dosage reduction to the minimally effective dose, drug holiday (usually with sertraline or citalopram), or switching to bupropion, nefazodone, or mirtazapine, all of which have low incidence of sexual side effects, can be used. Agents that are useful as an antidote for antidepressant-induced sexual dysfunction include both antiserotonergic and prodopaminergic agents. Drugs that act primarily through antiserotonergic pathways include cyproheptadine, dosed at 4 to 12 mg in the evening; mirtazapine, which may be dosed at 7.5 to 15 mg; and nefazodone,

Table 6-6 Comparison of Pharmacokinetic Parameters of SSRIs and Venlafaxine

	Citalopram	Fluoxetine	Fluvoxamine	Paroxetine	Sertraline	Venlafaxine XR
% protein bound	80	95	80	95	99	27
Peak plasma level (hour)	3-4	6-8	2-8	2-8	6-8	1-2
Parent t½ (hr)	35	48-72	15-19	21	26	5
Dose range (mg/day)	10-60	10-80	50-300	10-60	50-200	75-225
Absorption altered by fast or fed status	No	No	No	No	Yes	No
Linear pharmacokinetics	Yes	No	No	Yes	No	Yes

Adapted from Preskorn SH: *Clin Pharmacokinet* 32(suppl 1):15, 1997.

Box 6-3 Serotonin Syndrome

Serotonin syndrome likely to occur if SSRI combined with the following:
- MAO inhibitors—phenelzine, tranylcypromine
- MAOI (selective)—selegiline, moclobemide
- Tryptophan (serotonin precursor)
- St. John's Wort

Signs and symptoms of serotonin syndrome (most to least frequent):
- Mental status changes, including confusion or hypomania
- Restlessness or agitation
- Myoclonus
- Hyperreflexia
- Diaphoresis
- Shivering (or shaking chills)
- Tremor
- Diarrhea, abdominal cramps, nausea
- Ataxia or incoordination
- Headaches

MAOI, Monoamine oxidase inhibitor.

Box 6-4 Management of Antidepressant-Induced Sexual Dysfunction

- Wait and observe.
- Reduce current dosage.
- Institute a drug holiday.
- Substitute drugs as necessary.
- Use adjunctive agents.

---

which may be dosed at 50 to 150 mg in the evening. In addition, buspirone, at 5 to 15 mg two to three times daily may offset sexual side effects. Prodopaminergic agents include stimulants, for example, Dexedrine at 10 to 20 mg, and methylphenidate at 5 to 10 mg, amantadine at 100 to 200 mg, bromocriptine at 2.5 mg, or bupropion at 75 to 150 mg in the morning. Viagra at 25 to 100 mg may also be used on an as-needed basis.[31] Other agents, including bethanechol and yohimbine, have been reported to be useful in reversing anorgasmia.[51,53] Interestingly, many individuals experience more robust orgasmic function while taking SSRIs (and venlafaxine), and low dosages of some SSRIs (e.g., sertraline 25 to 50 mg) have been used to treat premature ejaculation. Further discussion of antidepressant-induced sexual dysfunction can be found in Chapter 13.

Treatment Implications

Therapeutic versus toxic levels. SSRIs have a low potential for overdose. Even high dosages have not resulted in fatalities. Toxic symptoms include nausea, vomiting, tremor, myoclonus, and irritability. Treatment is symptomatic and supportive.

Use in pregnancy. SSRIs are pregnancy category B drugs, indicating risks to the fetus have not been established. Nonetheless, it is believed that these drugs should be avoided during the first trimester as a prudent precaution. The long half-lives of fluoxetine and sertraline could also be significant factors in treating the pregnant patient. A general discussion of treating depression during pregnancy is found later in this chapter.

Use in the elderly. SSRIs are safe for use in the elderly because of their side effect profile. As with most medications, SSRI dosage should be reduced in the elderly. Their potential for weight loss warrants close monitoring in elderly patients. The half-life of paroxetine increases two to three times in the elderly; thus appropriate precautions are important.

Interactions. The effect of SSRIs on hepatic isoenzymes represents an important clinical characteristic. SSRIs can variably inhibit specific cytochrome P-450 isoenzymes. The inhibition is competitive and reversible and depends on the affinity of the SSRI and its concentration in relation to another substrate, for example, another drug. Therefore drug interaction may occur, resulting in significant elevations in drug concentrations and reduction in drug clearance.[46] Toxic effects of a variety of coadministered drugs can occur (Box 6-5). For example, coadministration of the SSRIs with the TCAs may result in potentially toxic blood levels, with as much as a tenfold increase in plasma levels.[46] The extent and duration of effect on drug metabolism will depend on the potency of cytochrome P-450 inhibition, the half-life of the drug, and its dose and duration of administration. The short to intermediate half-life agents, relative to fluoxetine, are less active inhibitors of metabolism of a coadministered drug; fluoxetine's influence may persist for 4 to 6 weeks after it is stopped. Thus switching from fluoxetine to a TCA (or an MAOI) may result initially in adverse or toxic effects or lead to a modest overdose of the TCA. Because of its long half-life, fluoxetine has the potential to interact with MAOIs for as long as 4 to 6 weeks after its discontinuation. Therefore the use of MAOIs during that interval after discontinuation or concomitantly is strictly forbidden. SSRIs should be used cautiously with CNS-active drugs. SSRIs, other than citalopram and fluvoxamine, are highly bound to plasma proteins, and combining these drugs with another tightly bound drug could cause a displacement in one or the other.

Patient education. Patients and their families should be instructed as follows concerning SSRIs:
- Although it is not clear that combining alcohol or OTC medications with SSRIs is harmful, the patient should be cautioned against use of alcohol and encouraged to discuss such decisions with the prescriber. An exception to OTC drugs is dextromethorphan, an agent found in cough syrup. This combination could trigger the serotonin syndrome.
- When sedation results from SSRIs, driving or operating hazardous machinery should be avoided.

Box 6-5 Drugs Metabolized by CYP Enzymes

CYP 1A2
Antidepressants: amitriptyline, clomipramine, imipramine
Antipsychotics: clozapine
Beta-blockers: propranolol, theophylline, R-warfarin

CYP 2C9/10
Phenytoin, S-warfarin, tolbutamide

CYP 2C19
Antidepressants: citalopram, clomipramine, imipramine
Barbiturates: hexobarbital, mephobarbital, s-mephenytoin
Benzodiazepines: diazepam
Beta-blockers: propranolol

CYP 2D6
Antiarrhythmics: encainide, flecainide, mexiletine, propafenone
Antipsychotics: haloperidol, perphenazine, risperidone, thioridazine
Beta-blockers: alprenolol, bufarolol, metoprolol, propranolol, timolol
Miscellaneous: debrisoquin, 4-hydroamphetamine, perhexiline, phenformin,
   sparteine
Opiates: codeine, dextromethorphan, ethylmorphine
SSRIs: fluoxetine, *N*-desmethylcitalopram, paroxetine
TCAs: amitriptyline, clomipramine, desipramine, imipramine, des-
   methyclomipramine, nortriptyline, trimipramine
Other antidepressants: venlafaxine, the mCPP metabolite of nefazodone and
   trazodone

CYP 3A3/4
Analgesics: acetaminophen, alfentanil, codeine, dextromethorphan
Antiarrhythmics: amiodarone, disopyramide, lidocaine, propafenone,
   quinidine
Anticonvulsants: carbamazepine, ethosuximide

SSRIs, Selective serotonin reuptake inhibitors; *TCAs,* tricyclic antidepressants.

- Pregnancy or breast-feeding should be discussed with the primary health care provider because the effects of SSRIs during these developmental stages are of concern. A discussion of antidepressant therapy and pregnancy is found later in this chapter.

Treatment Issues

The possibility of adverse effects upon discontinuation of a TCA is well documented.[50] Recent reports have described apparent discontinuation-emergent signs and symptoms occurring upon cessation of SSRI treatment. Symptoms are similar to those observed earlier with TCAs, including dizziness, headache, nausea, vomiting, diarrhea, movement disorders, insomnia, irritability, visual disturbance, lethargy, anorexia, tremor, electric shock sensations, and lowered mood.[50] The risk for these events appears to be related to drug half-life; thus fluoxetine, with its long half-life, is associated with fewer discontinuation-emergent adverse events than are shorter-acting agents such as fluvoxamine and paroxetine. The implication of SSRI "discontinuation syndrome" is to taper SSRIs over a minimum of 1 to 2 months, especially those with shorter half-lives (less than 60 hours). Unfortunately, noncompliance or forgetfulness, abrupt termination of treatment, scheduled drug holidays, rapid tapering of a dose of an SSRI (or a TCA such as clomipramine) may all contribute to the symptoms associated with discontinuation syndrome. In addition to short half-life of the drug and its active metabolites, the potency of the reuptake inhibition and anticholinergic properties may also contribute to these signs and symptoms, as shown in Box 6-3. The relative risk of SSRI withdrawal syndrome has been reported to be 30.8% with clomipramine, 20% with paroxetine, 14% with fluvoxamine, 2.2% with sertraline (and presumably citalopram), and 0% with fluoxetine.[16]

Long-term therapy with SSRIs, as well as with other antidepressants, needs to be continued for at least 4 to 6 months after recovery from an acute episode. Many patients will need maintenance treatment for a year or longer depending on the severity and course of their illnesses and their history or family histories. Long-term therapy is often compromised by poor patient compliance. Issues affecting patient compliance with SSRIs include drug interactions, sustained adverse effects such as gastrointestinal or sexual side effects (as previously discussed), and weight gain. Weight decreases with short-term SSRI treatment may be followed by increases as an individual's depression improves and improvement in appetite occurs with treatment success. Citalopram has been associated with minimal weight gain in longitudinal studies up to 12 months. The relative percentage of patients with a 7% or greater weight gain after 6 months include fluoxetine (6.8% of patients), sertraline (4.2% of patients), and paroxetine (25.5% of patients). Thus paroxetine may possess greater risk of weight gain with longitudinal therapy.

VENLAFAXINE

Venlafaxine (Effexor) is a structurally novel antidepressant (see Figure 6-3) that causes clinically significant inhibition of serotonin and norepinephrine reuptake. It is also a weak inhibitor of dopamine reuptake at higher dosages. It is unique, promoting rapid onset of noradrenergic subsensitivity and acts as an atypical serotonin reuptake inhibitor (see Table 6-4). Venlafaxine has no impact on alpha-adrenergic, histaminergic, or cholinergic receptors.[17]

Venlafaxine is absorbed rapidly and is 98% bioavailable (see Table 6-6). Food delays absorption but does not change the overall absorption. Half-life and protein binding are shorter and lower respectively. It is metabolized to O-desmethylvenlafaxine, which possesses similar biochemical and clinical properties to venlafaxine and has a half-life of about 11 hours.

Because venlafaxine lacks affinity for histaminergic, cholinergic, and alpha-adrenergic receptors, common side effects associated with TCAs do not occur. The most common side effect is nausea, which may be severe and persistent. However, most patients build tolerance over a few weeks. An extended-release version of venlafaxine has reduced the risk of adverse effects caused by fluctuations in plasma levels and has allowed once-daily dosing. Common side effects include somnolence, dry mouth, dizziness, constipation, nervousness, sweating, and anorexia. Elevation in blood pressure in some patients (approximately 2% to 5%) has occurred with large doses, for example, 225 mg or greater; hence patients should be monitored and screened before starting this drug. Venlafaxine is not a potent inhibitor of cytochrome P-450 enzymes. This property, together with low protein binding, reduces the potential for drug interaction. Venlafaxine has little effect on lithium, benzodiazepines, or ethanol and is unlikely, in contrast to fluvoxamine, fluoxetine, and paroxetine (or nefazodone), to interfere with hepatic isoenzymes.

Venlafaxine is reported to have a more rapid onset of action once therapeutic dosages are achieved.[28,40] However, overall efficacy rates are similar to those of other antidepressants. Venlafaxine is effective in a broad range of depressive illnesses but is especially useful in the more treatment-resistant, chronically depressed patients; hence melancholia, bipolar depression, depression with attention deficit hyperactivity disorder (ADHD), depression in the medically ill, and depression with general symptoms of anxiety are most appropriate for venlafaxine.[36] As previously mentioned, venlafaxine does not have as great a potential for drug interactions as some of the SSRIs, but the associated side effects are similar to those of the SSRIs. Other side effects, at dosages of 75 and 150 mg or greater, most likely stem from its noradrenergic properties.

BUPROPION

Bupropion (Wellbutrin) is a novel antidepressant agent that is not a TCA, an SSRI, or an MAOI (see Figure 6-3). Bupropion's exact mechanism of action is thought to result from norepinephrine and dopamine reuptake inhibition or enhancement (see Table 6-4).[2] Clinical tests indicate that orthostatic hypotension, cardiovascular conduction problems, anticholinergic effects, daytime sedation, and other typical effects of TCAs are not seen with this compound. However, bupropion is "activating," and agitation is sometimes produced. Bupropion is prescribed as a second-line agent in cases of treatment-resistant depression because of its novel mechanism of action. Bupropion is quite useful in bipolar depression and in patients with comorbid ADHD. Bupropion is contraindicated in patients with seizure disorders and not recommended for patients with diagnosis of either bulimia or anorexia. As discussed in Chapter 12, bupropion (Zyban) is indicated for use in smoking cessation. Bupropion, as with the other antidepressants, should not be given in combination with the MAOIs because of the potential for drug interaction and hypertensive crisis.

Bupropion is rapidly absorbed, with a half-life of about 8 to 15 hours. Several metabolites are active.[54] A sustained-release version of bupropion has enabled once-daily or twice-a-day dosing schedules. More common side effects include agitation, insomnia, gastrointestinal upset, and headache. The incidence of sexual side effects and long-term weight gain are low with bupropion. Bupropion (as discussed) may also be prescribed as an antidote for SSRI-induced sexual dysfunction; low dosages of 75 to 150 mg are sometimes effective. Bupropion is dosed two or three times a day, with no more than 450 mg/day or 150 mg/dose, to prevent adverse effects and seizure risk. The substained-release formulation is dosed once or twice daily in most cases. Initial dosing is 75 mg twice daily or 100 to 150 mg daily (sustained release), with most patients responding to dosages of 225 to 450 mg. Elderly and debilitated patients may (or may not) require reduced dosages and should be titrated conservatively. Overdosage may result in grand mal/generalized seizures, hallucinosis, tachycardia, and signs of neurotoxicity.

NEFAZODONE

Nefazodone (Serzone) is chemically related to trazodone (see Figure 6-3) but lacks the alpha-adrenergic blockade that accounts for trazodone's orthostasis, priapism, and certain cardiovascular effects, such as risk of atrial arrhythmia (see Table 6-4). Nefazodone is also less sedating than trazodone. Nefazodone is a selective $5HT_2$ receptor antagonist and also inhibits presynaptic reuptake of serotonin and norepinephrine. Nefazodone has a pharmacologic profile that is distinct from SSRIs, TCAs, MAOIs, and venlafaxine. The potent blockade of $5HT_{2A}$ receptors is the most distinct difference between nefazodone and most other new antidepressants. Nefazodone does not significantly bind to histaminergic, cholinergic, or alpha-adrenergic receptors and therefore is not associated with TCA-like side effects.

Nefazodone is rapidly absorbed, is extensively metabolized, and has an active metabolite (see Table 6-3). It has a half-life between 2 and 4 hours. Twice-daily dosing results in a steady state within 5 days. Initial dosing is at 50 to 100 mg twice daily for the first week, with titrations in 100-mg increments occurring not more than weekly. Most patients respond with 300 to 500 mg/day. The amount of nefazodone may be increased up to 600 mg/day, but with nonlinear plasma concentrations resulting, titrations should be conservative. Elderly and debilitated patients usually (but not necessarily) require a lower dosage (approximately 150 to 300 mg). Nausea is the most common side effect, with dizziness, insomnia, headache, asthenia, and agitation occurring in a small percentage of patients.

Nefazodone has been shown to be equally efficacious compared with imipramine, sertraline, fluoxetine, and paroxetine. Significant improvements with anxiety and sleep may occur within the first 2 weeks of therapy. Nefazodone has novel effects on sleep, reducing insomnia and nighttime awakenings. Full antidepressant response occurs after several weeks, similar to other antidepressants. Tolerability is usually excellent. As a therapeutic response is achieved, dosing adjustments may allow lower dosages during the day and the majority of drug dosed at bedtime. The incidence of sexual dysfunction in men and women is comparable to that seen with placebo.

Nefazodone is metabolized by 3A3/4 and inhibits P-450 3A3/4 (see Box 6-5). Hence drugs that inhibit 3A4 (e.g., ketoconazole) may alter nefazodone metabolism, and drugs that induce 3A4 (e.g., carbamazepine) may reduce plasma levels of nefazodone. Nefazodone, through inhibition of 3A4, can also increase levels of several drugs, including cisapride. Because of its potential for cardiotoxicity, cisapride is contraindicated with nefazodone. Alprazolam and triazolam concentrations may be increased twofold to threefold, and a 50% reduction in dosage of these drugs is warranted when coadministered with nefazodone. Coadministration of an MAOI is contraindicated with nefazodone. Other drugs that may be affected include antihypertensives but not propranolol, haloperidol, or lorazepam. Nefazodone is very safe in overdosage. Symptoms include nausea, vomiting, and somnolence. Overall, nefazodone has a low incidence of side effects and lacks the sexual side effects, nervousness, and insomnia seen with the SSRIs and venlafaxine. Thus it should be considered a first-line agent for the treatment of depression.[3]

MIRTAZAPINE

Mirtazapine (Remeron) is a relatively new antidepressant, demonstrating efficacy over placebo in several clinical studies. As with many of the other atypical new-generation antidepressants, mirtazapine is devoid of side effects often observed with the classical TCAs or the second-generation SSRIs. Mirtazapine has a unique structure and mechanism of action, different from that of TCAs, SSRIs, and MAOIs, and could be best described as a noradrenergic and specific serotonergic antidepressant (see Figure 6-3 and Table 6-4). Mirtazapine is a $5HT_2$ antagonist, or blocking agent, similar to nefazodone, but is also a potent and direct alpha-2-adrenoreceptor antagonist, causing enhancement of both noradrenergic and serotonergic transmission. Its neurochemical profile is shown in Table 6-4.

Mirtazapine has no substantial affinity for dopaminergic receptors and low affinity for central and peripheral muscarinic cholinergic receptors. In contrast to TCAs, mirtazapine has a low affinity for the alpha-1-adrenoreceptor. In fact, these receptors are stimulated rather than blocked as a result of the enhancement of noradrenergic transmission by mirtazapine. Mirtazapine, despite having significant interactions with histamine receptors, is less sedating than imipramine. As the dosage of mirtazapine is increased beyond 15 mg, the noradrenergic activation and subsequent enhancement of arousal may functionally counteract the sedating consequences of its antihistaminergic properties. This concurs with a relatively low incidence of transient sedation observed in clinical studies of mirtazapine use in depressed patients.[56] Mirtazapine may promote deep sleep, similar to nefazodone, which may or may not be caused by interactions with histamine receptors. Indeed, several studies implicate serotonergic $5HT_2$ receptors, probably the $5HT_{2A}$ subtype, rather than histamine receptors in the control of deep sleep.

Mirtazapine's blockade of $5HT_2$ and $5HT_3$ receptors is also associated with anxiolytic properties; the $5HT_{2A}$ effects may account for its low potential to (1) interfere with sleep, (2) be anxiogenic as sometimes seen with the SSRIs, (3) promote sexual dysfunction, or (4) cause gastrointestinal stimulation or upset. Such side effects occur in 15% to 30% of patients treated with SSRIs, venlafaxine, and the MAO inhibitors. Mirtazapine's efficacy is comparable to other antidepressants, with double-blind controlled studies showing response rates up to 70%. As with other antidepressants, full antidepressant response may take several weeks.

The most commonly reported adverse events associated with mirtazapine are somnolence (54%), increased appetite (17%), weight gain (12%), and dizziness (7%). Because of its pharmacologic profile, mirtazapine may improve anxieties and sleep disturbances in as little as 1 to 2 weeks, with minimal effect on libido and low incidence of gastrointestinal upset. Mirtazapine presumably does not significantly inhibit P-450 enzymes (2D6, 1A2, 3A4) in vitro; formal drug interactions studies have not been conducted, and it is not possible to make definitive statements about the risks of coadministration of mirtazapine with other drugs. Mirtazapine has a long half-life of 35 hours, enabling once-daily dosing(see Table 6-3). Bedtime dosing initially at 7.5 to 15 mg is followed by titration, if necessary, after 1 to 2 weeks.[13,57] Coadministration with an MAOI or use within 14 days of initiating or discontinuing therapy with an MAOI is not recommended. Mirtazapine has rarely (2 of 2796 patients) been associated with agranulocytosis or severe neutropenia. The relative safety of mirtazapine in overdose is similar to that of nefazodone and the SSRIs.

Overall, mirtazapine represents a superb and relatively unique addition to the antidepressant armamentarium. As with nefazodone and bupropion, mirtazapine has been used as an antidote for SSRI-induced sexual dysfunction. It may be preferentially used with patients with sleep disturbance, poor appetite, or pain because of its pharmacologic profile. In addition, mirtazapine represents a reasonable choice in patients who are medically ill and taking multiple medications because of the assumption that it will not interfere with the drug metabolism of other medications.[57]

MONOAMINE OXIDASE INHIBITORS

MAOIs, another class of antidepressant, are prescribed as third-line agents after SSRIs or other new generation agents or TCAs have been tried. An argument can still be made that MAOIs are particularly effective in treating atypical depression, for example, depression characterized by mood reactivity, interpersonal hypersensitivity, hypersomnia, and compulsions (e.g., excessive eating). MAOIs may also be effective in treating certain types of anxiety syndromes, including panic, agoraphobia, social anxiety, or posttraumatic stress disorder (PTSD). The third-class status afforded the MAOIs is generally related to their potential for serious adverse reactions. Although many expert clinicians think the fear of MAOIs is unwarranted, the reluctance to use them seems to be the norm.

In general, the MAOIs can be divided into the nonselective MAOIs, phenelzine (Nardil) and tranylcypromine (Parnate), and the selective MAOIs, selegiline (Eldepryl) and moclobemide (Manerix) (see Figure 6-4 and Table 6-7). These drugs block monoamine oxidase, the major enzyme involved in the metabolic decomposition and thus the inactivation of norepinephrine, serotonin, and dopamine. The increased level of these neurotransmitters in the PNS and CNS can be dramatic. According to the biogenic amine theory of depression, depressed individuals have a deficiency of these neurotransmitters. MAOIs help restore the "normal" amount of neurotransmitters by slowing the deactivation of the monoamines. This mechanism is in contrast to mechanisms of TCAs and other agents, which achieve the normal level or restore the relative deficiency by preventing the reuptake of amines, increasing the release of amines, or directly affecting the postsynaptic receptor. Generally, a period of 10 days to 4 weeks is required for the antidepressant effects of the MAOIs to occur, but as with the other antidepressants, the physiologic action (the inhibition of monoamine oxidase) occurs rapidly. This phenomenon suggests that factors other than low levels of specific neurotransmitters are involved in the pathogenesis of depression.

Pharmacokinetics

MAOIs are well absorbed from the gastrointestinal tract and are given orally. They are metabolized in the liver, and metabolites are excreted in the urine. Table 6-7 gives the usual doses for these drugs.

Side Effects

MAOIs induce PNS and CNS side effects.

Peripheral nervous system effects. In the PNS, the slow release of norepinephrine causes decreased heart rate, decreased vasoconstriction, and hypotension. MAOIs also inhibit monoamine oxidase in the liver, which may lead to elevated levels of other drugs that are normally metabolized in the liver by a monoamine oxidase.

Hypotension is the most common nontherapeutic effect. The slowdown in the release of norepinephrine is the presumed mechanism of action of MAOIs. Unlike the TCAs, reflex tachycardia does not occur in response to orthostatic hypotension because the slowed release of norepinephrine prevents the heart rate from reflexively speeding up. Thus hypotension combined with the failure of compensatory increased heart rate may lead to heart failure in predisposed individuals. Interestingly, pargyline (Eutonyl) is an MAOI that is not used as an antidepressant but rather as an antihypertensive agent.

MAOIs may also cause anticholinergic effects such as dry mouth, blurred vision, urinary hesitancy, and constipation, although constipation occurs to a lesser extent than observed with TCAs. Hepatic and hematologic dysfunctions may rarely occur and are potentially serious. Blood cell counts and liver function tests should be obtained before therapy begins; symptoms indicating bone marrow suppression or liver dysfunction should be investigated.

Central nervous system effects. Because MAOIs increase the availability of biogenic amines in the brain, CNS hyperstimulation may also occur, causing

Table 6-7 Monoamine Oxidase Inhibitors

Drug	Class	Dosage range (mg/day)	MAOI diet	Special characteristics
Phenelzine	Nonselective	30-90	Yes	Atypical depression; anxious, phobic, obsessional patients
Tranylcypromine	Nonselective	20-60	Yes	Direct stimulant effect, often rapid onset; useful in fatigued, anergic patients
Selegiline	Selective MAO-B	5-10	No	10 mg/day or more requires dietary restriction
Moclobemide	Selective MAO-A	300-600	No	Minimal hypotension, excitation, and sexual effects; efficacy similar to that of other MAOIs but terminates more rapidly after discontinuation

MAOI, Monoamine oxidase inhibitor.

agitation, acute anxiety, restlessness, insomnia, and euphoria. Full schizophrenic episodes as a response to MAOIs may also develop in individuals with quiescent schizophrenia. Hypomania is also a common effect.

Treatment Implications

Therapeutic versus toxic levels. As with the TCAs, an intensification of the effects already discussed may occur with overdosage of MAOIs. A lethal dose of MAOIs may be achieved at only 6 to 10 times the usual daily dose. Careful monitoring should occur when medications are being ingested. As noted with the antipsychotic agents, cheeking and hoarding of these drugs could be disastrous, and these possibilities should be considered in individuals at risk. When an MAOI overdose is suspected, the following actions should be taken:
1. Emesis and gastric lavage, which are particularly helpful if performed early
2. Monitoring of vital signs
3. External cooling, which is particularly warranted when high fever occurs
4. Standard treatment of hypotension

Use in pregnancy. MAOIs should be given during pregnancy only when the anticipated benefit justifies the potential risk to the fetus and should be avoided altogether in the first trimester. A full review of antidepressant therapy during pregnancy is presented later in this chapter.

Use in the elderly. Monoamine oxidase does not appreciably decline with aging; therefore use of MAOIs does not present the same age-related risks associated with other antidepressants more dependent on the P-450 and other hepatic metabolizing enzymes. On the other hand, because of strict dietary and OTC-MAOI interactions concerns, only meticulously compliant patients should be prescribed these drugs. Deciding whether elderly depressed individuals would be able to adhere to a rigorous MAOI regimen is an important decision.

Side effect interventions. Several important side effects associated with MAOIs and appropriate interventions are listed in Box 6-6.

Interactions. MAOIs have a number of serious interactions. Potentially lethal interactions may occur with both drugs and foods and are listed in Boxes 6-7 and 6-8 and in Table 6-8. Drug and food interactions should be guarded against, particularly with compounds that have the potential to cause hypertension, anticholinergic effects, or sympathomimetic effects. Sympathomimetic drugs are classified as direct acting, indirect acting, and mixed acting, that is, having both direct and indirect properties. Indirect-acting and mixed-acting sympathomimetics may cause serious and sometimes fatal hypertension and should be avoided. Direct-acting sympathomimetics act by adding new norepinephrine to the body, whereas indirect agents release existing epinephrine or norepinephrine from the neuron. Because MAOIs increase the amount of stored norepinephrine in the peripheral nervous system, the potential for these indirect- or mixed-acting sympathomimetics to release relatively large amounts of norepinephrine makes crucial the avoidance of these interacting drugs. Even small amounts may trigger a hypertensive crisis. Typical indirect- and mixed-acting sympathomimetics include amphetamines, cocaine, methylphenidate, dopamine, and ephedrine. OTC weight-loss and stimulant products containing phenylephrine, phenylpropanolamine, and pseudoephedrine, which are mixed- or

Box 6-6 Side Effects and Interventions for MAOIs

Central nervous system hyperstimulation
Reassure the patient. Assess for developing psychosis, hypomania, or seizures. When symptoms warrant, withhold the drug and notify the physician.

Hypotension
Monitor blood pressure frequently and intervene to prevent falls and injuries; having patient lie down may help return blood pressure to normal.

Anticholinergic effects
See the teaching section for Amitriptyline drug profile in Part II for the appropriate nursing interventions.

Hepatic and hematologic dysfunction
Blood cell counts and liver function tests should be performed. When dysfunction is apparent, MAOI should be discontinued.

MAOI, Monoamine oxidase inhibitor.

Box 6-7 Contraindications with MAOIs

Sympathomimetic drugs should not be combined with MAOIs.
Tyramine-containing foods must not be ingested by the patient who is taking MAOIs.
MAOIs are contraindicated as follows:
- In the patient with a history of stroke or cardiovascular disease
- In the patient with a pheochromocytoma, a tumor that secretes pressor substance
- In the patient undergoing elective surgery (because of the hypotensive potential of combined MAOIs and anesthesia)

MAOIs should not be given in combination with the following:
- Other MAOIs
- TCAs
- Meperidine (Demerol)

Hypertensive crisis is a major concern. If it occurs, the nurse should respond as follows:
- Discontinue MAOIs and contact the physician.
- Know that therapy to reduce the blood pressure is warranted, and know that phentolamine (Regitine) 5 mg intravenously is the appropriate drug.
- Manage fever by external cooling.
- Institute supportive nursing care as indicated.

MAOIs, Monoamine oxidase inhibitors; *TCAs,* tricyclic antidepressants.

Box 6-8 Tyramine-Rich Foods to Avoid While Taking MAOIs

Alcoholic beverages
Beer and ale
Chianti and sherry wine

Dairy products
Cheese: cheddar, bleu, brie, and
    mozzarella
Sour cream
Yogurt

Fruits and vegetables
Avocados
Bananas
Fava beans
Canned figs

Meats
Bologna
Chicken liver
Fish, dried
Liver
Meat tenderizer
Pickled herring
Salami
Sausage

Other foods
Caffeinated coffee, colas, and tea (large
    amounts)
Chocolate
Licorice
Soy sauce
Yeast

MAOIs, Monoamine oxidase inhibitors.

Table 6-8 Drugs to Avoid While Taking MAOIs

Drugs	Interaction
Anticholinergic drugs	Compound anticholinergic response
Anesthetics (general)	Deepen CNS depression
Antihypertensives (diuretics, beta-blockers, hydralazine)	Compound hypotensive effect
CNS depressants	Intensify CNS depression
Meperidine	CNS depression; deaths have occurred
Guanethidine, methyldopa, reserpine	Produce severe hypertension
Sympathomimetics (mixed- and indirect-acting) Amphetamines, methylphenidate, dopamine, phenylpropanolamine (in many over-the-counter medications)	Precipitate hypertensive crisis, cardiac stimulation, arrhythmias, cerebrovascular hemorrhage
Sympathomimetics (direct-acting) Epinephrine, norepinephrine, isoproterenol	Same as for mixed- and indirect-acting sympathomimetics, but theoretically should not produce as severe a reaction
Cyclic and newer antidepressants	Same as for epinephrine, norepinephrine, isoproterenol; possibly serotonin syndrome

MAOIs, Monoamine oxidase inhibitors; *CNS,* central nervous system.

indirect-acting sympathomimetics, should be avoided altogether. Direct-acting sympathomimetics (norepinephrine, epinephrine, and isoproterenol) theoretically should not trigger the release of existing norepinephrine. As previously noted, MAOIs should not be given in combination with TCAs except in unusual refractory cases of depression, in hospitalized patients, or in patients who are closely monitored. Use with other antidepressants (SSRIs, venlafaxine, bupropion, and nefazodone) should also be avoided.

The initial symptoms of hypertensive crisis are palpitation, tightness in the chest, stiff neck, and a throbbing, radiating headache. Extremely high blood pressure with elevation of heart rate is common. Cardiovascular consequences have included myocardial infarctions, cerebral hemorrhage, myocardial ischemias, and arrhythmias. Diaphoresis and pupillary dilation are also prominent signs. Anticholinergic effects may be present to a greater extent when other anticholinergic drugs are given in concert with the MAOIs. Typical anticholinergic side effects are similar to those for TCAs.

Because MAOIs inhibit monoamine oxidase in the liver, some drugs, particularly CNS depressants, are not metabolized there; with these drugs, serum levels may be achieved more rapidly and may be high enough to seriously depress the CNS. Meperidine (Demerol) is specifically contraindicated; a marked potentiation of this drug can occur. Deaths have been attributed to this combination.

Hypotensive drugs are also potentiated by the MAOIs; hence these are relatively contraindicated.

Food-drug interactions center on the amino acid tyramine, a precursor to dopamine, norepinephrine, and epinephrine. Tyramine is found in many foods commonly consumed in a North American diet. In fact, all high-protein foods that have undergone protein breakdowns by means of aging, fermentation, pickling, or smoking should be avoided. Hypertension and hypertensive crisis can develop from these food-drug combinations by the mechanism previously discussed. General guidelines for avoiding interactions involving MAOIs include the following:

1. Sympathomimetic drugs should not be combined with MAOIs.
2. Tyramine-containing foods should not be ingested by the patient taking MAOIs.
3. MAOIs should not be given in combination with another MAOI or with a TCA except in unusual refractory patients and then under close supervision.
4. MAOIs should not be given in combination with meperidine.
5. If a hypertensive crisis is suspected, the following measures should be instituted:
   - Discontinue the MAOI.
   - Have phentolamine (Regitine) available. Phentolamine 5 mg intravenously reduces blood pressure.
   - Some clinicians recommend that their patients carry nifedipine (10 mg) to be taken sublingually for a hypertensive emergency.
   - Manage fever by external cooling.
   - Provide supportive care as indicated.

Patient education. Because combining MAOIs with a variety of interactants is a serious matter, it is important to be consistent in teaching both the patient and his or her family about these drugs (see Table 6-8 and Boxes 6-7 and 6-8). Teaching should include the following general points:
   - A "lag time" of 10 days to 4 weeks occurs before a full therapeutic effect is experienced.
   - Driving should be avoided if sedation is pronounced.

- The patient should inform all medication prescribers when he or she is taking MAOIs.
- Foods containing large amounts of tyramine should be avoided.
- Headaches, palpitations, and stiff neck may indicate hypertensive crisis and should be reported immediately.

SPECIFIC MONOAMINE OXIDASE INHIBITORS

A list of MAOIs used to treat depression is found in Figure 6-4 and Table 6-7. Phenelzine (Nardil) is the most studied and most effective MAOI in depressed individuals with atypical features on clinical examination. Phenelzine is also the most sedative MAOI. A clinical response is generally experienced or begins to be experienced in about 4 weeks. Tranylcypromine (Parnate) is the most effective MAOI for treatment of severe or endogenous depression. A clinical effect may be experienced rapidly, in about 10 days, which is faster than with the other MAOIs. Tranylcypromine is also the most stimulating MAOI. As mentioned previously, pargyline is not used as an antidepressant.

Phenelzine and tranylcypromine are irreversible, nonselective inhibitors of MAO-A and MAO-B. MAO-A is primarily serotonergic. Selective inhibition of MAO-B occurs with selegiline (used in treating Parkinson's disease) at dosages lower than 10 mg, which allows the drug to be used without dietary restriction.[69] It is metabolized to three active compounds, including amphetamine and methamphetamine, which may account for its therapeutic action. A favorable antidepressant response may occur at these smaller doses, although a more robust response occurs at larger doses of 30 to 50 mg (where the selective MAO-B inhibition is lost and dietary restrictions are needed). Patients with anergic depression and bipolar depression may be responsive to low-dose therapy at 10 to 15 mg.

Moclobemide and brofaromine, both of which are investigational drugs, known as *RIMAs*, are reversible, selective inhibitors of MAO-A (elevates serotonin). Moclobemide (Manerix, Aurorex), not available in the United States, is a reversible inhibitor of MAO-A, with antidepressant efficacy similar to that of fluoxetine.[63] Fewer adverse effects (e.g., hypotension, sexual dysfunction, or hypertensive reactions) occur with the use of moclobemide. Divided doses of 300 to 600 mg are usually therapeutic. Brofaromine is similar to moclobemide but also inhibits the reuptake of serotonin. Neither of these agents requires dietary restriction; they show promise but are still under investigation.

NOREPINEPHRINE REUPTAKE INHIBITORS

A new line of antidepressant medications is being developed with regard to the noradrenergic system. This development is occurring in the context of many newly identified adrenoreceptors: alpha-1, alpha-2A, alpha-2B, alpha-2C, beta-1, beta-2, and beta-3. The development of selective agonists and antagonists and the examination of regional expression in binding patterns to these adrenoreceptors have resulted in research on neuronal localization (presynaptic and postsynaptic). The evidence of the role of norepinephrine in depression includes the following: (1) abnormal urinary/plasma/cerebrospinal fluid MHPG (3-methoxy-4-hydroxyphenylglycol), (2) elevated beta adrenoreceptors on lymphocytes and in suicide victims, (3) decreased platelet alpha-2-adrenoreceptor binding sites for alpha-2 agonists and decreased epinephrine-induced platelet aggregation, (4) blunted growth hormone response to clonidine, (5) elevated levels of tryosine hydroxylase in the locus ceruleus of suicide victims, and (6) decreased levels of tyrosine hydroxylase in rats following chronic antidepressant administration.

With regard to the development of antidepressants that are more or less selective for norepinephrine, reboxetine (Vestra) is under development for the treatment of depression. Reboxetine is the most selective norepinephrine reuptake blocker that has been developed thus far. It may have very useful effects in depressive individuals with defects in norepinephrine function and may have utility in the treatment of major depression in both older and younger adults. Studies of reboxetine in younger adults have yielded little or no adverse effects on cognition or motor function, more rapid improvement in social functioning, and possibly greater or equal efficacy than that seen with SSRIs in severe depression (melancholia). In older or medically ill patients, reboxetine has generally been well tolerated (better than imipramine) and is safer in patients with cardiac disease. Response rates are comparable to imipramine. Side effects are usually mild to moderate in nature, with early response predicting long-term outcome.[34,42]

Initial studies of reboxetine suggest that symptoms that improve in direct relation to noradrenergic antidepressants include loss of interest, loss of pleasure, loss of energy, loss of appetite, lack of concentration, depressed mood, worthlessness, guilt, and somatic anxiety. An illustration of reboxetine with respect to its relationship to other agents, including desipramine, venlafaxine, paroxetine, and citalopram, is shown in Figure 6-5.

Reboxetine, thought to be close to receiving U.S. Food and Drug Administration (FDA) approval, has linear pharmacokinetics, is metabolized by CYP-3A4, has no active metabolites, and has a half-life of 12 to 24 hours, reaching steady state usually within 3 to 5 days. Because reboxetine has no effect on cytochrome P-450 3A4 activity at therapeutic dosages, clinically significant interactions with CYP-3A4 substrates, such as oral contraceptives, steroids, alprazolam, triazolam, nifedipine, and lidocaine, are unlikely. Certainly, inhibitors of cytochrome P-450 3A4 (erythromycin, ketoconazole, or nefazodone) may increase reboxetine plasma concentrations. Reboxetine does not potentiate the CNS effects of alcohol. However, potential for tyramine-like effect when given with an MAOI inhibitor is significant. As with other antidepressants, concomitant use of an MAOI and reboxetine should be avoided. Overall, the in vivo and in vitro studies support findings of low potential for drug interactions with reboxetine. Common side effects include dry mouth, constipation, insomnia, sweating, dizziness, nausea, urinary hesitancy, urinary

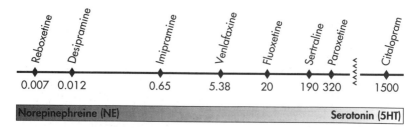

Figure 6-5 Ratio of inhibition of major selective serotonin reuptake inhibitors (SSRIs). (Data from Richelson E, Pfenning M: Blockade by antidepressants and related compounds of biogenic amine into rat brain synaptosomes: most antidepressants selectively block norepinephrine reuptake, *Eur J Pharmacol* 104:277, 1984.)

retention, and tachycardia at placebo-adjusted rates of less than 10% to 15%, with the exception of dry mouth. Increases in supine blood pressure after reboxetine administration are minimal or not clinically significant.[18] Daytime somnolence, anxiety, agitation, or nervousness also occurs in relatively low rates of less than 2% to 5%.

The starting dose of reboxetine is 4 mg twice daily with a maximum dose of 10 mg daily. Elderly patients are started on 2 mg daily, with a maximum dose of 6 mg. Other norepinephrine reuptake inhibitors, such as tamoxetine, may have additional utility in treating apathy and amotivational behavior in dementia as well as attention deficit disorder in children, adolescents, and adults. Whether reboxetine and other norepinephrine reuptake inhibitors will be available and made available in the United States remains to be seen. However, their clinical utility and potential for certain patient populations is of great interest to clinicians and psychopharmacologists alike.

TREATMENT ISSUES WITH ANTIDEPRESSANTS
Efficacy and Drug Selection Criteria

Antidepressant pharmacotherapy requires careful consideration of the selection and use of a specific agent and its long-term potential for treatment success. Antidepressant treatment options include tricyclic and heterocyclic antidepressants, MAOIs, SSRIs, and other new generation atypical agents discussed in this chapter. The clinical limitations of antidepressants include delays in their onset of full response, efficacy rates of 50% to 80%, the potential for side effects and toxicity, and compliance issues. Selection of an antidepressant requires some understanding and consideration of the agent's safety, tolerability, efficacy, the price of the drug and payer source, convenience of dosing and titration, and spectrum of effect. These considerations have been discussed with respect to both older- and newer-generation antidepressants. Generally, first-line treatment will incur the use of an SSRI or other new generation atypical agent (Box 6-9). Augmentation of that antidepressant may be necessary or prudent to enhance the antidepressant effect (discussed later).

Box 6-9 Antidepressant Strategy

First line	
First choice	SSRI or atypical/novel antidepressant
Second choice	If one of the above is not effective, select an alternative from the other class
For nonresponders/partial responders	Augmentation (see Table 6-10)
Second line	Dual-mechanism antidepressant (e.g., bupropion or venlafaxine)
For treatment-refractory patients	Combination
Third line	ECT-MAOIs-TCAs-experimental agents

SSRI, Selective serotonin reuptake inhibitor; *ECT*, electroconvulsive therapy; *MAOIs*, monoamine oxidase inhibitors; *TCAs*, tricyclic antidepressants.

Treatment Resistance

Despite a clinician's best effort to select and use an antidepressant (with or without the concomitant use of other agents), 20% to 35% of patients diagnosed and treated will fail to respond to an adequate trial of a particular antidepressant. Approximately 10% to 15% of patients will show treatment resistance after two adequate trials of an antidepressant, again with or without augmentation. When patients have failed to respond to adequate trials of an antidepressant medication, selection of agents with dual or multiple mechanisms (e.g., bupropion or venlafaxine) have been promulgated in the literature. However, definitive studies involving treatment-refractory patients are relatively scarce. In some cases, combinations of antidepressant medications with disparate mechanisms of action may be used to achieve a greater rate of success in treatment-resistant cases. ECT and MAOIs, thought to be the more powerful antidepressant treatments, may also be used in such cases of treatment-resistant depression.

Dosing Strategies

As first-line agents, SSRIs have flat dose-response curves, similar overall efficacy, relatively benign adverse effect profiles, safety in overdose, and variable side effects and potential for drug interactions as discussed. SSRIs generally have a flat dose-response; that is, the starting dose (or no more than one or two titrations) is usually therapeutic.

Non-SSRI antidepressants tend to yield increased rates of response with upward titrations. Patients can gradually accommodate to unwanted side effects as the dosage is titrated. Once an optimal dose is achieved or a therapeutic response is experienced, the patient who is tolerating the antidepressant medication may be given a single dose of tricyclic or heterocyclic agents with equal therapeutic efficacy.

Trazodone, nefazodone, mirtazapine, bupropion, and venlafaxine are continued on a once- or twice-daily regimen. A short half-life or an ongoing potential for adverse effects prompts a divided dosing schedule. A single bedtime dose may not be desirable in elderly patients or in patients sensitive to the adverse effects of the antidepressant. These individuals may better tolerate the drug when the dose is divided throughout the day. With more sedating agents, patients may benefit from a similarly divided dosage schedule in order to alleviate anxiety without the need to add an anxiolytic medication to the regimen. Coadministration of antianxiety or antipsychotic agents may sometimes be necessary while awaiting the therapeutic response of an antidepressant. In the event that a benzodiazepine is used concurrently, short- to intermediate-acting agents are the best choice, for example, lorazepam or alprazolam (see Chapter 7). For patients with paranoid ideation and delusional thinking, concomitant treatment with an antipsychotic agent, for example, risperidone, is preferable (see Chapter 5).

Common Problems with Antidepressant Treatment

Two common problems with antidepressant medications are the prescription of inadequate doses and the discontinuation of drug treatment before the patient has recovered from the immediate depressive symptoms. Premature discontinuation of an antidepressant medication is a common cause for relapse in depressed patients.[48] Although a 4-month course of medication may be appropriate with the first episode of depression, it is more reasonable to plan for a 6- to 12-month course, followed by cautious tapering, particularly in an individual with a previous episode or a positive family history. As previously discussed, antidepressant medication should not be

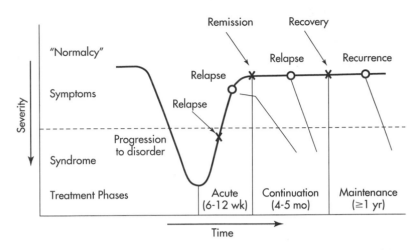

Figure 6-6 Phases of treatment for depression. (From Kupfer DJ: *J Clin Psychiatry* 52(suppl 5): 28, 1991; and Depression Guideline Panel: *Depression in primary care. Vol 2: Treatment of major depression. Clinical Practice Guideline No. 5,* 1993.)

withdrawn abruptly, and the dosage should be tapered, preferably over several weeks. Continuation therapy and maintenance (Figure 6-6) can prevent relapse and recurrence.[38]

Another continuing problem in achieving a prompt, satisfactory response to antidepressant drugs is the inability to predict which patient will respond optimally to which type or class of antidepressant agent. Thus a treatment algorithm is necessary to systematically approach partial or nonresponders (see Box 6-9).

The routine measurement of plasma concentration is generally not necessary for effective therapy. However, if the patient fails to respond and is indeed taking the medication, it is generally appropriate to increase the dosage and evaluate the response. Most evidence, with the exception of evidence pertaining to the SSRIs, supports a linear relationship between plasma concentration and therapeutic response, although a therapeutic window for nortriptyline and possibly desipramine has been suggested in the literature.[6] Table 6-9 provides a comparison of SSRIs relative to dose plasma concentration and other characteristics. Table 6-5 suggests some generally accepted ranges of plasma levels of older agents.[49] Monitoring the plasma level of TCAs may help the noncompliant patient understand the reason for nonresponse and give added emphasis to restructuring of a therapeutic relationship. Inadequate data exist to support reliable statements regarding the correlation of therapeutic response and plasma levels for newer generation antidepressants.

Augmentation Strategies

As noted, approximately 10% to 15% of patients will show treatment resistance after two adequate trials of an antidepressant with or without augmentation, yet only limited data exist to guide treatment in such instances. Augmentation or potentiation with adjunctive drugs can be useful for partial responders to an antidepressant or in cases of nonresponse (Box 6-10). Lithium may potentiate a response (50% of nonresponders will respond) in a matter of 2 to 3 weeks, usually at levels of 0.5 to 0.9 mEq/L. Thyroid supplementation is an augmentation strategy. T_3 (triiodothyronine

Table 6-9 Relationship of Dose, Plasma Level, Potency, and Serotonin Uptake Inhibition

SSRI	Minimum effective dose (mg/day)	Plasma level (ng/ml)	In vitro potency	5HT uptake inhibition
Citalopram	40	85	1.8	60%
Fluoxetine	20	200	6.8	80%
Fluvoxamine	150	100	3.8	70%
Paroxetine	20	40	0.29	80%
Sertraline	50	25	0.19	80%

Adapted from Preskorn SH: *Clin Pharmacokinet* 32(suppl 1):15, 1997.

Box 6-10 Antidepressant Augmentation

Lithium: 0.4 to 0.8 mEq/L
Thyroid hormone: 25 to 50 μg T_3
Trazodone: 50 to 150 mg
Buspirone: 15 to 45 mg
Ritalin: 10 to 60 mg
Beta-blockers: 2.5 to 15 mg pindolol
Hormones: estrogens
Antiepileptics: 600 to 3000 mg gabapentin

[Cytomel]) appears to be more effective than T_4 (thyroxine [Synthroid]), and results in relatively rapid response.[33] Augmentation therapy with buspirone or pindolol may also be useful. These drugs tend to stimulate $5HT_{1A}$ receptors.[7] Psychostimulants (e.g., methylphenidate, dextroamphetamine, or pemoline) may also be useful adjuncts. For example, methylphenidate at a dosage of 10 mg twice daily is started and titrated up to 30 mg twice daily in divided doses given early in the day. Another strategy is the use of low-dose heterocyclics, for example, desipramine 10 to 25 mg or trazodone 50 to 150 mg, combined with an SSRI.[70]

Antidepressant combination therapy has been used in patients who are treatment resistant with some success. Generally, these strategies involve the combination of SSRIs or venlafaxine with approximately one third the usual doses of TCAs, bupropion, or $5HT_2$ blockers (i.e., nefazodone or mirtazapine). There is no evidence that these strategies are faster, more effective, or better tolerated, but some patients seem to respond to this so-called rationale polypharmacy.

Essentially, there are no studies to support the combined use of TCAs and MAOIs. In the experience of one of the authors (DGF), this combination is not more effective than an MAOI alone.

Comorbid Anxiety

Other principles in using antidepressants may relate to individuals with comorbid depression and anxiety. Antidepressants are effective for both mood and anxiety symptoms. Benzodiazepines, as previously stated, are effective adjunctively for anxiety- and antidepressant-induced stimulation but ineffective as monotherapy for depression. The general tendency in patients with anxiety symptoms is to start with a lower dosage and titrate slowly to minimize the potential for hypersensitivity when initiating antidepressant therapy; however, it is important to aim for an effective dosage level.

Continuation Therapy

Factors that may affect the success rates of continuation therapy include the tolerability of the medication, dosing schedule, half-life, (shorter half-lives increase the risk of discontinuation syndrome), side effects, and drug-drug interactions. Certainly, reinforcement from the prescriber and support from the family or other social supports will improve the likelihood of a successful therapeutic response as well as continuation therapy.

Psychotherapy combined with antidepressant medication may significantly improve outcome and is a subject of ongoing study. Cognitive therapy and other psychosocial interventions, including social skills training, dynamic psychotherapy, general psychotherapy, supportive therapy, group therapy, interpersonal psychotherapy, and self-help groups, have all been reported as useful interventions in combination with pharmacotherapy. Other strategies that will enhance outcome include the formation of a therapeutic alliance, education of the patient and the family regarding the illness and antidepressant therapy, discussion of the benefits and risks of treatment, involvement of the patient in medication decisions, and relief of adverse effects with adjunctive therapy. Barriers in the recovery of individuals receiving antidepressant therapy include poor compliance, bereavement, social isolation, occult self-medication, and lack of a support system. More sedating antidepressants may be problematic over time because of the potential to increase side effect burdens such as daytime drowsiness and fatigue.

The Role of Electroconvulsive Therapy

Finally, ECT may be an effective strategy for treatment-resistant depression, especially in cases of psychotic or endogenous depression. Some nonpsychotic depressed patients have a more favorable response when a low-dose neuroleptic is added to the antidepressant regimen.[59] Chapter 14 provides a full discussion of this issue.

ALTERNATIVE TREATMENTS FOR DEPRESSION
St. John's Wort

St. John's Wort is licensed and used primarily in Europe for the treatment of mild to moderate depression. Its use in depressive disorder remains somewhat controversial; however, St. John's Wort has gained in popularity as an alternative treatment for depression. A full discussion of St. John's Wort is found in Chapter 18. Generally, St. John's Wort is unregulated and not approved in the United States for the treatment of depression. The most effective preparation containing hypericin, the active ingredient, and the most effective dosages of St. John's Wort are unknown. No data as to which types of depression are most responsive to St. John's Wort exist. No long-term maintenance or relapse prevention data are available, and no comparison studies with newer antidepressants have been completed. However, the National Institutes of Health is conducting multicenter, placebo-controlled trials, and comparisons with SSRIs are ongoing.

S-Adenosylmethionine

S-adenosylmethionine (SAMe) was first discovered in 1953 in Italy. Reports that SAMe could treat depression were widely disseminated in Europe in the early 1970s, and in 1977, it became commercially available for that purpose. SAMe was not available in the United States until the spring of 1999.

SAMe is a ubiquitous methyl-donor molecule located throughout the body. It plays a key role in numerous metabolic pathways that involve the transfer of methyl groups. SAMe is formed in the body by a combination of adenosine triphosphate (ATP) and the amino acid methionine. SAMe then donates its methyl group to any of a wide range of molecules and is subsequently transformed to homocysteine.

The mechanism by which SAMe might treat depression is a mystery. Possible hypotheses include that it (1) increases the synthesis of neurotransmitters such as serotonin and norepinephrine, (2) increases the responsiveness of neurotransmitter receptors, and (3) increases the fluidity of cell membranes of phospholipids.[11] Oral SAMe has a very low bioavailability estimated to be less than 1%, so its usefulness as an oral agent is open to question. Parenterally administered SAMe does appear to cross the blood-brain barrier. There have been more than 40 trials evaluating SAMe for depression; almost all have involved parenteral formulations. Only five trials have tested oral forms of SAMe. These studies were methodologically flawed and extremely small, involving 15 patients, 17 patients, and 23 patients, respectively. Some articles claim that SAMe has a faster onset of action than TCAs, but the results from the two clinical trials comparing oral SAMe with TCAs do not support this. Numerous trials that have tested parenteral dosing of SAMe have generally shown it to be effective with a faster onset of effect. However, given SAMe's questionable absorption from the gastrointestinal tract, it is not valid to extrapolate this data to the oral use of SAMe.

The primary adverse effects associated with the use of SAMe include mania, manifested by pressured speech and a display of grandiose ideas. These patient's thought processes return to normal when SAMe is discontinued. SAMe otherwise appears to be well tolerated, without anticholinergic or antihistaminergic side effects. Some patients taking oral SAMe have reported nausea.

Because homocysteine levels have been implicated in the development of coronary atherosclerosis, the fact that SAMe is transferred to homocysteine raises some safety concerns.[21] It is unknown whether the administration of SAMe raises homocysteine levels in the human heart or if it has an effect on the risk and development of coronary artery disease. Certainly, SAMe should be used cautiously in patients with coronary artery disease and is contraindicated in patients with a history of mania or bipolar disorder.

Studies testing parenteral forms of SAMe have used a wide variety of dosages, ranging from 45 to 400 mg/day. Parenteral SAMe is not commercially available in the United States. The five oral trials have used 1600 mg/day in two equal doses. Oral SAMe is available in 200-mg tablets. Distributor instructions typically recommend 400 mg twice daily, but this dose has never been tested in trials. Thus, at dosages thought to be effective, SAMe is significantly more expensive than common pharmaceutical agents (Table 6-10).

Overall, the preponderance of the evidence suggests that intramuscular or intravenous SAMe may be effective in treating serious depression. However, SAMe is very poorly absorbed, and little data would support the efficacy of oral SAMe—even at dosages of 1600 mg/day. Moreover, SAMe may be potentially harmful because it may induce mania or increasing levels of homocysteine. Thus oral SAMe cannot be currently recommended for the treatment of depression because of its uncertain absorption, high cost, and significant potential for causing mania.

Table 6-10 Retail Cost of Pharmacologic Therapies for Depression

Therapeutic agent	Usual dosage	Cost (30-day supply)
St. John's Wort	300 mg tid	$15
Desipramine (Norpramin)	150 mg qd	$44
Sertraline (Zoloft)	50 mg qd	$71
Paroxetine (Paxil)	20 mg qd	$74
Fluoxetine (Prozac)	20 mg qd	$81
SAMe	800 mg bid	$240

Average cost based on phone survey of national pharmacy chains and online nutritional supplement distributors, October 1999.

SIGNIFICANT ISSUES RELATED TO WOMEN AND ANTIDEPRESSANT THERAPY
Antidepressants during Pregnancy and Lactation

The use of antidepressant drugs in pregnancy is an important issue in psychopharmacologic management of depression (and anxiety). Basic questions remain about whether antidepressant drugs are safe for women to take during pregnancy and lactation, whether some antidepressants are safer than others, and to what extent children of women who took antidepressants during pregnancy have a greater incidence of anomaly or developmental difficulties. Certainly, studies of both TCAs and SSRIs have yielded little evidence that those drugs contribute to congenital abnormalities, premature birth, or low birth weight.

Although initial studies had suggested some possible problem with drugs such as fluoxetine, more recent studies with better design and analysis have yielded more favorable results with respect to a lack of adverse effect of SSRIs during pregnancy. For example, Cohen and others, assessed birth outcomes following prenatal exposure to fluoxetine in 31 newborns.[15] A nonstatistically significant trend toward a higher risk of neonatal complications was associated with longer exposure to fluoxetine. However, a longer duration of treatment was also associated with more severe depression or anxiety, both of which may have contributed to poor neonatal outcome. Goldstein and others prospectively identified 123 infants exposed to fluoxetine during all three trimesters and failed to find an association between fluoxetine exposure and neonatal complications.[26] Of 796 women who took fluoxetine during the first trimester, spontaneous abortions occurred in 110 (13.8%) of the pregnancies; malformations, deformations, and disruptions were reported in 34 (5%) of the remaining 686 pregnancies. These rates are consistent with those found in historic reports of surveys concerning newborns.

In another series of studies by Nulman and associates involving assorted antidepressant agents, 80 women who had taken TCAs during pregnancy were not found to have increased risk of hazardous effects.[43] Another review of the children of 55 women who took fluoxetine while pregnant and another 84 children whose mothers had not been exposed to an agent demonstrated no adverse impact on the children's global IQs in language and behavioral development assessed between 16 and 86 months of postnatal age.[43] Moreover, no significant differences were observed in these children in the areas of temperament, mood, arousability, activity level, distractibility, behavioral problems, or scores on neurobehavioral tests.

The literature on antidepressant drugs during lactation indicates that serum drug levels of antidepressants in infant plasma are relatively low and often immeasurable, with no or little adverse effects reported in mothers taking amitriptyline, nortriptyline, desipramine, and clomipramine. Similar findings of very low plasma levels of antidepressants in infants of mothers taking sertraline and fluvoxamine have been reported.[65,68] Other reports of paroxetine, citalopram, and fluoxetine have indicated relatively undetectable levels of antidepressant in the infants of mothers taking those agents at usually effective doses. Generally, antidepressants prescribed during lactation are best dosed at bedtime, with avoidance of nighttime breast-feeding to minimize or reduce the possibility of secretion of antidepressant into breast milk. Thus daytime breast-feeding with bottle-feeding at night and nighttime dosing of the antidepressant may minimize the potential for crossover of antidepressant into breast milk and thus introduction into the infant. Depression in a mother may adversely effect the development of cognition, language, and behavior in infants and young children. Thus, when a pregnant woman is depressed, perinatal risks rise. Current evidence suggests that in most cases, treating depression is better for both the mother and offspring than allowing the mother's depression to remain untreated or to recur because an antidepressant was withdrawn. The need for systematic behavioral assessments and longitudinal developmental follow-up of breast-fed babies and an expanded database on mother and infant serum levels are certainly needed.

Antidepressant Therapy of Premenstrual Dysphoric Disorder

A recent use for the antidepressant medications has been in premenstrual dysphoric disorder (PMDD), which affects about 3 million American women. This clinical syndrome, described in Box 6-11, is characterized by a minimum of five symptoms involving mood stability, mood tension, mood swings, irritability, decreased interest, difficulty concentrating, fatigue, changes in appetite, sleep, a sense of being overwhelmed, or physical symptoms together with the onset of symptoms 1 to 2 weeks before menses, with significant functional impairment. Treatment of PMDD has occurred with many pharmacologic treatments, including hormones, vitamins, diuretics, and most recently, psychotropic medications, primarily antidepressants.[66,67] Psychotropic agents with the greatest utility and effectiveness in the treatment of PMDD are antidepressant agents that preferentially block serotonin reuptake. Clomipramine and the SSRIs fluoxetine, paroxetine, and sertraline have been the most studied in this area. These agents in typically effective antidepressant doses have been found to be useful in diminishing or resolving symptoms of PMDD. Treatment has been successful with both continuous dosing and pulse dosing 5 to 10 days before the onset of menses (during the late luteal phase). Clinical trials have shown that in addition to providing symptomatic relief, antidepressant treatment has

---

Box 6-11 Premenstrual Dysphoric Disorder

Diagnostic criteria
- Minimum of five symptoms:
    Low mood, tension, mood swings, irritability, decreased interest,
        difficulty concentrating, fatigue, changes in appetite, changes in sleep
        patterns, sense of being overwhelmed, physical symptoms
- Symptoms begin 1 to 2 weeks before menses.
- At least one symptom is a mood symptom.
- Symptoms cause functional impairment.

caused dramatic improvement in functioning in individuals with PMDD.[22,58,61,66] Fluoxetine (under the trade name Sarafem) at dosages of 20 to 60 mg has received FDA approval for the treatment of PMDD. Other SSRI antidepressants may also receive approval as studies are completed and reviewed. The only other agent that has shown promise in the treatment of PMDD is alprazolam.[52] However, not all trials using alprazolam have been successful, and concerns about the dependence potential and sedative adverse effects of alprazolam eliminate its applications in this disorder.

Binge Eating and Bulimia Nervosa

Another disorder that affects primarily women is binge eating or bulimia nervosa involving repeated episodes of rapidly binge eating large amounts of food with compensatory behaviors to prevent weight gain. Self-induced vomiting; the misuse of laxatives, diet pills, and diuretics; fasts; very strict diets; and vigorous exercise are examples of typical compensatory behaviors. At least two binge eating and purging or severe compensatory behavior episodes per week for a minimum of 3 months are necessary to establish the diagnosis of bulimia. Unrelenting concern with weight and body shape occur, and subtypes of the bulimia are specified as *purging* or *nonpurging* type. The individual with purging-type bulimia, who uses self-induced vomiting or misuses laxatives or diuretics, is contrasted to the individual with nonpurging-type bulimia, who engages in other inappropriate behaviors such as excessive exercise or fasting and does not ordinarily self-induce vomiting or misuse laxatives or diuretics. A more thorough discussion of this topic may be found in Reference 37, Chapter 8.

Controlled studies indicate that bulimia may be treated with TCAs, the SSRIs fluoxetine and fluvoxamine, and MAOIs. Common problems include medication compliance and the maintenance of therapeutic levels in the face of persistent vomiting. Fluoxetine and the TCAs have been the best studied and the most often used antidepressants for this condition. The results of antidepressant medication trials are similar to short-term outcomes with cognitive-behavioral psychotherapies. However, many patients who do not respond to psychologic approaches alone will benefit from medication; symptoms are reduced in 70% to 90% of patients and approximately one third become abstinent.[41] More recently, fluvoxamine in standard antidepressant doses has also been found to be effective in the acute treatment of binge eating disorder, a newly described eating disorder characterized by recurrent episodes of binge eating without purging behaviors.[32]

ANTIMANIC AND MOOD-STABILIZING DRUGS: LITHIUM

Lithium was discovered in 1817 by Arfwedson, who named the drug after the Greek word for stone. Lithium was initially used in the United States as a salt substitute for cardiac patients but was quickly removed from the market after some of these individuals died of toxic effects. John Cade, an Australian physician, used lithium salts experimentally in mania to produce sedation; he also used lithium preparations to treat epilepsy because of the apparent anticonvulsant action.[10]

Lithium, as a treatment for mental illness, spread to England and Denmark and then throughout Europe before eventually coming to the United States, which became the last country to authorize the therapeutic use of lithium (in 1970).

Precisely how lithium achieves its normalizing effects in mania is not known; however, the lithium ion substitutes for the sodium ion, thereby compromising the ability of neurons to release, activate, or respond to neurotransmitters. Lithium also has serotonergic properties, enhances acetylcholine formation, effects norepinephrine, stabilizes calcium channels, and decreases neuronal activity via effects on second messenger systems, all of which may add to its therapeutic profile. Although indicated for the treatment of mania and maintenance in patients with bipolar disorder, lithium is prescribed for a variety of other psychiatric disorders.

Pharmacokinetics

Lithium is well absorbed from the gastrointestinal tract and is normally given in oral tablets, capsules, or concentrates. Peak blood serum levels are reached in 1 to 4 hours. More than 95% of the amount ingested is excreted unchanged by the kidneys; that is, it is not metabolized. It is not bound to plasma protein. The plasma half-life is approximately 24 hours; hence the steady state is achieved in 4 to 5 days. Renal insufficiency or disease lengthens the half-life, necessitating reduction in dosage. Absorption and excretion of lithium are closely linked to those of sodium. When dietary sodium intake increases, serum levels of lithium are likely to drop because lithium is excreted more rapidly. Conversely, when sodium in the diet decreases or when sodium is lost in ways other than through the kidney (e.g., sweating or diarrhea), lithium serum levels increase. Because a therapeutic serum level of lithium is not much lower than a toxic serum level, such considerations are significant. Diet and activity levels should not change abruptly.

Lithium is manufactured primarily in 300-mg capsules or tablets (lithium carbonate). A 450-mg, sustained-release preparation is available. Lithium is effective in as many as 80% of patients; however, it takes 1 to 2 weeks to begin to achieve a clinical response. Lithium dosage is based on both the clinical response and lithium serum levels (Table 6-11). The typical dosage for acute mania is 600 mg three times per day, usually producing a serum level of 1.0 to 1.5 mEq/L. Desirable serum levels for maintenance are 0.6 to 1.2 mEq/L, which can be maintained on an average dose of 900 to 1200 mg/day. Lithium serum levels greater than 1.5 mEq/L usually result in toxic effects.

Pharmacologic Effect

Although no consensus exists regarding the antidepressant efficacy of lithium carbonate, some studies have indicated its beneficial effect in patients with depressed mood.[44] As previously discussed, lithium carbonate, in conjunction with antidepressants, may be useful in many patients who have not responded to adequate trials of antidepressants. Controlled studies have confirmed the ability of lithium to augment a therapeutic response.[30,47]

The efficacy of lithium in the treatment of acute mania has been well documented. Perhaps the major disadvantage of lithium in the treatment of acute mania is that improvement is gradual. It may take up to 3 weeks to adequately control manic symptoms. Thus antipsychotic agents such as olanzapine or potent benzodiazepines such as lorazepam or clonazepam may be necessary alone or in combination to achieve rapid control of psychotic or agitated behavior. Lithium serum levels are ideally obtained approximately 12 hours after the administration of the last dose. Clinical observations and well-documented compliance should coincide with this practice.

Considerable evidence supports the use of lithium for prophylaxis of recurrent depression in persons with bipolar illness. Lithium may also be useful for recurrent depression in patients who do not have a manic component to their mood disorder. Perhaps the most interesting and important application of lithium in depression is its potential to facilitate a therapeutic response to therapy.

Table 6-11 Medical Evaluation of New Patients with Manic
(or Major Depressive) Episodes

	Inpatients	Outpatients
First-line tests	■ *Complete physical examination* ■ *Serum levels of lithium, carbamazepine, selected tricyclics** ■ *Thyroid function if not obtained recently* ■ *CBC and general chemistry screen* ■ Urinalysis if starting lithium ■ ECG in patients older than 40 ■ Urine toxicology for substance abuse ■ Pregnancy test if relevant*	■ *Serum levels of lithium, valproate, carbamazepine, selected tricyclics** ■ *Thyroid functions if not obtained recently* ■ *CBC and general chemistry screen* ■ Urinalysis if starting lithium ■ Complete physical examination ■ Pregnancy test if relevant
Second-line tests		■ Urine toxicology for substance abuse ■ ECG in patients older than 40

Further recommendations:
■ When necessary, mood stabilizers and other medications used for bipolar disorder can usually be started before test results are available if the patient has been in good general health. If clinical judgment determines an urgent need, medication can be started even before laboratory specimens have been obtained.
■ CT or MRI, and EEG, are second-line options in the evaluation of treatment-resistant patients. They are not needed routinely without a specific clinical reason.
■ Clinicians should rely on their own judgment in two areas in which there is no consensus: obtaining ECGs in patients younger than 40 and obtaining a general medical consultation before treatment.

From Treatment of bipolar disorder. Steering Committe. The Expert Concensus Guidelines Series, *J Clin Psychiatry* 57(suppl 12A):3, 1996.
CBC, Complete blood count; *ECG*, electrocardiogram; *CT*, computed tomography; *MRI*, magnetic resonance imaging; *EEG*, electroencephalogram.
Note: **Bold italic** type represents assessment of choice.
*See Table 6-5.

Side Effects

Lithium, an ion interchangeable with sodium, has a variety of physiologic and pathophysiologic actions in various organ systems. Thus it is important to ascertain whether the patient is in good health and whether there are any medical contraindications to lithium. In addition, it is important to determine whether the patient has sufficient renal function to clear the ion adequately so that lithium intoxication may be prevented. Serum creatinine or blood urea nitrogen levels should be obtained. For patients consuming a low-salt diet or taking diuretics, baseline electrolyte values should also be determined. A baseline electrocardiogram (ECG) is necessary because lithium often produces repolarization (ST-segment and T-wave) changes in the ECG. About 20% of patients taking lithium have a T-wave flattening or inversion at therapeutic blood levels that does not indicate underlying heart disease. Patients who develop lithium intoxication may show a variety of cardiovascular abnormalities, including arrhythmia, conduction disturbance, and hypotension. Because lithium is associated with the development of a euthyroid goiter, hyperthyroidism with or without thyroid gland enlargement or abnormalities in serum determinations of thyroid function warrant baseline measurements of thyroid function. Lithium administration is often associated with weight gain, partially related to fluid retention and increased caloric intake. The patient should be considered at risk for this nontherapeutic effect. Lithium often produces benign reversible leukocytosis; white blood cell counts of 12,000 to 15,000 cells/mm^3 are commonly observed during therapy. This condition does not indicate hematologic disease, and lithium need not be discontinued.

Because lithium is a simple ion whose entry into the body is governed by the same physiologic mechanisms as sodium, lithium reaches virtually all body tissues. Lithium's side effects are linked primarily to serum blood levels. Blood levels greater than 1.5 mEq/L can be toxic, and generally, levels above 2.0 mEq/L induce toxic signs and symptoms. Common side effects include nausea, dry mouth, diarrhea, and thirst. Drowsiness, mild hand tremor, polyuria, weight gain, a bloated feeling, sleeplessness, and headaches are other relatively common side effects. A lithium tremor tends to be irregular in rhythm and amplitude and affects the fingers. Jerky motions of the flexion and extension of fingers are also commonly associated with lithium therapy. These tremors often disappear spontaneously when the dose is held constant for the first 2 to 3 weeks of lithium treatment. Sometimes, reducing the dosage of lithium or advising the patient to take smaller doses several times throughout the day alleviates this unwanted effect. However, when the tremor is persistent and severe enough to cause inconvenience to the patient's daily activities, a beta-blocking agents such as propranolol, metoprolol, and nadolol may be effective as an antidote.[72] The use of slow-release lithium preparations may reduce the severity of lithium tremor and other side effects by reducing serum blood level peaks. Side effects unrelated to serum levels include weight gain, a metallic taste, headache, edema of the hands and ankles, and pruritus. Lithium, even in therapeutic levels, can affect thyroid gland function. In some patients, thyroid hormone therapy may be required. Lithium may also impair the mental or physical capabilities required for driving.

Polyuria and polydipsia develop in many patients taking lithium. These symptoms are generally benign and are not indicative of renal or metabolic disease. Patients who develop renal changes in association with therapeutic doses of lithium have not been reported to develop renal failure. However, lithium should not be prescribed unless there is both a reasonable clinical indication of its necessity and the likelihood that it will benefit the patient therapeutically. It may add somewhat to the safety of long-term lithium management and provide reassurance to the patient and the clinician to measure urine osmolality once or twice yearly, after a 12-hour period of fasting. This practice is of course in addition to periodic determinations of lithium serum levels.

During lithium treatment, patients who develop edema of the ankle or lower legs generally show normal renal, cardiovascular, and hepatic function. This edema may disappear spontaneously or may respond favorably to 25 to 50 mg twice a day of spironolactone, an aldosterone inhibitor that normalizes tubular reabsorption of sodium. Patients with edema may also respond to an intermittent dose of a thiazide diuretic, for example, hydrochlorothiazide 50 mg daily or every other day. If hydrochlorothiazide is administered regularly, serum potassium and supplemental oral potassium levels need to be monitored. Weight gain may be caused in part by fluid retention, but variable changes in glucose metabolism may also be an important mechanism. Patients should be educated about this possibility and taught to maintain adequate fluid and salt intake during the course of any rapid weight loss. Moreover, it is often appropriate to measure lithium serum concentration more frequently in individuals who are on a weight-reducing diet.

Lithium therapy may be associated with the development of goiter (approximately 3%) in the presence of normal thyroid function tests and a euthyroid state. This condition is usually associated with an increased thyroid-stimulating hormone level and an enlarged thyroid gland as it attempts to maintain a euthyroid state. Nonetheless, hypothyroidism (approximately 5%) may be induced by lithium treatment, and monitoring is recommended. This occurrence does not indicate that the dosage needs to be changed or the medication discontinued; however, proper evaluation and replacement therapy with an appropriate thyroid hormone regimen may be necessary in conjunction with lithium treatment.

Dermatologic reactions may occur with lithium. Acne may worsen; psoriasis may exacerbate. Occasionally, a maculopapular rash, with or without pruritus, may emerge during the course of lithium treatment. Hair loss may also occur and may be limited to the scalp or may affect other body regions.

Many patients taking lithium have gastrointestinal complaints, most commonly burning sensations and persistent indigestion. Taking lithium at mealtime or with a snack often alleviates these symptoms. Mild diarrhea is occasionally associated with therapeutic doses of lithium but is more apt to occur in the presence of excessive lithium serum concentration. Vomiting is a major risk because it contributes to dehydration, which in turn may worsen lithium intoxication. Patients who have nausea, vomiting, or other flulike symptoms during lithium therapy should be advised to discontinue lithium and maintain adequate fluid intake for a short time.

Lithium intoxication is a common problem; when it is suspected, the drug should be discontinued and blood samples sent for determinations of lithium serum concentration and serum creatinine and electrolyte levels. Specific interventions include adequate hydration, antiemetics as necessary, and monitoring of serum levels of electrolytes, lithium, and creatinine, which in turn can guide the rate and nature of fluid replacement. An ECG should also be obtained because of the possibility of cardiac arrhythmia. A patient with lithium intoxication may also develop central neurotoxicity, including confusion, stupor, and the potential for seizure.

Treatment Implications

Therapeutic versus toxic levels. Therapeutic lithium serum levels are 0.6 to 1.2 mEq/L. At serum levels above 1.5 mEq/L, adverse reactions usually occur. Typically, the higher the serum levels, the more severe the reaction. Mild to moderate toxic reactions occur at levels of 1.5 to 2.0 mEq/L, and moderate to severe reactions occur at 2.0 to 3.0 mEq/L. Diarrhea, vomiting, drowsiness, muscular weakness, and lack of coordination can be early signs of lithium intoxication. At higher levels, ataxia, giddiness, tinnitus, blurred vision, and a large output of dilute urine may be seen. At serum levels above 3 mEq/L, multiple organs and organ systems may be involved, leading to coma and death.[60] Although patients with serum levels as high as 10 mEq/L have survived, serum levels should not be allowed to exceed 2 mEq/L.

There is no antidote for lithium poisoning. When supportive intervention is available, discontinuing the drug may be enough. In acute overdose, gastric lavage has been used successfully. Parenteral normal saline solution infused over 6 hours (1 to 2 L) may provide enough volume to prevent hypovolemia and to restore blood pressure and enough sodium to counteract lithium's ill effects, enhancing renal excretion for serum levels below 2.5 mEq/L. Forced diuresis may be necessary for patients with lithium poisoning, and mannitol may be used. Acetazolamide, which alkalinizes the urine, may also be given to increase lithium excretion in the case of an acute overdose. In some severe cases, hemodialysis has been found to be helpful.

Use in pregnancy. Cessation of lithium during pregnancy is suggested because of its relationship to Epstein's anomaly and other cardiovascular teratogenic effects in the first trimester. However, lithium is less teratogenic than the anticonvulsant alternatives (i.e., valproate and carbamazepine). If antimania treatment is essential during this time, treatment with olanzapine or thioridazine may be beneficial. These drugs, when used instead of lithium, also carry unknown risks when prescribed in the second and third trimesters. Dosages of lithium should be reduced as much as 50% before the delivery because of the potential for neonatal intoxication resulting from high serum levels of lithium in the mother.[14]

Use in the elderly. Because of age-related changes, renal clearance of lithium is decreased. Furthermore, age-related changes also cause elderly patients to respond to treatment at lower serum levels (0.4 to 0.8 mEq/L versus 0.6 to 1.2 mEq/L in younger adults). Elderly patients are more susceptible to side effects (e.g., polydipsia, polyuria) and to adverse responses such as CNS toxicity.

Side effect interventions. Because lithium has a narrow therapeutic index, lithium serum levels should be determined frequently. Levels are determined twice weekly in most acute-care treatment units. Once the patient's condition is stabilized, monthly and then quarterly serum level determinations are adequate. Blood is usually drawn before administration of the first dose of lithium in the morning (usually 8 to 12 hours after the last dose). However, laboratory tests alone are not sufficient to evaluate the patient's status with respect to lithium therapy and are not a substitute for clinical monitoring.

Interactions. Familiarity with the drugs that can elevate lithium serum levels is essential (Box 6-12). Diuretics, with the exception of acetazolamide, increase sodium excretion, thereby elevating serum lithium levels. Nonsteroidal antiinflammatory agents (e.g., ibuprofen) increase serum levels of lithium by reducing renal elimination. Switching to a low-salt diet also elevates lithium serum levels. Some drugs decrease serum lithium levels and pose problems of inadequate treatment and symptom exacerbation. This decrease may occur in one of two ways: by increasing lithium excretion or by decreasing lithium absorption. Drugs that increase lithium excretion include acetazolamide, caffeine, and alcohol. Lithium also prolongs the paralyzing effect of some neuromuscular-blocking agents that may be given before surgery or used during ECT. Appropriate measures should be taken in these cases.

Lithium and antipsychotic or anxiolytic drugs are often combined. Antipsychotics are prescribed with lithium because lithium's clinical response time is delayed at least 1 to 2 weeks. Antipsychotic agents are prescribed to produce an immediate

Box 6-12 Mood Stabilizers and Clinical Applications

Lithium
: Mixed manic episode
Mania with rapid cycling
Add-on in manic episode that has partially responded to valproate
Switch to in manic episode that has shown no response to valproate
When using a mood stabilizer alone to treat depression
When mood stabilizer must be given in a single bedtime dose
Patients with liver disease, excessive alcohol use, cocaine use, or older than 65
During first 2 months, check serum level every 1-2 weeks
For the long term, check serum level every 3-6 months, check thyroid yearly, and check renal function every 6-12 months

Valproate
: Classic euphoric mania
Mixed manic episode
Mania with rapid cycling "secondary" mania
When mood stabilizer must be started rapidly using a loading dose
Add-on in manic episode that has partially responded to lithium
Add-on, or switch to, in manic episode that has shown no response to lithium
Long-term maintenance in patients who do not tolerate lithium because of "flat" feeling
Patients with structural central nervous system disease, renal disease, substance use, or older than 65
During first 2 months, check serum level every 1-2 weeks, and CBC and LFTs monthly
For the long term, check serum level every 3-6 months, and check CBC and LFTs every 6-12 months

Carbamazepine
: Add-on, or switch to, in manic episode that has shown no response to lithium
Long-term maintenance in patients who do not tolerate lithium because of "flat" feeling
Patients with structural central nervous system disease, renal disease, substance use, or older than 65
During first 2 months, check serum level every 1-2 weeks, and CBC and LFTs monthly
For the long term, check serum level every 3-6 months, and check CBC and LFTs every 6-12 months

CBC, Complete blood count; *LFTs,* liver function tests.

neuroleptic or antipsychotic effect. A potential problem with this combination that has not been mentioned is that the antiemetic properties of the antipsychotic agent may potentially mask the early signs of lithium intoxication (nausea and vomiting). Furthermore, the combination of lithium and haloperidol has resulted in irreversible CNS toxicity resulting in brain damage.

Box 6-13   Patient Guidelines for Taking Lithium

To achieve a therapeutic effect and to prevent toxic effects of lithium, patients taking lithium should be advised of the following:

1. Lithium must be taken on a regular basis, preferably at the same time each day. If a patient is taking lithium, for example, on a three-times-daily schedule and forgets a dose, he or she should wait until the next scheduled time to take the lithium but should not take twice the amount at that time because lithium intoxication could occur.

2. When lithium treatment is initiated, mild side effects such as a fine hand tremor, increased thirst and urination, nausea, anorexia, and diarrhea or constipation may develop. Most of the mild side effects are transient and do not represent toxic effects of lithium. Also, in some patients who are taking lithium, some foods such as celery and butter have an unappealing taste.

3. Serious side effects of lithium that necessitate its discontinuance include vomiting, extreme hand tremor, sedation, muscle weakness, and vertigo. If any of these occur, the prescribing clinician should be notified immediately.

4. Lithium and sodium compete for elimination from the body through the kidneys. An increase in salt intake increases lithium elimination, and a decrease in salt intake decreases lithium elimination. Thus it is important that the patient maintain a balanced diet and salt intake. If the patient wishes to alter his or her diet, he or she should first consult with the prescribing clinician.

5. Various situations can require an adjustment in the amount of lithium administered to a patient, for example, the addition of a new medication to the patient's drug regimen, a new diet, or an illness with fever or excessive sweating.

6. Blood should be drawn in the morning for determination of lithium levels, approximately 10 to 14 hours after the last dose was taken.

Patient education. The patient and family alike must be familiar with the nontherapeutic effects of lithium and the symptoms of minor and major toxic effects (Box 6-13). Side effects associated with lithium should be reviewed, and in individuals of childbearing age, appropriate measures should be taken with regard to the risks of lithium treatment during pregnancy. Avoidance of driving until the patient is stabilized on a regimen of lithium is also reasonable. The interventions outlined in Box 6-14 should also be considered in applicable cases.

ALTERNATIVE ANTIMANIC AND MOOD-STABILIZING DRUGS
Valproate

Sodium valproate, valproic acid, and related compounds such as divalproex (Depakote) have been used since the 1960s as antiepileptic agents. Divalproex received FDA approval in 1995 and is indicated for the primary treatment of mania.[8] A more complete review of the pharmacologic effects, pharmacokinetics, side effects, and treatment implications are found in Chapter 9.

Box 6-14 Interventions for Patients Taking Lithium

Prepare the patient for expected side effects in a nonanxious manner.
Discuss which side effects should subside (nausea, dry mouth, diarrhea, thirst, mild hand tremor, weight gain, bloatedness, insomnia, and light-headedness).
Identify the side effects that require immediate notification of the physician (e.g., vomiting, severe tremor, sedation, muscle weakness, and vertigo).
Suggest taking lithium with meals to reduce nausea.
Suggest drinking 10 to 12 glasses of water per day to reduce thirst and to maintain normal fluid balance.
Advise patient to elevate feet to relieve ankle edema.
Advise patient to maintain a consistent dietary sodium intake but to increase sodium if there is a major increase in perspiration.

**Box 6-15 General Medical Conditions
That Cause Secondary Mania**

Anoxia	Stroke
Hyperthyroidism	Brain tumor
Hemodialysis	Multiple sclerosis
Lyme disease	Normal pressure hydrocephalus
Hypercalcemia	Medications
AIDS	Other neurologic disorder

AIDS, Acquired immunodeficiency syndrome.

Compared with lithium, divalproex showed significantly better response in cases with clinical presentations of mixed mania and rapid cycling. Valproate and carbamazepine are effective in treating mania secondary to general medical conditions (secondary mania) (Box 6-15). The advantages and disadvantages of valproate and lithium are compared in Table 6-12.

The various formulations of valproate differ with respect to absorption and potential side effects. Valproic acid formulations are rapidly absorbed. Divalproex in the form of an enteric-coated or sprinkle tablet is more slowly absorbed (2 versus 4 hours). Common side effects of valproate, shown in Table 6-11, include gastrointestinal upset, somnolence, tremor, and dizziness. These dose-related side effects can be avoided or reduced by using the enteric-coated formulations. Other possible adverse effects are shown in Table 6-12. Hepatitic toxicity and acute pancreatitis rarely occur. These are thought to be dose related and are most likely to emerge in younger children.

The bioavailability of valproate is 100% at therapeutic concentrations, with up to 90% to 95% protein binding. The drug may be displaced by other drugs, such as carbamazepine or warfarin, causing adverse or toxic side effects. The metabolism of valproate is complex; valproate has several active metabolites. Divalproex has a

Table 6-12 Advantages and Disadvantages of Mood Stabilizers

Advantages	Disadvantages
Valproate	
Rapid onset	Transient hair loss
Can be used as initial treatment	Weight gain
High quality of clinical studies (acute mania)	Tremors, gastrointestinal upset
	Dose-related thrombocytopenia
Divalproex formulation well tolerated; minimal effects on cognition	Rare hepatotoxicity, pancreatitis
Effective in bipolar disorder subtypes	
Lithium	
More than 40 years of clinical experience	Nonresponse in 30% to 50% of cases
Most effective for euphoric mania and hypomania	Narrow therapeutic index
	Slow onset of action
Can reduce mortality by decreasing suicide	Side effects very common
Inexpensive	High rate of noncompliance
	Less effective in bipolar subtypes
Carbamazepine	
More rapid onset than lithium	Stimulates own oxidative metabolism (autoinduction)
May be effective in difficult-to-treat cases	
May be effective as adjunctive therapy in acute mania	Blood dyscrasias, skin reactions
	Complex drug interactions
Generally well tolerated	Sedation, poor coordination
	Hyponatremia (poorly tolerated by elderly)

half-life of 6 to 16 hours and reaches steady state in 2 to 5 days. Induction of microsomal enzymes, for example, P-450, may lead to lower plasma concentrations, as occurs with coadministration of phenobarbital or carbamazepine. These drugs, along with phenytoin (Dilantin), aspirin, and alcohol, represent the more significant observed drug interactions. Compared with lithium and carbamazepine, the potential for drug interaction is less.

As with lithium, the use of valproate requires an initial evaluation and ongoing monitoring. Valproate, or divalproex, is initially dosed at 250 mg two or three times a day and titrated at 250 to 500 mg every 3 days (see Table 6-11). A more rapid onset of effect occurs with valproate than with lithium when therapeutic concentrations of 50 to 100 µg/ml are achieved. Oral loading of valproate at 20 mg/kg/day (in divided doses) has resulted in a rather quick response in some cases (5 to 7 days).[35] A rapid titration using this technique is depicted in Box 6-16.

Carbamazepine

Carbamazepine (Tegretol) is an effective alternative treatment for manic episodes when lithium or valproate is ineffective, contraindicated, or not tolerated (see Box 6-12 and Table 6-12). Carbamazepine is chemically related to the TCAs. Patients with rapid-cycling bipolar disorder or secondary mania may respond especially well to carbamazepine, and at times, carbamazepine may be given in combination with lithium, valproate, or other mood-stabilizing drugs. Although the mechanism of

---

Box 6-16 Divalproex: Rapid Titration

For a 70-kg person*

Day 1:	250 mg tid
Day 2:	250 mg tid and 500 mg hs
Day 3:	500 mg tid
Day 5:	Check plasma level

*20 mg/kg/day after titration.

---

antimanic action of carbamazepine is unknown, early work focused on its ability to inhibit kindling.

Carbamazepine is absorbed erratically, with bioavailability of 75% to 85%. Although plasma concentrations of carbamazepine correlate to its anticonvulsant effect, the relationship of blood level to antimanic activity is less clear. Initial dosages of 250 mg two or three times daily are titrated slowly to achieve levels of 8 to 12 µg/ml (see Table 6-11). The side effects of carbamazepine are compared with those of lithium in Tables 6-11 and 6-12. Nausea, anorexia, and occasional vomiting may occur with carbamazepine, particularly when the drug is administered on an empty stomach or when relatively large doses are used. Sedation and drowsiness are common side effects that may be minimized by lowering initial dosages and with slower titration or dosing regimens of three times a day. An extended-release version of carbamazepine has allowed once- or twice-daily dosing regimens. As with valproate, the sedative effects of carbamazepine may be useful in managing acute agitation and psychoses with mood cycling. A more complete review of carbamazepine can be found in Chapter 9.

The most serious and rare side effect of carbamazepine is agranulocytosis; mild to moderate leukopenia, anemia, and thrombocytopenia may also occur. A baseline evaluation should be performed before starting carbamazepine. Complete blood cell counts and examination of the blood smear should be performed weekly during the first month of therapy and may be performed at progressively longer intervals during the course of treatment. Complete blood counts and other appropriate laboratory tests in patients receiving maintenance therapy with carbamazepine should be monitored every 3 to 4 months during treatment. For patients who benefit from carbamazepine but have mild leukopenia, anemia, or thrombocytopenia, periodic monitoring may be acceptable

Toxic effects of carbamazepine, as well as excessive drowsiness, may occur with coadministration of nefazodone and other agents that inhibit CYP-450 3A4. Carbamazepine induces its own metabolism through microsomal induction (Figure 6-7). Carbamazepine may also increase serum lithium concentration and decrease serum concentrations of a number of drugs, including valproate and neuroleptics.

Benzodiazepines and Atypical Antipsychotics for Mania

Clonazepam (Klonopin) is a benzodiazepine with potent anticonvulsant properties and is used as a treatment or an adjunct for the treatment of acute mania. Clonazepam may obviate or reduce the need for the adjunctive use of neuroleptic agents; except for considerable drowsiness, minimal adverse effects are seen in patients receiving clonazepam at dosages of 2 to 16 mg/day.[12]

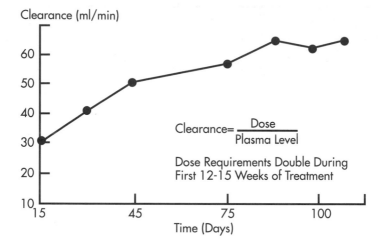

Figure 6-7 Carbamazepine autoinduction after initiation of treatment.

Lorazepam is also useful in providing sedation in cases involving acute mania and overactivity.

Olanzapine (Zyprexa) and possibly other atypical antipsychotics may be useful alone in the treatment of acute mania or as adjuncts to mood stabilizers. Clinical trials involving olanzapine at dosages of 15 to 45 mg have demonstrated good efficacy for mania. It has received recent approval from the FDA for the treatment of mania.

Clozapine (Clozaril) has been used successfully in the treatment resistant mania and for prophylaxis in bipolar mood disorder. Dosages similar to those used in schizophrenia (100 to 600 mg), have been effective. Clozapine treatment may obviate the need for other mood stabilizers and is more effective than ECT in treatment of refractory cases. Slow titration with hematologic monitoring is required, as discussed in Chapter 5.

Miscellaneous Agents for Acute Mania in Bipolar Disorder

Calcium channel blockers. Calcium channel blockers have been studied in the treatment of bipolar disorder. These agents presumably work by blocking the influx of calcium into brain tissue, which may decrease the release of a number of neurotransmitter systems. Flunarizine at dosages of 10 mg/day is reported to have prophylactic effects in patients with bipolar disorder. Nimodipine has been used in the treatment of refractory bipolar disorder and as an augmentor of carbamazepine.[45] Nimodipine, dosed up to 510 mg/day in three or four divided doses, has shown robust improvements in mania and has been used in patients with rapid-cycling bipolar disorder, and in combination with lithium.[20,27] Verapamil has been used most extensively in treating bipolar disorder at dosages of 160 to 480 mg/day. It is useful as an adjunct in combination with lithium or in combination with a neuroleptic such as olanzapine, or as an alternative to other mood stabilizers during pregnancy. Some studies suggest efficacy in the treatment of rapid-cycling bipolar disorder, the prophylaxis of bipolar disorder, secondary mania, and depression.[5,25] Verapamil may be more effective in lithium-responsive than in lithium-resistant patients.[19,62] Verapamil and other calcium channel blockers may prevent antidepressant-induced switches into mania. Bromocriptine is a dopaminergic agent that has been used in the treatment of severe mania and treatment-resistant bipolar disorder. Its biphasic effect is hypothesized to act on presynaptic autoreceptors to inhibit dopaminergic transmission at lower dosages, while acting as a dopamine postsynaptic receptor agonist at high dosages. Dosages of 7.5 to 15 mg/day have been used with responses seen in 2 to 14 days.[55] Rebound psychiatric and physical symptoms have been reported on acute discontinuation; thus verapamil should be tapered slowly.

Gabapentin. Gabapentin (Neurontin) is an anticonvulsant agent that is used in the treatment of bipolar disorder. Gabapentin is dosed up to 3600 mg/day, with usual dosing at 900 to 1800 mg/day in divided doses. Gabapentin has been effective in treating patients with mania or hypomanic symptoms as well as patients with treatment-refractory bipolar disorder. Open trials and case reports have demonstrated efficacy in rapid cycling. Gabapentin may be more effective in bipolar II disorder or when used as an adjunctive medication to another mood stabilizer. Mood-elevating properties are certainly present, and verapamil may actually induce mania itself. Sedation may be a beneficial effect during the manic phase when accompanied by anxiety or insomnia. Tremor can limit therapy, especially at higher dosages; other side effects include hypotension, ataxia, incoordination, gastrointestinal effects, increased appetite, and weight gain.

Lamotrigine. Lamotrigine (Lamictal) has been used in the treatment of bipolar disorder at dosages of 100 to 500 mg/day, beginning at 50 mg/day and gradually increasing every 2 weeks up to 250 mg twice daily. Lamotrigine is an anticonvulsant $5HT_3$ blocker; it stabilizes neural membranes and modulates the release of excitatory amino acids. Conservative dosing minimizes the potential for nausea; lower dosages are advised when combined with valproate because of the potential for elevated plasma levels and increased risk of rash. Lamotrigine has demonstrated efficacy in patients with rapid-cycling refractory bipolar disorder; efficacy has also been reported in depressed, hypomanic, manic, and mixed states. Antidepressant properties have suggested its use as an augmentor of antidepressant response and bipolar disorder. Significant adverse effects may be noted, including rash in approximately 10% of patients with increased risk in combination with valproate, with higher dosages, and in children. Stevens-Johnson syndrome has been reported in 1% to 2% of children and 0.1% of adults. Lamotrigine's activating effects may result in a switch to mania, especially with higher dosages. Agitation, insomnia, and cognitive blunting (a "spaced out" feeling) have been reported. Cardiovascular effects include restlessness, dizziness, and conduction changes.[23,25]

Topiramate. Topiramate (Topamax), another anticonvulsant GABA agonist, has been reported to be useful in bipolar disorder at dosages of 200 to 600 mg/day. Responses at low dosages of topiramate (25 mg twice daily) have been reported. Open-label studies suggest efficacy in acute mania as well as adjunctive use in combination with other mood stabilizers. Some efficacy in rapid cycling has also been suggested. Onset of side effects may be delayed by 1 to 2 weeks, suggesting the need to titrate dosages slowly. Adverse effects include weight loss, cognitive side effects, fatigue, dizziness, and parethesias.[25]

REFERENCES

1. American Psychiatric Association: *Diagnostic and statistical manual of mental disorders-TR*, ed 4, revised, Washington, DC, 2000, The Association.

2. Ascher JA and others: Bupropion: a review of its mechanism of antidepressant activity, *J Clin Psychiatry* 56:395, 1995.

3. Ayd FJ Jr: *Lexicon of psychiatry, neurology and the neurosciences*, Baltimore, 1995, Williams & Wilkins.

4. Baldesserini RJ: *Chemotherapy in psychiatry*, Cambridge, Mass, 1985, Harvard University.

5. Bennet J and others, *J Clin Psychopharmacol* 17(2):141, 1997.

6. Bernstein JG: *Handbook of drug therapy in psychiatry*, ed 3, St Louis, 1995, Mosby.

7. Blier P, Bergeron R: Effectiveness of pindolol with selected antidepressant drugs in the treatment of major depression, *J Clin Psychopharmacol* 15:217, 1995.

8. Bowden CL and others: Efficacy of divalproex vs lithium and placebo in the treatment of mania, *JAMA* 271:918, 1994.

9. Brown WA, Harrison W: Are patients who are intolerant to one serotonin selective reuptake inhibitor intolerant to another? *J Clin Psychiatry* 56:1, 1995.

10. Cade JFJ: Lithium salts in the treatment of psychotic excitement, *Med J Aust* 2:349, 1949.

11. Carney MW, Toone BK, Reynoldo EH: S-adenosylmethionine and affective disorder, *Am J Med* 83:95, 1987.

12. Chouinard G: Antimanic effects of clonazepam, *Psychosomatics* 26(12):7, 1985.

13. Claghorn JL, Lesem MD: A double-blind placebo-controlled study of ORG 3770 in depressed outpatients, *J Affect Disord* 34:165, 1995.

14. Cohen LS: Psychotropic drug use in pregnancy, *Hosp Community Psychiatry* 40:566, 1989.

15. Cohen LS and others: Birth outcomes following prenatal exposure to fluoxetine. Poster presented at the 150th Annual Meeting of the American Psychiatric Association, San Diego, Calif, May 17-22, 1997.

16. Coupland NT, Bell CJ, Potokar JP: Serotonin reuptake inhibitor withdrawal, *J Clin Psychopharmacol* 16(5):356, 1996.

17. Cunningham LA and others: A comparison of venlafaxine, trazodone, and placebo in major depression, *J Clin Psychopharmacol* 14(2):99, 1994.

18. Denolle T and others. Hemodynamic effects of reboxetine in healthy male volunteers, *Clin Pharm Ther* 66:282, 1999.

19. Dubovsky SL, Buzan RD: Verapamil in bipolar disorder, *CNS Drugs* 4(1):47, 1995.

20. Dubovsky SL, Buzan RD: Novel alternatives and supplements to lithium and anticonvulsants for bipolar affective disorder, *J Clin Psychiatry* 58(5):224, 1997.

21. Eikelboom JW and others: Homocyst(e)ine and cardiovascular disease: a critical review of the epidemiologic evidence, *Ann Intern Med* 131:363, 1999.

22. Eriksson E, Hedberg MA, Andersch B, Sundblad C: The serotonin reuptake inhibitor paroxetine is superior to the noradrenaline reuptake inhibitor maprotiline in the treatment of premenstrual syndrome, *Neuropsychopharmacology* 12:169, 1995.

23. Fatemi SH and others: Lamotrigine in rapid-cycling bipolar disorder, *J Clin Psychiatry* 58(12):522, 1997.

24. Freud S: Mourning and melancholia. In *The complete psychological works of Sigmund Freud*, London, 1957, Hogarth.

25. Ghaemi SN, Katzow JJ, Desai SP: Lamotrigine in bipolar disorder, *Int Drug Therapy Newslett* 34(4):25, 1999.

26. Goldstein DJ, Sundell KL, Corbin LA: Birth outcomes in pregnant women taking fluoxetine (letter to editor). *N Engl J Med* 336:872, 1997.

27. Goodnick PJ: Nimodipine treatment of rapid cycling bipolar disorder, *J Clin Psychiatry* 56(7):330, 1995.

28. Guelfi JD, White C, Magni G: A randomized double-blind comparison of venlafaxine and placebo in inpatients with major depression and melancholia, *Clin Neuropharmacol* 15(suppl 1):323b, 1992.

29. Harsch HH, Holt RE: Use of antidepressants in attempted suicide, *Hosp Community Psychiatry* 39:990, 1988.

30. Heninger GR, Charney DS, Sternberg DE: Lithium carbonate augmentation of antidepressant treatment: an effective prescription for treatment-refractory depression, *Arch Gen Psychiatry* 40:1335, 1983.

31. Hirschfield RM: Care of the sexually active depressed patient, *J Clin Psychiatry* 60(suppl 17):32, 1999.

32. Hudson JI and others: Fluvoxamine in the treatment of binge-eating disorder: a multicenter placebo-controlled, double-blind trial, *Am J Psychiatry* 155(12):1756, 1998.

33. Joffe RT, Singer W: Thyroid hormone potentiation of antidepressants. In Amsterdam JD, editor: *Refractory depression: advances in neuropsychiatry and psychopharmacology,* vol 2, New York, 1991, Raven Press.

34. Katona C and others: Reboxetine versus imipramine in the treatment of elderly patients with depressive disorders: a double-blind randomised trial, *J Aff Disord* 55:203, 1999.

35. Keck PE and others: Valproate oral loading in the treatment of acute mania, *J Clin Psychiatry* 54(8):305, 1993.

36. Keltner NL: Venlafaxine: a novel antidepressant, *J Psychosoc Nurs Ment Health Serv* 33(1): 51, 1995.

37. Keltner NL and others: *Psychobiological foundations of psychiatry care,* St Louis, 1998, Mosby.

38. Kupfer DJ: Long-term treatment of depression, *J Clin Psychiatry* 52(suppl 5):28, 1991.

39. Meador-Woodruff JH: Psychiatric side effects of tricyclic antidepressants, *Hosp Comm Psychiatry* 41:84, 1990.

40. Mendels J and others: Efficacy and safety of b.i.d. doses of venlafaxine in a dose-response study, *Psychopharmacol Bull* 29:169, 1993.

41. Mitchell JE, Raymond N, Specker S: A review of the controlled trials of pharmacotherapy and psychotherapy in the treatment of bulimia nervosa, *Int J Eating Disorders* 14:229, 1993.

42. Mucci M: Reboxetine: a review of antidepressant tolerability, *J Psychopharmacol* 11(suppl): S33, 1997.

43. Nulman I and others: Neurodevelopment of children exposed in utero to antidepressant drugs, *N Engl J Med* 336:258, 1997.

44. Ortiz A, Dabbagh M, Gershon S: Lithium: clinical use, toxicology, and mode of action. In Bernstein JG, editor: *Clinical psychopharmacology,* ed 2, Boston, 1984, John Wright BPSG.

45. Pozzaglia PS and others, *J Clin Psychopharmacology* 18(5):404, 1998.

46. Preskorn SH, Magnus RD: Inhibition of hepatic P-450 isoenzymes by serotonin selective reuptake inhibitors: in vitro and in vivo findings and their implications for patient care, *Psychopharmacol Bull* 30:251, 1994.

47. Price LH, Charney DS, Heninger GR: Efficacy of lithium-tranylcypromine treatment in refractory depression, *Am J Psychiatry* 142:619, 1985.

48. Prien RF, Kupfer DJ: Continuation of drug therapy for major depressive episodes: how long should it be maintained? *Am J Psychiatry* 143:18, 1986.

49. Risch SC, Janowsky DS, Hyey LY: Plasma levels of tricyclic antidepressants and clinical efficacy. In Enna SJ, Malick JB, Richelson E, editors: *Antidepressants: neurochemical, behavioral, and clinical perspectives,* New York, 1981, Raven Press.

50. Rosenbaum JF and others: Selective serotonin reuptake inhibitor discontinuation syndrome: a randomized clinical trial, *Biol Psychiatry* 44:77, 1998.

51. Rothschild AJ: Selective serotonin reuptake inhibitor-induced sexual dysfunction: efficacy of a drug holiday, *Am J Psychiatry* 152:10, 1995.

52. Schmidt PJ, Grover GN, Rubinow DR: Alprazolam in the treatment of premenstrual syndrome: a double-blind, placebo-controlled trial, *Arch Gen Psychiatry* 50:467, 1993.

53. Segraves RT: Treatment-emergent sexual dysfunction in affective disorder: a review and management strategies, *J Clin Psychiatry* (Update Monogr) 1:1, 1994.

54. Settle EC and others: Safety profile of sustained-release bupropion in depression: results of three clinical trials, *Clin Ther* 21:3454, 1999.

55. Sitland-Marken PA and others: Psychiatric applications of bronocriptine therapy, *J Clin Psychiatry* 51(2):68, 1990.

56. Sitsen JMA, Zivkov M: Mirtazapine: clinical profile, *CNS Drugs* 4(suppl 1):39, 1995.

57. Stahl S and others: Meta-analyses of randomized, double-blind, placebo-controlled efficacy and safety studies of mirtazepine versus amitriptyline in major depression, *Acta Psychiatr Scand* 96(suppl 391):22, 1997.

58. Steiner M and others: Fluoxetine in the treatment of premenstrual dysphoria, *N Engl J Med* 332:1529, 1995.

59. Stern SI, Mendels J: Drug combinations in the treatment of refractory depression: a review, *J Clin Psychiatry* 42:368, 1981.

60. Sugarman JR: Management of lithium intoxication, *Fam Pract* 18:347, 1984.

61. Sundblad C, Modigh K, Andersch B, Eriksson E: Clomipramine effectively reduces premenstrual irritability and dysphoria: a placebo-controlled trial, *Acta Psychiatr Scand* 85:39, 1992.

62. Walton SA and others: Superiority of lithium over verapamil in mania: a randomized controlled single-blind trial, *J Clin Psychiatry* 57(11):543, 1996.

63. Williams R and others: A double-blind comparison of moclobemide and fluoxetine in the treatment of depressive disorder, *Int Clin Psychopharmacol* 7:155, 1993.

64. Winokur G: Types of depressive illness, *Br J Psychiatry* 120:265, 1972.

65. Wisner KL, Perel JM: Serum nortriptyline levels in nursing mothers and their infants, *Am J Psychiatry* 148:1234, 1991.

66. Yonkers KA: Treatment of premenstrual dysphoric disorder, *Curr Rev Mood Anxiety Disord* 1:215, 1997.

67. Yonkers KA and others: Symptomatic improvement of premenstrual dysphoric disorder with sertraline treatment: a randomized controlled trial, *JAMA* 278(12):983, 1997.

68. Yoshida K, Smith B, Channi Kumar R: Fluvoxamine in breast milk and infant development (letter to editor), *Br J Clin Pharmacol* 44:210, 1997.

69. Yu PH, Boulton AA: Clinical pharmacology of MAO-B inhibitors. In Kennedy SH, editor: *Clinical advances in monoamine oxidase inhibitor therapies*, Washington, DC, 1994, American Psychiatric Press.

70. Zajecka JM, Jeffriess H, Fawcett J: The efficacy of fluoxetine combined with a heterocyclic antidepressant in treatment-resistant depression: a retrospective analysis, *J Clin Psychiatry* 56(8):338, 1995.

71. Zimmerman PG: Tricyclic antidepressant overdose, *Am J Nurs* 97(10):39, 1997.

72. Zubenko GS, Cohen BM, Lipinski JF: Comparison of metoprolol and propranolol in the treatment of lithium tremor, *Psychiatry Res* 11:163, 1984.

CHAPTER 7

Anxiety Disorders

HISTORICAL CONSIDERATIONS

Anxiety is as old as mankind, and attempts to allay this subjective uneasiness by ingesting something are just as old. The earliest self-medicating strategy involved alcohol. Even today in the 21st century, alcohol is still the most commonly self-prescribed treatment for anxiety.

Many compounds historically used for anxiety were neither safe nor effective in long-term treatment (Box 7-1). For example, bromo seltzers were proclaimed efficacious at the turn of the 20th century, yet bromide dependency became a significant problem, and these products were withdrawn from the market.[30] Subsequently, barbiturates were developed as a potentially safe class of drugs; again, their development was followed by the recognition of adverse effects, including seizures and the potential for addiction, dependence, and withdrawal. Other agents, such as opioids and tincture of belladonna, were fraught with significant problems of abuse and dependence as well.

A major advance following barbiturates was the development of meprobamate in the mid-1950s. This drug was initially heralded as an effective and addiction-free agent. However, widespread use of meprobamate resulted in symptoms of addiction and withdrawal. The first benzodiazepine, chlordiazepoxide (Librium), appeared on the scene in the 1960s (Figure 7-1). Introduced with the promise of efficacy and safety, withdrawal symptoms were observed similar to those seen with meprobamate and the barbiturates. Finally, in 1986, buspirone (BuSpar), a structurally unique nonbenzodiazepine antianxiety drug, was introduced. This drug did not have the tolerance, dependency, or withdrawal symptoms associated with its predecessors. The development of anxiolytic compounds has improved safety and efficacy, yet the dangers of dependency and the complications associated with anxiolytic treatment persist with some agents. Drugs currently under study hold promise that anxiolytic compounds will someday be available without the adverse effects typical of this class of agents.

DIAGNOSTIC CONSIDERATIONS

Anxiety may represent a symptom, a syndrome, or a disorder, or it may be part of another psychiatric disorder, for example, major depression (Table 7-1). The current nomenclature suggests that anxiety may be experienced in anticipation of an unpleasant or stressful experience (anticipatory or situational anxiety), may be experienced as a component of a phobia, or may occur without an apparent external cause, as with panic anxiety. Obsessive-compulsive disorder (OCD) is a specific type of anxiety associated with intrusive thoughts and compulsive rituals. Posttraumatic stress disorder (PTSD) is characterized by symptoms that follow a psychologically distressing event. Generalized anxiety disorder (GAD) is characterized by unrealistic or excessive anxiety and worry focused on two or more life circumstances. The pharmacologic approach to generalized and other specific anxiety disorders is discussed in this chapter.

Box 7-1   Historical and Contemporary Anxiolytic Drugs

Historical (primarily)
Alcohol
Opioids
Belladonna
Barbiturates
Meprobamate
Phenothiazines
Bromo seltzers

Contemporary
Antihistamines
Beta-blockers
Benzodiazepines
Monoamine oxidase inhibitors
SSRI antidepressants
Buspirone
Cyclic antidepressants

SSRI, Selective serotonin reuptake inhibitor.

Table 7-1   DSM-IV Anxiety Disorders

1. Generalized anxiety disorder
2. Panic disorder without agoraphobia
3. Panic disorder with agoraphobia
4. Agoraphobia without a history of panic disorder
5. Specific phobia
6. Social phobia
7. Obsessive-compulsive disorder
8. Posttraumatic stress disorder
9. Anxiety disorder resulting from a general medical condition
10. Substance-induced anxiety disorder
11. Anxiety disorder not otherwise specified

Adapted from American Psychiatric Association: *Diagnostic and statistical manual of mental disorders-TR,* Washington, DC, 2000, The Association.

GENERALIZED ANXIETY DISORDER

GAD is manifested by unrealistic or excessive anxiety or worry about two or more life circumstances that persists for 6 months or longer. Diagnostic features are listed in Box 7-2. The symptoms of GAD may vary and are distinct from the types of anxiety associated with mood or psychotic disorders. Symptoms of anxiety may be generally described as psychologic or somatic (Boxes 7-3 and 7-4). Symptoms of anxiety disturb concentration, result in irritability or sleep disturbance, and if they persist, result in "chronic" anxiety. Essentially, the anxiety and worry are excessive, pervasive, and uncontrollable. The person finds it difficult to focus attention on the tasks at hand because worry and energies are directed toward seeking relief.

Especially noteworthy in primary care and ambulatory outpatient facilities are individuals who manifest mixed symptoms of anxiety and depression. This

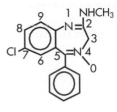

Chlordiazepoxide

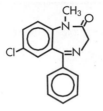

Diazepam

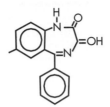

Oxazepam

Clorazepate

Lorazepam

Prazepam

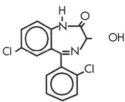

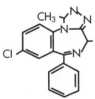

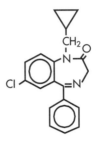

Halazepam

Alprazolam

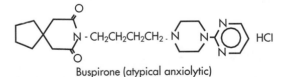

Buspirone (atypical anxiolytic)

Figure 7-1 Chemical structures of benzodiazepines and buspirone.

subsyndromal disorder may cause significant impairment or distress and is responsive to a pharmacologic agent. Clinically significant anxiety may be present as a result of a general medical condition or may be induced by specific substances such as medications or foodstuffs. It is often difficult to determine whether the anxiety exists primarily or secondarily; despite the presence of a general medical condition or substance use disorder, anxiety often becomes a focus of treatment (Table 7-2 and Box 7-5).

Box 7-2 Diagnostic Features of Generalized Anxiety Disorder

Excessive worry and apprehension
Difficulty controlling worry
Associated symptoms*
1. Restlessness/nervousness
2. Fatigue
3. Concentration difficulties
4. Irritability
5. Tension
6. Sleep disturbance

Modified from American Psychiatric Association: *Diagnostic and statistical manual of mental disorders-TR*, ed 4, Washington, DC, 2000, The Association.
*Three or more are needed to meet current diagnostic criteria.

Box 7-3 Psychologic Symptoms of Anxiety

The patient may be the following:
Anxious
Apprehensive
Compulsive
Fearful
Experiencing feelings of dread
Irritable
Intolerant
Nervous
Overconcerned

Panicky
Phobic
Preoccupied
Repetitive in motor activities
Feeling threatened
Wound up
Sensitive to shame
Worried

Box 7-4 Somatic Signs and Symptoms of Anxiety

Anorexia
Backache
"Butterflies" in stomach
Chest discomfort
Diaphoresis
Diarrhea
Dizziness
Dyspnea
Dry mouth
Faintness

Fatigue
Flushing
Headache
Hyperventilation
Light-headedness
Muscle tension
Nausea
Pallor
Palpitations
Paresthesia

Sexual dysfunction
Shortness of breath
Stomach pain
Sweating
Tachycardia
Tremulousness
Urinary frequency
Vomiting

Table 7-2 Drugs That Can Induce Anxiety*

Drug category	Example
Stimulants	Caffeine
Anorectics	Fenfluramine
Analgesics	Salicylates
Anticholinergics	Diphenhydramine
Hallucinogens	Cannabis
Sympathomimetics	Ephedrine
Steroids	Prednisone
Neuroleptics (akathisia)	Haloperidol
Diuretics	Acetazolamide

*Anxiety may emerge acutely or with long-term treatment.

Box 7-5 General Medical Causes of Anxiety

Cardiovascular disorders
Arrhythmias, especially paroxysmal
Atrial tachycardia
Angina pectoris
Mitral valve prolapse
Orthostatic hypotension
Myocardial infarction

Endocrine disorders
Hyperthyroidism
Hypothyroidism
Pheochromocytoma
Hypoglycemia
Carcinoid syndrome
Hypoparathyroidism
Insulinoma
Cushing's syndrome
Acute intermittent porphyria

Respiratory disorders
Chronic obstructive
  respiratory disease
Hypoxia resulting from any cause
Pulmonary embolism
Asthma

Neurologic disorders
Aura of migraine
Early dementia
Cerebral neoplasia
Delirium
Partial complex seizures
Demyelinating disease
Vestibular disturbance
Postconcussive syndrome
Withdrawal from sedative-
  hypnotics, caffeine, or nicotine

From Rosenbaum JF, Pollack MH. In Hackett TP, Cassem NH, editors: *Massachusetts General Hospital handbook of general hospital psychiatry,* ed 2, Littleton, Mass, 1987, PSG Publishing.

Treatment of Generalized Anxiety Disorder

The most efficacious treatment approach to GAD skillfully combines pharmacotherapy, psychotherapy, and behavioral techniques in the context of general medical management. Benzodiazepines are the most widely prescribed agents for general symptoms of anxiety. These agents are most appropriately prescribed with situational or acute anxiety or in conjunction with another medication that will be used long term. Benzodiazepines are sometimes prescribed in a cavalier fashion, providing the patient with a quick fix. Unfortunately, this strategy may serve to alleviate distress but

Table 7-3   Comparison of Benzodiazepines and Buspirone

Benzodiazepines	Buspirone
Rapid onset of therapeutic effect	Delayed onset of effect (full effect, 3-6 weeks)
Effective in many anxiety disorders	FDA approved for GAD only but used with success in other anxiety disorders
Can cause sedation	Does not cause sedation
May impair performance	Does not impair performance
Additive effects with alcohol	No additive effect with alcohol
May cause dependence and withdrawal	Does not cause dependence and withdrawal
Abuse potential	No abuse potential
Pharmacokinetic changes with age	No pharmacokinetic change with age
Associated with falls in elderly	Does not cause falls in elderly

Adapted from Reference 41.
FDA, Food and Drug Administration; *GAD,* generalized anxiety disorder.

may also diminish the patient's awareness of his or her stressors. Ultimately, these drugs may interfere with the patient's ability to adapt, to adjust lifestyle, or to improve coping behaviors. A haphazard pharmacologic approach may simply serve as a substitute for the time required to assist an anxious or unhappy individual to discover and modify the sources of his or her psychic pain. Thus benzodiazepines are best prescribed in short courses or single doses for acute situational anxiety.

Buspirone represents the first of a new generation of anxiolytic compounds that conceptually fall within a subtype of nonbenzodiazepine anxiolytics. The structural and pharmacologic properties of buspirone are unrelated to those of the benzodiazepines (see Figure 7-1 and Table 7-3). Buspirone is not a central nervous system (CNS) depressant, nor does it produce significant sedation, yet it alleviates many symptoms of GAD.

Benzodiazepines, buspirone, and certain antidepressant agents (e.g., venlafaxine [Effexor]) are the more efficacious agents for the treatment of general symptoms of anxiety. An anxious patient may feel uncomfortable and nervous and may have prominent physical signs and symptoms (see Box 7-4). In fact, severe anxiety is usually accompanied by a variety of somatic or autonomic nervous system manifestations, including dry mouth, tachycardia, palpitations, irregular heart rhythm, dizziness, diarrhea, abdominal pain, headache, and other neuromuscular symptoms. These physiologic, somatic, and autonomic manifestations may be present in each of the various subtypes of anxiety. Autonomic overactivity may not be fully responsive to benzodiazepines or antidepressant medications, whereas beta-adrenergic blocking drugs such as propranolol, metoprolol, atenolol, or pindolol may dramatically inhibit the physiologic manifestations of anxiety. This ability to inhibit physiologic anxiety has also made beta-blockers a popular "stage fright" antidote.

ANXIOLYTIC MEDICATIONS
BENZODIAZEPINES

Among anxiolytics, the benzodiazepines have dominated clinical practice for more than three decades. The structures of most of these agents are shown in Figure 7-1. The dosage range, dosage equivalencies, half-lives, and anxiolytic and sedative effects of benzodiazepines are provided in Table 7-4.

Table 7-4 Antianxiety Drugs: Usual Daily Dosage, Equivalent Doses, Half-Life, and Anxiolytic and Sedative Effects

	Usual daily dose (mg/day)	Equivalent dose (mg)	Half-life (hr)	Anxiolytic effect	Sedative effect
Benzodiazepines					
Short-acting	Triazolam (Halcion) 0.125-0.5	0.25	1.5-5	x	xxx
Intermediate	Alprazolam (Xanax) 0.75-4*	0.5	12-15	xx	x
Intermediate	Halazepam (Paxipam) 60-160*	40	14-100†	xx	-
Intermediate	Lorazepam (Ativan) 2-6*	1	10-20	xxx	xx
Intermediate	Oxazepam (Serax) 30-60*	15	5-20	xx	x
Intermediate	Temazepam (Restoril) 10-60	10	10-15	x	xxx
Long-acting	Chlordiazepoxide (Librium) 15-100*	25	5-30†	xx	—
Long-acting	Clonazepam (Klonopin) 0.5-10*	0.25	18-60†	xx	x
Long-acting	Clorazepate (Tranxene) 7.5-60*	10	30-100†	xx	—
Long-acting	Diazepam (Valium) 4-40*	5	20-80†	xxx	xx
Long-acting	Flurazepam (Dalmane) 15-30	15	3-150†	x	xxx
Long-acting	Prazepam (Centrax) 20-40*	10	30-100†	xx	—
Long-acting	Quazepam (Doral) 7.5-30*	7.5	30-150†	x	xxx
Nonbenzodiazepines					
	Buspirone (BuSpar) 15-40*		2-11†	xxx	—

Adapted from References 11 and 41; and previous edition of *Psychotropic drugs*, St Louis, 1997, Mosby.
x, Weak; *xx*, moderate; *xxx*, strong effect.
*Given in divided doses.
†With active metabolite.

Pharmacologic Effect

Many benzodiazepine agents used primarily to treat anxiety are helpful in inducing sleep and exert a dose-related depressant effect on the CNS (see Chapter 10). Benzodiazepines compete for gamma-aminobutyric acid (GABA) receptors in the brain and for specific benzodiazepine receptors responsible for the selective actions on neuronal pathways throughout the CNS. The anxiolytic potency of the various benzodiazepines correlates with their affinity for benzodiazepine receptors.

Benzodiazepines increase the affinity of GABA molecules for their specific receptor. GABA is a naturally occurring inhibitory neurotransmitter. Benzodiazepines increase the frequency with which anion (i.e., chloride) channels open in response to GABA.[22] The relationship of GABA to specific anxiolytic effects of benzodiazepines is not definitively known; however, the GABAergic action of benzodiazepines may at least partially account for their anticonvulsant and muscle relaxant effects. Benzodiazepines may also decrease norepinephrine and serotonin turnover rates. This mechanism may partially account for the antianxiety and sedative effects of the benzodiazepines.

Pharmacokinetics

Benzodiazepines differ from one another with respect to their pharmacokinetic profile. In general, benzodiazepines are completely absorbed and reach peak plasma levels 30 minutes to 4 hours after oral administration. Intravenously administered diazepam has an immediate effect but is absorbed unpredictably when injected intramuscularly. This erratic intramuscular absorption is observed with all benzodiazepines except lorazepam (Ativan). High-potency benzodiazepines (e.g., lorazepam and alprazolam) are also rapid acting.

Benzodiazepines are lipophilic and 85% to 90% bound to plasma proteins. The pharmacokinetics of benzodiazepines are often complex because many have active metabolites that dominate the course of their pharmacologic effect. Agents with slowly eliminated active metabolites have prolonged clinical actions and are categorized as long-acting benzodiazepines. Plasma levels that approach twice the level considered effective and safe may be associated with undesirable degrees of sedation or may begin to result in toxicity. Thus long-acting benzodiazepines should be given in two to four small single daily doses. Shorter-acting agents are also best given in two to four small portions as well to maintain steady plasma levels. This dosing strategy is especially important for the treatment of daytime anxiety, in which a minimal amount of oversedation is desirable and therapeutic.

Lorazepam, oxazepam (Serax), and alprazolam (Xanax) are exceptional benzodiazepines in that they have virtually no important pharmacologically active metabolites. However, all three of these agents ultimately rely on conjugation with glucuronic acid to form inactive metabolites. Because benzodiazepines rely heavily on hepatic mechanisms, they must be used cautiously in patients with liver disease because the ability to eliminate these agents may be significantly reduced by the liver disease. Oxazepam and lorazepam represent the safest benzodiazepines for patients with inefficient hepatic functioning.

Side Effects

The most commonly encountered nontherapeutic side effects of the benzodiazepines are sedation, decreased mental acuity, and some decrease in coordination. This may lead to occupational inefficiency, decreased productivity, and an increased risk of accidents. Combining these drugs with alcohol increases the risk of adverse effects. Autonomic, anticholinergic, and extrapyramidal side effects are rarely encountered. Liver damage, blood dyscrasias, and other end-organ toxic effects are also rare. Benzodiazepines may be associated with dysphoria, irritability, agitation, or otherwise "disinhibited" behavior. These reactions seem to be more characteristic of the benzodiazepines than of barbiturates or meprobamate.[6] Some other side effects of benzodiazepines may include weight gain, skin reactions, headache, impairment of sexual function, and menstrual irregularity. However, it is often difficult to determine whether these are symptoms of anxiety or drug side effects. In addition, when benzodiazepine doses are temporarily discontinued or dosage reduction occurs rapidly, it may be difficult to determine whether the patient has resurfacing anxiety or mild symptoms of drug withdrawal.

Perhaps the most serious unwarranted effect of the benzodiazepines and other sedative-hypnotics is their relative tendency to produce tolerance, physiologic dependence, and psychologic habituation. Tolerance can contribute to innocent self-medication and dose escalation. Furthermore, because of their ability to produce euphoria or intoxication, these drugs may have street value. The probability of becoming physiologically dependent or of developing tolerance depends largely on the daily dose and the duration of use. Physiologic dependence on some benzodiazepines (chlordiazepoxide and diazepam) has been studied extensively; however, the greatest risks of tolerance and dependence may be more significant with the relatively shorter-acting, high-potency benzodiazepines alprazolam and lorazepam.

Treatment Implications

Therapeutic versus toxic levels. Because benzodiazepines may decrease mental alertness, patients should be cautioned about driving or operating hazardous machinery. Fortunately, tolerance to most benzodiazepine side effects develops quickly. Blood pressure should be monitored; a drop of 20 mm Hg (systolic) on standing warrants clinical assessment. Therapeutic levels of benzodiazepines have a comfortable margin of safety compared with those of other sedatives. However, overdoses equivalent to approximately twice a monthly supply, or even less, when taken with alcohol, have led to death. Moreover, the use of long-acting benzodiazepines, as well as the use of intravenous diazepam or lorazepam to control seizures or cardiac arrhythmias, is occasionally complicated by respiratory depression, apnea, ventricular arrhythmias, or even cardiac arrest. Most deliberate overdoses seem to involve more than one agent; typically alcohol is involved. Thus it is difficult to assess or determine what supply of benzodiazepines would be considered safe. The continued use of benzodiazepines for longer than several weeks should be applied in the context of the critical appraisal of risks and benefits in individual cases.

Use in pregnancy. The safety of sedative tranquilizer use in pregnancy is not established. There is inconclusive evidence that benzodiazepines may be teratogenic, causing cleft lip and palate in the first trimester. The level of risk involved is probably below the overall level of risk for birth defects, and in general, the risk of toxic effects of benzodiazepines in pregnancy is low.

Use in the elderly. Benzodiazepines are commonly prescribed for elderly individuals. Several important age-related changes may cause benzodiazepines to have a greater effect in this population. First, pharmacodynamic considerations related to receptor sensitivity can cause these drugs to have a greater effect. Furthermore, pharmacokinetic differences in this population cause a different response in older persons compared with younger adults. The higher ratio of fat to muscle in this age group and reduction in phase I or oxidative metabolic proficiency tends toward the development of longer elimination half-lives, leading to drug accumulation. Hence relatively shorter-acting drugs without active metabolites (lorazepam, oxazepam, alprazolam) metabolized primarily by nonoxidative mechanisms should be prescribed for older individuals.

Interactions. Benzodiazepines tend to have low potential for pharmacokinetic interactions with most other drugs. The possible exceptions are the monoamine oxidase inhibitors (MAOIs), which potentiate the sedating effects of the benzodiazepines, and nefazodone (Serzone), which inhibits cytochrome P-450 enzymes involved in the metabolism of alprazolam and triazolam. Unlike barbiturates, the benzodiazepines have minor ability to induce their own hepatic metabolism. Benzodiazepines also have less potential for tolerance building and dose escalating. In other words, in contrast to the barbiturates, a sustained antianxiety or hypnotic effect does not require steadily increasing doses of the benzodiazepines. However, tolerance to the sedating effects and habituation may develop. Marked withdrawal symptoms are indicative of prolonged use at higher dosages. Withdrawal from benzodiazepines can manifest as anxiety, insomnia, anorexia, vertigo, tremor, irritability, tinnitus, headache, perceptual disturbances, depression, autonomic overactivity, and seizures.[41] High-potency, short-acting benzodiazepines present the greater risk of habituation and withdrawal, warranting a slow taper. Such risks of withdrawal are lessened or at least delayed with the use of long-acting benzodiazepines such as clonazepam.

Interactions between benzodiazepines and other agents may occur as previously noted for MAOIs and nefazodone. Phenytoin and digitalis preparations, when combined with the benzodiazepines, can also produce increased plasma levels via hepatic metabolic interactions. Alcohol and the MAOIs increase the intoxication potential of all benzodiazepines. Disulfiram and cimetidine, but apparently not other H_2-receptor blockers, lead to increased plasma levels of long-acting benzodiazepines such as chlordiazepoxide but not of shorter-acting benzodiazepines metabolized exclusively by conjugation (oxazepam and lorazepam). Antacids may decrease the absorption of benzodiazepines, especially clorazepate, chlordiazepoxide, and diazepam. In addition, the interaction between benzodiazepines and food may produce a differential effect on absorption. These effects may include an initial decrease in absorption followed by a gradual increase, particularly with diazepam.[6]

Patient education. Benzodiazepines have a great potential for both use and abuse. Consequently, it is important to teach the patient and his or her family about the associated risks and benefits. The clinician must instruct the patient and the family as follows:
1. Benzodiazepines are not used in response to the minor stresses of everyday life.
2. Over-the-counter drugs may potentiate the actions of benzodiazepines.
3. Driving should be avoided until tolerance develops.
4. Alcohol and other CNS depressants potentiate the effects of benzodiazepines.
5. Hypersensitivity to one benzodiazepine may mean hypersensitivity to another.
6. Benzodiazepine use should not be discontinued abruptly.

Treatment Issues

Diazepam and possibly other benzodiazepines have been known to result in disinhibition, a phenomenon often characterized by escalating agitation that may lead to violence or psychotic terror. This loss of behavioral control, sometimes associated with explosive or violent behavior, may occur during the course of benzodiazepine treatment. Some evidence suggests that oxazepam is least likely to have a disinhibiting effect.

Benzodiazepines possess well-known amnestic properties. This phenomenon has been observed during the treatment of patients and in various studies assessing the anesthetic use of benzodiazepines. Diazepam, for example, selectively impairs anterograde episodic memory and attention while sparing access to information in long-term memory.[42]

Alprazolam (and triazolam, discussed in Chapter 10) is structurally unique among the benzodiazepines, with a "triazolo" ring bearing a somewhat similar configuration to the tricyclic antidepressants (see Figure 7-1). Thus it is not surprising that alprazolam exerts antidepressant and antipanic effects. However, loss of behavioral control (disinhibition) may emerge in patients receiving alprazolam and may be connected with the antidepressant action or may simply parallel the disinhibiting effect of other benzodiazepines. Moreover, alprazolam has U.S. Food and Drug Administration (FDA) approval for use in treating anxiety with depressed mood and panic disorder (discussed later in this chapter). Not surprisingly, alprazolam has been reported to induce mania similar to that observed with conventional antidepressants (e.g., tricyclic antidepressants [TCAs]).[27] In contrast, clonazepam, differing somewhat in structure and having only partial benzodiazepine agonist effects, produces an antimanic effect, as discussed in Chapter 6.

The use of benzodiazepines in a manner conducive to the development of addiction is of great concern to patients and clinicians alike. Treatment should not be discontinued abruptly in patients who have taken high dosages for more than 3 months. This also applies to patients who are taking other sedative-hypnotic class agents such as barbiturates, meprobamate, and chloral hydrate. Recognizing the potential risks of dependency associated with the long-term use of these agents is important. In chronically anxious patients who need prolonged drug therapy, other agents are worthy of consideration, for example, buspirone or venlafaxine.

Patients with discrete panic attacks, phobic or social anxiety, OCD, or PTSD benefit primarily from antidepressants or other classes of drugs. Antidepressants that have significant sedating effects may provide some initial advantage in the treatment of the general symptoms of anxiety. Antipsychotic drugs have been both recommended and condemned for treating chronic anxiety. Because of the risk of tardive dyskinesia and other serious adverse effects, neuroleptics are best avoided for use in GAD.

Many sedating antihistamines have been used for the management of anxiety (and insomnia). These compounds exert some anticholinergic and other nontherapeutic effects. Hydroxyzine, diphenhydramine, and promethazine are examples of these drugs. Hydroxyzine, a moderately sedating nonphenothiazine antihistamine, has been popularly used in a regimen of 10 to 25 mg one to four times daily. However, all antihistamines produce antianxiety effects primarily through sedation and are therefore not recommended.

BUSPIRONE

Buspirone (BuSpar), which belongs to a chemical subgroup, the azapirones, is the first in a unique class of pure anxioselective agents. Differing substantially in both clinical and pharmacologic characteristics from the benzodiazepines, buspirone does not cause the sedation, hypnosis, anticonvulsant effects, nor muscle relaxant effects of the benzodiazepines. Three to six weeks are required for buspirone to achieve maximal anxiolytic effects. The anxiolytic action of buspirone may be caused in part by an active metabolite, 1-2 pyrimidinyl piperazine (1PP). The mechanism of buspirone's anxiolytic effect is uncertain but probably relates to its partial agonist effects at the serotonin $5HT_{1A}$ receptor postsynaptically and as a full agonist at these presynaptic receptors.[50] At high dosages, intrinsic dopaminergic activity theoretically occurs at cerebral, cortical, and midbrain levels. However, the drug primarily affects presynaptic dopamine autoreceptors. Buspirone has no significant neuroendocrine effects nor consequential antipsychotic effects. It does not affect GABA systems.

Buspirone is particularly useful in treating anxiety or mixed anxiety-depression because it poses few of the disadvantages associated with benzodiazepines, such as physical or psychologic dependence, and does not significantly interact with other compounds (with the exception of the MAOIs and haloperidol). Anxiety control is distinguished from the sedative and euphoric actions of older anxiolytic drugs. In particular, symptoms of worry, apprehension, irritability, difficulty with concentration and cognition, and an inability to cope are the focus of treatment. Consequently, improvement in target symptoms (e.g., decreased agitation, improved concentration, and improved function) is produced over 1 to 3 months. Patients taking regimens of buspirone often become less fearful, have fewer somatic symptoms, and are more interpersonally responsible than before treatment.

Pharmacokinetics

Buspirone is extensively metabolized, and after the first pass, as little as 1% to 4% becomes bioavailable. The main metabolite 1PP reaches relatively higher concentrations in the brain than does the parent compound buspirone itself. However, 1PP has only 1% to 20% of the potency of buspirone.[54] Buspirone is almost completely bound to plasma proteins (approximately 95%). The distribution half-life of 1PP is four times longer than that of buspirone; the distribution half-life of buspirone is short and difficult to fully establish. Food increases its bioavailability by decreasing first-pass metabolism. Buspirone is rapidly and completely absorbed and widely distributed to all tissues. The drug is excreted almost exclusively as metabolites.

Target symptoms in response to buspirone may begin to improve within days of initiation of an adequate dose, with the full effect occurring at an average of 3 to 6 weeks. The usual daily dose is 15 to 40 mg given in divided doses, with a range of 15 to 60 mg/day. Buspirone may be effective in mixed anxiety-depression or when cognitive and interpersonal problems exist.

Treatment Implications

Therapeutic versus toxic levels. The most remarkable aspect of buspirone is its safety. No reported deaths have resulted from overdosage of buspirone when it is taken alone. Early studies in which dosages of up to 2400 mg/day were used in patients with schizophrenia revealed no major untoward side effects. Common side effects associated with buspirone include headache, dizziness, light-headedness, and nausea, each of which can occur in 3% to 12% of patients.[21] Compared with the benzodiazepines, sedation seldom occurs with buspirone. In addition, objective measures of motor impairment are far more common with the benzodiazepines, and the additive effects seen when benzodiazepines are combined with alcohol are not observed with buspirone. Nonetheless, precautions against falls or driving are important should a sedative response occur with buspirone.

Interactions. As previously mentioned, drug interactions with buspirone are not observed; however, haloperidol does interact with buspirone in as much as serum levels of haloperidol increase. Cimetidine has been reported to increase the 1PP metabolite by 30%.[21] Interaction with MAOIs resulting in a hypertensive reaction has also been reported.

Use in pregnancy. No data exists regarding the use of buspirone during pregnancy.

Use in the elderly. Pharmacokinetics are not significantly different between younger patients and those older than 65.

Patient education. Buspirone has little potential for abuse; however, issues of safety and effective use should be considered when this agent is discussed with the patient. Patients should be taught the following:

- To avoid alcohol use and to inform the prescriber about prescription and nonprescription drugs he or she is taking
- To discuss pregnancy and breast-feeding with the prescriber
- To avoid driving or operating hazardous machinery if buspirone causes drowsiness, light-headedness, or dizziness

Treatment Issues

An important clinical implication is that buspirone cannot be substituted immediately for benzodiazepines; that is, their pharmacologic characteristics are dissimilar, and in clinical practice, buspirone takes many weeks to become fully therapeutic. Hence benzodiazepines must be gradually tapered while buspirone therapy is being initiated. The common complaint of insomnia, which may be present in patients with mixed anxiety-depression, may be appropriately treated with concomitant use of trazodone or other sedating compounds.

The anxioselectivity of buspirone, without antipsychotic effects, extrapyramidal side effects, and other sequelae of antipsychotic agents, implies that it cannot result in tardive dyskinesia despite its dopamine-related effects. Indeed, its serotonin-modulating effects, its intrinsic dopaminergic activity, and its presynaptic action theoretically alleviate tardive dyskinesia.

VENLAFAXINE

Venlafaxine extended release (Effexor XR) has recently been approved by the U.S. FDA as a first-line treatment for GAD (Table 7-5). Venlafaxine is the first FDA-approved product for the treatment of both depression and GAD. As noted, individuals diagnosed with GAD present with symptoms of excessive anxiety and worry that they find difficult to control. The intensity, duration, or frequency of this excessive anxiety and worry generally outweighs the actual possibility or effect of the circumstance causing the anxiety.[3] The anxiety and worry of GAD are not part of a more specific disorder, such as panic disorder, social phobia, or OCD. Furthermore, it is not related to concerns about other issues such as eating or gaining weight as seen in anorexia nervosa, neither is it caused by multiple physical complaints as seen in somatization disorder or hypochondriasis. In short, considerable variation exists among individuals who express symptoms or complaints of anxiety, and this may complicate accurate diagnosis and treatment of GAD. Nonetheless, patients with GAD often exhibit a wide variety of somatic complaints, including muscle trembling, twitching, or soreness; cold, clammy hands; dry mouth; sweating; nausea and/or diarrhea; and urinary frequency.

Venlafaxine has been shown to be well tolerated and significantly more efficacious than placebo when given once a day in the treatment of outpatients with GAD.[55] Venlafaxine is an inhibitor of both the serotonergic and norepinephrine reuptake transporters. The pharmacology of venlafaxine is discussed in greater detail in Chapter 6. Venlafaxine's mechanism of action differs considerably from other drugs indicated for the treatment of GAD. In 349 outpatients with long-term GAD (lasting 12 months or longer), venlafaxine showed significant rates of improvement at doses of 75 to 225 mg. Psychic anxiety was especially responsive at doses of 150 and 225 mg ($p = .01$). The most common adverse effects seen in studies of venlafaxine used for anxiety are nausea, insomnia, dry mouth, dizziness, and somnolence. Side effects

Table 7-5 Antidepressants Indicated for Anxiety

Agent	Class	Starting dose (mg)	Dosage range (mg/day)	Comment (FDA approval)
Clomi-pramine (Anafranil)	TCA	25-50	100-250	Approved for OCD 250 mg maximum dose because of increased risk of seizures
Fluvoxamine (Luvox)	SSRI	25-50	100-300	Approved for OCD
Paroxetine (Paxil)	SSRI	10-20	40-60	Approved for panic, OCD, and social anxiety
Sertraline (Zoloft)	SSRI	25	50-200	Approved for panic, OCD (adults and children), and PTSD
Venlafaxine (Effexor XR)	SNRI	37.5	75-225	Approved for generalized anxiety, 150- and 225-mg dosages are superior (possibly because of more potent norepinephrine reuptake)
Fluoxetine (Prozac)	SSRI	10-20	20-80	Approved for OCD

FDA, Food and Drug Administration; *TCA,* tricyclic antidepressant; *OCD,* obsessive-compulsive disorder; *SSRI,* selective serotonin reuptake inhibitor; *PTSD,* posttraumatic stress disorder; *SNRI,* selective serotonin norepinephrine reuptake inhibitor.

(as well as therapeutic response) are observed in a dose-response relationship in the range of 75 to 225 mg/day with once-a-day dosing. Fewer than 1% of the patients developed sustained increases in blood pressure that led to discontinuation. This phenomenon, discussed in Chapter 6, is an uncommon dose-related adverse effect. Overall, venlafaxine has proven to be a useful alternative to benzodiazepines and buspirone in the treatment of GAD. Venlafaxine offers low rates of discontinuation, convenient once-a-day dosing, and a reasonable rate of tolerance.

SPECIFIC ANXIETY DISORDERS

A number of specific anxiety disorders are distinct entities; these disorders appear to be individualized expressions of related biochemical and physiologic disturbances of brain function. For a comprehensive discussion, see *Psychobiological Foundations of Psychiatric Care,* by Keltner and others.[36] These disorders include panic disorders, OCD, phobias, and PTSD.

PANIC DISORDER

Patients with panic disorder have discrete episodes of intense fear, discomfort, or anxiety that may vary considerably in frequency and severity. During attacks, patients most commonly complain of shortness of breath, dizziness, palpitations, and sweating (Box 7-6). During a panic attack, patients may have a sense of impending doom, a fear of "going crazy," and a profound loss of control. Sometimes, these

Box 7-6 Clinical Features of Panic Disorder

1. Discrete and intense period of anxiety, apprehension, and distress
2. Associated symptoms
       Palpitations
       Sweating
       Trembling
       Dizziness or light-headedness
       Depersonalization or derealization
       Fear of going insane
       Dyspnea or a choking sensation
       Fear of dying
       Chest pain or discomfort
       Paresthesias
       Gastrointestinal upset
       Chills or hot flashes
3. Agoraphobia may occur with or without panic or vice versa

feelings are accompanied by feelings of depersonalization and derealization. Panic may be complicated by anticipatory anxiety, dependency, or agoraphobia. Rates of agoraphobia approach 90%; comorbid depression occurs in one third to one half of cases.[37]

The pharmacologic treatment alternatives for panic disorder are often best combined with other approaches, including behavioral techniques, psychotherapeutic intervention, and an attempt to identify any medical or physiologic contributors. Supportive psychotherapy together with pharmacotherapy may be beneficial, particularly with an emphasis on patient education about the disorder. Caffeine and other physiologic or environmental contributors to these attacks can be identified and discussed with the patient.

Currently, the biologic component of panic disorder is hypothesized to be increased sensitivity to augmented noradrenergic function with an impaired presynaptic noradrenergic regulation.[36] An association between the occurrence of mitral valve prolapse and panic disorder has been established. A subset of patients with atypical panic disorder may show hostility, irritability, severe derealization, and social withdrawal. Some of these patients may have evidence of partial complex seizure disorder and typically exhibit temporal lobe abnormalities on electroencephalogram. A therapeutic response may be observed with anticonvulsants such as carbamazepine, as well as with conventional treatments for panic.

Treatment

Four classes of drugs have proven therapeutically effective in managing panic disorder: benzodiazepines, TCAs or cyclic antidepressants, selective serotonin reuptake inhibitors (SSRIs), and MAOIs. Each class has advantages and disadvantages based on its therapeutic and side effect profiles.[8] The pharmacology of cyclic antidepressants, SSRIs, and MAOIs are reviewed in Chapter 6. Compared with placebo in patients with panic disorder, each of these classes of drugs can result in considerable benefit. Variations in efficacy between one drug and another may be evident between individuals. The SSRIs are the safest and represent effective treatment for panic.

Currently, two SSRIs, sertraline (Zoloft) and paroxetine (Paxil), are approved in the United States for the treatment of panic disorder. Starting doses, dosage ranges, and minimum effective doses are depicted in Table 7-5. With starting doses of 25 mg of sertraline or 10 mg of paroxetine and gradual titration to a minimum effective dose of 50 and 40 mg, respectively, reduction in the number of panic attacks can occur, with significant relief occurring as early as 2 weeks.[9] A full response may not occur for 6 to 12 weeks. Therefore the use of benzodiazepines for early symptom control and reduction of panic attacks is often well advised. Other SSRIs (fluvoxamine, citalopram, and fluoxetine) have demonstrated efficacy in clinical trials for panic disorder. A major issue in the use of SSRIs in the treatment of panic disorder concerns the residual avoidance behavior and other symptoms that may not robustly respond to drug therapy alone. Cognitive-behavioral therapy or behavioral techniques focusing on avoidant behavior are best combined with pharmacotherapy and psychoeducational approaches. Information on the nature of panic disorder and anxiety management skills (e.g., diaphragmatic breathing, cognitive restructuring, interoceptive exposure, and exposure) are also efficacious.[4]

Treating panic disorder with a benzodiazepine, either alprazolam or clonazepam, may be effective and is likely to provide immediate relief. Clonazepam has been effectively used to treat panic disorder, with good tolerability and effectiveness.[60] Alprazolam has received FDA approval for use in patients with panic disorder and has been found to be effective in a number of controlled studies.[38] However, clonazepam is equal or superior to alprazolam for treating panic disorder. Clonazepam, with its longer half-life and slower clearance, may be less likely than alprazolam to result in a withdrawal syndrome upon abrupt discontinuation. However, the longer half-life and slower clearance of clonazepam may produce a greater cumulative effect, which must be considered in each individual case.

Clonazepam is likely to be twice as potent as alprazolam (see Table 7-4) and therefore can be administered in smaller daily doses and can be taken once or twice daily, as opposed to the regimen of three or four doses per day for alprazolam. The average antipanic dose of alprazolam is approximately 3 mg/day, but 6 to 8 mg/day may be required to achieve a favorable response. Clonazepam exerts its antipanic effect at a daily dose of approximately 1.5 mg, although patients may require up to 4 to 6 mg/day. With either alprazolam or clonazepam, a low dosage should be used initially, with gradual upward titration as tolerated by the patient and as required to achieve symptom control. Alprazolam treatment may be started at a dosage of 0.25 mg three times daily, titrating at 0.25-mg increments every 1 to 3 days. Clonazepam treatment may be started at a dosage of 0.25 mg twice daily, with dosage increments of 0.25 mg every 1 to 2 days as tolerated. Because these benzodiazepines may produce drowsiness and impair performance, patients whose dosages are being titrated should be advised against such activities as driving and operating machinery until a stable dosage is established.

Tricyclic and cyclic antidepressants have been effectively used to treat individuals with panic disorder. Imipramine and, to a lesser extent, desipramine and clomipramine have been used in the United States to treat panic disorder.[4,14] Other cyclic antidepressants, including amitriptyline and trazodone, have also been reported to have antipanic effects. The dosages of tricyclic and cyclic agents to treat panic are comparable to those used in depressive illness (see Chapter 6). However, a lower dosage is initially prescribed with careful titration because a paradoxic effect caused by hypersensitivity may be observed in some individuals.

Clinical studies and extensive experience support the use of MAOIs to treat panic.

Phenelzine and tranylcypromine have been used effectively to manage panic disorder.[56] In treating panic with MAOIs, 1 to 3 weeks of pharmacotherapy are often required before significant reduction of panic symptoms is achieved.

When MAOIs are used, it is extremely important that the patient be educated regarding the dietary and medication restrictions, as previously discussed (see Chapter 6). Patients should receive this education in a nonthreatening and nonfrightening way, because many potential candidates will be terrified by the restrictions and cautions. Nonetheless, patients should be advised to go to the nearest hospital emergency department for evaluation and treatment if they experience signs or symptoms of a hypertensive reaction. Patients must also be advised and warned about headache, dizziness, and other symptoms that may be secondary to postural hypotension produced by the MAOIs. The patient's ability to monitor blood pressure at home may be helpful during the course of treatment or when the possibility of elevated blood pressure becomes a concern. It is of course important to measure each patient's blood pressure before initiating treatment with an MAOI and to monitor the blood pressure and pulse rate. A drop of 10 to 20 mm Hg in systolic pressure may occur in one half to two thirds of patients taking MAOIs. In some cases, moderately severe symptomatic postural hypotension may be counteracted by increased salt intake. The cautious administration of the salt-retaining steroid fluorocortisone in low dosages of 0.05 to 0.1 mg once or twice daily may also be a useful technique.

PHOBIC DISORDERS

Phobic disorders have become prominent with the increasing ability to provide pharmacologic and psychotherapeutic treatment. The two more common phobic disorders potentially amenable to pharmacotherapy are agoraphobia, which often occurs in association with panic attacks, and social phobia (social anxiety disorder).

Agoraphobia

Agoraphobia is characterized by intense fear of being in places or situations from which escape may be difficult or embarrassing, or fear of places where help may not be readily available (Box 7-7). Agoraphobic patients are often frightened to be away from their homes and may remain in the home, avoiding occupational, social, and other interpersonal interactions. Many agoraphobic patients attempt to participate in normal life situations and endure intense anxiety in the process. However, most severely agoraphobic patients are unable to travel on public transportation and experience great difficulty in stores, theaters, or other public places.

Box 7-7 Clinical Features of Agoraphobia and Social Phobia (Social Anxiety)

Agoraphobia	Social phobia
Fear of places	Fear of scrutiny
Fear of situations	Hypersensitivity to others
Avoidance of interactions	Extreme shyness
Avoidance of public places	Low self-esteem
Maintains access to help	Fear of embarrassment or humiliation

Agoraphobic patients, whether or not they experience panic attacks, may benefit from pharmacologic intervention. As with patients with panic disorder, patients with agoraphobia may be significantly helped by behavioral techniques, including exposure therapy and other types of interventions. These are most effective when combined with pharmacologic intervention. In most instances, optimizing the general medical and physiologic status of the patient enhances responsivity to pharmacologic intervention and may also be combined with psychotherapeutic interventions. The pharmacologic approach to agoraphobia has generally included the use of benzodiazepines, SSRIs, TCAs, and MAOIs. As with panic disorders, alprazolam at relatively high dosages between 3 and 6 mg/day may be effective. Imipramine dosed at 150 mg/day (in combination with behavioral techniques) has also been reported to be highly beneficial in treating agoraphobia.[45] Cyclic antidepressants that are strongly serotonergic (e.g., clomipramine or nefazodone) are generally thought to be more beneficial than noradrenergic agents. SSRIs have also been reported to be effective in the treatment of agoraphobia at dosages similar to those used to treat panic disorders.[26,56]

MAOIs, especially phenelzine, are effective in the treatment of agoraphobia.[52] Phenelzine is the preferred agent when an SSRI or cyclic antidepressant is ineffective. Bernstein suggests that MAOI use for the treatment of agoraphobic patients may produce greater relief of symptoms than do other antidepressants or benzodiazepine anxiolytics; however, the disadvantages of dietary and medication restrictions and the potential for postural hypotension must be assiduously evaluated in each case.[10]

Social Phobia (Social Anxiety Disorder)

Social phobia, or social anxiety disorder, is a common and limiting illness characterized by persistent fear of situations in which one is exposed to the scrutiny of others (see Box 7-7). Social anxiety should be considered in patients who present with depression, patients who report having anxiety in social settings, or patients who have a history of alcohol or drug abuse.[24] Individuals with social anxiety show hypersensitivity to negative evaluation, have low self-esteem, and may be shy. Individuals with social phobia fear that they will say or do something to embarrass or humiliate themselves or that others will notice that they are anxious. Consequently, people with social phobia often avoid situations in which they may be scrutinized and subject to intense distress. Not surprisingly, this results in considerable impairment of functioning and reduced quality of life. These individuals have few friendships, experience trouble dating, drop out of school, reject promotions at work, become demoralized and depressed, abuse alcohol, and develop other psychiatric comorbidities.[58]

Social phobia may be exclusively related to fear of public speaking but can be far more generalized and disabling. Recent epidemiologic surveys have demonstrated that social phobia is the third most common psychiatric disorder in the general population after major depression and alcohol dependence. It has lifetime, 12-month, and 30-day prevalence rates of 13.3%, 7.9%, and 4.5%, respectively.[44] Most individuals with social phobia who present for treatment have a "generalized" subtype. The mean age of onset for social phobia is 15.3 years. Given the high prevalence rate, early age of onset, associated psychiatric comorbidity, and impairment in social and occupational functioning, social anxiety needs to be considered a serious disorder that imparts a significant burden of suffering on affected individuals.[63]

Treatment

The patient with social phobia may respond well to pharmacologic interventions. Beta-blockers, high-potency benzodiazepines, SSRIs, MAOIs, and gabapentin (Neurontin) have been prescribed with success. Cognitive-behavioral therapy has also been shown to be effective in the treatment of social phobia, but this treatment may be unavailable to many patients who do not live in large urban areas or near academic centers. Thus pharmacotherapy is often the more practical treatment option.

The general aim of pharmacotherapy for social anxiety disorder is symptom relief by reducing autonomic and physiologic arousal, reducing anticipatory anxiety, diminishing catastrophic cognitions, and alleviating avoidance behaviors. Over time, such symptom reduction often leads to improvement in social and occupational functioning. Generally, establishing an effective pharmacologic regimen and response should precede any encouragement or effort to return the patient to normal function in all spheres of life.

Beta-blockers are commonly used primarily by musicians for treatment of performance anxiety. These individuals may not meet criteria for generalized social phobia. Controlled studies of propranolol and atenolol have been disappointing for the treatment of more generalized symptoms and are not significantly better than placebo in short-term studies.[23,61] It is possible that certain individuals will benefit from the use of beta-blockers over extended periods, whereas others may benefit from intermittent use of beta-blockers taken before specific performances. Dosages prescribed are propranolol 10 to 20 mg, three to four times a day; metoprolol 25 to 50 mg twice daily; or atenolol 50 to 100 mg once daily. Obviously, a careful history and assessment of blood pressure, pulse rate, heart, and lungs should precede the use of beta-adrenergic blocking agents. History of congestive heart failure, cardiac arrhythmia, and chronic obstructive pulmonary disease with asthma pose contraindications to treatment with beta-adrenergic blocking drugs.

Benzodiazepines alone or in combination with antidepressants may be effective in the treatment of social phobia. Clonazepam may be more effective than other benzodiazepines because of its serotonergic properties. However, only one controlled trial of clonazepam has been conducted in the treatment of social phobia.[17] In this 12-week study, 78% of the clonazepam group versus 20% of the placebo group were rated improved. Because of the high rates of comorbidity of social phobia with depression and substance abuse/dependence, as well as the lack of efficacy of benzodiazepines in the treatment of depression and their potential for abuse of those agents, enthusiasm for benzodiazepines usage has waned. Thus benzodiazepine treatment of social phobia is not considered a first-line choice.

Several large multicenter studies have convincingly shown that SSRIs are the first-line choice for treatment of social phobia (see Table 7-5). Fluvoxamine was the first SSRI to show efficacy in a controlled trial.[65] Stein and others completed a larger study that showed that an average dosage of 202 mg/day in 92 patients was effective in treating generalized social phobia.[57] Other studies have shown sertraline, dosed at 50 to 200 mg, is also an effective agent.[63] Blomhoff and colleagues, in Scandinavia, combined exposure therapy with sertraline treatment.[12] This combination resulted in even greater efficacy when compared with drug alone or other active treatments. Four controlled trials on the use of the SSRI paroxetine to treat social phobia have been completed, making it the most studied agent for this condition. Paroxetine has received FDA approval for treatment of social anxiety. In these studies, paroxetine in doses of 20 to 60 mg were used; however, the range of 40 and 60 mg was significantly more effective.[7,58] Like sertraline, paroxetine has been found to be significantly effective in reducing avoidance behaviors and social anxiety.

Several studies have documented the therapeutic efficacy of MAOIs, primarily phenelzine, in treating social phobia. The MAOI phenelzine was the first medication to show efficacy in treating social phobia.[25] Liebowitz and others found that after 8 weeks of treatment, phenelzine at mean dosages of 75 mg/day was more effective than atenolol or placebo.[43] MAOIs used to treat social phobia should be given in conventional antidepressant doses, as previously discussed. Although MAOIs, and particularly phenelzine, have long been considered the gold standard of drug treatment for social phobia, the dietary restrictions and the risk of significant life-threatening adverse events (e.g., hypertensive crises) associated with the use of these medications have resulted in a significant reluctance to use them as first-line treatments.[18] The RIMAs have shown little, if any, efficacy in the treatment of social phobia, making them a third- or fourth-line drug. These agents are not available in the United States.

Buspirone has not been documented to be effective in either panic, agoraphobia, or social phobia.[66] Nonetheless, this compound may be useful as an adjunct in treating anticipatory anxiety or may be useful when a patient is participating in behavioral therapy techniques, such as exposure or desensitization.

The anticonvulsant gabapentin (Neurontin) has been used effectively in the treatment of social phobia. The magnitude of anxiolytic effects of gabapentin is comparable to that of benzodiazepines. Pande and colleagues compared gabapentin at dosages of 900 to 3600 mg/day with placebo in a controlled trial involving 69 patients with social phobia.[51] A significant reduction in symptoms of social phobia was observed among patients taking gabapentin compared with patients receiving placebo, as evaluated by clinician- and patient-rated scales. With average doses of gabapentin at 2100 mg, adverse effects were minimal and included the known side effects of gabapentin (dizziness, dry mouth, somnolence, nausea, flatulence, and decreased libido). Thus gabapentin offers a favorable risk to benefit ratio for the treatment of patients with social phobia.

Other open-label studies of social phobia have included nefazodone, venlafaxine, bupropion, selegiline, clonidine, and valproate. Nefazodone has shown promise in treating symptoms of social anxiety, including the avoidance symptoms, at average dosages of 400 to 450 mg/day.[62] Venlafaxine may be effective at dosages of 75 to 300 mg/day.[1,35] Other open-label studies have used bupropion at dosages of 300 mg/day, selegiline at dosages of 10 mg/day, and valproate at dosages ranging from 500 to 1500 mg/day.[62]

Overall, accumulating evidence has supported the use of the SSRIs as first-line treatment for social phobia. However, several challenges remain in the pharmaco-therapy of social phobia. Because social phobia is believed to be a chronic, unremitting disorder, clinicians will need to consider the duration of treatment. As with other anxiety disorders, there is some evidence supporting the need for lifelong pharmacotherapy, given the significant relapse rates upon medication discontinuation. In addition, the known comorbidity with social phobia requires that further studies be conducted. Studies of longitudinal course and treatment are important given the early age of onset of social phobia and its subsequent interference with development and functioning.

OBSESSIVE-COMPULSIVE DISORDER

OCD is now recognized as a commonly occurring disorder that affects approximately 2% of the population. In the United States, 1 of every 50 adults has OCD, and twice that number have had it at some point in their lives. Clinical features of OCD are shown in Box 7-8. Worries, doubts, and superstitious beliefs are all common in

<hr>

Box 7-8 Clinical Features of Obsessive-Compulsive Disorder

Obsessions
1. Unrealistic recurring or persistent thoughts, impulses, or images; intrusive or distressing
2. Attempt to neutralize or suppress the thoughts, images, or impulses
3. Impairment or interference with daily routine, functioning, or relationships

Compulsions
1. Repetitive behaviors in response to an obsession, rigidly applied
2. Behavior or actions that serve to prevent or reduce distress
3. Impairment or interference with daily routine, functioning, or relationships

<hr>

everyday life, but when they become excessive, for example, hours of handwashing or driving around and around the block to check that an accident did not occur, a diagnosis of OCD is made. OCD has been referred to as *mental hiccups* that will not go away. Individuals with OCD usually present with both obsessions and compulsions, although a person with OCD may sometimes have only one or the other. Obsessions are thoughts, images, or impulses that occur repeatedly and make a person feel out of control. Obsessions are accompanied by uncomfortable feelings such as fear, disgust, doubt, or a sensation that things have to be done in a way that is "just so." People with OCD typically try to make their obsessions go away by performing compulsions. Compulsions are acts the person performs over and over again, often according to "certain rules." For example, a person may wash constantly, to the point that his or her hands become raw and inflamed, or a person may repeatedly check that the stove or iron is turned off because of an obsessive fear of burning the house down. Unlike compulsive drinking or gambling, OCD compulsions do not give a person pleasure. Rather, the rituals are performed to obtain relief from the discomfort caused by the obsessions. OCD symptoms by definition consume large periods of time (more than an hour per day) or significantly interfere with a person's work, social life, or relationships.

Treatment

Strategies for the treatment of OCD are aimed toward ending the current episode and preventing recurrences. Education is a crucial element of helping patients and families learn how to manage OCD and prevent its complications. Cognitive-behavioral psychotherapy is the key element of treatment for many patients with OCD. Pharmacotherapy, with an SSRI or other agent, is also beneficial for most patients.[29] Support groups may be invaluable to treatment. These groups provide a forum for mutual acceptance, understanding, and self-discovery. Participants develop a sense of camaraderie with other attendees because they have all lived with OCD. Similar groups are useful in social anxiety, as previously discussed, and PTSD.

In patients with OCD, symptoms worsen when coexisting symptoms of depression or other combined conditions develop. Depression is found in one third of patients upon presentation and in two thirds of cases over a lifetime. The effectiveness of antidepressant drugs in treating OCD lends further support to the possibility that this condition shares some common neurochemical or neurobiologic disturbances with depression.

Clomipramine (Anafranil) and the SSRIs have emerged as the more effective drug treatments of OCD (see Table 7-5). Other TCAs and the MAOIs continue to be used as therapeutic agents.[32] Buspirone, as an alternative treatment, is more often used as an adjunct to an SSRI. Alprazolam and other benzodiazepines may significantly exacerbate the symptoms of OCD because the patient may feel uncomfortable with sedation and other side effects. Patients with coexisting symptoms of depression are much more likely to benefit from the use of an SSRI or other antidepressant. Neuroleptic medications may be useful in treating psychotic features or refractory cases. Lithium has *not* been found to be therapeutic alone or as an adjunct in the treatment of OCD. Overall, conventional antidepressants remain the preferred pharmacologic agents.

Clomipramine (Anafranil) is the most serotonergic of the TCAs; at a dosage of approximately 100 to 200 mg/day, it is a potent antiobsessional agent.[15] Clomipramine is a TCA and is not a pure serotonin reuptake inhibitor. Its active metabolite desmethylclomipramine, a potent reuptake inhibitor of norepinephrine, may account in part for its clinical efficacy. Three carefully controlled, double-blind studies have shown clomipramine's preferential effectiveness in reducing obsessional symptoms.[2,31,48] Its effect may not be fully apparent until 5 to 10 weeks after treatment. Plasma level determinations may be helpful in avoiding dosages that are too high or too low, both of which seem to be connected to poor outcome. Combining clomipramine with behavioral exposure treatment is desirable, and the response to treatment is generally prolonged over several years. With the exception of dental problems that result from the reduced production of saliva (which can be prevented by careful oral hygiene), no serious long-term effects of clomipramine use have been described. At lower dosages of 50 to 100 mg/day, clomipramine may be used to augment the antiobsessional effects of SSRIs.

SSRI therapy, including the use of venlafaxine for OCD, is now considered the first-line approach to OCD. Fluoxetine, fluvoxamine, paroxetine, and sertraline have FDA approval for use in the treatment of OCD (see Table 7-5). Venlafaxine and citalopram have also shown efficacy in treating OCD.[28,33] Fluvoxamine is the most extensively studied; dosages of 200 to 300 mg/day are recommended.

Paroxetine, a high-potency SSRI with greater selectivity than fluvoxamine, has been compared with clomipramine with respect to its antiobsessional effects. A comparison of this drug with fluvoxamine and citalopram showed all three have good tolerability, and resulted in no drop outs, and minimal adverse effects.[49] Recommended starting dosages and dosage ranges with minimum effective dosages are noted in Table 7-5. The use of SSRIs, as opposed to clomipramine treatment of OCD, seems to improve the compliance with treatment, leading to global improvement of the pharmacologic management of this illness. Furthermore, with regard to the comparative efficacy of fluvoxamine, paroxetine, citalopram, sertraline, and fluoxetine, the results of meta-analyses suggest these drugs have similar antiobsessional efficacy.[28,53] Augmentation strategies with SSRIs have been developed using clomipramine, high-potency benzodiazepines (especially clonazepam), neuroleptics, or buspirone. More recently, gabapentin, beginning at 300 mg twice a day and increasing every few days to a target dosage of 1800 to 2400 mg/day, may relieve anxiety and chronic depression accompanying OCD and may modestly ameliorate the OCD symptoms.

There are no controlled studies using MAOIs in patients with OCD. However, a few case reports have alluded to a favorable response.[33] Generally, the MAOIs may be effective in patients with OCD who have associated panic or other forms of severe anxiety. Some patients with OCD have been reported to be responsive to lithium but in fact are responsive only if they have an underlying cyclothymia or manic-depressive illness.[59] Controlled trials have not been supportive of lithium's use in OCD.[46] Likewise, antipsychotic agents may be useful in patients with psychotic or refractory symptoms. Alprazolam or clonazepam may both be successful in patients with mixed anxiety-depression, possibly in part because of their effects on mood. Neither lithium, antipsychotics, nor the anxiolytics have been extensively studied in this population. Electroconvulsive therapy (ECT) is generally regarded as not useful in treating patients with OCD. Although a link between depression and OCD may be present, ECT has not been found to be effective, and no reports exist of successfully treating OCD with ECT.

Many patients with OCD have been referred for psychosurgery when severe illness is present and multiple therapeutic approaches have failed. The results of surgical intervention can be impressive.[5] Three main surgical approaches are used: orbital frontal, anterior cingulum, and stereotactic. Behavioral therapy after surgery is recommended. Recent psychosurgical research suggests that the cingulum is primarily involved.[5,47] According to Baer, at 2-year follow-up, approximately 25% to 30% of the patients who previously were unresponsive to medication and behavioral treatment were significantly improved with cingulotomy.[5] A comprehensive discussion of this topic, however, is beyond the scope of this text.

POSTTRAUMATIC STRESS DISORDER

PTSD has become increasingly recognized as a prevalent psychiatric disorder associated with significant distress, impairment, and disability in affected individuals. Recent survey data indicate that 60% to 70% of individuals in the United States have suffered a traumatic event and that 5% to 10% meet threshold criteria for PTSD (Table 7-6 and Box 7-9). PTSD is a heterogeneous disorder with a wide variety of clinical presentations. Generally, PTSD follows a traumatic event and is characterized by a reexperiencing of the trauma, persistent avoidance of associated stimuli, and persistent increased arousal symptoms that extend for 1 month or longer (usually longer).[3] Certain traumatic events seem to be more commonly associated with PTSD. Some of these events are being raped, badly beaten, or sexually assaulted; being involved in a serious accident; incurring significant injury; being shot or

Table 7-6 Prevalence Rates of Trauma and Posttraumatic Stress Disorder (PTSD)*

	Men experiencing event (%)	Men experiencing PTSD (%)	Women experiencing event (%)	Women experiencing PTSD (%)
Natural disaster	18.9	3.7	15.2	5.4
Criminal assault	11.1	1.8	6.9	21.3
Combat	6.4	38.8	0.0	—
Rape	0.7	65	9.2	49.5
Any trauma	60.7	8.1	51.2	20.4

From Kessler RC and others: Posttraumatic stress disorder in the National Comorbidity Survey, *Arch Gen Psychiatry* 52(12):1052, 1995.
*Overall prevalence rates are approximately 5% in men and 10% in women.

**Box 7-9 Selected Trauma Types and Overall Rate of
Posttraumatic Stress Disorder (PTSD) for Both Men and Women**

Selected traumas	PTSD rate
Sexual assault	24%
Beaten severely	22%
Serious accident or injury	17%
Shot or stabbed	15%
Sudden, unexpected death of friend or relative	14%

**Box 7-10 Posttraumatic Stress Disorder (PTSD)
Subtypes and Presenting Symptoms**

Depressive: restricted affect, guilt, decreased interest
Anxious-depressed: decreased sleep, concentration, interest
Anxious: restless, apprehensive, irritable, hypervigilant
Somatic: multiple somatic complaints, especially neuromuscular,
   cardiorespiratory, and gastrointestinal

---

stabbed; or having a sudden and unexpected death of a close friend or relative occur. Certainly, combat experience in veterans is commonly associated with PTSD. Psychosocial treatments for PTSD include group therapy, hypnotherapy, psychodynamic treatments, and cognitive-behavioral treatments. Diagnostic subtypes (Box 7-10), as well as comorbidity of PTSD with other psychiatric disorders, are now being considered with regard to treatment implications.

The TCAs and MAOIs have been demonstrated to be useful in placebo-controlled trials of the treatment of PTSD. More promising data from controlled clinical trials have involved the use of sertraline, fluoxetine, other SSRIs, and cyclic antidepressants.

A number of studies have shown that TCAs, MAOIs, and SSRIs, particularly fluoxetine and sertraline, provide good to moderate relief of PTSD symptoms and dramatic improvement in functioning (Table 7-7). Quality of life improves as well. Other open-label trials have suggested that the use of paroxetine, fluvoxamine, nefazodone, mirtazapine, olanzapine, cyproheptadine, and valproate may be effective in the treatment of PTSD.

The most impressive studies of PTSD pharmacotherapy involve fluoxetine and sertraline (sertraline is FDA approved for the treatment of PTSD). In one multicenter study of sertraline involving 12 U.S. centers, 208 patients showed good to moderate improvement in symptoms of PTSD in comparison to placebo-treated patients.[17] Reexperiencing and intrusive thoughts, avoidance and numbing, and hyperarousal were robustly responsive to sertraline at doses of 50 to 200 mg. A study of fluoxetine involved 53 civilians with PTSD who were treated for 12 weeks with up to 60 mg/day. Assessments of PTSD severity, disability, stress-vulnerability, and functioning showed robust improvements in 85% of the patients.[16] Brady and others

Table 7-7 Placebo-Controlled Studies of Posttraumatic Stress Disorder (PTSD)

Study	Drug	N	Population	Results
Davidson and others, 1990[19]	Amitriptyline	62	Combat	Superior
Kosten and others, 1991[39]	Imipramine Phenelzine	61	Combat	Superior (both)
Katz and others, 1995[34]	Bromafarine*	45	Mixed	Superior
van der Kolk and others, 1994[64]	Fluoxetine	47	Mixed	Superior (especially civilian)
Davidson and others, 1997[20]	Fluoxetine	64	Civilian	Superior
Davidson and others, 1997[20]	Sertraline	109	Civilian	Superior
Brady and others, 1995[13]	Sertraline	187	Civilian	Superior
Connor and others, 1999[16]	Fluoxetine	52	Civilian	Superior

*Bromafarine has not been effective in other studies and is not available in the United States.

evaluated the impact SSRIs had on PTSD with comorbid alcohol dependence.[13] Although limited by small sample size and open-label design, the study suggests that SSRI treatment (sertraline) may be useful in the treatment of PTSD complicated by alcoholism. The medication was well tolerated, and the subjects showed improvement in PTSD symptoms with decreased alcohol consumption.

A number of other medications have been used alone or as augmentors of antidepressants in the clinical pharmacotherapy of PTSD. This includes use of the anticonvulsive drugs carbamazepine, valproate, and gabapentin, as well as lithium, clonidine, and beta-blockers. The dosages of these drugs are comparable to those used in treating patients with other psychiatric conditions.

ETHNICITY AND CULTURAL ISSUES IN ANXIETY

Regarding ethnicity and cultural issues and the treatment of anxiety, benzodiazepines have demonstrated significant pharmacokinetic differences within two ethnic groups. Generally, Asians have shown slower metabolism of benzodiazepines, suggesting genetic factors are important. Moreover, Asians residing in different areas of the world when given diazepam and alprazolam have demonstrated this phenomenon consistently. Thus genetic factors appear to be more important than environmental factors in the control of benzodiazepine metabolism. In a recent study of the pharmacokinetics and pharmacodynamics of adinazolam, a triazolo-benzodiazepine, African-Americans were found to have decreased clearance resulting in significantly higher concentrations and greater drug effects on psychomotor performance. If this ethnic difference translates to other triazolo-benzodiazepines (e.g., alprazolam), it might explain the greater drug effects observed in some African-Americans. Future studies are necessary to sort out these discrepancies.[40]

REFERENCES
1. Altamura AC, Pioli R, Vitto M, Mannu P: Venlafaxine in social phobia: a study in selective serotonin reuptake inhibitor non-responders, *Int Clin Psychopharmacol* 14:239, 1999.
2. Ananth J and others: Clomipramine therapy for obsessive-compulsive neurosis, *Am J Psychiatry* 136:700, 1979.

3. American Psychiatric Association: *Diagnostic and statistical manual of mental disorders-TR,* ed 4, Washington, DC, 2000, American Psychiatric Press.
4. American Psychiatric Association: *Guidelines for panic disorder,* Washington, DC, 1996, American Psychiatric Press.
5. Baer L and others: Cingulotomy for intractable obsessive-compulsive disorder, *Arch Gen Psychiatry* 52:384, 1995.
6. Baldessarini RJ: *Chemotherapy in psychiatry,* Cambridge, Mass, 1985, Harvard University.
7. Baldwin D and others: Paroxetine in social phobia/social anxiety disorder, *Br J Psychiatry* 175:120, 1999.
8. Ballenger JC: Pharmacotherapy of the panic disorders, *J Clin Psychiatry* 47(suppl 6):27, 1986.
9. Ballenger JC and others: Double-blind, fixed dose, placebo-controlled study of paroxetine in the treatment of panic disorder, *Am J Psychiatry* 155:36, 1998.
10. Bernstein JG: *Drug therapy in psychiatry,* ed 3, Littleton, Mass, 1995, PSG Publishing.
11. Bezchlibnyk-Butler KZ, Jeffries JJ: *Clinical handbook of psychotropic drugs,* ed 7, Seattle, 1997, Hogrefe & Huber.
12. Blomhoff S and others: Treatment of generalized social phobia. Presented at 152nd Annual Meeting of the American Psychiatric Association; May 20, 1999, Washington, DC.
13. Brady KT, Sonne SC, Roberts JM: Sertraline treatment of comorbid posttraumatic stress disorder and alcohol dependence, *J Clin Psychiatry* 56:502, 1995.
14. Broocks A and others: Comparison of aerobic exercise, clomipramine, and placebo in the treatment of panic disorder, *Am J Psychiatry* 155(5):603, 1998.
15. Clomipramine Collaborative Study Group: Clomipramine in the treatment of patients with obsessive-compulsive disorder, *Arch Gen Psychiatry* 48:370, 1991.
16. Connor KM and others: Fluoxetine in posttraumatic stress disorder: randomised, double-blind study, *Br J Psychiatry* 175:17, 1999.
17. Davidson JRT and others: Treatment of social phobia with clonazepam and placebo, *J Clin Psychopharmacol* 13:423, 1993.
18. Davidson J, Turnbull CD: The effects of isocarboxazid on blood pressure, *J Clin Psychopharmacol* 6:139, 1986.
19. Davidson J and others: Treatment of posttraumatic stress disorder with amitriptyline and placebo, *Arch Gen Psych* 47(3):259, 1990.
20. Davidson JR and others: Response characteristics to antidepressants and placebo in posttraumatic stress disorder, *Int Clin Psychopharmacol* 12(6):291, 1997.
21. Domantay AG, Napoliello MJ: Buspirone for elderly anxious patients, *Int Med Certif* 3:1, 1989.
22. Enna SJ: Role of gamma-aminobutyric acid in anxiety, *Psychopathology* 17:15, 1984.
23. Falloon IR, Lloyd GG, Harpin R: The treatment of social phobia: real-life rehearsal with non-professional therapists, *J Nerv Ment Dis* 169:180, 1981.
24. Fones CSL, Manfro GG, Pollack MH: Social phobia: an update, *Harv Rev Psychiatry* 5: 247, 1998.
25. Gelernter CS and others: Cognitive-behavioral and pharmacological treatments of social phobias, *Arch Gen Psychiatry* 48:938, 1991.
26. Gloger S and others: Treatment of spontaneous panic attacks with clomipramine, *Am J Psychiatry* 138:1215, 1981.
27. Goodman WK, Charney DS: A case of alprazolam, but not lorazepam, inducing manic symptoms, *J Clin Psychiatry* 48:117, 1987.
28. Greist J and others: Double-blind parallel comparison of three dosages of sertraline and placebo in outpatients with obsessive-compulsive disorder, *Arch Gen Psychiatry* 52:289, April 1995.
29. Greist JH and others: Efficacy and tolerability of serotonin transport inhibitors in obsessive-compulsive disorder: a meta-analysis, *Arch Gen Psychiatry* 52(1):53, 1995.
30. Harvey SC: Hypnotics and sedatives. In Gilman AG, Goodman LS, Rall TW, editors, *The pharmacological basis of therapeutics,* ed 7, New York, 1985, Macmillan.
31. Insel TR and others: Obsessive-compulsive disorder: a double-blind trial of clomipramine and clorgyline, *Arch Gen Psychiatry* 40:605, 1983.

32. Jenike MA: Pharmacologic treatment of obsessive-compulsive disorders, *Psychiatr Clin North Am* 15(4):895, 1992.

33. Jenike MA, Baer L, Minichiello WE: *Obsessive-compulsive disorders: theory and management,* St Louis, 1986, Mosby.

34. Katz RJ and others: Pharmacotherapy of post-traumatic stress disorder with a novel psychotropic, *Anxiety* 1:169, 1994.

35. Kelsey JE: Venlafaxine in social phobia, *Psychopharmacol Bull* 31:767, 1995.

36. Keltner NL, Folks DG, Palmer CA, Powers R: *Psychobiological foundations of psychiatric care,* St Louis, 1998, Mosby.

37. Kessler RC and others: Lifetime panic-depression comorbidity in the national comorbidity survey, *Arch Gen Psychiatry* 55:801, 1998.

38. Klerman GL: Overview of the Cross-National Collaborative Panic Study, *Arch Gen Psychiatry* 45:407, 1988.

39. Kosten TR and others: Pharmacotherapy for posttraumatic stress disorder using a phenelzine or imipramine, *J Nerv Ment Dis* 79(6):366, 1991.

40. Lesser IM, Smith M, Poland RE, Lin KM: Psychopharmacology and ethnicity. In Friedman S, editor: *Cultural issues in the treatment of anxiety,* New York, 1997, The Guilford Press.

41. Lieberman JA, Tasman A: *Psychiatric drugs,* St Louis, 2000, WB Saunders.

42. Liebowitz MR and others: Pharmacotherapy of social phobia, *Psychosomatics* 28:305, 1987.

43. Liebowitz MR and others: Phenelzine vs atenolol in social phobia: a placebo controlled trial, *Arch Gen Psychiatry* 49:290, 1992.

44. Magee WJ and others: Agoraphobia, simple phobia, and social phobia in the National Comorbidity Survey, *Arch Gen Psychiatry* 53:159, 1996.

45. Mavissakalian M, Perel J: Imipramine in the treatment of agoraphobia: dose-response relationships, *Am J Psychiatry* 142:1032, 1985.

46. McDougle CJ and others: Neuroleptic addiction in fluvoxamine-refractory obsessive-compulsive disorder, *Am J Psychiatry* 147(5):652, 1990.

47. Mindus P and others: Capsulotomy and cingulotomy as treatments for malignant obsessive-compulsive disorder: an update. In Hollander E and others, editors: *Creative insights in obsessive-compulsive disorder,* London, England, 1994, John Wiley & Sons.

48. Montgomery SA: Clomipramine in obsessional neurosis: a placebo-controlled trial, *Pharmacol Med* 1:189, 1980.

49. Mundo E, Bianchi L, Bellodi L: Efficacy of fluvoxamine, paroxetine, and citalopram in the treatment of obsessive-compulsive disorder: a single-blind study, *J Clin Psychopharmacol* 17(4):267, 1997.

50. Neppe VM: Buspirone: an anxioselective neuromodulator. In VM Neppe, editor: *Innovative psychopharmacotherapy,* New York, 1989, Raven.

51. Pande AC and others: Treatment of social phobia with gabapentin: a placebo-controlled study, *J Clin Psychopharmacol* 119:341, 1999.

52. Phol R, Berchou R, Rainey JM: Tricyclic antidepressants and monoamine oxidase inhibitors in the treatment of agoraphobia, *J Clin Psychopharmacol* 2:399, 1982.

53. Piccinelli M, Pini S, Bellantuomo C, Wilkinson G: Efficacy of drug treatment in obsessive-compulsive disorder. A meta-analytic review, *Br J Psychiatry* 166:424, 1995.

54. Riblett LA and others: Pharmacology and neurochemistry of buspirone, *J Clin Psychiatry* 43:11, 1982.

55. Rickels K and others: Efficacy of extended-release venlafaxine in nondepressed outpatients with generalized anxiety disorder, *Am J Psychiatry* 157:968, 2000.

56. Sheehan DV: The treatment of panic and phobic disorders. In Bernstein JC, editor: *Clinical psychopharmacology,* ed 2, Boston, 1984, John Wright BPSG.

57. Stein MB and others: Paroxetine treatment of generalized social phobia (social anxiety disorder), *JAMA* 280(8):708, 1998.

58. Stein MB and others: Fluvoxamine in the treatment of social phobia: a double-blind, placebo-controlled study, *Am J Psychiatry* 156:756, 1999.

59. Stern TA, Jenike MA: Treatment of obsessive-compulsive disorder with lithium carbonate, *Psychosomatics* 24:671, 1983.

60. Tesar GE and others: Double-blind, placebo-controlled comparison of clonazepam and alprazolam for panic disorder, *J Clin Psychiatry* 52:69, 1991

61. Turner SM, Beidel DC, Jacob RG: Social phobia: a comparison of behavior therapy and atenolol, *J Consult Clin Psychol* 62:350, 1994.

62. Van Ameringen M, Mancini C, Oakman J: Nefazodone in the treatment of social phobia, *J Clin Psychiatry* 60:96, 1999.

63. Van Ameringen M, Swinson R, Walker JR, Lane RM: A placebo-controlled study of sertraline in generalized social phobia. Presented at the 19th National Conference of the Anxiety Disorders Association of America, March 25-28, 1999, San Diego, Calif.

64. van der Kolk BA and others: Fluoxetine in posttraumatic stress disorder, *J Clin Psychiatry* 55(12):517, 1994.

65. van Vliet LM, Den Boer J, Westenberg HGM: Psychopharmacological treatment of social phobia: a double-blind placebo controlled study with fluvoxamine, *Psychopharmacology* 115:128, 1994.

66. van Vliet LM and others: Clinical effects of buspirone in social phobia: a double-blind placebo-controlled study, *J Clin Psychiatry* 58:164, 1997.

CHAPTER 8

Dementia and Delirium

Dementia and delirium are major health problems; in 1991, the United States spent $100 billion on patients with cognitive loss. Approximately 60% of nursing home residents have some type of cognitive impairment. Unfortunately, clinicians may be less interested in dementia and delirium compared with their interest in other health care problems for the following several reasons:

1. Lack of diagnostic precision
2. Lack of effective treatment
3. Many time-consuming complaints from the family
4. Problems in finding adequate care and disposition for these cases

Caregiver families are often unhappy with the quality of medical care provided by the health care system to patients with dementia. This chapter addresses the key issues in recognition and management of dementia and delirium, with emphasis on drug therapy.

DEMENTIA SYNDROMES
DISEASE DEFINITION

Dementia comes from the Latin phrase *de mens* or "out of mind." Dementia is the loss of multiple intellectual functions as a result of the death or permanent dysfunction of neurons. This definition distinguishes dementia from isolated cognitive losses, such as aphasia after a stroke. Patients with dementia develop myriad cognitive symptoms that appear confusing to clinicians, health care professionals, and family caregivers. Recognition of these symptoms may serve to prevent unnecessary behavioral problems in patients with dementia and ease the burden of care for health care professionals and families.

The essential features of dementia are multiple cognitive deficits that include memory impairment and at least one of the following:

1. Aphasia or communication problems
2. Apraxia or inability to perform previously learned motor tasks
3. Agnosia or inability to recognize previously learned sensory input
4. A disturbance in executive functioning, or the inability to think abstractly and to plan, initiate, sequence, monitor, and stop complex behavior

The order of onset and relative prominence of the cognitive disturbances and associated symptoms vary with the specific type of dementia.

Memory impairment is generally a prominent early symptom of dementia. Individuals have difficulty learning new material or develop memory impairment, for example, misplacing valuables such as wallets and keys or forgetting food cooking on the stove. In more severe dementia, previously learned information and material may be forgotten, including the names of loved ones. Dementia can result in difficulties with spatial tasks such as navigating around the house or in the immediate neighborhood. Poor judgment and poor insight are common as well. Individuals may exhibit no awareness of their memory loss or other cognitive difficulties. They may have difficulties with problem solving, make unrealistic assessments of their abilities, and make plans that are not congruent with their deficits and prognosis. They may also underestimate the risks involved in activities such as driving.

A diagnosis of dementia requires that a cognitive deficit be sufficiently severe to cause impairment in occupational or social functioning and represent a decline from a previous level of functioning. The nature and degree of impairment is variable and often depends on the particular social setting of the individual. For example, mild cognitive impairment may significantly impair an individual's ability to perform a complex job but not a less demanding one. A number of associated features of dementia include difficulties with behavior and daily functioning. Individuals with dementia may show disinhibited behavior, including inappropriate jokes, neglect of personal hygiene, undue familiarity with strangers, or disregard for conventional rules of social conduct. Individuals may become agitated or violent and strike out at others. Suicidality may develop, especially in mildly impaired individuals who are more likely to have insight into their deficits and be capable of formulating and carrying out a plan of action.

Anxiety is commonly seen with dementia. Individuals will often manifest "catastrophic reactions," or overwhelming emotional responses to relatively minor stressors such as changes in routine or environment. Depressed mood is also common, as are sleep disturbances independent of depression. Psychosis, including delusions, especially those involving themes of abandonment, infidelity, or suspiciousness (e.g., the belief that misplaced possessions have been stolen), can occur. Misidentifications of familiar people as unfamiliar or vice versa may occur. Hallucinations may develop in all sensory modalities, but visual hallucinations are more commonly observed. Some individuals will exhibit a peak period of agitation or other behavioral disturbance during the evening hours, referred to as *sundowning*.

Delirium is often superimposed on dementia because the underlying brain disease increases susceptibility to the effects of medications, concurrent general medical conditions, or other adverse factors. Individuals with dementia are vulnerable to psychosocial stressors that may exacerbate their intellectual deficits and associated problems. Dementia may be accompanied by motor disturbances, including gait difficulties, slurred speech, or a variety of abnormal movements. Other neurologic symptoms such as myoclonus, seizures, and fasciculations may be present.

EVALUATION AND DIAGNOSIS

The differential diagnosis of dementia is described in detail in DSM-IV.[3] A major differential consideration in dementia is delirium. Delirium is characterized by the reduced ability to maintain and shift attention appropriately; the cognitive deficits in delirium tend to fluctuate, whereas those of dementia tend to be stable or progressive. An amnestic disorder is characterized by memory impairment without significant impairment of other cognitive domains.

Major depressive disorder may be associated with complaints of poor memory and concentration with reduction in intellectual abilities demonstrated by history or mental status examination. This clinical presentation is the "dementia syndrome of depression," or depressive pseudodementia. The assessment of clinical course, onset of the depressive and cognitive symptoms, and other clinical features help distinguish depression from dementia (Table 8-1). However, even when the onset of depressive symptoms precedes or coincides with the onset of cognitive symptoms and resolves with antidepressant treatment, as many as half of the patients with these symptoms will later develop irreversible dementia within 3 to 5 years.[2]

Table 8-1 Diagnostic Features Distinguishing Depression and Dementia

Major depression	Dementia
Depressive symptoms	Euthymia
Subacute onset	Insidious onset
History of depression more common	History of depression less common
Aphasia, apraxia absent	Aphasia, apraxia present
Orientation intact	Orientation impaired
Concentration impaired	Recent memory impaired
Patient emphasis on memory complaint	Patient minimizes memory complaint
Patient gives up on testing	Patient makes effort on testing

Box 8-1 Underlying Causes of Cognitive Impairment

D	Drug toxicity
E	Eyes/ears, sensory impairment
M	Metabolic disturbance or endocrinopathy
E	Emotional disturbances, especially depression
N	Normal-pressure hydrocephalus or nutritional deficiency
T	Toxins, tumors, trauma to the head
I	Infection
A	Atherosclerosis including vascular disease

Dementia must be distinguished from age-related or mild cognitive impairment that occurs as a result of physiologic aging but that is nonprogressive and does not lead to functional impairment. Of course, many patients with mild cognitive impairment go on to develop a dementia syndrome.

The evaluation of dementia begins with a thorough clinical history. A mental status and neurologic and physical examinations are the other critical first steps in the evaluation of dementia. An important consideration is to review medications—both prescription and over-the-counter—consumed by the patient. Many patients will arrive with a bag full of medicines.

Mental Status Examination

The basic dementia evaluation outlined in Box 8-1 identifies treatable, reversible, and arrestable causes of cognitive decline. Numerous neuropsychologic batteries can identify cognitive loss, but the Mini-Mental State Examination (MMSE) remains a simple, cost-efficient instrument for the screening and assessment of cognitive impairment (Table 8-2).[19] This brief cognitive screen can be performed in 20 minutes or less by a clinician or staff member. MMSE scores can monitor the progression of symptoms or the efficacy of treatment. The 7-minute screen developed by Solomon and Pendlebury is designed to quickly identify patients with Alzheimer's disease (AD) and related disorders.[51] The neurocognitive battery consists of four individual tests of orientation, memory, clock drawing, and verbal fluency. When compared with normal subjects, patients with dementia are

Table 8-2 The Mini-Mental State Examination

I. Orientation (maximum score = 10)	Date (e.g., February 1) -----------	1 ___
Ask "What is today's date?" Then ask	Year------------------------------	2 ___
specifically for parts omitted: e.g., day,	Month-----------------------------	3 ___
month, year	Day (e.g., Monday) ---------------	4 ___
"Can you also tell me what season it is?"	Season----------------------------	5 ___
Ask "Can you tell me the name of this	Hospital--------------------------	6 ___
hospital?"		
"What floor are we on?"	Floor -----------------------------	7 ___
"What town (or city) are we in?"	Town/City ------------------------	8 ___
"What county are we in?"	County ---------------------------	9 ___
"What state are we in?"	State -----------------------------	10 ___

I. Orientation (maximum score = 10)

Ask "What is today's date?" Then ask specifically for parts omitted: e.g., day, month, year

"Can you also tell me what season it is?"

Ask "Can you tell me the name of this hospital?"

"What floor are we on?"

"What town (or city) are we in?"

"What county are we in?"

"What state are we in?"

	Date (e.g., February 1) -----------	1 ___
	Year------------------------------	2 ___
	Month-----------------------------	3 ___
	Day (e.g., Monday) ---------------	4 ___
	Season----------------------------	5 ___
	Hospital--------------------------	6 ___
	Floor -----------------------------	7 ___
	Town/City ------------------------	8 ___
	County ---------------------------	9 ___
	State -----------------------------	10 ___

II. Registration (maximum score = 3)

Ask the subject if you may test his/her memory. Then say "ball," "flag," "tree" clearly and slowly, about one second for each. After you have said all three words, ask subject to repeat them. This first repetition determines the score (0-3), but keep saying them (up to 6 trials) until the subject can repeat all three words. If (s)he does not eventually learn all three, recall cannot be meaningfully tested.

"ball"----------------------------	11 ___
"flag"----------------------------	12 ___
"tree"----------------------------	13 ___
Record number of trials: ___	

III. Attention and calculation (maximum score = 5)

Ask the subject to begin at 100 and count backward by 7. Stop after 5 subtractions (93, 86, 79, 72, 65). Score one point for each correct number.

If the subject cannot or will not perform this task, ask him/her to spell the word "world" backwards (D, L, R, O, W). The score is one point for each correctly placed letter, e.g., DLROW = 5; DLORW = 3. Record how the subject spelled "world" backwards. _____

     D L R O W.

"93" ------------------------------	14 ___
"86" ------------------------------	15 ___
"79" ------------------------------	16 ___
"72" ------------------------------	17 ___
"65" ------------------------------	18 ___
	OR
Number of correctly	
placed letters -----------------------	19 ___

IV. Recall (maximum score = 3)

Ask the subject to recall the three words you previously asked him/her to remember (learned in Registration)

"ball"---------------------------	20 ___
"flag"---------------------------	21 ___
"tree"---------------------------	22 ___

V. Language (maximum score = 9)

Naming: Show the subject a wristwatch and ask "What is this?" Repeat for pencil. Score one point for each item named correctly.

Watch--------------------------	23 ___
Pencil--------------------------	24 ___

Repetition: Ask the subject to repeat, "No ifs, ands, or buts." Score one point for correct repetition.

Repetition-----------------------	25 ___

From Folstein MF, Folstein SE, McHugh PR: "Mini-Mental State": a practical method of grading the cognitive state of patients for the clinician, *J Psychiatr Res* 12:189, 1975.

Continued

Table 8-2 The Mini-Mental State Examination—cont'd

3-Stage Command: Give the subject a piece of blank paper and say, "Take the paper in your right hand, fold it in half and put it on the floor." Score one point for each action performed correctly.	Takes in right hand ---------------- 26 ____ Fold in half ------------------------- 27 ____ Puts on floor------------------------- 28 ____
Reading: On a blank piece of paper, print the sentence "Close your eyes" in letters large enough for the subject to see clearly. Ask subject to read it and do what it says. Score correct only if s(he) actually closes his/her eyes.	Closes eyes ------------------------- 29 ____
Writing: Give the subject a blank piece of paper and ask him/her to write a sentence. It is to be written spontaneously. It must contain a subject and verb and make sense. Correct grammar and punctuation are not necessary.	Writes sentence -------------------- 30 ____
Copying: On a clean piece of paper, draw intersecting pentagons, each side about 1 inch, and ask subject to copy it exactly as it is. All 10 angles must be present and two must intersect to score 1 point. Tremor and rotation are ignored. e.g.,	Draws pentagons ------------------ 31 ____

Score: Add number of correct responses. In section III, include items 14-18 or item 19, not both (maximum total score 30).
Rate subject's level of consciousness: ____(a) coma, (b) stupor, (c) drowsy, (d) alert

significantly more impaired in each of the four tests included in the 7-minute screen. The battery correctly identifies 92% of patients with dementia and 96% of normal subjects. Other brief screening tools for dementia assessment include Six-Item Blessed Orientation-Memory Concentration Test, Clock Drawing Task, and the Functional Activities Questionnare.[26,33,60] A listing of cognitive, behavioral, and functional measures used in clinical trials include the MMSE, the Alzheimer's Disease Assessment Scale–cognitive subscale, the Mattis Dementia Rating Scale, and the Severe Impairment Battery.

Laboratory Evaluation

Laboratory tests for dementia should include a complete blood cell count, erythrocyte sedimentation rate, serum electrolytes, blood glucose, blood urea, liver functions, serum vitamin B_{12} concentration, thyrotropin levels, free thyroid index, and serologic test for syphilis. Computed tomography (CT) or magnetic resonance imaging (MRI) of the brain should be requested if a diagnosis is not established by history and laboratory assessment. Electroencephalography, lumbar puncture, heavy metal screen, human immunodeficiency (HIV) tests, or other specialized evaluations

---

Box 8-2 Causes of Dementia

Major causes
Alzheimer's disease
Vascular disease
Lewy body dementia
Frontotemporal dementia
Alcohol-related

Less common causes
Prion disease
Corticobasilar degeneration
Huntington's disease
Progressive supranuclear palsy
Parkinson's disease
HIV/AIDS

Rare causes
Normal-pressure hydrocephalus
Progressive subcortical gliosis
Cerebral vasculitis
Multiple sclerosis
Wilson's disease
Metachromatic leukodystrophy
Pick's disease
Keef disease
Storage diseases
Whipple's disease
Mitochondrial disease

HIV, Human immunodeficiency virus; *AIDS,* acquired immunodeficiency syndrome.

---

are requested when clinical findings suggest the need. Genotype testing for the E4 allele of apolipoprotein does not predict which individuals will develop AD and does not contribute to the routine diagnostic evaluation of a patient with dementia. However, this test may increase the diagnostic confidence in a patient already diagnosed with AD. As shown in Box 8-2, diagnosis (and management) of disorders characterized by cognitive impairment requires assiduous evaluation for possible underlying causes. Medications that may contribute to cognitive impairment are noted in Table 8-3.

Prevalence and Clinical Course of Dementia

Estimates of the prevalence of dementia vary with the definition, the specific threshold criteria, and the clinical setting in which the study occurs. Clearly, the prevalence rates of dementia increase dramatically with advancing age. The syndrome affects approximately 5% to 8% of individuals older than 65; 15% to 20% of individuals older than 75; and 25% to 50% of individuals older than 85.[27] AD is the most common form of dementia, affecting 50% to 75% of the total number of individuals with dementia, with the greater proportion in the higher age ranges (i.e., older than 75). Vascular dementia is probably the next most common dementia, perhaps at 10% to 15%. The remaining types of dementia account for a much smaller fraction of the total, although Lewy body dementia has been suggested to be more prevalent (approximately 10% to 15%) than previously realized.[48]

The mode of symptom onset and subsequent course of dementia depend on the underlying cause. Classically, AD has an insidious onset and gradual decline, whereas vascular dementia is characterized by an abrupt onset and stepwise deterioration. Both disorders are common, and the two may coexist, although only one diagnosis may be established during an individual's life. Other dementias may be progressive, static, or remitting. The reversibility of a dementia is a function of the underlying pathologic condition and the availability and timely application of effective treatment.

Table 8-3 Medications That May Cause Cognitive Impairment

Antiarrhythmic agents	Disopyramide, quinidine, tocainide
Antibiotics	Cephalexin, cephalothin, metronidazole, cipro-floxacin, ofloxacin, norfloxacin, cefuroxime
Anticholinergic agents	Benztropine, homatropine, scopolamine, tri-hexyphenidyl, orphenadrine, atropine, meclizine
Antidepressants	amitriptyline, imipramine, desipramine, fluoxetine, trazodone, doxepin
Anticonvulsants	Phenytoin, valproic acid, carbamazepine
Antiemetics	Promethazine, hydroxyzine, metoclopramide, prochlorperazine
Antihypertensive agents	Propranolol, metoprolol, atenolol, verapamil, methyldopa, prazosin, nifedipine, diltiazem
Antineoplastic agents	Chlorambucil, cytarabine, interleukin-2, spirohydantoin mustard
Antimanic agent	Lithium
Antiparkinsonian agents	Levodopa, pergolide, bromocriptine
Antihistamines/decongestants	Phenylpropanolamine, diphenhydramine, chlor-pheniramine, brompheniramine, pseudoephedrine
Cardiotonic agents	Digoxin
Corticosteroids	Hydrocortisone, prednisone, dexamethasone
Histamine$_2$-recptor antagonists	Cimetidine, ranitidine, famotidine, nizatidine
Immunosuppressive agents	Cyclosporine, interferon
Narcotic analgesics	Codeine, hydrocodone, oxycodone, meperidine, propoxyphene
Muscle relaxants	Baclofen, cyclobenzaprine, methocarbamol, carisoprodol, chlorzoxazone
Nonsteroidal antiinflammatory agents	Acetylsalicylic acid, ibuprofen, indomethacin, naproxen, sulindac, diflunisal
Radiocontrast agents	Metrizamide, iothalamate, iohexol, diatrizoate
Sedatives	Alprazolam, diazepam, lorazepam, phenobarbital, butabarbital, chloral hydrate, triazolam, butalbital

STAGES OF DEMENTIA

Primary degenerative or progressive dementias are generally staged according to the level of functional impairment; the same categories may be used to describe the degree of severity of any dementia. The ability to perform a specific function depends on baseline skills, cognitive deficits, and the social environment. Thus the severity of illness should be assessed in the context of past functioning in several domains. Individuals with mild impairments show borderline functioning in several areas but definite impairment in none. Such individuals are not considered demented but should be evaluated over time; many will progress to a dementing disorder, some may return to normal functioning, and others may remain in a questionable state of "mild cognitive impairment." Individuals with mild dementia are likely to have difficulties with balancing a checkbook, preparing a complex meal, or managing a difficult medication schedule. Those with moderate dementia have difficulties with simpler food preparation, household cleanup, and yard work and may require some assistance with some aspects of self-care, for example, reminders to use the bathroom, help with fasteners, or help shaving. Those with severe dementia require considerable assistance with personal care, including feeding, grooming, and toileting. In profound dementia, patients become largely oblivious to their surroundings and are almost totally dependent on caregivers. The terminal phase of dementia generally results in the individual becoming bedridden, requiring constant care, with susceptibility to accidents and infectious diseases that often prove fatal.

Symptom Progression

The clinical progression of dementia may be divided into three phases: early, middle, and late. The classic dementia syndrome of AD includes impairment of learning new information; poor recall of remote material; impaired naming and verbal comprehension; deterioration in constructional and visual spatial abilities; and poor calculations, abstracting, and judgment. Amnesia is the common early symptom of dementia. Fluency of verbal output, repetition skills, and the ability to read aloud are retained until later in the disease. Motor and sensory functions are also spared throughout most of the course of the illness. In the final phases, there is total abolition of intellectual function, progressive loss of ambulation and coordination, dysphagia, and incontinence. Aspiration pneumonia, sepsis associated with urinary tract infection or decubitus ulcers, or an independent age-related disease usually accounts for the death of the patient.

SPECIFIC DEMENTIA SYNDROMES

A number of specific dementia syndromes have been identified and differentiated from the most common form of dementia—AD. AD is a dementia with insidious onset, gradual progression, and deterioration in functioning. Various patterns of deficits are seen, but the disorder most commonly begins with deficits in recent memory and mild anomia, followed by other neurocognitive deficits that develop after several years. The diagnosis of AD is made only after other causes for the dementia have been excluded by careful history, physical and neurologic examination, and laboratory tests. Identification of underlying causes of cognitive impairment are considered part of the dementia evaluation or workup (see Box 8-2). Most commonly, drug toxicity, depression, thyroid disease, B_{12} deficiency, and normal-pressure hydrocephalus are found during a comprehensive evaluation. A definitive diagnosis of AD depends on the microscopic examination of the brain, generally at autopsy, which reveals numerous characteristics of senile plaques and neurofibrillary tangles widely distributed in the cerebral cortex. A clinical diagnosis of AD conforms to the pathologic diagnosis up to 93% of the time.[27]

Alzheimer's Disease

A comprehensive discussion of the risk factors and epidemiology of AD is beyond the scope of this chapter; the reader is referred to Keltner and others.[27] Known risk factors for AD include advancing age, family history of AD, genetic factors, and to a lesser extent, head injury and the history of or presence of depression. Onset generally occurs in late life, most commonly after age 65, but in rare instances, the disorder may occur as early as age 40. The incidence of AD increases with age and is estimated at 0.5% per year from age 65 to 69, 1% per year from age 70 to 74, 2% per year from age 75 to 79, 3% per year from age 80 to 84, and 5% per year from age 85 onward.[22] AD is arbitrarily termed *early onset* if symptoms of cognitive decline begin at or before age 65, and *late onset* if they begin after age 65 (Box 8-3).

Box 8-3 Cognitive Symptoms of Early, Middle, and Late Stages of Alzheimer's Disease

Early stage

Forgetfulness for faces, names, and conversations

Subtle decline in performing work or activities of daily living (trouble learning new routines, slowing of work performance, and decreased output)

Subtle personality changes (decline in social graces and withdrawal from social contacts)

Early language problems (difficulty expressing complex ideas, shortening of phraseology)

Repetitiveness

Anxiety, worry, and depression concerning the decline of these abilities

Early-middle stage

Pervasive memory problems (forgetting major, important items and "forgetting to remember")

Inability to work in one's customary job

Paranoia, apathy, or delusions

Need for supervision in household chores

Difficulties in naming objects

Disorientation outdoors, especially in relatively unfamiliar places

Definite decline in personal grooming

Occasional incontinence

Needing reminders to bathe and assistance in dressing

Late-middle stage

Frequent disorientation indoors

Needing supervision in bathroom

Very limited vocabulary and comprehension

Disorders of sleep-wakefulness cycle

Extremes of emotional reactivity

General withdrawal from all social contacts

State of "living in the past"

Purposeless hyperactivity or energy

Late stage

Dissolution of personality

Lack of recognition

Severe language impairment

Inability to feed oneself

Incontinence

Severe motor deficits

Modified from Kokmen E: Etiology, diagnosis, and management of dementia, *Campr Ther* 15(9):59, 1989.

Note: The order, intensity, and duration of symptoms vary considerably among patients.

AD affects 4 to 5 million people in the United States and is the most common cause of long-term care. This age-related disease results from a degenerative process characterized by deposits of amyloid and other abnormal proteins in the brain. Inflammatory and immune mechanisms are involved in neuronal destruction.[1] Furthermore, complementary components are known to attack and are found around neurons and neurofibrillary tangles. Thus anti-inflammatory and immunosuppressive drugs are being investigated as possible treatments of AD.

Although numerous changes in various neurotransmitter systems have been documented in the brains of patients with AD, accumulating evidence suggests that dysfunction of the cholinergic system is crucial in the development of memory loss and related cognitive problems.

Vascular Dementia

Vascular dementia (VD) is a dementia resulting from the effects of one or more strokes or other vascular disease. Abrupt onset and stepwise deterioration occur in the context of cerebral vascular disease, documented by history, focal neurologic signs and symptoms, and/or imaging studies. Patchy cognitive deficits, depending on which region of the brain has been destroyed, are observed. Neurologic signs and symptoms include extensor plantar response, pseudobulbar palsy, gait abnormalities, exaggeration of deep tendon reflexes, and weakness of an extremity. Structural imaging studies usually indicate multiple vascular lesions of the cerebral cortex and subcortical structures.

The onset of VD may occur at any time in late life but becomes less common after age 75, whereas the incidence of AD continues to rise after age 75. Because AD and VD (including strokes) are both common and often coexist, a mixed dementia may be seen. Also, small strokes may lead to the increased clinical expression of AD per se. Early treatment of hypertension and other risk factors associated with VD may prevent further progression of vascular dementia.

Many types of VD exist, including multiinfarct dementia, ministroke dementia, Binswanger's disease, and subcortical arteriosclerotic leukoencephalopathy. Each type has a specific history or medical literature that lacks diagnostic precision because few patients have a single specific type of vascular disease. Most vascular dementia involves multiple types of ischemic brain injury.

The clinical symptoms of VD are often indistinguishable from those of AD. Clinical symptoms of vascular dementia often fluctuate, and psychiatric symptoms are common. Patients often have preexisting cardiovascular disease, hypertension, diabetes, and a history of smoking. A detailed medical history is therefore important to determine the risk for VD.

Lewy Body Dementia

Lewy body dementia (LBD) is a recently characterized disorder that shares some similarities with AD. However, LBD tends to have earlier and more prominent visual hallucinations, parkinsonian features, and a more rapidly evolving course. Patients are notably sensitive to extrapyramidal side effects (EPSEs) of antipsychotic medications. The neuropathology of this dementia subtype is marked by the presence of Lewy inclusion bodies in the cerebral cortex. The disorder is likely to come to psychiatric attention because of the patient's prominent psychotic symptoms and sensitivities to antipsychotic medications.

Parkinson Disease—Associated Dementia

Another form of dementia with parkinsonism is dementia resulting from Parkinson's disease (PD). PD is a slowly progressive neurologic condition characterized by tremor, rigidity, bradykinesia, and postural instability; its onset is typically in middle to late life. In approximately one third to two thirds of cases, PD is accompanied by a dementia that is more common late in the course of the illness. This dementia has insidious and slow progression and is characterized by cognitive and motor slowing, executive dysfunction, and impairment in memory retrieval.

Frontotemporal Dementia

Frontotemporal dementia (FTD) is characterized by changes in personality, executive dysfunction, deterioration of social skills, emotional blunting, behavioral disinhibition, and prominent language abnormalities. Pick's disease is a type of FTD that occurs in fewer than 1% of dementia cases. Difficulties with memory, apraxia, and other features of dementia usually follow later in the course of FTD. As the dementia progresses, apathy or extreme agitation and aggressive behavior may emerge. Individuals develop severe problems with language, attention, or behavior, making cognitive assessment difficult. These dementias are difficult to distinguish from atypical AD; the diagnosis is confirmed at autopsy. FTD most commonly manifests itself in individuals 50 to 60 years of age, although it can develop in older individuals.

Miscellaneous dementia syndromes. Other progressive dementias include Huntington's disease, Creutzfeldt-Jakob disease, and acquired immunodeficiency syndrome (AIDS) dementia associated with the HIV virus. *AIDS dementia complex* describes a variable mixture of cognitive, motor, and behavioral abnormalities that develops in patients with AIDS. Approximately 60% of individuals infected with HIV who develop AIDS will also develop dementia. Dementia may be the presenting symptom in some HIV-infected individuals. The rate of progression and symptom constellation vary from patient to patient. Early symptoms include difficulties with concentration, memory, and conceptualization. As the dementia progresses, patients develop apraxia, hyperreflexia, dysarthria, and frontal lobe dysfunction. Patients with late-stage AIDS dementia demonstrate apathy, withdrawal, and unresponsiveness. Some evidence suggests that high-dose AZT administration may slow the progression of HIV dementia; formal treatment trials are under way.

General medical conditions can cause dementia, including those that cause structural brain lesions (e.g., normal pressure hydrocephalus). These dementias may be potentially amenable to treatment (see Box 8-1). It is critical that clinicians caring for individuals with dementia be familiar with general medical and other neurologic causes of dementia to ensure that the diagnosis is accurate and that potentially treatable conditions are identified.

TREATMENT OF DEMENTIA—NONPHARMACOLOGIC APPROACHES
General Treatment Principles

The treatment of dementia is multimodal. It is guided by the stage of illness and focused on the specific symptoms manifested. Management of dementia includes the skillful combination of education and support for the caregiver, nonpharmacologic and behavioral interventions, the use of medications for cognitive and behavioral symptoms, and supplemental therapies (e.g., gingko biloba, bright light, or exercise).

Dementia management has four major components: (1) treating the cognitive deficit in selected patients, (2) ameliorating associated behavioral disturbances, (3) reducing the consequences of disability, and (4) addressing the needs of the caregiver. In addition, patients with coexisting general medical conditions or psychiatric disorders contributing to the cognitive impairment will require treatment of that underlying disorder. Untreated or undertreated general medical problems such as chronic obstructive pulmonary disease (COPD) disease may worsen the patient's distress and confusion.

Psychosocial Approaches to Dementia

The principal goals of supportive care for dementias of all types are to maintain the patient's socialization in a safe but stimulating environment and to counsel the family. Agitation, paranoid thinking, and irrational behavior can be prevented to some degree by providing patients with nonstressful, familiar, and constant surroundings; schedules that are both regular and structured encourage patients to continue physical and mental activities within their capacities. Measures that can help patients orient themselves within their home environments include prominently displaying clocks and calendars, supplying night-lights, posting bulletin boards displaying such items as schedules of daily activities and pictures of family members, putting labels on commonly used items, and addressing notes to patients about simple safety measures. Activities that may improve cognitive function include listening to the radio or looking at newspapers or television, doing chores, engaging in physical exercise, attending structured social events, and participating in discussion and reminiscences. A patient can cope better when household activities—meals, walks, chores—occur at the same time every day. Familiarity with an environment can make a patient's life less stressful; thus a patient should be surrounded by familiar objects. Discouraging naps can lessen the chances of nighttime wandering. Patients who have progressed beyond the earliest stages of dementia should not be permitted to drive because of disease-associated disorientation and impairment of judgment, as well as decreased reaction time and visual perception.

Most patients, especially those in the last stages of AD, will eventually require institutional care. Incontinence and disruptive behavior are the most common factors that influence families' decisions to seek a long-term care facility. What constitutes appropriate care for people with dementia is still an evolving body of knowledge.

Home-based dementia care addresses the needs of the patient and the caregiver who provides assistance 24 hours per day. Care of the caregiver is an essential aspect of the total management of dementia. Family members provide most of the care, a stressful undertaking. Increased rates of depression, psychotropic medication use, and stress-related illnesses are found among AD caregivers. Community resources such as assisted home care, day care, respite care, and extended residential care may reduce the burden. Participation in dementia support groups can help immensely, but some caregivers may require formal counseling or psychotherapy.

Caregivers require detailed information and constructive realistic suggestions for each phase of the patient's dementia. They need information on the basic disease process, medications and side effects, monitoring for new medical or dental problems, organization of legal or financial issues, preparation for long-term care, and considerations for end-of-life planning. Extensive, consumer-friendly literature for family caregivers is available through The Alzheimer's Association and through texts such as *The 36 Hour Day*.

The successful management of patients with dementia requires a broad range of tasks that are grouped under the term *psychiatric management*.[4] These interventions help maximize a patient's level of functioning and ensure safety and comfort for both patients and families in the context of living with a difficult disease. These psychosocial and psychotherapeutic interventions are used to address memory, executive function, language, judgment, and spatial abilities. It is often helpful to track cognitive status with a simple examination such as the MMSE.[19]

Behavioral Disturbances

Behavioral disturbances associated with dementia can be a source of extreme psychologic distress to the patient, especially when coupled with the awareness that one's mental faculties are being irreversibly lost. A systematic approach is necessary to evaluate and treat behavioral complications. The evaluation should begin with the identification and specification of target symptoms. Once these are characterized, clinicians should perform a comprehensive medical examination to determine whether the behavioral problem is caused by an underlying general medical disorder. Agitation, for instance, may be caused by an infection, medication side effects, an occult hip fracture, pain, or loss of sleep. At the same time, psychiatric and mental status examinations should be conducted to evaluate whether symptoms are caused by a recurrent or new-onset identifiable disorder such as depression or mania. Following this evaluation and the treatment of relevant abnormalities, the remaining behavioral disturbances may be addressed on a symptomatic basis.

The initial approach may include modulating the environment and addressing factors that aggravate the behavior, such as a noisy roommate, excessively bright light, or other factors. A consistent daily routine is followed, optimizing the social and physical stimulation with techniques such as validation, encouragement, support, and reminiscence. Educating those who are providing care for the patient and using other techniques such as simple communication, avoidance of fatigue, the use of distraction, or seeking additional help or respite when necessary are also important. All of these behavioral techniques help maximize functioning and independence, enhance communication, and modulate behavior. These nonpharmacologic approaches are best exhausted before psychotropic drugs are used; the drug therapies should be guided by the specific diagnosis and target symptoms.

TREATMENT OF DEMENTIA—PHARMACOLOGIC APPROACHES
Agitation

Agitation and *aggressive behavior* are terms that are difficult to conceptualize precisely. The two syndromes overlap and thus are generally applied to a host of nonspecific behaviors that include such manifestations as wandering, pacing, uncooperativeness, and verbal outbursts (Table 8-4). *Aggression* is often defined as hostile actions directed at others, objects, or oneself and may be physical, verbal, or sexual.

Benzodiazepines. The use of benzodiazepines in the treatment of agitation in dementia has not been well studied. Benzodiazepines are best given in single doses or short courses when sedation or immediate anxiolytic effects are desirable. Patients with coexisting anxiety, extrapyramidal symptoms, sleeping problems, and tension may benefit from benzodiazepine therapy. Benzodiazepines may cause side effects, including sedation, confusion, amnesia, ataxia, and disinhibition, which are associated with an increase in confusion, agitation, and amnestic effects. Patients can become dependent on benzodiazepines or develop withdrawal symptoms when treatment is abruptly stopped. Short-acting benzodiazepines (e.g., lorazepam and oxazepam) are preferred agents because they are more easily metabolized and

Table 8-4   Agitation in Dementia

Physical	Verbal	Aggressive behaviors	
Pacing	Complaints	Hitting	Threats
Inappropriate disrobing	Attention seeking	Pushing	Accusations
Wandering	Negativism	Teasing	Name calling
Handling things inappropriately	Repeated questions	Spitting	Obscenities
Restlessness	Repeated phrases	Kicking	
Stereotypy	Screaming	Scratching	
		Biting	

Adapted from References 11 and 55.

unlikely to accumulate over time. Generally, these drugs have limited utility in treating agitation associated with dementia.

Buspirone. Buspirone, a nonbenzodiazepine anxiolytic, has been shown to have some benefit in treating agitation in dementia. Agitation, aggressive behavior, apprehension, and persistent anxiety, as well as drug-induced EPSEs, have improved at dosages of 15 to 60 mg in divided doses.

Mood stabilizers. Mood stabilizers are a recent addition to the armamentarium for the treatment of agitation in dementia. Individuals with agitation, sleep disturbances, and abnormalities of speech and motor behavior may benefit from treatment with anticonvulsants. The GABAergic effects of mood stabilizers may have an ameliorating effect on agitation and disruptive behaviors in dementia.

Lithium has limited utility in treating agitation in dementia. It may be used to augment the response to another drug. Serum levels of 0.4 to 0.8 mEq/L are recommended. Neurologic and EPSEs may occur at therapeutic doses in the elderly demented patient.

Carbamazepine is effective in the treatment of agitated dementia. Few "pure" studies exist, and carbamazepine is often used in combination with other drugs. Usual dosages to achieve levels of 4 to 12 µg/ml are recommended. Adverse effects, drug interactions, and autoinduction make carbamazepine difficult to use in this group of patients. Dosage and titration may take several months to reach an optimal dose, limiting its utility.

The use of valproate or divalproex has been effective in both acute and chronic agitation in dementia. The quality of clinical reports with divalproex supports its use as a first-line agent. Dosages to achieve therapeutic levels of 50 to 100 µg/ml are recommended. Valproate is superior in cases involving dysphoria and mood cycling. Tolerability, lower potential for drug-drug interaction, and the utility of valproate's more rapid titration are helpful.

Gabapentin may be useful in agitated patients with dementia. Tolerability and lack of drug interactions make this an appealing drug, especially in combination with other drugs. A wide range of dosages, from 600 to 3600 mg/day, may be used. Lamotrigine has not been reported to be useful in treating agitation in dementia. Theoretically, it could be useful, especially in those cases of dementia involving mood disturbance or self-injurious behavior—in view of the inhibitory effects on glutamate.

Overall, mood stabilizers address a wide range of disruptive behaviors, including agitation, aggression, combativeness, shouting, hyperactivity, and disinhibition associated with mood disturbance or psychosis.[59] Patients already taking Dilantin

Table 8-5 Selected Antipsychotic Medications for Agitation in Dementia

Drug	Initial dose (mg/day)	Typical range (mg/day)
Thioridazine	10-25	50-150
Haloperidol	0.25-0.5	1-4
Fluphenazine	0.25-0.5	1-4
Thiothixene	0.5-1	2-8
Risperidone	0.25-0.5	1-3
Olanzapine	2.5-5	5-15
Quetiapine	12.5-2.5	75-200
Clozapine	6.25-12.5	25-200

Adapted from References 18 and 56.

and phenobarbital for anticonvulsant effects are preferably switched to divalproex or possibly augmented with gabapentin to control breakthrough seizures or behavioral symptoms. Once the "new" agent is therapeutic, the "old" agent may be gradually tapered over several weeks.

Antipsychotics. Conventional antipsychotic medications have commonly been used as first-line agents for the treatment of behavioral disturbance in dementia. A meta-analysis of published studies demonstrated that although the magnitude of the effect varies, typical antipsychotic drugs produce modest improvements in some target symptoms and are most effective for the treatment of psychotic features.[45] No single typical antipsychotic medication is more efficacious than another; thus drug choice is guided by the side effect profile of the compound. Of the conventional antipsychotics, the high-potency agent haloperidol and the low-potency agent thioridazine have been most commonly used in the treatment of agitation, aggression, and psychosis in patients with dementia (Table 8-5). Antipsychotics have demonstrated efficacy in the treatment of symptoms such as hallucinations, delusions, paranoia, and excessive suspiciousness. However, significant side effects are reported, including the development of tardive dyskinesia and neuroleptic malignant syndrome. Thus these drugs should be initiated at low dosages and increased slowly.

More recently, atypical antipsychotics have been introduced. These drugs include clozapine, risperidone, olanzapine, quetiapine, and ziprasidone A growing body of evidence supports their utility in the treatment of dementia.[18] The initial dosage and typical range of dosages for some of these medications are shown in Table 8-5.

Antidepressants. A number of antidepressants have been useful in treating agitation and aggression associated with dementia. Trazodone, a serotonergic antidepressant with alpha-2 blocking effects, may reduce symptoms of irritability, anxiety, restlessness, and affective disturbance. Repetitive behaviors, verbal aggression, negativism, resistance to care, and unwarranted accusations have been reported to be improved in response to trazodone.[54] Low dosages, 25 to 50 mg/day, or larger dosages up to 150 mg to enhance sleep, are used and may address "sundowning" symptoms as well. Common side effects include orthostatic hypotension (at higher dosages), sedation, confusion, and delirium.

Serotonin neurotransmission is linked to agitation, aggression, and psychosis in dementia. Consequently, selective serotonin reuptake inhibitors (SSRIs), by restoring serotonergic function, are expected to improve some signs and symptoms of dementia. Of the few clinical investigations, the most promising have involved sertraline and citalopram.[10,21,33,34] Citalopram at dosages of 20 to 30 mg/day and sertraline at dosages of 25 to 100 mg/day have demonstrated efficacy in open-label studies, with few side effects. Improvements were seen in agitation, aggression, psychosis, and appetite.

Depression

Depression occurs in approximately 30% to 40% of patients with dementia, with a higher prevalence among those with mild to moderate, rather than severe, cognitive impairment. The treatment of depression may be complicated by the questionable efficacy and side effects of antidepressant drugs. Patients with AD, because of cholinergic deficit, may be more vulnerable to the anticholinergic side effects of tricyclic antidepressants (TCAs). Thus the antidepressant selected should produce minimal anticholinergic activity to prevent further decreases in cognitive function. Selective serotonin reuptake inhibitors (SSRIs), venlafaxine, bupropion, and nefazodone are preferred. Monoamine oxidase inhibitors (MAOIs) may also be used for patients who are refractory to first-line agents. MAOIs have few anticholinergic effects; the most problematic side effects are hypotension and insomnia or sedation.

Cognitive Symptoms

Successful pharmacologic management of cognitive impairment is limited by our understanding of the pathogenesis and pathophysiology of the underlying disease. None of the drugs now being used for dementia treatment have proven to be efficacious in a large percentage of patients. The fact that dementias include several subtypes partly explains this. Following is a discussion of classes of drugs that have been studied for use in treating the most common form of dementia, AD, and related disorders in some cases).

Cholinergic enhancers: tacrine, donepezil, rivastigmine, and so on. Cholinergic neurons are selectively destroyed early in the course of AD. Acetylcholinesterase, the substrate of acetylcholinesterase inhibitors, is located in the synaptic space and in the synaptic membranes of the neurons of the cholinergic system (Figures 8-1 and 8-2). All layers of the cerebral cortex receive cholinergic innervation; the density of cholinergic projections is highest in the upper regions of the cortex. The limbic areas, which include the amygdala and the hippocampus, also have this high density of cholinergic axons; paralimbic regions have the next highest density of cholinergic fibers. The primary visual cortex also has cholinergic projections, but these are the least abundant. Two classes of cholinergic receptors are recognized on the basis of their responses to specific agonists and antagonists—muscarinic and nicotinic. Three types of muscarinic receptors have been identified pharmacologically, and five types have been shown to exist on the basis of molecular cloning experiments.[38]

Muscarinic receptors use G-proteins for transduction; nicotinic receptors use ligand-gated ion channels for signal transduction. The M-1 receptor is the most common muscarinic subtype in the cerebral cortex. The highest concentrations of M-1 receptors are found in the dentate gyrus, hippocampus, anterior olfactory nucleus, cerebral cortex, olfactory tubercle, and nucleus accumbens. The M-2 receptor is found in brain areas with abundant cholinergic neurons, including the basal forebrain. The M-2 receptor is a presynaptic autoreceptor that governs cholinergic release. Nicotinic receptors are most abundant in the thalamus,

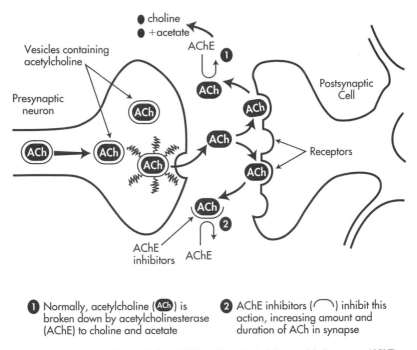

① Normally, acetylcholine (ACh) is broken down by acetylcholinesterase (AChE) to choline and acetate

② AChE inhibitors (⌒) inhibit this action, increasing amount and duration of ACh in synapse

Figure 8-1 The release of acetylcholine *(ACh)* and its hydrolysis by acetylcholinesterase *(AChE)*. Inhibition of acetylcholinesterase can increase the availability of acetylcholine in the brain. (Adapted from Cummings JL: *Understanding and treating Alzheimer's disease: a primer,* 1997, Lisai Inc. and Pfizer, Inc.)

periaqueductal gray, and substantia nigra. Intermediate levels of M-2 receptors are found in cerebral cortex, and low levels are found in the hippocampus and amygdala.

The cholinergic hypothesis predicts that drugs that potentiate central cholinergic function should improve cognition and perhaps behavioral problems experienced with AD. Approaches to the treatment of cholinergic deficit in AD, most of which initially focused on the replacement of acetylcholine precursors, failed to increase central cholinergic activity. Other studies investigated the use of cholinesterase (ChE) inhibitors that reduce the hydrolysis of acetylcholine (ACh), for example, physostigmine. Although various ChE inhibitors have been developed as treatments for AD, the pharmacologic activities of these agents differ. For example, tacrine (Cognex) and donepezil (Aricept) are mixed-type reversible inhibitors of ChE. These compounds inhibit ChE via noncompetitive mechanisms (i.e., blockade of the deacetylation process) and competitive mechanisms. Carbamates such as rivastigmine (Exelon) and physostigmine (Antilirium) are pseudoirreversible ChE inhibitors and actually cleave the enzyme, resulting in a covalent modification of the enzyme. This inhibition is noncompetitive with ACh and is irreversible. However, this association of the carbamate is transient because of the rapid metabolism and rapid rate of decarbamoylation that regenerates ChE. Another compound, metrifonate, inhibits ChE irreversibly. This is a prodrug that is converted to *dichlorvos,* an organophosphorous ChE inhibitor with a very long duration of inhibition and a half-life of 52 days.

The selectivity of ChE enzyme inhibition plays a crucial part in determining the

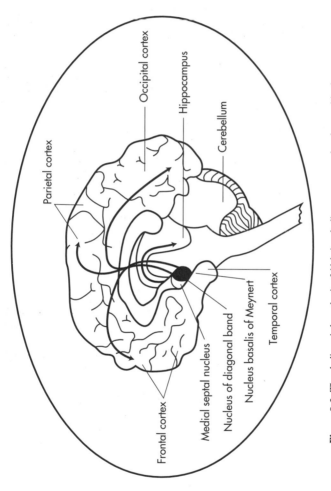

Figure 8-2 The cholinergic hypothesis of Alzheimer's disease proposes that the cognitive loss associated with this disease is related to decreased cortical cholinergic neurotransmission and that increasing the transmission may enhance cognitive function. (Adapted from Cummings JL: *Understanding and treating Alzheimer's disease: a primer*, 1997, Lisai Inc. and Pfizer, Inc.)

therapeutic profile of any ChE inhibitor. All ChE inhibitors possess greater or lesser degrees of selectivity. Some agents that inhibit acetylcholinesterase (AChE) in the neural tissue may also inhibit butyrocholinesterase (BChE) in the periphery. BChE inhibition may be associated with unwanted peripheral side effects, although to date, this remains an unproved empirical finding.

The ChE inhibitors are the best developed and most widely used drugs for the treatment of AD. They exert their effects by inhibiting ChE in the brain, thereby increasing the available levels of ACh. ChE inhibitors appear to have similar actions in improving symptoms of memory and cognitive loss. ChE inhibitors directly increase central cholinergic function by reducing the breakdown of ACh, thereby increasing the effective amount of ACh within the synapse. In normal physiologic functioning, ACh is synthesized from choline and acetylcoenzyme A within the neuron and released into the synapse. Here, it interacts with nicotinic and muscarinic ACh receptors and remains active until its rapid hydrolysis by the ChE enzyme.

At present, there are three ChE inhibitors—tacrine, donepezil, and rivastigmine—approved by the U.S. Food and Drug Administration (FDA) for use in the United States. Metrifonate is currently under review, and several other agents are being studied. Differences in study design among trials do not allow a direct comparison between these agents; however, all have demonstrated modest improvement in cognitive function in patients, with good tolerability among the second-generation inhibitors. A summary of the trials for selected ChE inhibitors can be found in Farlow.[16] Ongoing studies of these agents are occurring to determine whether long-term advantages exist in tolerability and durability, one compared with the other.

Tacrine (Cognex) is a first-generation ChE inhibitor with a half-life of approximately 3 hours, requiring four-times-daily dosing. Donepezil (Aricept) is a reversible inhibitor that can be dosed once daily by virtue of its 70-hour plasma half-life.

Pseudoirreversible inhibition occurs with the carbamate compounds, which interact with the catalytic subsite of the active site. Physostigmine, a first-generation carbamate ChE inhibitor, has a very short half-life of inhibition of approximately 30 minutes, which limits its usefulness. Second-generation carbamates that are derivatives of physostigmine have longer half-lives; rivastigmine (Exelon), for example, has a half-life of inhibition of 10 hours, whereas its plasma half-life is approximately 2 hours. These drugs form carbamoylated complexes with the ChE, which are hydrolyzed very slowly. This makes the ChE molecule unavailable for further enzymatic action for several hours.[15] Because of this slowly hydrolyzed bond, the half-life of ChE inhibition of these compounds, for example, as seen with rivastigmine, outlasts the plasma half-lives.

Irreversible inhibition is produced by the organophosphorous compounds that result in an essentially permanent covalent bond. ChE function is restored mainly by the synthesis of new enzyme. Metrifonate, an organophosphate that has been used as an antihelminthic for many years, is not a ChE inhibitor itself but is a prodrug that is nonenzymatically converted to an organophosphorous metabolite by spontaneous hydrolysis. The complex produced by phosphorylation of ChE is extremely stable, resulting in ChE inhibition that can last for several weeks.[7]

In addition to the differing mechanisms of ChE inhibition, ChE inhibitors are metabolized and excreted in a variety of ways that affect their efficacy and tolerability. Tacrine is metabolized extensively via the cytochrome P-450 system, mainly by the 1A2 isoenzyme, with multiple metabolites—some of which are also active ChE inhibitors. Dose-related hepatotoxicity of tacrine and its metabolite, velnacrine, is a limiting factor for the use of this drug. Donepezil is partly excreted unchanged in the urine; the remainder is metabolized into four major metabolites, at least one of which inhibits ChE with the same potency as its parent compound. Although it is metabolized via the 2D6 and 3A4 isoenzymes of cytochrome P-450, no significant hepatotoxicity is seen with donepezil. Metabolites of donepezil are excreted through both renal and fecal pathways. Rivastigmine and other carbamate ChE inhibitors are metabolized in their interaction with ChEs; they are hydrolyzed just as acetylcholine is, albeit more slowly. The breakdown products are rapidly excreted in the kidney with no hepatic involvement; therefore no opportunity for drug-drug interactions exists with other drugs metabolized by cytochrome P-450. The organophosphorous inhibitors, such as DDVP, the active product of metrifonate, also have no involvement with the cytochrome P-450 system; the entire inhibitor-enzyme complex is gluconurated and excreted renally.

The most common side effects of ChE inhibitors are those related to the inhibition of peripheral ChEs such as BChE. Adverse effects include nausea, vomiting, diarrhea, facial flushing, sweating, rhinorrhea, bradycardia, and leg cramping. Thus a major goal of ChE inhibition therapy is to selectively inhibit central nervous system ChE, that is, to choose drugs that concentrate in the brain. As previously discussed, tacrine inhibits all types of ChEs nonspecifically and indeed has a much higher affinity for BChE than AChE. This contributes to peripheral cholinergic side effects at intermediate levels of ChE inhibition. Donepezil exhibits a relatively high degree of selectivity for neuronal AChE as opposed to peripheral BChE.[49] Rivastigmine is the most brain-region selective for AChE, especially in the cortex and hippocampus, and produces relatively little inhibition of peripheral ChEs.[5]

Tacrine. Tacrine (Cognex) was the first agent approved by the FDA for treating mild to moderate dementia of the Alzheimer's type. In patients with mild to moderate AD, tacrine demonstrated improvement compared with placebo as measured by the Alzheimer's Disease Assessment Scale–cognitive subscale (ADAS-cog), the clinician-based Global Impression of Change (CBIC), and the Caregiver-Rated Impression of Change (CGIC).[14] Dosing of tacrine in protocols has ranged from 40 to 160 mg/day in four divided doses usually given between meals. Higher dosages are not recommended because of concerns about hepatotoxicity and adverse effects. Blood monitoring is required every other week for the first 18 weeks after initiation of tacrine therapy to monitor alanine aminotransferase levels (ALT) and for 6 weeks after each successive dosage increase. Common side effects include gastrointestinal upset and agitation. Approximately 25% to 30% of cases will show ALT elevations that require withdrawal from the drug. Interestingly, about two thirds of these patients, who show elevated liver enzymes requiring drug discontinuation, are able to resume treatment after a rechallenge with tacrine. The recommended modifications with ALT elevations are available in the package insert for Cognex. Overall, 30% to 60% of individuals show improvement in cognitive function or maintain their present levels of cognitive function for extended periods ranging from 6 to 36 months.

Donepezil. Donepezil (Aricept) was the second cholinesterase inhibitor approved (in 1996) for symptoms of AD. Donepezil has several advantages over tacrine; its long half-life of 70 hours supports once-daily dosing and encourages compliance, as do the minimal adverse effects. With donepezil, once-daily dosage produces significant dose-related improvements in cognition and global functioning in more than 80% of patients. Some patients show measurable improvement; others simply do not deteriorate in cognition as expected. In either event, such response is viewed positively considering the progressive and degenerative nature of the disease. One 30-week randomized double-blind study of donepezil (5 or 10 mg/day) versus placebo showed statistically significant improvements at both 5 and 10 mg ($p = .001$) with respect to the ADAS-cog and the CBIC.[41,46] This clinical improvement was correlated with donepezil plasma concentrations and ChE inhibition.[40] The general thesis is that ChE inhibition will delay progression of symptoms and improve patients on an average of 6 to 12 months and up to 36 months equivalent of deterioration, with some patients showing more or less improvement.

Donepezil at 5 and 10 mg/day is well tolerated with no evidence of hepatotoxicity and an incidence of side effects at 5 mg/day similar to that of placebo. Cholinergic side effects are mild, transient, and resolve with continued treatment. As with the other available ChE inhibitors, including tacrine, the incidence of side effects is reported to be slightly increased in patients treated with the higher 10-mg dosage. No significant drug-drug interactions have been noted, although donepezil may interact with drugs that depend on the same metabolic pathways (e.g., carbamazepine, phenytoin, dexamethasone, and phenobarbital); ketoconazole and quinidine have been shown to inhibit the metabolism of donepezil in vitro. Donepezil does not appear to interact with theophylline, cimetidine, warfarin, or digoxin. Donepezil has the potential to cause bradycardia in patients with underlying cardiac conduction problems. Syncope has been noted in some patients. Dropout rates because of adverse effects were 16% for the 10-mg group and 6% for the 5-mg group. Rapid titration produces a higher incidence of cholinergic side effects in which nausea and vomiting are moderately severe but transient. However, 4- to 6-week titrations produce side effects comparable to those for the low-dose group. Abrupt discontinuation of donepezil produces no adverse events, but treatment benefit gradually diminishes over 6 weeks.

Rivastigmine. Rivastigmine (Exelon) has been approved for the treatment of AD. Rivastigmine is a ChE inhibitor. Clinical trials of rivastigmine were conducted with patients with concomitant diseases taking multiple medications.[52] The average patient age was 74.5 years old, in contrast with tacrine and donepezil trials that were conducted in somewhat younger and otherwise healthy patients with mild to moderate AD.[12] Observed adverse effects were mild to moderate in more than 3000 patients. Most side effects occurred during fixed dose escalation, resulting in discontinuation rates of 29% in the high-dose group. However, slower individualized titration will likely improve tolerance. The most common adverse effects at 6 to 12 mg include nausea (20%), vomiting (16%), and dizziness (14%). With rivastigmine's prolonged duration of action of approximately 10 hours, together with a plasma half-life of approximately 2 hours, the most effective dosing regimen is twice daily with optimal dosages at 6 to 12 mg/day. Rivastigmine's mechanism is pseudoreversible; cessation of medication allows recovery of acetylcholinesterase function within 24 hours. No drug interactions have been noted; concomitant antacids, beta-blockers, calcium antagonists, antidiabetic agents, antihypertensives, nonsteroidal antiinflammatory drugs (NSAIDs), estrogens, analgesics, antianginal agents, and antihistamines are well tolerated. As previously discussed, rivastigmine is not metabolized by cytochrome P-450, as are donepezil and tacrine: therefore clinically relevant drug reactions are unlikely. Rivastigmine is not associated with hepatotoxicity, and monitoring of liver functions is not required.

Metrifonate. At the time of this writing, the current new drug application for the approval of metrifonate is on hold pending further investigation of a small number of cases involving respiratory paralysis.[6]

Xanomeline. Xanomeline is a relatively selective cholinergic M-1 agonist. Postsynaptic cholinergic neurons in the cortex are relatively well preserved in AD. Thus the advantage of direct muscarinic agonists, such as with xanomeline, is that intact presynaptic neurons are not required, although AD may result in disruption of the coupling between the M-1 receptors and second messenger systems. One multicenter trial demonstrated that xanomeline 75 mg three times daily was superior to placebo in the treatment of cognitive and noncognitive symptoms of AD.

Table 8-6 Cholinergic-Enhancing Agents, Approved or in Phase III Evaluation

Drug	Dosing	Mechanism of action	Stage of development
Tacrine	80-160 mg qid	AChE inhibitor	FDA approved
Donepezil	5-10 mg qd	AChE inhibitor	FDA approved
Rivastigmine	6-12 mg bid	AChE inhibitor	FDA approved
Metrifonate	0.3-0.65 mg/kg qd	AChE inhibitor	Phase III
Xanomeline	75 mg tid	M-1 agonist	Phase III
Galantamine	Unknown	(AChE inhibitor; nicotinic modulator	Phase III

AChE, Acetylcholinesterase; *FDA,* Food and Drug Administration.

Significant improvement in behavior was noted in individuals with symptoms such as vocal outbursts, suspiciousness, delusions, agitation, and hallucinations.[9]

Other cholinesterase inhibitors. Information comparing acetylcholinesterase inhibitors currently approved or under investigation is shown in Table 8-6. Galantamine is a modulator of nicotinic cholinergic receptors as well as an acetylcholinesterase inhibitor. The primary benefit of acetylcholinesterase inhibitors is the enhancement of cognition and the global improvement in functioning seen in individuals with signs and symptoms of AD. Cholinergic agents may also improve behavioral disturbances associated with disturbances of cholinergic function in AD. Thus cholinergic agents may have behavioral benefits for all patients, even those who do not improve cognitively; cholinergic agents may also reduce neuropsychiatric symptoms late in the course of the disease when cognitive enhancement may be limited.[13] Whether acetylcholinesterase inhibitors have a psychotropic role that is independent of their cognitive effects is a subject of ongoing study.

Other indications for cholinergic enhancers. ChE inhibitors and other cholinergic enhancers may be useful for patients with Lewy body dementia or Parkinson's disease with dementia. Other neurologic disorders with cholinergic deficits, including Pick's disease, cerebellar atrophy, progressive supranuclear palsy, parkinsonian dementia complex of Guam, alcoholism with Wernicke's encephalopathy, Creutzfeldt-Jakob disease, subacute sclerosing panencephalitis, dementia pugilistica, and traumatic brain injury, may also benefit from cholinergic enhancers. Patients with vascular dementia may have lesions that interrupt projections from the nucleus basalis and produce a cortical cholinergic deficit, or they may have mixed AD plus vascular disease, in which case they are potentially responsive to ChE inhibitors.[30] In AD, as well as in related disorders, patients who exhibit substantial cognitive improvement usually have a concomitant behavioral response, but behavioral and cognitive responses may be disassociated.

Alternative medications for Alzheimer's disease

Memantine, a leading prescription drug for dementia in Germany, is now being developed for dementia for use in the United States. A 32-center U.S. study of 252 patients compared with placebo showed that memantine slowed progression of moderately severe Alzheimer's disease over 6 months and slowed deterioration of neuropsychologic test scores and daily living activities. Memantine has its mechanism of action through NMDA receptor antagonism, which presumably decreases neuronal damage secondary to excitatory amino acids. Thus memantine could potentially be combined with acetylcholinesterase inhibitors or other drugs to treat patients with Alzheimer's disease.

Other approaches for cognitive symptoms

Vitamin E. Considerable interest has been expressed in vitamin E (alpha-tocopherol) as a treatment for AD and other dementias because of its antioxidant properties. Vitamin E has been shown to slow nerve cell damage/death in animal models and cell cultures associated with amyloid deposition.[8]

A single clinical trial has been conducted concerning vitamin E and AD.[42] In this placebo-controlled, double-blind, multicenter trial of 341 moderately impaired patients randomized to either 1000 international units of vitamin E twice daily, 5 mg of selegiline twice daily or both versus placebo, vitamin E alone and selegiline alone were equivalent in delaying the advent of poor outcome (defined as death, institutionalization, or significant functional decline) over the course of 2 years. Combined treatment performed somewhat worse than either agent alone, but the difference was not statistically significant. The benefit observed among individuals with vitamin E (or selegiline) was equivalent to approximately 7 months' delay in reaching any of the endpoints designated as poor functional outcome. No improvement was observed compared with baseline, but decreased rates of functional decline were observed with active treatment compared with placebo. No data are available concerning the role of vitamin E in AD with mild or severe impairment or in other dementing illness. However, vitamin E has been used clinically for other indications, with relatively low rates of toxicity at dosages between 400 and 3000 IU/day. Vitamin E is safe and well tolerated; at high dosages, it has been noted to worsen blood coagulation defects in patients with vitamin K deficiency.[25] However, given vitamin E's lack of medication interactions and general safety and tolerability, its use in combination with a ChE inhibitor is well advised. Efficacy data reported by Sano and colleagues was at a high dosage of 2000 IU/day.[42] Because of the association of vitamin E and worsening of coagulation defects, vitamin E is best limited to conventional dosages of 400 to 800 IU/day in populations at risk for bleeding (i.e., those with vitamin K deficiency).

Selegiline. Selegiline, also known as deprenyl, is a selective MAO-B inhibitor licensed in the United States for the treatment of Parkinson's disease. Selegiline is used as a dementia medication in some European countries and by some clinicians in the United States as well. Selegiline may act as an antioxidant or neuroprotective agent, slowing the progression of AD. Because of its effects on catecholamine metabolism, it could also act in a variety of other ways. Generally, selegiline has shown both cognitive and noncognitive improvements in five double-blind randomized trials looking at its effects in dementia.[4] One of selegiline's principal side effects is orthostatic hypotension, which may interfere with the patient's tolerance of the medication. Otherwise, patients appear to tolerate selegiline, with a slightly higher rate of falls and syncope reported in some clinical studies. Selegiline is activating, which is helpful for some patients but may lead to anxiety or irritability in others. The dosage of 5 to 10 mg/day is relatively selective for MAO-B and does not fully inhibit MAO-A, so a tyramine-free diet and avoidance of sympathomimetic agents are not required. The 10-mg dose ceiling, however, should be emphasized given the potential for symptoms of hypertensive crisis and other MAOI adverse effects that occur at higher dosages. More significant adverse effects of medication interactions, including severe mental status changes, seizures, and even death, have been noted in combination with meperidine, SSRIs, and TCAs. Selegiline is generally contraindicated for patients who are taking any of these agents. The limited data concerning its role in AD necessitates further study regarding its utility in other related dementias.

Antiinflammatory agents. Antiinflammatory agents may have significant impact on the course of AD, reducing the rate of decline secondary to the damage and destruction that occurs as a result of an associated inflammatory response. For individuals who are exposed to NSAIDs, the relative risk of the onset of symptoms of AD may be decreased significantly.[53] NSAIDs, especially the cyclooxygenase-2 (COX-2) inhibitors (e.g., rofecoxib, celecoxib) are now under investigation to determine their usefulness in AD.

Estrogens. An association between biologic markers of estrogen status such as serum levels of estradiol and decreased risk of cognitive decline has been suggested, with support of the hypothesis that estrogen per se is protective in AD. Women who choose to take estrogen are typically younger, are more educated, and lead more healthful lifestyles. Thus the lower risk of cognitive impairment attributed to estrogen may be because of these other factors.

Estrogen has direct biologic effects on neurotransmitters modulating acetylcholine, serotonin, and monoamine oxidase. It has direct effects on neurons, resulting in synaptic regulation and dendritic sprouting. Favorable lipid alterations and the facilitation of normal amyloid metabolism are seen in the context of adequate levels of estrogen. Estrogens may have significant impact on prevention of cerebral ischemia with respect to vasodilation, platelets, and oxidative stress. Estrogen replacement therapy users show increased positron emission tomography (PET) blood flow on memory tasks and decreased white matter changes on structural MRI.[36,43]

Serum estrogens are lower in AD. Women with lower estrogen levels, when compared with aged-matched controls, may be at increased risk for AD with a lifetime risk of one in three at age 65. Current studies support the hypothesis that estrogens prevent cognitive decline and the onset of symptoms of dementia.

The apolipoprotein E4 (ApoE4) allele significantly increases the susceptibility to cognitive impairment with aging. An association has been noted between ApoE4 and gender, with women having ApoE4 at higher risk for AD. Perhaps estrogen modifies the association between ApoE4 and the risk of cognitive decline. Recent studies support the notion of an interaction between estrogen and the ApoE4 genotype; ongoing and recently completed trials are evaluating the effects of estrogen on cognitive function in persons with AD. Thus far, it is known that in women who are E4 negative, estrogen is associated with less cognitive decline versus those who are E4 positive, in whom no association is observed.

The National Institute of Aging cooperative study of 120 hysterectomized AD women older than 60 has now been completed. This study was a 15-month study of estrogen at two dosage levels versus placebo to determine whether any therapeutic benefit could be derived from estrogen. Unfortunately, the study did not show significant therapeutic benefit of estrogen after diagnosis of AD that is, as a treatment for AD.[31] Some individuals have speculated that raloxifene (Evista) may be beneficial in dementia syndromes. Raloxifene is a selective estrogen receptor modulator that serves as an antagonist on the breast and uterus, and an agonist on bone and lipids. Its role on the central nervous system is questionable, especially given the lack of evidence that it crosses the blood-brain barrier. Nonetheless, an ongoing randomized trial of 7700 postmenopausal women is being conducted as a part of a dementia ancillary treatment study.

Metabolic enhancers/vasodilators. Hydergine, a compound of ergoloid mesylates, previously termed a *vasodilator* but now classified a *metabolic enhancer,* is approved by the FDA for treating dementia; however, its mechanism of action is currently unknown, and controlled trials have found this agent to be of no benefit.[44] The peripheral vasodilator nicergoline, another ergot drug, ameliorated disorientation in 30% of patients in a multicenter, double-blind placebo trial, but this drug is not available in the United States. The calcium channel blocker nimodipine, which is specific for the brain vasculature, is currently under investigation in patients with AD. Its potential benefit in treating AD may reside in its ability to reduce focal ischemia.

Nootropics. Nootropics are drugs that enhance neuronal metabolic activity. One avenue of research has focused on increasing nerve cell function so that neurotransmitter synthesis is increased. The mechanisms of action of nootropics responsible for improving memory are uncertain but are thought to include stimulation of phospholipid turnover and protein synthesis, and subsequent enhancement of cholinergic transmission. Potentially beneficial nootropics include piracetam and the related drug oxiraceptam. As previously stated, disruption of other neurotransmitter systems such as the serotonergic and noradrenergic systems has been documented in patients with AD. Attempts to increase their synthesis and thus improve symptoms by using an MAOI or an SSRI have yielded only mild or nonsignificant improvements.

Ginkgo. Ginkgo biloba, a living fossil tree dating back almost 200 million years, has been reported to have antioxidative and cognitive enhancing properties. Ginkgo is an herbal extract that has been used primarily in Europe to alleviate symptoms associated with numerous cognitive disorders. Its use in dementia is based on positive results from a few controlled trials, most of which have not included standard assessments of cognition and behavior. The efficacy and safety of ginkgo has been evaluated in AD and multiinfarct dementia in a 52-week randomized double-blind, placebo-controlled, parallel group, multicenter study.[28] Patients with mild to severe dementia without other significant medical conditions were treated with 120 mg/day of ginkgo versus placebo. Using the ADAS-cog along with global evaluation by the clinician, relative improvement in cognitive performance and social functioning were noted in a significant number of patients over a 6- to 12-month period. The 309 patients involved in this study showed that approximately 25% patients had at least a 4 point improvement in the ADAS-cog compared with 14% of those receiving placebo (p = .005). Adverse effects did not differ between placebo- and ginkgo-treated subjects. Although modest, the cognitive improvements induced by ginkgo were objectively measured and were of sufficient magnitude to be recognized by the caregivers who participated in this study.

The mechanism of action of ginkgo in the central nervous system is only partially understood, but the main effects seem to be related to its antioxidant properties, which require the synergistic action of the flavonoids and the terpenoids (ginkgolides and balobalide), and the organic acids that are principal constituents of ginkgo. These compounds, to varying degrees, act as scavengers for free radicals, which have been considered the mediators of cell damage observed in AD.

DELIRIUM

The management of delirium, as previously defined, may require any of three therapeutic tasks. The first fundamental task is assessment to determine the underlying physiologic or anatomic disturbances thought to be causal (Table 8-7). Generally, this phase of treatment requires a diligent clinical evaluation. Medications must also be assiduously evaluated, in particular their accumulative doses and temporal relationship to the onset of the delirium. A high index of suspicion is warranted for any of the classes of medications listed in Box 8-4.

The second therapeutic task is to provide general supportive measures, including both environmental measures and physiologic stabilization (Box 8-5). Ideally, these therapeutic principles will obviate the need for pharmacologic intervention or prolonged physical restraint. However, the effective use of psychotropic drugs is indicated when behavioral disturbances, psychomotor agitation, or psychosis predominates the clinical picture.

The third therapeutic task involves selecting one or more pharmacologic agents that will result in symptomatic relief, effectively treat the underlying cause, or both.

Table 8-7 Underlying Conditions Commonly Associated with Delirium

Type	Disorder
Central nervous system disorder	Head trauma
	Seizures
	Postictal state
	Vascular disease (e.g., hypertensive encephalopathy)
	Degenerative disease
Metabolic disorder	Renal failure (e.g., uremia)
	Hepatic failure
	Anemia
	Hypoxia
	Hypoglycemia
	Thiamine deficiency
	Endocrinopathy
	Fluid or electrolyte imbalance
	Acid-base imbalance
Cardiopulmonary disorder	Myocardial infarction
	Congestive heart failure
	Cardiac arrhythmia
	Shock
	Respiratory failure
Systemic illness	Substance intoxication or withdrawal
	Infection
	Neoplasm
	Severe trauma
	Sensory deprivation
	Temperature dysregulation
	Postoperative state

Box 8-6 outlines pharmacologic considerations and lists specific medications for each of the three categories of delirium. Cases categorized as withdrawal from alcohol, sedative-hypnotic agents, or a similar agent are best treated with a benzodiazepine such as lorazepam. However, delirium precipitated by anticholinergic drugs requires withdrawal of the offending agents, and individuals with urgent problems may also benefit from using an anticholinesterase agent such as physostigmine (Antilirium). Conventional antipsychotic drug treatment should be avoided or minimized in cases of anticholinergic delirium because of the potential for additional anticholinergic effects and the possible lowering of the seizure threshold.

GENERAL PRINCIPLES OF TREATMENT IN DELIRIUM

The general approach to the treatment of delirium includes the following:
1. Coordinating care for the patient
2. Identifying the etiology (identification and correction of the etiologic factors)
3. Initiating interventions for acute conditions, including a review of the patient's medications and discontinuation of those that are nonessential, keeping needed medications at the lowest dosage possible

---

Box 8-4 Classes and Examples of Medications That Induce Delirium

Anticholinergics: benztropine, trihexyphenidyl
Anticonvulsants: barbiturates, phenytoin
Antidiabetics: insulin, oral hypoglycemics
Antihypertensives: clonidine, methyldopa
Antiparkinsons: levodopa, carbidopa
Cancer chemotherapeutics: procarbazine, nitrogen mustard
Cardiovascular agents: digoxin, lidocaine
Corticosteroids: prednisone, prednisolone
Gastrointestinal agents: cimetidine, belladonna
Narcotic analgesics: opioids, synthetic narcotics
Nonnarcotic analgesics: salicylates, propoxyphene
Psychotropics: anxiolytics, antidepressants

Box 8-5 Nonpharmacologic Treatment of Delirium

Environmental manipulation
Arrange consistent, supportive nursing care.
Minimize personnel.
Place family member or significant other at bedside.
Use orienting remarks and devices such as calendars or clocks.
Place in a well-lighted room with window.
Provide familiar objects such as personal belongings and photographs.

Supportive measures
Effect fluid and electrolyte balance.
Maintain nutritional and vitamin status.
Obtain visual or hearing aids.
Provide moderate sensory input.
Encourage physical activity or ambulation.
Apply physical restraints as necessary.

---

4. Providing other disorder specific treatment, for example, treating disorders such as hypoglycemia, hypoxemia, hypothermia, hypertension, thiamine deficiency, withdrawal, and anticholinergic-induced or other substance-induced delirium
5. Monitoring and ensuring safety
6. Assessing and monitoring psychiatric status, including depression, suicidal ideation or behavior, hallucinations, delusions, aggressive behavior, agitation, anxiety, disinhibition, affective lability, cognitive deficits, and sleep disturbance
7. Assessing individuals' and families' psychologic and social characteristics
8. Establishing and maintaining alliances

Box 8-6   Pharmacologic Treatment of Delirium

Sedative-hypnotic, similar agent, or alcohol withdrawal
1. Maintain fluid and electrolyte balance.
2. Replace or provide nutritional and vitamin requirements.
3. Provide effective sedation with a benzodiazepine agent: chlordiazepoxide (Librium) 25 to 50 mg orally or intramuscularly every 4 to 6 hours or lorazepam (Ativan) 1 to 2 mg orally or intramuscularly every 6 to 8 hours.

Anticholinergic-induced delirium
1. Withdraw offending anticholinergic agent(s).
2. Counteract severe cases with physostigmine (Antilirium) 1 to 2 mg slowly intravenously; may be repeated every 30 to 60 minutes.

Multifactorial or miscellaneous variables
1. Withdraw offending agent(s) or treat underlying cause(s).
2. Enhance sleep with short-half-life hypnotic*†: triazolam (Halcion) 0.25 to 0.5 mg, zolpidem (Ambien) 0.5 to 10 mg, temazepam (Restoril) 15 to 30 mg orally at bedtime, or chloral hydrate 500 to 1000 mg orally at bedtime.
3. Treat "sundowning" or disruptive behavior with high-potency antipsychotic†: haloperidol (Haldol) or fluphenazine (Prolixin) hydrochloride 1 to 2 mg orally (concentrate) or intramuscularly 2 to 4 times daily, Risperdal 0.25 to 0.5 mg 2 to 4 times daily, or olanzapine 2.5 to 5 mg 1 to 2 times daily.

*Hypnotics can potentially worsen the clinical course and diminish cognition.
†Dosage must be adjusted individually; geriatric patients may be started on a regimen of half doses.

---

9. Educating patients and families regarding the illness
10. Providing postdelirium management

When possible, means other than restraints, such as sitters, should be used to prevent the delirious patient from harming himself or herself, others, or the physical environment. Restraints themselves can increase agitation and carry the risk of injury. They should be considered only when other means of control are not effective or appropriate.[23]

DRUGS TO TREAT DELIRIUM
Antipsychotics

The primary symptomatic treatment of delirium may require pharmacologic intervention. High-potency antipsychotic medications (e.g., haloperidol) are most commonly used, although other pharmacologic and somatic interventions may be used in particular instances. Intramuscular formulations of the newer atypical antipsychotic agents (e.g., olanzapine, ziprasidone) are anticipated and will likewise be useful when they become available. For somatic treatments, other than haloperidol, no large, prospective trials or studies exist. Information regarding these treatments comes mainly from small case reports or open-label studies.

Antipsychotics have been the medication of choice in the treatment of delirium. Haloperidol, a high-potency agent with no anticholinergic side effects, minimal cardiovascular side effects, and no active metabolites, has generally been considered the antipsychotic medication of first choice in the treatment of delirium. Droperidol, a butyrophenone with rapid onset of action and relatively short half-life that is more sedating than haloperidol, has been found to be an effective treatment for patients with agitation with or without delirium.[37] Droperidol may have advantages of a more rapid onset of action and shorter half-life than haloperidol; droperidol is associated with greater sedation and hypotensive effects.[20] Very little study of newer antipsychotic medications such as risperidone, olanzapine, and quetiapine have occurred in the treatment of delirium, although a few case reports of the use of risperidone have appeared.[35,50]

Antipsychotics, when prescribed in delirium, may result in neurologic side effects, including EPSEs, tardive dyskinesia, and neuroleptic malignant syndrome.

Few studies have determined the optimal dosages of antipsychotic medications in the treatment of delirium. Generally, dosages of haloperidol in the range of 1 to 2 mg every 2 to 4 hours as needed is suggested. Low dosages, as low as 0.25 to 0.5 mg every 4 hours, are more useful for older or elderly patients. On the other hand, high haloperidol dosages of up to 500 mg/day intravenously have been reported and are associated with minimal effects on heart rate, respiratory rate, blood pressure, pulmonary artery pressure, or EPSEs.[29,39] Haloperidol, used in the treatment of delirium, has been reported to lengthen the cardiac QT interval, which can lead to fatal arrhythmias and sudden death. This serious event has usually been associated with higher intravenous dosages but has been reported with lower-dose oral haloperidol.[24] Other side effects of antipsychotic medications include a lowered seizure threshold, galactorrhea, elevations in liver enzyme levels, inhibition of leukopoiesis, and withdrawal movement disorders.

Benzodiazepines

Little evidence supports the use of benzodiazepines alone for general cases of delirium. However, some cases of delirium may be significantly benefited by benzodiazepine use, especially when related to alcohol or benzodiazepine withdrawal. Other circumstances in which benzodiazepines may be useful include situations in which there is a need for medication that can raise the seizure threshold or when anticholinergic side effects or akathisia associated with antipsychotics would seriously exacerbate a patient's condition. As noted in Chapter 11, the combination of antipsychotics and benzodiazepines for the treatment of delirium may decrease medication side effects and potentially increase clinical effectiveness in special populations, for example, severely ill cancer patients or AIDS patients. The adverse effects of benzodiazepines have been discussed with respect to their use in treating agitation in dementia. Benzodiazepines are generally contraindicated in treating delirium from hepatic encephalopathy resulting from accumulation of glutamine, which is related chemically to GABA. Benzodiazepines should also be avoided in patients with respiratory insufficiency, as with treating agitation in dementia; lorazepam and oxazepam are preferred agents.

Cholinergic Agents

Anticholinergic mechanisms have been implicated in the pathogenesis of medication-induced delirium. In addition, anticholinergic mechanisms may be involved in delirium from hypoxemia, hypoglycemia, thiamine deficiency, traumatic brain injury, and stroke.[57] Thus cholinergic medications have been used in a limited fashion to treat delirium, almost exclusively in the case of delirium associated with anticholinergic medications. Physostigmine, a centrally active cholinesterase inhibitor, has been used most often, with tacrine and donepezil receiving less attention. Side effects of cholinesterase inhibitors are caused by cholinergic excess, and these include bradycardia, nausea, vomiting, salivation, and increased gastrointestinal acid. Clearly, donepezil is the best tolerated of the currently available cholinesterase inhibitors and has been used in acute delirium in dosages of 5 mg.[58] Physostigmine is usually administered parenterally in doses ranging from 0.16 to 2.0 mg or with continuous intravenous infusions of 3 mg/hr.

Vitamin Replacement Therapy

Certain vitamin deficiencies are commonly described in delirium. Thus some deliria may reverse in response to vitamin repletion. In general, any patient with delirium who has a reason to be vitamin B deficient, for example, alcoholic or malnourished patients, should be given multivitamin replacement therapy.

Oxygen Therapy

Hypoxia, fatigue, and the metabolic consequences of overexertion may exacerbate delirium. Hypercatabolic conditions may accompany cases of agitated delirium, such as that seen with hyperdynamic heart failure, adult respiratory distress syndrome, and hyperthyroid storm. For these patients who are unresponsive to other pharmacologic interventions, a paralytic agent and mechanical ventilation may be useful. This improves oxygenation and reduces skeletal muscle exertion. The patient is generally heavily sedated in this instance.

Analgesics

Morphine or other opioids are used as an important palliative treatment in cases of delirium where pain is an aggravating factor.[47] However, some opioids can exacerbate delirium, particularly through their metabolites, which possess anticholinergic activity. Among the opioids, meperidine and fentanyl are particularly anticholinergic.

TREATMENT ISSUES IN DELIRIUM

Decisions regarding the care of patients with delirium are often complex because of the risks associated with treatments. Treatment decisions are sometimes made quickly because of the seriousness of underlying general medical conditions. Unfortunately, delirium intermittently affects consciousness, attention, and cognition and can impair a patient's decisional capacity. Although the presence of delirium does not necessarily imply that a patient is incompetent or lacks capacity to give informed consent, a formal assessment is essential to determine the patient's understanding about proposed interventions and the consequences of a decision to be made.

Decision-making guidelines have been suggested for patients with delirium who lack decisional capacity or competence to give informed consent.[17] Often, treatment is needed urgently and the risks and benefits of treatment can be considered accordingly. In medical emergencies, the first alternative under the common law doctrine of implied consent is to treat the patient with delirium without informed consent. In nonemergency situations, input or consent from surrogates, including interested and involved family members, can be obtained. Opinions of other clinicians can be useful in decision making, as can consultation with hospital administrators, risk managers, or legal counsel. All assessment of a patient's decisional capacity or competence and the reasons for particular courses of action should be well documented in the patient's medical record. For decisions that involve significant risks or substantial disagreements among family members, a court-appointed guardian can be sought if time permits. In more emergent cases, an urgent hearing with a judge may be required.

REFERENCES

1. Aisen PS, Davis KL: Inflammatory mechanisms in Alzheimer's disease: implications for therapy, *Am J Psychiatry* 48:1105, 1994.
2. Alexopoulos G and others: The course of geriatric depression with "reversible dementia": a controlled study, *Am J Psychiatry* 150:1693, 1993
3. American Psychiatric Association: *Diagnostic and statistical manual of mental disorders,* ed 4, Washington, DC, 1994, American Psychiatric Association.
4. American Psychiatric Association Practice Guidelines: Practice guideline for the treatment of patients with Alzheimer's disease and other dementias of late life, *Am J Psychiatry* 154(suppl): 5, 1997.
5. Anand R, Gharabawi G, Enz A: Efficacy and safety results of the early phase studies with Exelon (ENA-713) in Alzheimer's disease: an overview, *J Drug Dev Clin Pract* 8:1, 1996.
6. Bayer/Metrifonate-2: testing delayed for at least 3 mos (press release). Leverkusen, Germany: Dow Jones News; September 23, 1998.
7. Becker RE and others: Cholinesterase inhibitors as therapy in Alzheimer's disease: benefit to risk considerations in clinical application. In Becker R, Giacobini E, editors: *Alzheimer disease: from molecular biology to therapy,* Boston, 1997, Birkhauser.
8. Behl C, Davis J, Cole G, Shubert D: Vitamin E protects nerve cells from beta-amyloid protein toxicity. *Biochem Biophys Res Commun* 186:944, 1992.
9. Bodick NC and others: Effects of xanomeline, a selective muscarinic receptor agonist, on cognitive function and behavioral symptoms in Alzheimer disease, *Arch Neurol* 54:465, 1997.
10. Burke WJ and others: The use of selective reuptake inhibitors for depression and psychosis complicating dementia, *Int J Geriatr Psychiatry* 12:519, 1997.
11. Cohen-Mansfield J, Billig N: Agitated behaviors in the elderly. I: a conceptual review, *J Am Geriatr Soc* 34:711, 1986.
12. Corey-Bloom J, Anand R, Beach J: A randomized trial evaluating the efficacy and safety of ENA 713 (rivastigmine tartrate), a new acetylcholinesterase inhibitor, in patients with mild to moderately severe Alzheimer's disease, *Int J Geriatr Psychopharm* 1:55, 1998.
13. Cummings JL: Cholinesterase inhibitors: a new class of psychotropic compounds, *Am J Psychiatry* 157:4, 2000.
14. Davis KL and others: Tacrine collaborative study group: a double-blind, placebo-controlled multicenter study of tacrine for Alzheimer's disease, *N Engl J Med* 327:1253, 1992.
15. Enz A, Floersheim P: Cholinesterase inhibitors: an overview of their mechanisms of action. In Becker R, Giacobini E, editors: *Alzheimer disease: from molecular biology to therapy,* Boston, 1997, Birkhauser.
16. Farlow MR: Cholinesterase inhibitors—pharmacology and efficacy. In: *Alzheimer's disease: management and expectations,* Greenwich, Conn, 1998, Scientific Exchange.
17. Fogel B, Mills M, Landen J: Legal aspects of the treatment of delirium, *Hosp Comm Psychiatry* 37:154, 1986.
18. Folks DG: Neuroleptics in the treatment of agitation in dementia. In Klein DL, Hay DG, editors: *Treatment of agitation in dementia,* Washington, DC, 2000, American Psychiatric Press.
19. Folstein MF, Folstein SE, McHugh PR: "Mini-Mental State": a practical method for grading the cognitive state of patients for the clinician, *J Psychiatr Res* 12:189, 1975.
20. Frye MA and others: Continuous droperidol infusion for management of agitated delirium in an intensive care unit, *Psychosomatics* 36:301, 1995.

21. Geldmacher DS, Waldman AJ, Doty L: Fluoxetine in dementia of the Alzheimer's type: prominent adverse effects and failure to improve cognition, *J Clin Psychiatry* 55:161, 1994.

22. Herbert LE and others: Age-specific incidence of Alzheimer's disease in a community population, *JAMA* 273:1354, 1995.

23. Inouye SK, Chapentier PA: Precipitating factors for delirium in hospitalized elderly persons: predictive model and interrelationships with baseline vulnerability, *JAMA* 275:852, 1996.

24. Jackson T, Ditmanson L, Phibbs B: Torsades de pointes and low-dose oral haloperidol, *Arch Intern Med* 157:2013, 1997.

25. Kappus H, Diplock AT: Tolerance and safety of vitamin E: a toxicological position report, *Free Radic Biol Med* 13:55, 1992.

26. Katzman R and others: Validation of a short orientation-memory-concentration test of cognitive impairment, *Am J Psychiatry* 140:734, 1983.

27. Keltner NL and others: *Psychobiological foundations of psychiatric care*, St Louis, 1998, Mosby.

28. LeBars PL and others: A placebo-controlled, double-blind randomized trial of an extract of ginkgo biloba for dementia, *JAMA* 278:1327, 1997.

29. Levenson JL: High dose intravenous haloperidol for agitated delirium following lung transplantation, *Psychomatics* 36:66, 1995.

30. Mendez M, Younesi F, Perryman K: Use of donepezil for vascular dementia: preliminary clinical experience, *J Neuropsychiatry Clin Neurosci* 11:268, 1999.

31. Mulnard RA and others: Estrogen replacement therapy for treatment of mild to moderate Alzheimer disease: a randomized controlled trial. Alzheimer's disease cooperative study, *JAMA* 283:1007, 2000.

32. Nyth AL, Gottfries CG: The clinical efficacy of citalopram in treatment of emotional disturbances in dementia disorders: a Nordic multicentre study, *Br J Psychiatry* 157:894, 1990.

33. Pfeiffer RI, Kurosaki TT, Harrah CH: Measurement of functional activities in older adults in the community, *Gerontology* 37:323, 1982.

34. Pollock BG and others: An open pilot study of citalopram for behavioral disturbances of dementia: plasma levels and real-time observations, *Geriatric Psychiatry* 5:70, 1997.

35. Ravona-Springer R, Dolberg OT, Hirschmann S, Grunhaus L: Delirium in elderly patients treated with risperidone: a report of three cases (letter), *J Clin Psychopharmacol* 18:171, 1998.

36. Resnick M, Burton B: Droperidol vs haloperidol in the initial management of acutely agitated patients, *J Clin Psychiatry* 45:298, 1984.

37. Resnick SM and others: Effects of estrogen replacement therapy on PET cerebral bloodflow on neuropsychological performance, *Horm Beh* 34:171, 1998.

38. Richelson E: Cholinergic transduction. In Bloom FE, Kupfer DJ, editors: *Psychopharmacology: the fourth generation of progress,* New York, 1995, Raven Press.

39. Riker RR, Fraser GL, Cox PM: Continuous infusion of haloperidol controls agitation in critically ill patients, *Crit Care Med* 22:433, 1994.

40. Rogers SL, Friedhoff ST, and the Donepezil Study Group: The efficacy and safety of donepezil in patients with Alzheimer's disease: results of a US multicenter, randomized, double-blind, placebo-controlled trial, *Dementia* 7:293, 1996.

41. Rosen WG, Mohs RC, Davis KL: A new rating scale for Alzheimer's disease, *Am J Psychiatry* 141:1356, 1984.

42. Sano M and others: A controlled trial of selegiline, a-tocopherol, or both as treatment for Alzheimer's disease, *N Engl J Med* 336(17):1216, 1997.

43. Schmitt F and others: The severe impairment battery: concurrent validity and the assessment of longitudinal change in Alzheimer's disease, *Alzheimer Dis Assoc Disord* 11(suppl 2):S1, 1997.

44. Schneider LS, Olin JT: Overview of clinical trials of Hydergine in dementia, *Arch Neurol* 51:787, 1994.

45. Schneider LS, Pollock VE, Lyness SA: A meta-analysis of controlled trials of neuroleptic treatment in dementia, *J Am Geriatr Soc* 38:553, 1990.

46. Schneider LS and others: Validity and reliability of the Alzheimer's disease cooperative study-clinical global impression of change, *Alzheimer Dis Assoc Disord* 11(suppl 2):S22, 1997.

47. Shapiro BA and others: Practice parameters for intravenous analgesia and sedation for adult patients in the intensive care unit: an executive summary, Society of Critical Care Medicine, *Crit Care Med* 23:1596, 1995.

48. Shergill S, Mullan E, D'Ath P, Katona C: What is the clinical prevalence of Lewy body dementia? *Int J Geriatr Psychiatry* 9:907, 1994.

49. Shintani EY, Uchida KM: Donepezil: an anticholinesterase inhibitor for Alzheimer's disease, *Am J Health Syst Pharm* 54(2):2805, 1997.

50. Sipahimalani A, Sime RM, Masand PS: Treatment of delirium with risperidone, *Int J Geriatr Psychopharmacol* 1:24, 1997.

51. Solomon PR, Pendlebury WW: Recognition of Alzheimer's disease: the 7 minutes screen, *Fam Med* 30(4):265, 1998.

52. Spencer CM, Noble S: Rivastigmine: a review of its use in Alzheimer's disease, *Drugs Aging* 13:391, 1998.

53. Stewart WF, Kawas C, Corrada M, Metter EJ: Risk of Alzheimer's disease and duration of NSAID use, *Neurology* 48:626, 1997.

54. Sultzer DL and others: A double-blind comparison of trazodone and haloperidol for treatment of agitation in patients with dementia, *Am J Geriatr Psychiatry* 5:60, 1997.

55. Tariot PN, Blazine L: The psychopathology of dementia. In Morris JC, editor: *Handbook of dementing illness,* New York, 1994, Marcel Dekker.

56. Tariot PN and others: *Behavioral disorders in dementia,* Bethesda, Md, 1998, American Association for Geriatric Psychiatry Education and Research Foundation.

57. Trzepacz PT, Wise MG: Neuropsychiatric aspects of delirium. In Yudofsky SC, Hales RE, editors: *American Psychiatric Press textbook of neuropsychiatry,* Washington, DC, 1997, American Psychiatric Press.

58. Wengel SP, Burke WJ, Roccaforte WH: Donepezil for postoperative delirium associated with Alzheimer's disease (letter to the editor), *J Am Geriatr Soc* 47:379, 1999.

59. Wengel SP, Folks DG: Mood stabilizers. In Klein DL, Hay DG, editors: *Treatment of agitation in dementia,* Washington, DC, 2000, American Psychiatric Press.

60. Wolf-Klein GP and others: Screening for Alzheimer's disease by clock drawing, *J Am Geriatr Soc* 37:730, 1989.

CHAPTER 9

Seizure Disorders

Epilepsy is the most common seizure disorder, with an incidence somewhere between 0.5% and 1% of the U.S. population (higher rates of 2% to 3% have been reported).[15,41] Approximately 150,000 new diagnoses of epilepsy are made each year in the United States, obtained from the approximate 300,000 Americans seeking medical attention for seizures.[15,41] Overall, it is estimated that about 2 million individuals with epilepsy are being treated in the United States.[2] Approximately 17% of these individuals are younger than 17 years of age, and 1.5% to 2% are older than 75.[16] In some nonindustrialized countries, as many as 5.7% of the population have epilepsy.[40] Worldwide, as many as 50 million people are affected.[38,40]

According to McKenna, Kane, and Parrish, about 7% of the patients diagnosed with epilepsy have a persistent psychosis.[29] When this level of disorder (7%) is compared with the morbidity rate for schizophrenia in the general population (about 1%), it appears a relationship exists between epilepsy and psychosis.[5,18,42,45] These data suggest that more than 100,000 individuals suffer from both a psychosis and a seizure disorder in this country. Because seizure disorders among a psychiatric population are relatively common, antiepileptic drug information is an important part of both the mental health and the primary care clinician's resources.

EPILEPSY

The Neuroepidemiology Branch of the U.S. National Institute for Neurological Disorders and Strokes defines *epilepsy* as two or more afebrile seizures unrelated to acute metabolic disorders or to withdrawal from drugs or alcohol. *Active epilepsy* is defined as a seizure within the past 5 years or the current use of an antiepileptic drug assuming a correct diagnosis. Individuals who have experienced only febrile or neonatal seizures are not included under this diagnosis.

Epilepsy is a condition in which abnormal electrical activity in a particular area of the brain (i.e., a *focal area*) occurs and spreads to and involves other parts of the brain.[8] The abnormal electrical activity has varying effects; hence several distinguishable forms of epilepsy are recognizable. Onset is most common during childhood (90 per 100,000) or after age 65 (130 to 170 per 100,000); however, onset is not limited to these particular stages of life.[16] Epilepsies may be broadly categorized as either acquired or idiopathic (70% in the United States).[37] It should be noted that seizures and epilepsy are not synonymous.[12] Seizures are a symptom of epilepsy and can also occur because of alcohol withdrawal, hypoglycemia, anoxia, and fever, to name a few causes.[36] The extent of genetic influence is unknown, but it is generally acknowledged that a genetic predisposition for epilepsy exists. Treatment is aimed at controlling seizure activity, and for many individuals, this entails a lifelong dependence on antiepileptic therapy.

Categories of Seizures

Epileptic seizures are grouped according to characteristic physical and neurologic signs (Table 9-1). Each subtype also has a characteristic electroencephalogram (EEG) pattern.[19] Seizures are divided into two broad categories: partial seizures and generalized seizures. If an aberrant electrical discharge is confined to a local area, the seizure is partial or focal. If the electrical aberration spreads from a focal area to affect the entire cerebrum, it is classified as a generalized seizure. The diagnosis of each of these seizure types can be refined to include several subtypes.

Table 9-1 Characteristics of Common Epileptic Seizure Classifications

Seizure type	Comments
Partial seizures	Most common seizure type (accounts for about 70% of adults and 40% of children with epilepsy); electroencephalographic changes initially are localized, may evolve into other seizure types
Simple partial seizures	Typically no loss of consciousness; motor symptoms (jacksonian); sensory symptoms (visual, auditory, gustatory, and hallucinations) and somatosensory symptoms (tingling); autonomic symptoms (pallor, sweating, vomiting, and flushing)
Complex partial seizures	Consciousness is impaired at onset of seizure or later; cognitive, affective, perceptive, and psychomotor symptoms can occur
Generalized seizures	Involve symmetric (both hemispheres) distribution of abnormal brain discharge; bilateral motor changes; consciousness may be totally impaired
Nonconvulsive seizures	
Absence seizures	Abrupt loss of consciousness, usually lasting <10 seconds; usually begin in childhood, often stop spontaneously during teenage years; mild clonic component; atonic component; diminution of muscle tone; automatisms; autonomic components
Myoclonic seizures	Single or multiple jerks, typically lasting 3-10 seconds; sudden, brief, shocklike contractions, generalized or confined
Atonic seizures	Sudden diminutions of muscle tone ("drop attacks")
Convulsive seizures	
Tonic-clonic	Consciousness lost abruptly; series of muscle spasms lasting 3-5 minutes from onset to recovery; postictal state may last from a few minutes to about half an hour, often characterized by confusion, dizziness, sleepiness, and "glazed" look
Status epilepticus	Could apply to any prolonged or repetitive seizure but most often applied to repetitive or fused tonic-clonic seizures which last 30 minutes or longer; a medical emergency requiring immediate drug intervention to prevent brain damage or death resulting from impaired ventilation

Partial seizures. Partial seizures are more common than generalized seizures, accounting for approximately 70% of all seizures in adults and 40% of all seizures in children.[10] As defined, partial seizures typically begin in a focal area. Abnormal brain activity can spread to other parts of that cerebral hemisphere or even to the other hemisphere.[10] Partial seizure subtypes include simple partial seizures (no loss of consciousness) and complex partial seizures (consciousness impaired). Partial seizures may evolve into generalized seizures.

Simple partial seizures. Simple partial seizures do not impair consciousness, and because electrical abnormality is localized, symptoms depend on the area affected. Symptoms may be primarily motor, sensory, or autonomic. Motor symptoms include localized jerks, focal jerks that "march" to involve other muscles (sometimes referred to as *jacksonian seizures*), and speech involvement. Sensory symptoms (visual, auditory, gustatory, and hallucinations) and somatosensory symptoms (tingling) also develop. Autonomic symptoms are particularly distressing and include pallor, sweating, vomiting, flushing, tachycardia, hypotension, and hypertension. Automatic behaviors can include lip smacking and repetitive movements.

Complex partial seizures. Complex partial seizures are also known as *psychomotor* or *temporal lobe seizures.* Consciousness is impaired, and violent behavior may be a major component of seizure activity. Complex partial seizures typically begin as a perceived aura. A number of cognitive, affective, perceptive, and psychomotor symptoms can occur. Déjà vu, fear and anxiety, hallucinations, and automatic behaviors (automatisms) are commonly present.

Generalized seizures. Generalized seizures involve a symmetric distribution of abnormal electrical activity in the brain. Generalized seizures include a number of nonconvulsive seizures, which primarily cause unresponsiveness and amnesia, and convulsive seizures, which cause unconsciousness and major convulsions. Nonconvulsive seizures include absence seizures, myoclonic seizures, and atonic seizures. Tonic-clonic seizures and status epilepticus are major types of convulsive seizures.

Nonconvulsive seizures: absence, myoclonic, atonic. Absence seizures are characterized by a sudden loss of responsiveness. Often, the loss of consciousness is so brief (10 seconds) that those around the person are unaware of a change. Absence seizures may occur hundreds of times per day. Eye blinking is a common manifestation. A variant of absence seizure is the true petit mal seizure, which produces a distinct EEG pattern. Absence seizures typically start in childhood and remit during the teenage years. For a description of myoclonic and atonic seizures, see Table 9-1.

Convulsive seizures: tonic-clonic, status epilepticus. Tonic-clonic (grand mal) seizures are characterized by intense, repetitive tonic-clonic (tonic [muscle rigidity] -clonic [muscle jerking]) contractions of the whole body. Abnormal brain activity is symmetric, with most brain pathways involved. Seizures may typically last between 3 and 5 minutes, and prolonged seizure activity can result in brain hypoxia. A number of other physical consequences may result.

Status epilepticus is a seizure type in which continuous tonic-clonic convulsions occur for 30 minutes or longer. Status epilepticus is a medical emergency that requires immediate attention and has a mortality rate of 6% to 20% if untreated.[4] Neuronal necrosis and permanent cerebral injury result from prolonged refractory status epilepticus.[11,20] Several drugs given intravenously have been used successfully to stop these seizures, including the benzodiazepines diazepam and lorazepam.[20]

COMMONLY PRESCRIBED ANTIEPILEPTIC DRUGS

Antiepileptic drugs (AEDs) suppress the start of seizure activity and reduce the spread of seizure activity. The straightforward goals for AED treatment of epilepsy are as follows: (1) control seizure activity, (2) keep side effects of AED therapy to a minimum, and (3) attempt maintenance with a regimen of one drug (monotherapy) if possible. Unfortunately, between 20% and 30% of patients with epilepsy have intractable epilepsy, causing them numerous social and psychologic difficulties.[33,48] Five major categories of AEDs may be distinguished, and when added to the noncategorized agents, a substantial number of individual drugs are at the clinician's disposal. The most commonly used antiepileptics include phenytoin, phenobarbital, carbamazepine, valproic acid, and certain benzodiazepines. These drugs will receive primary attention in the following discussion. A number of other important, although less often used, AEDs are discussed as well. Some of these drugs have rather broad indications (used for several seizure types), whereas others have limited application (used for one seizure type).

Careful medical evaluation is needed before an AED is prescribed. Based on an evaluation that includes an EEG, a specific seizure type may be identified and an AED selected (Tables 9-1 and 9-2). General principles of administration are found in Box 9-1.

Based on information found in Table 9-2, it is obvious more than one drug may control seizure activity. However, one drug may be preferred over another based on criteria found in Box 9-2. In addition, because more than one seizure type may be present, determining whether a given drug might exacerbate a particular seizure pattern is a secondary consideration in selecting the correct AED. Table 9-3 presents examples of selected AEDs and their proposed mechanism of action.

PHENYTOIN

Phenytoin (Dilantin) is a hydantoin. It is effective in treating tonic-clonic and complex partial seizures but not effective for absence seizures. Phenytoin is the most widely used hydantoin, but two other hydantoins, ethotoin and mephenytoin, are available. Because phenytoin controls seizures without causing sedation, it appears that central nervous system (CNS) depression is not a prerequisite for seizure control.[35]

Pharmacologic Effects

The main site of action of hydantoins is the motor cortex. Phenytoin inhibits the spread of abnormal brain electrical activity by normalizing abnormal fluxes of sodium across the nerve cell membrane during or after depolarization. This inhibition stabilizes a state of hyperexcitability. Hydantoins also decrease activity of brainstem centers responsible for the tonic phase of grand mal seizures.[31] Phenytoin depresses cardiac electrical conduction, making it useful therapeutically for patients with arrhythmias.

Pharmacokinetics

Phenytoin is slowly absorbed from the gut after oral administration (Table 9-4). The bioavailability can vary from as much as 10% to 90% among the different brands of phenytoin. Peak serum levels are reached in 1.5 to 3 hours when the promptly absorbed form is used; the extended-acting form reaches peak levels in 4 to 12 hours.

Table 9-2 Seizure Types Amenable to Specific Antiepileptic Drugs (AEDs)

Antiepileptic drug	Seizure type
Most commonly used AEDs	
Hydantoins	
Phenytoin (Dilantin)	Tonic-clonic (first line), complex partial, status epilepticus (second line)
Ethotoin (Peganone)	Tonic-clonic, complex partial
Mephenytoin (Mesantoin)	Tonic-clonic, focal, jacksonian
Barbiturates	
Phenobarbital	Tonic-clonic, simple partial, complex partial, status epilepticus (second line)
Mephobarbital (Mebaral)	Tonic-clonic, absence seizures
Benzodiazepines	
Clonazepam (Klonopin)	Lennox-Gastaut, akinetic, myoclonic, absence seizures (?)
Diazepam (Valium)	Status epilepticus (first line)
Lorazepam (Ativan)	Status epilepticus (first line)
Others	
Carbamazepine (Tegretol)	Tonic-clonic, complex partial, mixed seizures
Valproic acid (Depakene)	Absence seizures (first line), tonic-clonic, myoclonic, complex partial
Other important AEDs	
Succinimides	
Ethosuximide (Zarontin)	Absence seizures
Methsuximide (Celontin)	Absence seizures
Phensuximide (Milontin)	Absence seizures
Oxazolidinediones	
Trimethadione (Tridione)	Absence seizures
Paramethadione (Paradione)	Absence seizures
Other	
Primidone (Mysoline)	Tonic-clonic, partial seizures
Newer AEDs	
Gabapentin (Neurontin)	Partial seizures (adjunctive)
Lamotrigine (Lamictal)	Partial seizures (adjunctive), may have implications for generalized seizures
Vigabatrin (Sabril)	Partial seizures (primarily adjunctive), infantile spasms
Topiramate (Topamax)	Partial seizures (adjunctive), partial-onset seizures in children (?), tonic-clonic (?), drop attacks in Lennox-Gastaut (?)
Tiagabine (Gabitril)	Partial seizures (adjunctive)
Oxcarbazepine (Trileptal)	Tonic-clonic, partial seizures
Zonisamide	Partial seizures, generalized seizures
Felbamate (Felbatol)	Tonic-clonic, partial epilepsy, Lennox-Gastaut in children (adjunctive)
Rarely used AEDs	
Acetazolamide (Diamox)	Tonic-clonic (adjunctive), absence (adjunctive), myoclonic (adjunctive)
Magnesium sulfate	Prophylaxis for preeclampsia, seizures related to eclampsia, alcohol withdrawal
Paraldehyde	Seizures associated with alcohol withdrawal

Box 9-1 General Rules for Using Antiepileptics

1. When possible (i.e., when there is not great urgency, as there is during status epilepticus), start with a low dosage and gradually increase until a therapeutic steady state is reached. This approach is more important with some AEDs than with others (see Table 9-5).
2. Give AEDs on time in order to achieve a steady state and to maintain the drug's therapeutic effect.*
3. Understand AED dosage varies among individuals; accordingly each dosage must also be individualized.
4. Understand the patient's history, including baseline pretreatment laboratory test results.
5. When an AED is to be discontinued, do so gradually to decrease the possibility of withdrawal-related seizures (i.e., status epilepticus).† Other caregivers should be made aware of the patient's drug regimen so that they may provide fully informed care of their own.
6. Monitor the patient's laboratory results, including serum drug levels, hematologic responses to drugs, and trough levels. Indications for drawing serum levels include therapeutic failure, noncompliance (may be as high as 50%), toxicity, and drug interactions. In general, serum drug level determinations are overused.‡
7. Attempt to use a single drug if possible. Patients receiving combination therapy have twice as many adverse responses as patients receiving monotherapy.

AED, Antiepileptic drug.
*From Woodward ES: *J Neurosurg Nurs* 14:166, 1982.
†From Callaghan N, Garrett A, Goggin T: *N Engl J Med* 318(15):942, 1988.
‡From Pellock JM, Willmore LJ: *Neurology* 41(7):961, 1991.

Box 9-2 Considerations in Initiating Antiepileptic Therapy

1. Size of the patient
2. Expense of the drug
3. Allergic response to the drug, if any
4. Childbearing potential
5. Tolerance to side effects

Phenytoin is seldom administered by intramuscular injection because it is stored in tissue and released slowly. Absorption can take up to 5 days (for the intramuscular form), which necessitates a 50% dosage adjustment when switching between oral and intramuscular routes of administration. When switching from oral to intramuscular modes, the dosage must be increased by 50%. Conversely, when switching from intramuscular to oral routes, the dosage must be decreased by 50%. Obviously, if the health care provider does not understand the difference between oral and parenteral forms of this drug, overdosing or underdosing can occur. Fosphenytoin (Cerebyx) is a phenytoin prodrug more suitable for injection.

Table 9-3 Proposed Mechanism(s) of Action for Selected Antiepileptic Drugs (AEDs)

AEDs that normalize sodium channel activity
Phenytoin
Carbamazepine
Valproic acid
Lamotrigine
Topiramate?
Oxcarbazepine
Zonisamide

AEDs that prevent GABA reuptake
Valproic acid (?)
Tiagabine

AEDs that enhance effect of GABA
Phenobarbital
Valproic acid
Benzodiazepines
Topiramate (?)
Zonisamide (?)

AED that is a GABA receptor agonist
Phenobarbital

AED that increases release of GABA
Gabapentin (?)

AED that inhibits GABA-transaminase
Vigabatrine

AEDs that normalize specific calcium channels
Valproic acid
Ethosuximide
Zonisamide

Table 9-4 Pharmacokinetic Comparison of Major Antiepileptic Drugs (AEDs)

Agent	Therapeutic serum level (μg/ml)	Half-life (hr)	Protein binding (%)	Peak serum levels (hr)
Phenytoin	10-20	Average = 22	~90	1.5-3 (prompt) 4-12 (extended)
Phenobarbital	15-40	Average = 80*	40-60	
Carbamazepine	4-12	12-17†	75	4-5
Valproic acid	50-100	6-16	90-95	<4
Diazepam		20-80	98	0.5-4
Ethosuximide	40-100	40-60 (adults)		3-7
Gabapentin	>2	5-8	Minimal	2-3
Lamotrigine	>2	25	55	1.5-4
Topiramate		21	13-17	~2

*Half-life is reduced after enzyme induction.
†After sustained dosage.

The therapeutic serum level is 10 to 20 µg/ml. Four to seven days of use are needed before a steady state is reached based on an average half-life of 22 hours. However, the half-life is almost tripled in some individuals (up to 60 hours), so reaching a steady state can take significantly longer.

Phenytoin is metabolized in the liver by cytochrome P-450 2C9/10 isoenzymes. The breakdown of phenytoin is nonlinear, meaning significant spikes in plasma concentrations (up to 50%) can occur with modest increases in dosage (just 10%). This occurs because phenytoin can saturate liver enzymes. High serum levels can also occur at normal doses when the patient has impaired liver function or congenital deficiencies in hepatic enzymes or in the presence of certain drugs (see Interactions discussion). Plasma protein binding is approximately 90%. Phenytoin is excreted in the urine, with a small amount (1% to 5%) excreted unchanged.

Oral administration. Phenytoin is available for oral administration in chewable tablets (pediatrics), capsules, suspensions, and extended-acting forms. The extended-acting form is the only one available for once-a-day dosage. Oral therapy in adults usually begins with a dosage of 100 mg three times daily. However, a loading dose of 1 g (given over 4 hours) can be given to hospitalized patients with good hepatic functioning. See Table 9-5 for specific dosing information.

Parenteral administration. Intramuscular phenytoin is given to patients who cannot tolerate oral administration or when a risk of seizure is suspected during or soon after surgery. Intramuscular use is absolutely not indicated for status epilepticus because of the slow absorption by this route; thus careful attention to the appropriate dosage must be observed.

Intravenous (IV) use of phenytoin for status epilepticus is warranted in many situations; however, diazepam and lorazepam are first-line drugs for status epilepticus, whereas phenytoin is typically given only in combination with diazepam because of its (phenytoin's) slow onset of action.[11,20] Diazepam aborts only the seizure in progress and is not appropriate for continuous use as an AED. Close scrutiny of IV phenytoin (at no more than 50 mg/min) is advised because of its narrow therapeutic index and because of cardiovascular (i.e., hypotension, cardiovascular collapse) and CNS depression associated with faster rates of administration. Maintenance dosages of 100 mg every 6 to 8 hours to prevent breakthrough seizures are warranted. Other dosing information is found in Table 9-5. Fosphenytoin was developed as an alternative and is soluble at a more physiologic pH. It can be given intravenously at a faster rate than phenytoin and intramuscularly with less tissue damage. It can be used for status epilepticus. Fosphenytoin 75 mg is equivalent to 50 mg of phenytoin.

Side Effects

The most common side effects of phenytoin are those involving the CNS—sluggishness, ataxia, nystagmus, confusion, and slurred speech. Dizziness, insomnia, nervousness, and fatigue occur less often. Phenytoin is considered the least sedating AED.

Peripheral side effects include those involving the blood, the gastrointestinal (GI) tract, connective tissue, and the skin. Hematologic effects such as leukopenia, agranulocytosis, megaloblastic anemia, and coagulation deficits in newborns have been reported. Nausea, vomiting, and constipation are the major GI effects. Gingival hyperplasia (overgrowth of gums down over the teeth) is a fairly common side effect of phenytoin use in children and in those who practice poor oral hygiene. Psychiatric patients and individuals with developmental disabilities seem to be susceptible to gingival hyperplasia. Other connective tissue problems include enlarged lips, coarsened facial features, and excessive growth of body hair. Skin reactions can range from the embarrassing, such as worsening of acne in a teenager, to the potentially fatal exfoliative dermatitis, lupus erythematosus, or Stevens-Johnson syndrome. Other skin reactions include a mild measlelike rash (2% to 5%). Other adverse responses include hepatitis and liver damage, hyperglycemia, edema, chest pain, numbness and paresthesia, photophobia, pulmonary fibrosis, osteomalacia caused by enhanced vitamin D metabolism, and lymphadenopathy (as severe as Hodgkin's disease).

Table 9-5 Dosage for Selected Antiepileptics (in Order of Appearance in Text)

Drug and clinical implications	Dosage
Phenytoin (Dilantin)	
Tonic-clonic and complex partial seizures	Oral: *Adults:* 100-200 mg tid or qid; Dilantin Kapseals (extended form) can be given once daily; *children:* 5 mg/kg/day; children >6 may require minimum adult dosage (300 mg/day)
Status epilepticus	IV: *Adults:* give a loading dose of 10-15 mg/kg; IV rate should not exceed 50 mg/min (in elderly patients, 25 mg/min); initial dose should be followed by maintenance dose of 100 mg orally or IV 6-8h; *children:* give 15-20 mg/kg slowly (not more than 1-3 mg/kg/min); use normal saline to avoid precipitation
Phenobarbital	
Tonic-clonic and partial seizures	Oral: *Adults:* 60-100 mg/day; *children:* 3-5 mg/kg/day in divided doses
Status epilepticus	IV: *Adults:* 15-18 mg/kg slowly (no faster than 60 mg/min); do not exceed 30 mg/kg; *children:* same 15-18 kg/mg over 10-15 min
Carbamazepine (Tegretol)	
Tonic-clonic, complex partial, and mixed seizures	Oral: *Adults and children >12:* 200 mg bid at first, then increase by 200 mg/day every 7 days if needed; maintenance dose usually 800-1200 mg/day in divided doses; adult dose rarely exceeds 1200 mg/day; *children 12-15:* should not receive more than 1000 mg/day; *children 6-12 yr:* 100 mg bid at first, then increase by 100 mg/day every 7 days, if needed; maintenance dose is usually 400-800 mg/day in divided doses; do not exceed 1000 mg/day
Valproic acid (Depakene) and derivatives	
Absence, tonic-clonic, complex partial, and myoclonic seizures	Oral: *Adults and children:* 15 mg/kg/day at first, then increase weekly by 5-10 mg/kg/day up to a maintenance dose of 20-60 mg/kg/day in divided doses
Diazepam (Valium)	
Status epilepticus	IV: *Adults:* 5-10 mg at 2-5 mg/min up to a maximum dose of 30 mg; may repeat in 2-4 hr; *children >5:* 1 mg every 3-5 minutes, up to 10 mg; *children 1 month to 5 yr:* 0.2 to 0.5 mg slowly every 2-5 minutes, up to 5 mg

Table 9-5 Dosage for Selected Antiepileptics (in Order
of Appearance in Text)—cont'd

Drug and clinical implications	Dosage
Lorazepam (Ativan) Status epilepticus	IV: *Adults:* 4 mg administered as a 2-minute IV push; may be repeated in 5-10 minutes if needed; maximum dose 8 mg; *infants and children:* 0.1 mg/kg over 25 minutes; maximum 4 mg at a single dose
Clonazepam (Klonopin) Lennox-Gastaut, akinetic, and myoclonic seizures	Oral: *Adults:* 0.5 mg tid at first, then increase every 3 days by 0.5-1.0 mg until seizures are controlled; 20 mg/day is the maximum dose; *children <10:* 0.01-0.03 mg/kg/day in divided doses at first, then increase by no more than 7.5 mg/week; maximum dose is 60 mg/day; not recommended for children <9 yr
Ethosuximide (Zarotin) Absence seizures	Oral: *Adults and children >6:* 500 mg/day at first, then increase by 250 mg/day every 4 to 7 days until seizures are satisfactorily controlled; *children 3-6:* 250 mg/day at first, then increase by 250 mg/day every 4 to 7 days (20 mg/kg/day is typical optimal dose); no person should receive more than 1.5 g/day
Primidone (Mysoline) Tonic-clonic and partial seizures	Oral: *Adults:* 125-250 mg bid to qid; *children <8:* half of the adult dose
Gabapentin (Neurontin) Adjunctive for partial seizures	Oral: *Adults and children >12:* 900-1800 mg/day in three divided doses; spacing should not exceed 12 hr between doses
Lamotrigine (Lamictal) Adjunctive for partial seizures and Lennox-Gastaut	Oral: *Adults:* adults taking an enzyme-inducing AED (carbamazepine, phenytoin, or phenobarbital) begin at 50 mg/day and then gradually increase to 150-250 mg bid; if taken with an enzyme inhibitor (e.g., valproic acid), begin with 25 mg qod and then gradually increase to between 50 and 75 mg bid
Vigabatrine (Sabril) Partial epilepsy	Oral: *Adults:* 0.5-1 g/day and titrated upward on a weekly basis to 2-3 g/day
Topiramate (Topamax) Adjunctive for partial seizures	Oral: *Adults:* begin at 50 mg/day and then incrementally increase to 200 mg bid

AED, Antiepileptic drug.

Continued

Table 9-5 Dosage for Selected Antiepileptics (in Order of Appearance in Text)—cont'd

Drug and clinical implications	Dosage
Tiagabine (Gabitril) Adjunctive for partial seizures	Oral: *Adults:* begin at 4 mg qd and increase by 4-8 mg weekly up to 30-56 mg/day in 2-4 divided doses; *children 12-18:* begin at 4 mg qd; can be increased by 4 mg/wk up 32 mg/day in 2-4 divided doses
Oxcarbazepine (Trileptal) Tonic-clonic and partial seizures	Oral: *Adults:* begin at 300-600 mg/day in 2-3 divided doses and can slowly increase to 900-3000 mg/day in 2-3 divided doses; *children:* start at 10 mg/kg/day and increase to 30 mg/kg/day as needed and/or tolerated
Zonisamide Generalized and partial seizures	Oral: *Adults:* begin at 100-200 mg/day and increase about every 2 wk as needed; maintenance dosages are 400-600 mg/day in 2 divided doses

CNS side effects are particularly debilitating for elderly patients because of the high susceptibility to falls and a tendency to misjudge situations, that is, forgetting that a medication was taken and then ingesting an extra dose. Megaloblastic anemia can be countered with folic acid; however, excessive doses of folic acid can lower phenytoin serum levels to a subtherapeutic range. Discontinuance of phenytoin can reverse lymph node involvement.

Treatment Implications

Therapeutic versus toxic levels. The typical therapeutic dosage of phenytoin ranges from 300 to 600 mg/day given in several doses or, if the extended-acting form is used, once per day. Toxic serum levels can occur at normal dosage levels for a variety of reasons, for example, impaired liver function, enzyme deficiencies, or drug interactions. Therapeutic serum levels range from 10 to 20 µg/ml. A toxic level of phenytoin occurs at serum levels above 20 µg/ml. Symptoms can include far-lateral nystagmus, ataxia, dysarthria, tremor, slurred speech, and nausea and vomiting. Diminished mental capacity occurs at serum levels above 40 µg/ml. Serum levels above 50 µg/ml may cause seizures. At serum levels above 100 µg/ml, the same symptoms are intensified, and hypotension, circulatory and ventilatory failure, coma, and death can occur. The estimated lethal dose in an adult is 2 to 5 g.[31] Death is caused by respiratory and circulatory failure.

Treatment for overdose and toxic effects are driven by the principle of further reducing drug absorption. Induced emesis, repeated gastric lavage and suctioning, and activated charcoal are interventions useful in interrupting phenytoin absorption. Because there is no known antidote, supportive measures for respiratory and circulatory systems should be used. Hemodialysis may be useful because phenytoin is not completely bound to plasma proteins.

Use in pregnancy. Expectant women treated for epilepsy have a higher propensity for experiencing seizures caused by poor phenytoin absorption during pregnancy. Phenytoin has been implicated in congenital defects, that is, cleft lip, cleft palate, and heart malformations.[9] In addition, children of women taking phenytoin are susceptible to coagulation defects caused by lower levels of vitamin K–dependent clotting factors, which can lead to hemorrhage. Prophylactic administration of vitamin K (phytonadione) to the mother at 1 month before delivery and to the newborn at birth (about 1 mg intramuscularly) can prevent the development of this hematologic disorder. Hematologic studies should be routinely acquired. Breast-feeding is not appropriate for women taking phenytoin because this drug is excreted in breast milk. Prudent treatment dictates use of monotherapy if possible and the lowest effective dosage.

Side effect interventions. CNS symptoms are most troublesome for elderly patients. These individuals should be observed closely to prevent falls or other problems associated with impaired judgment. Evaluation of mood, affect, and memory provide data from which interventions can be formulated.

Hematologic disorders can be minimized through careful assessment for fever, sore throat, malaise, or bruises. The patient should be instructed to self-assess for these signs and to report them. A contraindication for phenytoin use is the presence of bone marrow depression or a blood dyscrasia.

Nausea, vomiting, and other GI problems are reduced when phenytoin is given with meals. Gingival hyperplasia, coarsening of facial features, and other connective tissue consequences of phenytoin therapy can cause disfigurement; hence supportive measures are warranted. Thorough oral hygiene can reduce the severity of gingival hyperplasia.

Because skin rashes can range from mild, measlelike conditions to serious skin disorders such as exfoliative dermatitis and lupus erythematosus, phenytoin should be discontinued when a rash appears. Finally, acne is a common adverse reaction to phenytoin among teenagers and young adults, and its potential to lower self-esteem should not be underestimated by those responsible for care. If an AED besides phenytoin will control seizures, a change is indicated.

Parenteral phenytoin can cause cardiovascular effects such as hypotension, circulatory collapse, depression of cardiac conductility, and cardiac arrest. Patients with a history of sinus bradycardia, sinoatrial or second- or third-degree atrioventricular block, or Adams-Stokes syndrome should not be given this drug. When status epilepticus is being treated, monitoring the patient's blood pressure and respirations while giving IV phenytoin slowly (50 mg/min) reduces the likelihood of triggering a cardiovascular response.

Interactions. Many drugs interact with phenytoin (Box 9-3). These interactions can generally be categorized as those that cause an increase or decrease in phenytoin serum levels, those that cause a decrease in the action of the interacting drug, and those interactants with unpredictable effects.

Drugs that increase phenytoin serum levels or phenytoin effects (potential toxic effects). Other drugs increase the effect of phenytoin by one of the following means:

1. Inhibiting phenytoin metabolism
2. Displacing phenytoin from plasma protein-binding sites, leading to excessive levels of free (and active) phenytoin

Interactants that inhibit metabolism include acute alcohol ingestion, allopurinol, benzodiazepines (e.g., diazepam), H_1-receptor blocking antihistamines, disulfiram,

---

Box 9-3   Drug Interaction for Most Antiepileptics

Drugs affecting antiepileptics	Drugs affected by antiepileptics
Alcohol	Folic acid
Antacids	Meperidine (Demerol)
Aspirin	Oral anticoagulants
Carbamazepine	Oral contraceptives
Cimetidine (Tagamet)	Steroids
Disulfiram (Antabuse)	Theophylline
Erythromycin	Vitamins D and K
Fluoxetine (Prozac)	
Phenobarbital	
Phenytoin	
Propoxyphene (Darvon)	
Rifampin	
Valproate	

Modified from Ramsey RE and others: *Clinical issues in the management of epilepsy*, Miami, 1993, University of Miami.

---

isoniazid, phenacemide, phenylbutazone, succinimides (e.g., ethosuximide), sulfonamides, and valproic acid. Diazepam and ethosuximide are AEDs that might be prescribed along with phenytoin, so a downward adjustment in the dosage of phenytoin should be made. Disulfiram, a major drug treatment for chronic alcoholism, necessitates a low starting dosage of phenytoin, monitoring of serum levels of phenytoin, and careful assessment of the patient. Drinking alcohol when taking phenytoin leads to higher serum levels of the drug because alcohol successfully competes for liver enzymes. Valproic acid and salicylates increase phenytoin serum levels by displacing phenytoin from plasma protein-binding sites.

Drugs that decrease phenytoin serum levels (potential seizure breakthrough). A number of drugs decrease the serum levels of phenytoin by means of the following distinct mechanisms:

1. Increasing phenytoin metabolism
2. Decreasing its absorption
3. Unknown mechanisms

Phenobarbital, carbamazepine, alcohol (chronic use), and theophylline decrease phenytoin serum levels by increasing its breakdown in the liver. Antacids block phenytoin absorption. Folic acid (sometimes given prophylactically to prevent megaloblastic anemia), antineoplastics, influenza vaccine, and calcium gluconate decrease phenytoin serum levels by unknown mechanisms.

Interactant effects that are decreased by phenytoin. The effects of corticosteroids, oral anticoagulants, oral contraceptives, quinidine, and vitamin D are all compromised by phenytoin. Dangers of these interactive patterns include decreased corticosteroid effect; increased blood clotting; pregnancy, spotting, and breakthrough bleeding; reduced antiarrhythmic action; and increased risk of osteomalacia, respectively. Assessment should address these issues. Increasing the level of estrogen in the contraceptive may improve efficacy, and instructing the patient to seek medical help should a pregnancy be expected is a prudent measure to ensure optimal benefit. In addition, fluid retention lowers the seizure threshold; because retention occurs with the use of contraceptives, alternative birth control methods should be considered. Increasing the quinidine dosage can maintain its antiarrhythmic quality, and encouraging more vitamin D in the diet can forestall skeletal problems. Psychotropic drugs whose metabolism is enhanced by phenytoin include clonazepam, haloperidol, and methadone.

Interactants that behave unpredictably. Several drugs may either increase or decrease phenytoin serum levels. Two AEDs, phenobarbital and valproic acid, may cause phenytoin serum levels to rise or fall. Consequently, monitoring of laboratory data is important. Paradoxically, phenytoin can have the same effect on these two drugs; that is, their effects may increase or decrease.

Patient education. Patient teaching should focus on helping the patient maximize the therapeutic benefits of phenytoin while preventing or minimizing its serious side effects. The patient should be familiar with the desired action of the drug, the importance of taking the drug on time and as prescribed (i.e., maintaining therapeutic serum levels), the difference in efficacy between oral and parenteral routes, and the need to notify the clinician when certain side effects occur. Side effects that must be punctually reported include sore throat, fever, malaise, petechiae, and bruising. The other major issues in patient teaching are meticulous oral hygiene (brushing and flossing) to reduce gingival hyperplasia, warnings against driving when CNS symptoms such as dizziness or sedation occur, care when rising (to reduce the risk of falls), avoidance of prescription drugs that interact with phenytoin (all health care providers should be aware of phenytoin therapy), and consumption of alcohol. Generally, it is advisable for individuals taking AEDs to wear a medical identification bracelet.

Young women should be made aware of the potential for congenital defects should they become pregnant, and those desiring to become pregnant should first talk with their physicians. Individuals who have GI tract effects as a result of taking phenytoin should be encouraged to take the drug with their meals because doing so enhances absorption and decreases GI tract upset.

Patients should be advised not to abruptly discontinue phenytoin because of the potential for status epilepticus.

Related Hydantoins

The two other hydantoins successfully used to treat epilepsy are ethotoin (Peganone) and mephenytoin (Mesantoin). Ethotoin is indicated for the treatment of tonic-clonic and psychomotor seizures. It is contraindicated in patients with known hepatic abnormalities or hematologic disorders. Mephenytoin is used to treat tonic-clonic, focal, and jacksonian seizures but is not usually prescribed unless other, safer AEDs have been attempted first.

PHENOBARBITAL

Phenobarbital is a long-acting barbiturate. Many individual barbiturates are available, but only long-acting ones have antiepileptic potential. Phenobarbital is the prototypical long-acting barbiturate. Mephobarbital (Mebaral) is a related drug.

Although barbiturates have been used for nearly a century as sedatives, at subsedation dosages, only a few have been found to possess antiepileptic qualities. All barbiturates have antiepileptic properties at high dosages. It is phenobarbital's ability to inhibit seizures without inducing sedation that makes it beneficial.

Pharmacologic Effects

Phenobarbital's antiepileptic effect is caused by its ability to bind to gamma-aminobutyric acid (GABA) receptors. In fact, a specific barbiturate site on that receptor has been identified. Phenobarbital and other barbiturates both enhance the inhibitory effects of GABA and mimic GABA. This results in prolonged opening of chloride channels, thus inhibiting neuronal firing. This slows the response of nerves to seizure-causing stimuli and also slows the spread of abnormal electrical activity. The net effect is to raise the seizure threshold, that is, diminish the likelihood of a seizure. Oral phenobarbital is effective in treating tonic-clonic and partial seizures but not absence seizures. Parenteral phenobarbital can be used to stop status epilepticus when diazepam or phenytoin is ineffective or unavailable. Phenobarbital can produce a paradoxic effect—excitement—in children.

Pharmacokinetics

Phenobarbital is usually given orally, absorbed in varying degrees, and uniformly distributed to all tissues. Onset of action after an oral dose varies from 20 to 60 minutes. Phenobarbital is metabolized in the liver by the hepatic microsomal enzyme system, but 25% to 50% of its molecules are excreted unchanged in the urine. Nonetheless, phenobarbital has a dramatic effect on hepatic enzymes by increasing the synthesis of those enzymes (enzyme induction). Specifically, barbiturates increase the synthesis of porphyrin, a precursor to P-450 enzymes. The net effect is to expedite the metabolism of those drugs, including phenobarbital, that are metabolized by these liver enzymes. This mechanism produces tolerance to many effects and contributes to drug interactions. Tolerance to phenobarbital's antiepileptic activity and to its lethal effects is slight. Phenobarbital has the lowest lipid solubility and the longest duration of action of all barbiturates.

The therapeutic plasma level for phenobarbital is 15 to 40 µg/ml. It has a half-life of 80 hours (a range of 53 to 118 hours) initially and takes 16 to 21 days to reach a steady state. Half-life reduction occurs after enzyme induction. Phenobarbital is 40% to 60% bound to plasma proteins.

The low dosages associated with phenobarbital therapy seldom produce physical dependence or withdrawal symptoms. Elderly patients may require a reduced dosage. Patients who have status epilepticus or other acute seizures, for example, those caused by cholera, eclampsia, or meningitis, can be given IV phenobarbital (see Table 9-5). Phenobarbital is not the first choice for these emergency situations; diazepam and lorazepam are. The high dosages of phenobarbital needed to stop these seizures can cause CNS, respiratory, and cardiovascular depression.

Oral administration. Phenobarbital is available in a variety of oral forms: tablets, capsules, and elixirs. Long-term antiepileptic therapy is typically accomplished by means of oral phenobarbital use.

Parenteral administration. Parenteral use should be avoided unless oral administration is not feasible or a prompt antiepileptic response is needed. IV phenobarbital can be used to treat status epilepticus and other emergency convulsive states. A vein must always be used because interarterial injection can lead to a gangrenous condition caused by vessel spasm. The phenobarbital must be injected slowly, at a rate no faster than 60 mg/min. The onset of action after IV injection is about 5 minutes. Intramuscular phenobarbital should be injected into large muscles (gluteus maximus or vastus lateralis), where there is less risk of injecting into a peripheral nerve trunk or artery.

Side Effects

Phenobarbital is an inexpensive and effective drug with relatively few serious side effects. CNS depression is the most common side effect of phenobarbital. However, because seizure control is a long-term if not a lifetime concern, many of the side effects associated with phenobarbital become tolerated by the patient. An important contraindication is a history of porphyria (excessive hepatic formation of porphyrins) because, as noted, phenobarbital induces the synthesis of porphyrins. Hypotension and respiratory depression are potential adverse responses to high oral dosages or to rapid IV infusion.

Barbiturates at low dosages can cause excitability in children and elderly individuals.

Treatment Implications

Therapeutic versus toxic levels. The therapeutic serum phenobarbital level is 15 to 40 µg/ml. Serum phenobarbital levels of more than 40 µg/ml may be toxic. Although toxic doses vary among individuals, usually 1 g of phenobarbital taken orally can cause serious toxic effects and ingesting 2 to 10 g can be lethal.

A tolerance to many of the barbiturate effects, but not to the antiepileptic effects, develops with long-term use of phenobarbital. Therefore, although an increased amount of barbiturate may be needed for sedation, an increase is not required for continued seizure control. Significant tolerance to lethal levels does not develop either. Hence, in those individuals taking barbiturates for sedation, the therapeutic dose inches closer to the lethal dose. At toxic levels, respiratory and CNS depression, tachycardia, hypotension, hypothermia, and coma can occur. In cases of severe overdose, apnea, circulatory collapse, respiratory arrest, and death have been reported.

Treatment for overdose consists of maintenance of a patent airway and assistance with ventilation and oxygenation if needed. Gastric lavage can be used to empty the stomach. Monitoring vital signs and fluid balance is important. When renal function remains normal, forced diuresis and alkalinizing of the urine help eliminate the phenobarbital (because of the significant levels excreted unchanged).

Use in pregnancy. Phenobarbital has been implicated in congenital defects.[9,31] Withdrawal symptoms can occur in infants born to mothers who took barbiturates in their last trimester, and a coagulation defect in infants has been associated with maternal barbiturate use.

Side effect interventions. CNS effects such as drowsiness can impair driving and put the patient at risk in many situations, so the patient must be appropriately educated. Should an older patient or a child have paradoxic excitement after taking phenobarbital, precautions to prevent injury should be instituted. Patient assessment data should include information about a history of porphyria. Resuscitation equipment should be readily available when IV phenobarbital is given.

Interactions. Drugs that depress the CNS are the chief interactants with phenobarbital, so the patient who requires phenobarbital in conjunction with another CNS depressant should be observed carefully. Interactants can be categorized into two groups: drugs that increase the effects of barbiturates and drugs whose effects are decreased by barbiturates.

Drugs that increase effects of barbiturates (toxic effects). CNS depressants such as benzodiazepines, opioids, anesthetics, antihistamines, antipsychotics, and alcohol enhance the depressant effects of barbiturates. Alcohol and barbiturates should never be combined. Alcohol can reduce the antiepileptic effect of phenobarbital and dramatically increase the level of CNS depression. Deaths each year are attributed to the combination of barbiturates and alcohol.

Other AEDs also interact with phenobarbital. Because multiple-drug therapy is common in treating seizure disorders, it is important to recognize potential problems and to develop protocols for evaluating them. Valproic acid, for example, interacts with phenobarbital through a mechanism referred to as *selective metabolism.* The hepatic microsomal enzyme system selectively metabolizes valproic acid, delaying the metabolism of phenobarbital. Phenobarbital serum levels may increase by 40%, clearly presenting a serious risk of toxic effects.

Drugs whose effects are decreased by phenobarbital. Many drugs are compromised by coadministration with phenobarbital. The induction of hepatic microsomal enzymes that more speedily metabolize these drugs is responsible for their shortened response in the body. Most notably reduced in effect are clonazepam, digitoxin, oral anticoagulants, oral contraceptives, and TCAs. Although the effect of phenobarbital on phenytoin is not precisely known, it is thought that phenytoin metabolism is accelerated and consequently renders the drug less effective. The concurrent use of these two AEDs is common, so frequent monitoring of serum levels of both drugs is appropriate. Other drugs whose effects are decreased include griseofulvin, quinidine, doxycycline, and monoamine oxidase inhibitors.

Patient education. Patient teaching focuses primarily on health and safety. Patients should be warned to avoid driving or operating hazardous machinery and to avoid combining phenobarbital, alcohol, and other CNS depressants. Other teaching concerns include the reporting of side effects and adverse responses. Although hematologic side effects are uncommon, symptoms such as sore throat, fever, and bleeding should be reported so that the development of blood dyscrasias can be prevented.

Related Barbiturate: Mephobarbital

Mephobarbital is used to treat both tonic-clonic and absence epilepsy. It has two major advantages over phenobarbital. First, mephobarbital can be used to treat absence seizure, whereas phenobarbital cannot. Second, mephobarbital causes less drowsiness and sedation in adults and less excitability in children than does phenobarbital. This second feature accounts for the predominant rationale for prescribing mephobarbital.

CARBAMAZEPINE

Carbamazepine (Tegretol) is a major AED that is finding considerable use. It is structurally related to the TCAs (see Chapter 6), and some patients taking this AED testify to improved mood. Furthermore, carbamazepine is used successfully for patients with bipolar disorder and for those with schizophrenia. Both disorders demonstrate seizure-related phenomena and respond to carbamazepine.[7] Although carbamazepine is an effective AED, some clinicians are reluctant to prescribe it because of its potentially toxic effects.

Pharmacologic Effect

Although its exact mechanism of action is unknown, carbamazepine is thought to reduce high-frequency action potentials, thus preventing the spread of seizures.[31] The mechanism for doing this appears to be related to normalizing sodium channel activity (and sodium influx) similar to that of phenytoin. Carbamazepine is indicated for complex partial, tonic-clonic, or mixed seizures. It is not effective in controlling absence seizures. Carbamazepine also affects acetylcholine, norepinephrine, dopamine, and GABA systems, no doubt accounting for its various uses (see Chapter 6), for example, pain relief in persons with trigeminal neuralgia and restless leg syndrome, posttraumatic stress disorder, schizophrenia, and bipolar disorder.[21]

Pharmacokinetics

Carbamazepine is slowly but adequately absorbed from the GI tract. Peak serum levels are reached within 4 to 5 hours on average after oral administration but are delayed in some individuals up to 12 hours. Carbamazepine is bound to serum proteins (75%). It is metabolized in the liver by the P-450 isoenzymes 2D6 and 3A4 to an active metabolite. Initially, the half-life in drug-naive patients ranges from 25 to 65 hours, but after sustained dosage, the half-life is reduced to 12 to 17 hours as a result of autoinduction. A steady state is achieved within 2 to 4 days. Carbamazepine is eliminated through urinary (72%) and fecal (28%) excretions. Table 9-5 contains dosage information. Carbatrol and Tegretol-XR are long-acting formulations that provide continuous seizure protection related to stable serum levels. These formulations can be administered less often, enhancing compliance.

Side Effects

Common side effects of carbamazepine include drowsiness, dizziness, fatigue, headache, unsteadiness, nausea, and diplopia. Most of these diminish with time or when the dosage is reduced. Less common adverse reactions include activation of latent psychosis, confusion in elderly patients, hepatic and renal damage, cardiovascular complications, and hyponatremia. Skin rashes occur in up to 15% of individuals taking carbamazepine. Most can be treated with an antihistamine. Severe skin reactions (e.g., Stevens-Johnson syndrome, exfoliative dermatitis) require drug discontinuation.

A number of hematologic reactions occur with carbamazepine, some quite serious. Cases of fatal agranulocytosis (1 in 50,000 persons) and fatal aplastic anemia (1 in 200,000 persons) have been reported. Although the absolute incidence of these side effects is low, it is significantly greater than that for the general public. In general, patients taking carbamazepine experience neutropenia. Besides rare occurrences of agranulocytosis and aplastic anemia, thrombocytopenia (5%), increased prothrombin time, and transient leukopenia (10%) are potential effects of this drug.[26] Patients with a history of bone marrow depression or other preexisting hematologic abnormality should not receive this drug.

Treatment Implications

Therapeutic versus toxic levels. Therapeutic serum levels are 4 to 12 µg/ml. Levels above 12 µg/ml are potentially toxic. A toxic dose of carbamazepine ranges from 5 g in small children to 30 g in adults. The first signs of overdose appear within

1 to 3 hours of administration and tend to be neuromuscular. Muscle restlessness, twitching, exaggerated reflexes, and finally, reflex depression are among the initial indications of overdose. Large overdoses lead to respiratory difficulties; cardiovascular symptoms such as arrhythmias, tachycardia, and hypotension or hypertension; and seizures.

Although there is no specific antidote for carbamazepine overdose, supportive care and elimination of the drug from the body can save the patient's life. Supportive care might include elevating the patient's legs when hypotension develops, monitoring blood pressure, continuing surveillance of vital signs until full recovery, and intubating for respiratory difficulty.

Gastric lavage, even after several hours have passed, can help the patient recover from overdose. If alcohol is involved, gastric lavage is even more significant. Unless otherwise indicated, vomiting should be induced immediately after discovering an overdose. Activated charcoal given through a nasal gastric tube is warranted as well. Hemodialysis in cases of severe overdose, replacement therapy in small children, and the administration of an osmotic-based diuretic to hasten renal excretion are other interventions for carbamazepine poisoning. Parenteral diazepam or phenobarbital is indicated to control acute seizures brought on by carbamazepine overdose, but they may cause additional respiratory depression.

Use in pregnancy. Carbamazepine is not recommended for use during pregnancy. Breast-feeding is usually discouraged because breast milk can contain a level of the drug as high as 60% of the mother's drug serum level.[46]

Side effect interventions. Complete blood cell counts, hepatic and renal function tests, and eye examinations should be performed before carbamazepine therapy begins and routinely thereafter. If a significant abnormality in any of the preceding areas should develop, the patient's condition should be monitored carefully or the drug discontinued and a new AED ordered to prevent exacerbation of seizure activity. Because fatal agranulocytosis has been reported, when carbamazepine is discontinued based on hematologic grounds, blood levels should be determined regularly, perhaps as often as daily. In the elderly patient, confusion and CNS symptoms necessitate special attention.

Interactions. Carbamazepine interacts with many drugs. Carbamazepine is metabolized by P-450 2D6 and also induces this isoenzyme. Induction of 2D6 can decrease the plasma levels and half-lives of other drugs metabolized by this system. When given with drugs such as phenytoin, phenobarbital, or primidone, an increase in the respective doses of these drugs may be necessary because carbamazepine speeds their metabolism.

Drug serum levels decreased by carbamazepine. Carbamazepine decreases the effect of acetaminophen, barbiturates, some benzodiazepines, clozapine, corticosteroids, Coumadin, doxycycline, felbamate, haloperidol, isoniazid, methadone, oral contraceptives (risking breakthrough bleeding and possibly pregnancy), phenytoin, propranolol, succinimides, theophylline, tricyclic antidepressants, and valproic acid.

Drug serum level increased by carbamazepine. Carbamazepine possibly increases the effect of phenytoin.

Drugs that increase serum levels of carbamazepine. Cimetidine, diltiazem, erythromycin, fluoxetine, fluvoxamine, flu vaccine, *grapefruit juice*, isoniazid, nefazodone, propoxyphene, ritonavir, trazodone, valproic acid, and verapamil augment the effect of carbamazepine. Although increased serum carbamazepine levels will not require the clinician to abandon these combinations, careful monitoring of the patient is indicated should any of these drugs be ordered concurrently with carbamazepine.

Drugs that decrease serum levels of carbamazepine. Charcoal, phenobarbital, phenytoin, primidone, and theophylline decrease the effect of carbamazepine.

In addition, because the interactions of carbamazepine/lithium and carbamazepine/haloperidol can cause a neurotoxic condition, such combinations should be used with caution. It is thought that carbamazepine interacts with clozapine to potentiate bone marrow suppression.

Patient education. As with other AEDs, carbamazepine may cause GI tract upset, so the patient is advised to take the drug with food to prevent nausea and vomiting. Because drowsiness, dizziness, and blurred vision can complicate driving, precautions should also be taken. Because of the seriousness of hematologic reactions, the patient should notify the physician or nurse when any of the signs and symptoms of blood dyscrasia are present; these symptoms include sore throat, bruising, bleeding, fever, and chills.

VALPROIC ACID AND DERIVATIVES

Valproic acid and its derivatives, sodium valproate and divalproex sodium, are commonly prescribed AEDs. It was first synthesized in 1882 but not approved as an AED until 1978.[26] Valproic acid is a drug of choice for absence seizures. It is also effective for tonic-clonic, myoclonic, and complex partial seizures as well. Valproic acid is used for bipolar disorder and is probably more effective than carbamazepine for that condition (see Chapter 6).

Pharmacologic Effects

Valproic acid inhibits the spread of abnormal discharges through the brain. Although the precise nature of this action is not known, three or four mechanisms may be responsible: (1) an increase in GABA by either decreasing GABA metabolism or reducing its reuptake, (2) an increased postsynaptic response to GABA, (3) an increase in the resting membrane potential (sodium channel regulation), and/or (4) suppression of calcium influx through specific calcium channels.[23,26,31]

Pharmacokinetics

Valproic acid is rapidly absorbed after oral ingestion, whether taken in capsule or syrup form. Peak serum levels occur in less than 4 hours. Concurrent food intake and use of the enteric-coated form, divalproex sodium, slows absorption. Valproic acid is rapidly distributed in the body and is highly bound to serum proteins (90% to 95%). However, as serum levels rise, protein binding declines, causing nonlinear increases in free molecules. Patients with hypoalbuminemia are at even greater risk of having an excessive free fraction of the drug. The therapeutic serum level is 50 to 100 µg/ml. Valproic acid is metabolized mostly in the liver and excreted in the urine. The serum half-life is relatively short, 6 to 16 hours. In children with immature livers and older patients with cirrhosis or acute hepatitis, valproic acid has a prolonged half-life (67 hours and 25 hours, respectively). Table 9-5 contains dosage information.

Side Effects

Valproic acid causes relatively few serious side effects. This quality and its broad clinical utility are responsible for its growing acceptance as a major AED. Some GI tract symptoms are common during early therapy, but these disappear after continued use. Also, prescription of the enteric-coated form reduces GI tract discomfort. Up to 50% or so of the patients taking valproic acid gain weight. At therapeutic levels, only phenytoin causes less drowsiness than valproic acid.

Fatal hepatic failure, although rare, has been associated with valproic acid and is most likely to occur in children younger than 2 years of age. Valproic acid is often given with other AEDs, which confounds efforts to know the true extent of hepatotoxicity. Nonetheless, valproic acid and its derivatives are contraindicated in patients with liver disease and in children most at risk (those younger than 6 months of age). Valproic acid is also not given adjunctively to children younger than 3 years of age. Other adverse reactions can include emotional upset, some alopecia, and musculoskeletal weakness.

Treatment Implications

Therapeutic versus toxic levels. Therapeutic serum levels of valproic acid are 50 to 100 µg/ml. At serum concentrations above this level, CNS depression and coma develop. These events are most likely to result when valproic acid and phenobarbital are given concurrently. Restlessness and visual hallucinations are also symptoms of overdosage. Because valproic acid is absorbed quickly, treatment is supportive unless it begins soon after the drug was ingested. If little time has elapsed, gastric lavage and forced emesis can reduce absorption and should be attempted. If absorption has occurred, support of respiratory and cardiovascular systems is most appropriate. Hemodialysis has been used. Naloxone (Narcan), the narcotic antagonist, may reverse the CNS depressant effects of valproic acid; however, because naloxone could also reverse antiepileptic effects, it should be used cautiously.

Use in pregnancy. Valproic acid is teratogenic and should not be used unless other AEDs have been found ineffective (it is in category D). The Centers for Disease Control and Prevention estimate a risk of 1% to 2% for spina bifida in infants of mothers taking this drug.[31] Only when the risk to the mother's health is otherwise so great that withholding valproic acid could be deemed irresponsible should this drug be prescribed. Breast-feeding is considered compatible with valproic acid use.[3]

Side effect interventions. Serious side effects of valproic acid are uncommon. Drowsiness typically disappears after continued use. Hepatotoxicity, although potentially fatal, can be averted by testing hepatic function before treatment and by screening certain groups of patients, that is, infants and children younger than 2 years and individuals with liver dysfunction. GI tract problems are alleviated by taking this drug with food.

Interactions. Valproic acid interacts with several drugs. It potentiates the actions of other CNS depressants such as alcohol and barbiturates by inhibiting hepatic metabolism of those agents or displacing them from protein-binding sites (e.g., alcohol is displaced). Some seizure disorders may best be treated with a combination of valproic acid and clonazepam; however, evidence also indicates a potential for decreased efficacy of both drugs. Carbamazepine decreases valproic acid levels, as does acyclovir.

Drugs that increase serum levels of valproic acid. Chlorpromazine increases the half-life of valproic acid, as does aspirin. Because valproic acid inhibits platelet aggregation, use with aspirin and warfarin can cause prolonged bleeding and warrants close monitoring. Other drugs that increase valproic acid levels include cimetidine, erythromycin, felbamate, fluoxetine, fluvoxamine, and phenothiazines.

Drug serum levels increased by valproic acid. Free phenytoin serum levels are increased by valproic acid (as a result of protein-binding displacement), as are the plasma levels of phenobarbital (inhibition of hepatic metabolism) and ethosuximide. Phenobarbital serum levels are increased by as much as 40% when valproic acid is given concurrently; consequently, when given together, the amount of phenobarbital should be reduced. A similar interaction may occur with the related AEDs mephobarbital and primidone. Other drugs that have increased serum levels include amitriptyline, chlordiazepoxide, clonazepam, diazepam, and nortriptyline.

Patient education. It is important to teach the patient the following:
1. To take valproic acid with food if GI tract upset occurs
2. To swallow tablets or capsules whole (do not chew) to prevent irritation of the mouth and throat
3. To take the drug at bedtime to minimize effects of drowsiness and to be cautious when driving
4. To notify those monitoring for diabetes because valproic acid may give false-positive blood and urine ketone values

Related Drugs

Valproate (Depakene syrup) is the sodium salt of valproic acid, and the enteric-coated divalproex sodium (Depakote) is a compound containing equal portions of valproic acid and valproate. Dosages are equivalent. Noticeable differences are the more rapid absorption when the syrup is used and the delayed absorption with the enteric-coated divalproex. Divalproex may reduce GI tract irritation. Depacon is an IV alternative to oral valproic acid.

BENZODIAZEPINES: DIAZEPAM, LORAZEPAM, CLONAZEPAM

The benzodiazepines are primarily prescribed for their antianxiety properties and are thoroughly reviewed in Chapter 7. However, three benzodiazepines indicated for treating seizure disorders are discussed here.

Diazepam Indication: Status Epilepticus

Diazepam (Valium) is a drug of choice for treating status epilepticus (continuous tonic-clonic seizures lasting 30 minutes or longer). Diazepam is effective about 95% of the time in controlling these life-threatening seizures. Diazepam is also used adjunctively to treat other types of epilepsy.

A dose of 5 to 10 mg of diazepam (rate no faster than 2 to 5 mg/min) given intravenously stops most seizures within 5 minutes. Because the serum levels fall rapidly, it may be necessary to repeat the dose to maintain a seizure-free state. Typically, repeated doses at 10- to 15-minute intervals may be required. No more than 30 mg of diazepam should be given to treat a single episode of status epilepticus.[31] If a second episode of status epilepticus occurs within 2 to 4 hours, this protocol can be repeated.[31] Because of residual metabolites of diazepam, caution should be used. All IV injections of diazepam must be administered slowly (no more than 5 mg/min) to prevent thrombosis, phlebitis, and venous irritation. Children and infants have a significantly lower dosage restriction than do adults (see Table 9-5).

Because of the short-lived effect of diazepam, a phenytoin infusion (18 mg/kg or less at a rate no faster than 50 mg/min) can be hung to follow the first dose of diazepam, thereby avoiding repeated doses of diazepam.

If diazepam is used exclusively (up to 30 mg) and seizures are refractory to treatment, an IV phenytoin drip can be provided. A phenobarbital drip (at 100 mg/min) is the next option but should not follow diazepam because of the synergistic effect of these drugs in depressing respirations. For seizures still not controlled, a paraldehyde infusion can be considered. As a final resort, anesthesia coupled with a neuromuscular blocker can be administered to stop refractory status epilepticus.

Although the discussion of diazepam as a drug of choice for status epilepticus is informative, the real-life task of starting an IV line in a patient with this type of seizure is no easy matter. Should starting the IV line become impossible, an alternative is to inject the drug into a large muscle or to give it rectally. Diastat is a rectal gel formulation approved for home management of selected refractory patients.

Diazepam can be given orally as an adjunct to chronic treatment of convulsive disorders (10 mg four times a day) when the possibility of withdrawal seizures is likely.

Because diazepam has a wide therapeutic index, it is a safe drug when given alone. When mixed with other CNS depressants, however, diazepam can cause severe CNS depression. This fact is of slight clinical importance when diazepam is being used to treat the life-threatening emergency status epilepticus, but it becomes more significant when the drug is used adjunctively to treat other seizure forms. In either situation, support for ventilation and monitoring of blood pressure are critical precautions. Pharmacokinetics, side effects, and clinical implications for diazepam use are discussed in Chapter 7.

Lorazepam Indication: Status Epilepticus

Lorazepam (Ativan) is also a drug of choice for status epilepticus. Many clinicians prefer it over diazepam because it has a longer duration of action. Whereas diazepam, with its short duration, must be given frequently, lorazepam's antiepileptic effect lasts for 24 hours or longer. Lorazepam is given via IV push (4 mg over 2 minutes). A detailed discussion of lorazepam, including pharmacokinetic parameters, can be found in Chapter 7.

Clonazepam Indication: Lennox-Gastaut

Clonazepam (Klonopin) is effective in treating Lennox-Gastaut syndrome (a variant form of absence seizure) and akinetic and myoclonic seizures. It may also be effective in treating absence seizures not responsive to the succinimides. It is not effective for tonic-clonic or partial seizures. As with other benzodiazepines, its mechanism of action is probably related to enhancing the effects of GABA-mediated neuronal inhibition. Approximately one third of the patients taking clonazepam have breakthrough seizures, indicating a development of tolerance to this drug. Dosage adjustment can restore drug effectiveness. Therapeutic serum levels for clonazepam are 20 to 80 ng/ml. Clonazepam and valproic acid used concurrently can stimulate absence status epilepticus (prolonged absence seizures) and tonic seizures. Dosage information is found in Table 9-5. See Chapter 7 for a detailed discussion of benzodiazepines.

Oᴛʜᴇʀ Iᴍᴘᴏʀᴛᴀɴᴛ Aɴᴛɪᴇᴘɪʟᴇᴘᴛɪᴄ Dʀᴜɢs

This section covers antiepileptics that are not as commonly prescribed and that are considered second-line drugs, newer AEDs, or rarely used drugs for which antiepileptic properties are secondary uses.

ETHOSUXIMIDE

Ethosuximide (Zarontin) is from the succinimide family of AEDs. The succinimides are chemically distinct from the hydantoins and the long-acting barbiturates. Ethosuximide's contribution to antiepileptic therapy lies in its effectiveness in treating absence seizures (see Table 9-2). Up to 80% to 90% of these seizures are controlled in newly diagnosed patients.[23] Ethosuximide is not effective in the treatment of tonic-clonic or partial seizures.

Pharmacologic Effects

Ethosuximide decreases absence seizures by interfering with calcium conductances. It does not alter sodium channel activation, nor does it increase GABA inhibition. Ethosuximide is not the first drug of choice for absence seizures in adults; valproic acid is. Nonetheless, ethosuximide remains an important drug.

Pharmacokinetics

Ethosuximide is readily absorbed in the GI tract, and peak serum levels are reached within 3 to 7 hours (see Table 9-4). Ethosuximide, because of a long half-life of 40 to 60 hours in adults and 30 hours in children, can be given in once-a-day dosages. Steady state is achieved in 5 to 10 days in adults. It is extensively metabolized to inactive metabolites and excreted in the urine.

Ethosuximide is available in oral forms (capsules and syrup). It can be used adjunctively with other AEDs in patients with seizures other than absence seizures; however, because ethosuximide can increase the risk of tonic-clonic seizure breakthrough, higher dosages of the concurrent AED may be required. Used alone, ethosuximide can increase the risk of tonic-clonic seizures in some patients.

Side Effects

The common complaint associated with ethosuximide is GI tract upset. Nausea, vomiting, cramps, diarrhea, and anorexia are common but can be reduced by taking the medication with meals. Psychiatric and CNS symptoms (dizziness and drowsiness) can occur in some patients. Succinimides have been reported to cause abnormal hepatic and renal function in humans, so monitoring studies of these functions is consistent with good care. Giving ethosuximide to a patient with impaired liver functioning prolongs the already long half-life, increasing the risk of long-lasting toxic effects. Hematologic effects, which are uncommon but significant, and dermatologic effects occur in a few patients.

Treatment Implications

Therapeutic versus toxic levels. The therapeutic serum level of ethosuximide is 40 to 100 µg/ml. Toxic effects occur when the serum level is higher than 100 µg/ml. The most severe reactions to overdose are myopia, vaginal bleeding, CNS depression, and systemic lupus erythematosus. Overdoses are treated symptomatically, and patient care is supportive.

Use in pregnancy. Although, in general, AEDs are known to contribute to fetal abnormalities, ethosuximide seems to be a drug that can be given safely without the risk of significant defects in newborns. With appropriate monitoring, women have been able to take ethosuximide during pregnancy. This drug is not recommended for use during lactation.

Interactions. Ethosuximide does not interact in a significant way with any other drugs; however, excessive sedation could result from concurrent administration with a CNS depressant, for example, alcohol. Other interactions are noted in the drug profiles in Part 2 of this book.

Patient education. Patients who have any of the GI tract symptoms mentioned previously should be advised to take ethosuximide with food or milk. Because of the long half-life of ethosuximide and its once-a-day dosing, patients who miss a day of medication should not take a double dose the next day. To do so could substantially raise the serum level of ethosuximide and in turn cause intensified side effects and toxic reactions.

Patients taking ethosuximide should be advised to avoid alcohol and to refrain from abrupt discontinuance of this drug. Abruptly ceasing use increases the risk of seizures. Because ethosuximide can cause drowsiness, driving a car or operating hazardous machinery should be limited until the drug is well tolerated. Patients should report symptoms that indicate blood dyscrasias to the physician.

Related Succinimides

The two related succinimides are methsuximide (Celontin) and phensuximide (Milontin). Methsuximide is as effective as ethosuximide in treating absence seizures; however, it is slightly more toxic. Toxicity occurs when serum levels exceed 40 µg/ml. Other information can be found in Part 2 of this book.

Phensuximide is thought to be slightly less effective than either ethosuximide or methsuximide. Peak serum levels of the drug are reached within 4 hours, and its half-life is about 8 hours. Significant genitourinary tract side effects not associated with the other succinimides (i.e., urinary frequency, renal damage, and hematuria) have been reported to be caused by phensuximide. Also, a harmless urinary effect is pinkish, red, or red-brown urine. Regardless of the patient's age, the total daily dose may vary from 1 to 3 g.

TRIMETHADIONE

Trimethadione (Tridione) is an oxazolidinedione. The oxazolidinediones are AEDs normally used only when other drugs have proven ineffective. Trimethadione was introduced in 1946 and was the first drug developed to treat absence seizures. Although effective, it is not a first- or second-line drug of choice because it causes serious side effects and has been proven to be the most teratogenic AED. The exact nature of trimethadione's antiepileptic effect is not known. Trimethadione causes several serious side effects, and occasionally, patients taking a regimen of trimethadione have died. Prominent among the adverse responses are hepatic impairment, nephrosis, blood dyscrasias, exfoliative dermatitis, systemic lupus erythematosus, lymphadenopathy, and a myasthenia gravis–like syndrome.

PRIMIDONE

Primidone (Mysoline) is related to the barbiturates and is used alone or in conjunction with other AEDs to control tonic-clonic and partial seizures but not absence seizures. Two metabolites of primidone, phenobarbital and phenylethylma-lonamide, are responsible for the drug's antiepileptic properties. When a barbiturate is indicated, primidone is not a first-line drug because it is responsible for significant side effects (see Part 2). Emotional disturbances, including paranoid thinking and mood fluctuations, have also been reported in some patients. Some side effects, such as ataxia and vertigo, disappear after continued use. Adults and children are started on a regimen of primidone at modest dosages (100 mg at bedtime and 50 mg at bedtime, respectively); then dosages are carefully elevated over the next 10 days to arrive at a therapeutic maintenance dosage. Primidone has a half-life of 3 to 12 hours, but the active metabolites noted previously extend the half-life up to 118 hours. Details on dosages are given in both Table 9-5 and the psychotropic drug profiles found in Part 2. Adults are never given more than 2 g/day. Bioequivalence among brands of primidone is not supported by clinical experience, so switching products is not recommended. Therapeutic serum levels are reached at 5 to 12 µg/ml.

NEWER ANTIEPILEPTICS

Since 1993, a number of AEDs have been developed. Brief summaries of their indications, mechanisms of action, and pharmacokinetic profiles are presented next.

Gabapentin

Gabapentin (Neurontin) was approved in early 1994 as an adjunctive treatment for partial seizures in adults and adolescents older than 12.[22,30] This drug is similar to GABA in structure but with molecular alterations to make it more lipophilic and hence better able to penetrate the blood-brain barrier.[36] It does not directly join to GABA receptors but apparently increases GABA release from presynaptic neurons.

Absorption of gabapentin is dose dependent at high dosages.[1] Food does not alter absorption. It reaches peak serum levels in 2 to 3 hours. It has a relatively short half-life of 5 to 8 hours. It is not protein bound to any extent. It is not measurably metabolized and therefore is excreted as an unchanged molecule in the urine. Patients with decreased kidney function should be given smaller doses of this drug. Therapeutic serum levels are greater than 2 µg/ml.

Gabapentin is well tolerated and typically produces mild side effects. The most common of these are somnolence, dizziness, ataxia, and nystagmus.[31] More serious side effects reported include choreoathetosis, exacerbation of Lennox-Gastaut epilepsy, and dystonic movement disorders.[26] Gabapentin does not induce hepatic enzymes, nor does it inhibit them. Gabapentin has no drug interactions with other AEDs, so it can be used adjunctively when appropriate. Antacids reduce the bioavailability of gabapentin, and cimetidine increases it. Dosage information is found in Table 9-5.

Lamotrigine

Lamotrigine (Lamictal) was approved in late 1994 (in the United States) as an adjunctive treatment for partial seizures and may have implications for more general-ized seizures.[44] In 1997, its use was expanded to include treatment for Lennox-Gastaut syndrome and adult monotherapy.[27] It can be prescribed for patients older than 16 years of age. It blocks sustained repetitive firing of neurons by prolonging the inactivation of sodium channels.[28] It does not affect normal synaptic conduction.

Lamotrigine is rapidly absorbed, has a 90% bioavailability, reaches peak plasma levels in 1.5 to 4 hours, and is moderately bound to plasma proteins (55%). When patients are prescribed lamotrigine alone, its half-life is 25 hours. When combined with enzyme inducers such as carbamazepine, phenytoin, and phenobarbital, the half-life can decrease (to 10 hours). When given with enzyme inhibitors such as valproic acid, the half-life can increase (to 60 hours).[23,36] The dosage of lamotrigine is modified when given adjunctively with valproic acid, for obvious reasons. Therapeutic serum levels are greater than 2 μg/ml.

Side effects are usually mild. Common complaints include diplopia, somnolence, dizziness, ataxia, and blurred vision. Rashes occur in about 10% of patients and are usually of little significance; however, deaths have resulted from severe skin reactions. These severe skin reactions occur in 0.1% of adults and 1% to 2% of children taking lamotrigine.[26] If rash develops, lamotrigine should be discontinued. Other serious side effects include encephalopathies, hepatic failure, leukopenia, and cardiovascular problems.

Vigabatrin

Vigabatrin (Sabril) was first developed in the 1970s.[6,13] Vigabatrin is known to be effective for partial epilepsy and infantile spasms. This efficacy is thought to be caused by vigabatrin's irreversible inhibition of GABA-transaminase, the degradative enzyme for GABA. This action increases brain GABA levels and decreases GABA-transaminase.

Vigabatrin is rapidly absorbed with or without food intake. It has a high bioavailability and is not bound to plasma proteins. It has a half-life of 5 to 8 hours; however, because of its irreversible inhibition of GABA-transaminase, its half-life can be extended. It is excreted unchanged by the kidney, so individuals with renal insufficiency will not only eliminate vigabatrin more slowly but also should require lower dosages. Because it is not metabolized, the CYP-450 interactions often associated with other AEDs are not a concern. Vigabatrin can (but may not) reduce serum levels of phenytoin by 15% to 30% via some unknown mechanism.

CNS complaints such as drowsiness (13% to 40%), fatigue, and headache are relatively common. Weight gain has been reported, but rashes are not common in patients taking vigabatrin. A relatively high incidence of psychiatric disorders (e.g., depression, psychosis) has been associated with vigabatrin use.[25] Vigabatrin is typically initiated at 0.5 to 1 g/day and titrated upward at that dose on a weekly basis until reaching 2 to 3 g/day. Withdrawal is titrated in a similar fashion to reduce the risk of withdrawal-related seizures.

Topiramate

Topiramate (Topamax), a new AED, is approved for adjunctive therapy of partial seizures.[14] Topiramate may also be useful in treating partial-onset seizures in children, tonic-clonic seizures, and drop attacks associated with Lennox-Gastaut syndrome. Its mode of action is unknown, but it is thought that three separate mechanisms contribute to its antiepileptic capabilities: (1) sodium channel normalization, (2) GABA potentiation, and (3) antagonism of non-NMDA glutamate receptors.

Absorption of topiramate is rapid and is not hampered by food. It has a bioavailability of 80%. Peak plasma concentrations are reached in about 2 hours. The average half-life of this drug is about 21 hours. Steady state is reached within 4 days if the patient has normal renal function. Plasma protein binding is between 13% and 17%, and about 70% of the average dose of topiramate is excreted via the kidney unchanged because it is not extensively metabolized. Renal disease reduces clearance of this drug.

Common side effects of topiramate include somnolence, dizziness, ataxia, nervousness, abnormal vision, psychomotor slowing, speech disorders, memory problems, confusion, diplopia, and anorexia. Topiramate is a pregnancy category C drug because it has been shown to cause development toxicity in animal studies.

Interactions with topiramate are few and typically not severe. Digoxin levels are reduced with topiramate, oral contraceptives may lose their effectiveness, and use with carbonic anhydrase inhibitors may increase the risk for kidney stones. Topiramate levels are reduced with phenytoin, carbamazepine, and valproic acid.

The typical daily dosage begins at 50 mg/day and then is incrementally increased to 200 mg two times per day.

Tiagabine

Tiagabine (Gabitril) has been recently approved for adjunctive treatment of partial seizures.[39] Its effectiveness as an AED is related to its ability to inhibit the reuptake of GABA into presynaptic neurons and surrounding glial cells. The net effect is greater availability of GABA for postsynaptic cells, thus prolonging the GABA-mediated inhibition.

Tiagabine is rapidly and completely absorbed, with a bioavailability of about 90%. Food slows absorption but does not alter the extent of bioavailability. Peak serum levels are achieved between 1 to 2.5 hours. It is likely metabolized by the CYP-450 isoenzyme 3A. Other drugs metabolized by this isoenzyme (e.g., carbamazepine, phenytoin, primidone, phenobarbital) can decrease the half-life of tiagabine from 7 to 9 hours to 4 to 7 hours. Steady state is achieved within 2 days. Tiagabine does not alter serum concentrations in other drugs. Tiagabine is 96% bound to plasma proteins. Common side effects of tiagabine include somnolence, asthenia, dizziness, headache, nausea, and nervousness. Most are mild to moderate in severity. Dosage for tiagabine ranges from 30 to 56 mg/day.

Oxcarbazepine

Oxcarbazepine (Trileptal) is a new AED that is chemically similar to carbamazepine with similar efficacy but without the toxic effects of that drug.[43] Because of similarities in structure, it is suspected that oxcarbazepine's mechanism of action is similar to that of carbamazepine, that is, normalization of sodium channels reducing high-frequency action potentials.

Oxcarbazepine is almost completely absorbed, with food having little effect on bioavailability. Several metabolic steps are involved in oxcarbazepine's reduction. It is converted to an active metabolite, MHD (10,11,dihydro-10-hydoxy-5H-dibenzo(b,f)azepine-5-carboxamide), and because only minuscule amounts of oxcarbazepine can be found in peripheral blood, the effects of oxcarbazepine are attributed to this metabolite. Oxcarbazepine is considered a prodrug of MHD.

Pharmacokinetic information is based on MHD. Peak serum levels occur within 4 to 6 hours. The half-life of this metabolite is between 8 and 10 hours. Therapeutic serum levels are thought to be 25 μg/ml. Hepatic microsomal enzyme induction and autoinduction are much less dramatic compared with carbamazepine. Because of these factors, certain AEDs may have increased serum levels when coadministered with oxcarbazepine as opposed to carbamazepine.

Common side effects of oxcarbazepine include somnolence, headache, dizziness, nausea, rash, gum hyperplasia, tremor, and diplopia.

Monotherapy for adults typically begins at 300 to 600 mg/day in two or three divided doses. Upward dosing is incremental and eventually may reach 900 to 3000 mg/day in two or three divided doses.

Zonisamide

Zonisamide is considered a broad-spectrum AED with apparent efficacy for both partial and generalized seizures.[24] An antimanic effect has also been reported.[32] It is thought to have this broader application based on three mechanisms of action: (1) the ability to regulate sodium channels, (2) the ability to suppress calcium influx through specific calcium channels, and (3) the ability to modulate GABA-mediated neuronal inhibition.[47]

Zonisamide has a rapid and complete absorption, with peak serum levels occurring in 2 to 5 hours. It does not bind significantly to plasma proteins. Its half-life is estimated at 63 to 69 hours, with steady state achieved within 7 to 10 days. Zonisamide is metabolized in the liver, with some molecules excreted via the kidney unchanged. The CYP-450 enzymes are involved in zonisamide's metabolism, but the role of specific isoenzymes is still to be established. Drug-drug interactions are probably related to CYP induction. For example, carbamazepine and phenytoin decrease the serum levels of zonisamide. Common side effects of zonisamide include somnolence, ataxia, anorexia, confusion, abnormal thinking, nervousness, fatigue, and dizziness. The recommended initial dosage of zonisamide is 100 to 200 mg/day for adults, with dosage increases about every 2 weeks. Maintenance dosage is typically 400 to 600 mg/day for adults in two divided doses. Blood levels of 20 to 30 μg/ml appear to be effective.

Felbamate

Felbamate (Felbatol) was approved in 1993 for adjunctive or monotherapy in adults with partial or tonic-clonic seizures and as an adjunctive therapy for children with Lennox-Gastaut syndrome.[22] By mid-1994, an unusually high incidence of aplastic anemia (eventually 34 cases reported, with 13 deaths) and hepatic failure (eventually 18 cases reported) developed.[34] Felbamate was allowed to remain on the market. Nonetheless, a sharp decline in use occurred, and today just over 10,000 patients take the drug worldwide.[34]

RARELY USED ANTIEPILEPTICS
Acetazolamide

Acetazolamide (Diamox) is a diuretic that inhibits the enzyme carbonic anhydrase. This mechanism alkalinizes the urine, causing mild systemic acidosis. This reduction in blood pH reduces seizures in some individuals. Acetazolamide is used adjunctively to treat absence, tonic-clonic, and myoclonic seizures. There is convincing evidence that acetazolamide is an effective agent for treating refractory bipolar illness as well.[17]

Magnesium Sulfate

Patients with lowered levels of magnesium (patients with eclampsia and alcohol withdrawal syndrome) are subject to seizures. Magnesium sulfate given intramuscularly (preferred) or intravenously can prevent these seizures. Because low serum magnesium levels are ongoing in these conditions, it may be necessary to administer magnesium sulfate frequently.

Paraldehyde

Historically, paraldehyde has been used to control seizures associated with alcohol withdrawal. New drugs are now being used for this purpose; however, paraldehyde remains a viable agent for treating status epilepticus when other drugs have failed. It is administered intramuscularly or intravenously.

REFERENCES

1. Andrews CO, Fischer JH: Gabapentin: a new agent for the management of epilepsy, *Ann Pharmacother* 28(10):1188, 1994.
2. Begley CE and others: Cost of epilepsy in the United States: a model based on incidence and prognosis, *Epilepsia* 35(6):1230, 1994.
3. Bezchlibnyk-Butler KZ, Jeffries JJ: *Clinical handbook of psychotropic drugs*, ed 7, Seattle, 1997, Hogrefe & Huber.
4. Borgsdorf LR, Caldwell JW: *Clinical therapeutics: a disease-oriented approach to pharmacology and therapeutics*, Bakersfield, Calif, 1985, Kern Medical Center.
5. Bredkjaer SR, Mortenson PB, Parnas J: Epilepsy and non-organic non-affective psychosis. National epidemiologic study, *Br J Psychiatry* 172:235, 1998.
6. Buchanan N: Vigabatrin use in 72 patients with drug-resistant epilepsy, *Seizure* 3(3):191, 1994.
7. Carpenter WT and others: Carbamazepine maintenance treatment in outpatient schizophrenics, *Arch Gen Psychiatry* 48(1):69, 1991.
8. Commission on Classification and Terminology of the International League Against Epilepsy: Proposal for revised clinical and electroencephalographic classification of epileptic seizures, *Epilepsia* 22:489, 1981.
9. Dalessio JD: Seizure disorders and pregnancy, *N Engl J Med* 312:559, 1985.
10. Delgado-Escueta AV, Treiman DM, Walsh GO: The treatable epilepsies, *N Engl J Med* 308:1508, 1576, 1983.
11. Delgado-Escueta AV and others: Management of status epilepticus, *N Engl J Med* 306:1337, 1982.
12. Engel J, Starkman S: Overview of seizures, *Emerg Med Clin North Am* 12(4):895, 1994.
13. French JA: Vigabatrin, *Epilepsia* 40(suppl 5):S11, 1999.
14. Glauser TA: Topiramate, *Epilepsia* 40(suppl 5):S71, 1999.
15. Hauser WA: Recent developments in the epidemiology of epilepsy, *Acta Neurol Scand Suppl* 162:17, 1995.
16. Hauser WA, Annegers JF, Kurland LT: Prevalence of epilepsy in Rochester, Minnesota: 1940-1980, *Epilepsia* 32:429, 1991.
17. Hayes SG: Acetazolamide in bipolar affective disorders, *Ann Clin Psychiatry* 6(2):91, 1994.
18. Hyde TM, Weinberger DR: Seizures and schizophrenia, *Schizophrenia Bull* 23(4):611, 1997.
19. Jallon P: Electroencephalogram and epilepsy, *Eur Neurol* 34(suppl 1):18, 1994.
20. Jordan KG: Status epilepticus: a perspective from the neuroscience intensive care unit, *Neurosurg Clin North Am* 5 (4):671, 1994.
21. Keltner NL, Folks DG: Alternatives to lithium in the treatment of bipolar disorder, *Perspect Psychiatric Care* 27(2):36, 1991.
22. Laxer KD: Guidelines for treating epilepsy in the age of felbamate, vigabatrin, lamotrigine, and gabapentin, *West J Med* 161(3):309, 1994.
23. Lehne RA: *Pharmacology for nursing care*, ed 3, Philadelphia, 1998, WB Saunders.
24. Leppik IE: Zonisamide, *Epilepsia* 40(suppl 5):S23, 1999.
25. Levinson DF, Devinsky O: Psychiatric adverse events during vigabatrin therapy, *Neurology* 53(7):1503, 1999.
26. Lieberman JA, Tasman A: *Psychiatric drugs*, Philadelphia, 2000, WB Saunders.
27. Matsuo F: Lamotrigine, *Epilepsia* 40(suppl 5):S30, 1999.
28. Meldrum BS: Lamotrigine: a novel approach, *Seizure* 3(suppl A):41, 1994.
29. McKenna PJ, Kane JM, Parrish K: Psychotic syndromes in epilepsy, *Am J Psychiatry* 142:895, 1985.
30. Morris GL: Gabapentin, *Epilepsia* 40(suppl 5):S63, 1999.

31. Olin BR, ed: *Drug facts and comparisons,* St Louis, 1995, Wolters Kluwer.

32. Oommen KJ, Mathews S: Zonisamide: a new antiepileptic drug, *Clin Neuropharmacol* 22(4):192, 1999.

33. Patsalos PN, Sander JW: Newer epileptic drugs: towards an improved risk-benefit ratio, *Drug Safety* 11(1):37, 1994.

34. Pellock JM: Felbamate, *Epilepsia* 40(suppl 5):S57, 1999.

35. Putnam TJ, Merritt HH: Experimental determination of the anticonvulsant properties of some phenyl derivatives, *Science* 85:525, 1937.

36. Ramsey RE and others: *Clinical issues in the management of epilepsy,* Miami, 1993, University of Miami Press.

37. Roberts GW, Leigh PN, Weinberger DR: *Neuropsychiatric disorders,* London, 1993, Wolfe.

38. Rogawski MA, Porter RJ: Antiepileptic drugs: pharmacological mechanisms and clinical efficacy with considerations of promising developmental state compounds, *Pharm Rev* 42: 223, 1990.

39. Schachter SC: Tiagabine, *Epilepsia* 40(suppl 5):S17, 1999.

40. Senanayake N, Roman GC: Epidemiology of epilepsy in developing countries, *Bull WHO* 71(2):247, 1993.

41. Shorvon S: Epilepsy and driving, *Br Med J* 310(6984):885, 1995.

42. Smith PF, Darlington CL: The development of psychosis in epilepsy: a re-examination of the kindling hypothesis, *Behav Brain Res* 75(1-2):59, 1996.

43. Tecoma ES: Oxcarbazepine, *Epilepsia* 40(suppl 5):S37, 1999.

44. The Medical Letter: Lamotrigine for epilepsy, *The Medical Letter* 37(944):21, 1995.

45. Trimble MR: *The psychoses of epilepsy,* New York, 1991, Raven.

46. Vestermark V, Vestermark S: Teratogenic effect of carbamazepine, *Arch Dis Child* 66(5): 641, 1991.

47. White HS: Comparative anticonvulsant and mechanistic profile of the established and newer antiepileptic drugs, *Epilepsia* 40(suppl 5):S2, 1999.

48. Wilder BJ: The treatment of epilepsy: an overview of clinical practices, *Neurology* 45 (suppl 3):S7, 1995.

CHAPTER 10

Insomnia and Other Sleep Disorders

HISTORICAL CONSIDERATIONS

The pioneering work of sleep physiology involved Nathaniel Kleitman and his graduate students, Eugene Aserinsky and William Dement, at the University of Chicago.[3] Their studies of sleep led to technologic advances and the production of reliable electrographic recordings obtained from the human brain that allowed investigation of the neurophysiologic changes that occur on the wakefulness-to-sleep continuum. These investigators found that sleep, as it progresses through the nocturnal period, is not a unitary phenomenon and involves a sequence of sleep stages. Physiologic changes occur as one stage gives way to another; these stages alternate rhythmically throughout the night. Rapid eye movement (REM) sleep was identified as a state distinct from non-REM sleep.

The basic tool of sleep research is the simultaneous electrographic recording of multiple physiologic variables, now referred to as *polysomnography*. The study of sleep disturbances has become an interdisciplinary field, perhaps best illustrated in the area of sleep-induced breathing disorders, such as obstructive sleep apnea. Of all patients referred to sleep disorder centers in the United States, more than half exhibit disorders that reduce sleep. These disorders are a major cause of both social and work disability and contribute to systemic hypertension, cardiac arrhythmia, and other general medical consequences.

Depending on the nature of the problem, multidisciplinary clinicians work together to assess and diagnose the disorders in persons with disturbed sleep. The use of questionnaires, sleep diaries, histories and physicals, and laboratory examinations facilitates the basic clinical understanding of sleep disturbances. These assessment tools, together with the polysomnogram and pharmacologic interventions, are essential to the management of sleep disorder.

DIAGNOSTIC CONSIDERATIONS

Epidemiologic surveys suggest that 20% to 30% of adults report having sleep difficulties.[1] Approximately 7% of the population use sleeping agents to increase sleep, and about 1% use a prescription hypnotic 30 days or more per year. The incidence of excessive sleepiness ranges from 0.02% to 1% in the general population. Surveys of medical patients suggest that the rate of insomnia is 17% and the rate of hypersomnia is 3%. Age and disease tend to increase the prevalence rates of disturbed sleep.

Quality sleep normally requires good health, comfortable circumstances, and a lengthy daily period that is free of stressful obligations. Also freedom from the influence of stimulants and other drugs that negatively affect the structure of sleep is essential for quality sleep. In short, sleep is easily disrupted. The frenetic demands of a technologic culture may induce a briefer-than-normal average sleeping time. "Ad-lib" sleepers tend to sleep better than those whose obligations compel abbreviated sleep hours; short sleepers (those who require less sleep than normal) tolerate demanding work schedules better than those who require 8 hours or more of sleep. The impact of sleep loss precipitated by any of the aforementioned factors may extend into many areas of daily life. For example, consider the following facts:

1. People with chronic insomnia, and even those with occasional insomnia, doze off more often during the day.[1]
2. Insomniacs feel drowsy when driving and have more accidents.
3. Insomniacs take more naps during the day.
4. When asked to rate their ability to handle minor irritation, those with chronic or occasional insomnia report good to excellent ability significantly less often.
5. When asked about their ability to concentrate, insomniacs reported significantly worse ability to concentrate during the day.
6. Fifty-three percent of respondents with chronic insomnia report problems with memory, compared with 44% of those with occasional insomnia and 29% of those with no insomnia.
7. People with insomnia also report more problems in their relationships with spouses, families, and friends.[2]

Insomnia and other sleep disorders have gained widespread attention as an increasing number of individuals experience sleep deprivation. More than 80 types of sleep disorders affecting millions of Americans are identified by the International Classification of Sleep Disorders (ICSD). Both ICSD and the *Diagnostic and Statistical Manual of Mental Disorders,* fourth edition, distinguish between insomnia that is caused by (1) a general medical condition, (2) a medication or drug of abuse, (3) an underlying pathophysiology of sleep, (4) another mental disorder, (5) psychophysiologic or conditioned factors, or (6) circadian rhythm disturbances.

Insomnia Defined

Insomnia is the complaint of sleep insufficient to support good daytime functioning. Persistent insomnia without a coexisting general medical cause is called *primary insomnia.* Transient insomnia is relatively common, but persistent insomnia is not. Most individuals who come to sleep disorder clinics do so because of hypersomnia rather than insomnia.

Causes of Insomnia

Common, nonspecific disruptions of sleep may precipitate or aggravate insomnia. Thus many individuals can improve the quality of their sleep by instituting sleep hygiene (Box 10-1). When instituting a sleep hygiene program the clinician must carefully consider the patient's interests and motivations. Some aspects of good sleep hygiene, such as smoking cessation, are difficult to achieve. Other recommendations shown in Box 10-1 may be arduous or simply not possible.

Psychologic causes. Psychologic factors may disrupt sleep. Hypervigilance, anxiety, neuroticism, introversion, and insomnia all theoretically derive from common central nervous system (CNS) profiles of increased internal arousal.[17] Patients and clinicians alike are quick to attribute insomnia to psychologic problems. Specific psychiatric conditions may predispose persons to insomnia; mood and anxiety disorders, major psychoses, and dementia are often the cause. However, insomnia is not attributed to these conditions unless sleep hygiene measures are in place. Many patients have spent fruitless years seeking dependable sleep by means of anxiety reduction and psychotherapy while concomitantly working late, drinking coffee or alcohol, and sleeping late on weekends.

Box 10-1 Measures Used to Improve Sleep Hygiene

1. Arise at the same time each day.
2. Limit daily in-bed time to "normal" amount.
3. Discontinue use of drugs that act on the central nervous system, such as caffeine, nicotine, alcohol, and stimulants.
4. Avoid daytime napping except when sleep diary indicates a better night's sleep as a result.
5. Establish physical fitness with a routine of exercise early in the day, followed by other activity.
6. Avoid evening stimulation; substitute either listening to the radio or leisure reading for watching television.
7. Try a warm, 20-minute body bath or soak near bedtime.
8. Eat on a regular schedule; avoid large meals near bedtime.
9. Practice an evening relaxation routine.
10. Maintain comfortable sleeping conditions.
11. Spend no longer than 20 minutes awake in bed.
12. Adjust sleep hours and routine to optimize daily schedule and living situation.

Drug-related insomnia. Over-the-counter agents with CNS-stimulating actions may disrupt sleep, as may catecholamine reuptake blockers such as stimulating antidepressants (e.g., fluoxetine, protriptyline, bupropion), antiarrhythmic drugs, corticosteroids, thyroid preparations, and methysergide (Sansert). Diuretics may cause cramps, restless leg syndrome, or both. Sleeping pills paradoxically may worsen sleep. For example, short-acting hypnotic agents such as triazolam may cause agitation, amnestic episodes, early-morning awakening, or even next-day anxiety. These may merge together with next-night rebound insomnia, compounding sleeping difficulties. Thus the chronic administration of hypnotics may actually serve to diminish sleep quality.

Altered sleep schedule. A variety of sleep difficulties, including insomnia, may result from suboptimal sleep schedules or from general medical problems. In individuals who literally have their days and nights mixed up, a tendency may develop toward later arising times, which results in delayed sleep-phase syndrome. This syndrome is most likely to occur in individuals without regular morning obligations. Disruption of the circadian rhythms may follow. This condition, advanced sleep phase, is common in geriatric patients.[5] Treatment (discussed later) includes progressively shifting the sleep hours incrementally toward a desirable, fixed schedule.

Shift workers are at significant risk to sleep poorly. Some individuals who need little sleep may prefer night work and function well on the few hours of sleep that they are able to obtain. However, many shift workers sleep poorly and feel chronically fatigued. Workers on rotating shifts have the most difficulty with sleep because of the constant disruption of circadian rhythms. A potential partial solution is less frequent changing of shifts, for example, changing shifts monthly rather than weekly. Such a common-sense approach may result in less significant disturbances of sleep.

Individuals who are intolerant of shifting work schedules may develop chronic fatigue or become disabled, necessitating a change in occupation.

Physical causes of insomnia. Symptoms of disease or the direct effects of disease on sleep-regulating mechanisms can cause sleep disruption. Symptoms known to disrupt sleep significantly include itching, dyspnea, nocturia, diarrhea, angina, and migraine.

Disease states, such as in Parkinson's disease, unpredictable metabolism (e.g., liver disease), or cortical dysfunction (e.g., Alzheimer's disease), may directly disturb sleep because of the alteration of neurotransmitter systems. Other disease processes known to interfere with sleep include obstructive sleep apnea; cardiovascular disorders, especially angina; disorders with breathing impairment; and increased metabolic rate in concert with an endocrinopathy such as mild hyperthyroidism or diabetes. Esophageal reflux, chronic renal failure with uremia, other end organ failure, urinary frequency, fetal movements, and general discomfort women experience in the third trimester of pregnancy may cause diminished quantity and quality of sleep.

Environmental causes of insomnia. Inpatient hospitals or long-term care settings may be buzzing with constant activity and may have enforced sleeping positions, noises, and periodic crises, which hardly encourage adequate sleep. These clinical settings may sometimes actually exceed the Environmental Protection Agency guidelines for healthy noise levels.[10]

DRUGS USED TO TREAT INSOMNIA

Sleep disorders are categorized as insomnia, hypersomnia, or as one of several other sleep disorders. Insomnia and hypersomnia are conceptualized as being either primary (idiopathic) or secondary. Other sleep disorders include narcolepsy, the parasomnias, periodic leg movements (nocturnal myoclonus), and sleep apnea. All of these disorders may respond to pharmacologic intervention (Box 10-2).

Many drugs, including those used to treat insomnia, alter sleep and daytime function. They may mask wakefulness during sleep or diminish alertness during wakefulness. Changes in sleep may remain unnoticed by the individual, and even in the presence of daytime sedation, many patients are unaware of their impaired performances. Thus the effects that many drugs may have on the sleep-wakefulness continuum are clinically relevant. Moreover, many drugs modify REM activity; with the tricyclic antidepressants, this effect may even correlate with a response to therapy.

Transient Nature of Hypnotic Use

The use of hypnotics to relieve insomnia is at best a temporary strategy. All known hypnotics promote sleep and inhibit wakefulness. The effects on sleep and wakefulness should not be separated. Hypnotic drugs shorten the time that elapses before a person falls asleep (sleep latency), reduce nocturnal wakefulness, increase total sleep time, and decrease body movements during sleep. All hypnotics cause difficulty in arousal from sleep. Thus hypnotics are generally viewed as CNS depressants and are specifically viewed as sleep-promoting compounds. The benefit-to-risk ratio of a hypnotic must be considered with the knowledge that the aim of a good night's sleep is to improve the patient's vigor the following day. Rarely has this result been demonstrated as a consequence of the use of hypnotic drugs.

Box 10-2 Sleep Disorders Recognized by the American Sleep Disorders Association

I. Dyssomnias
Intrinsic sleep disorders
Psychophysiologic sleep disorders
Narcolepsy
Hypersomnias
Obstructive sleep apnea
Central nervous system sleep apnea
Periodic limb movement disorder
Restless leg syndrome
Extrinsic sleep disorders
Inadequate sleep hygiene
Environmental sleep disorder
Hypnotic-dependent sleep disorder
Stimulant-dependent sleep disorder
Alcohol-dependent sleep disorder
*Circadian rhythm
sleep disorders*
Jet lag
Work, shift-related
Delayed sleep-phase
Advanced sleep-phase

II. Parasomnias
Arousal disorders
Confusional-arousal disorder
Sleepwalking
Sleep terrors

Sleep-wake transition disorders
Sleep-starts disorder
Sleep-talking disorder
REM sleep-related disorders
Nightmares
Sleep paralysis
REM sleep behavior disorders

III. Psychiatric, Neurologic, and Other Medical Sleep Disorders
Psychiatric
Psychosis
Mood disorders
Anxiety disorders
Panic disorder
Alcoholism
Neurologic
Dementia
Parkinsonism
Epilepsy
Other medical disorders
Proposed sleep disorders
Fragmentary myoclonus
Menstrual-associated sleep
  disorders
Others

Strategies

The most appropriate and important management approaches to insomnia are removal or treatment of underlying causes and identification and alteration of poor sleep habits. Hypnotics, when prescribed, are generally administered in short courses and at low dosages; every-other-night therapy is often recommended. The emergence of nocturnal confusion, agitation, and restlessness, especially in older patients and children, must be assessed carefully. For younger or older patients (discussed in Chapters 20, 21, and 22), the approach includes combining an initial course of pharmacotherapy with nonpharmacologic approaches such as behavioral techniques and optimizing the patient's medical and physiologic status.

A useful approach to insomnia is to consider the duration of the complaint. Long-term insomnia (months or years), short-term insomnia (a week or so), and transient difficulties (periodic bouts of insomnia for 2 to 3 days) require different therapeutic strategies. The duration of the insomnia not only provides an indication of the origin of insomnia but also guides the use of hypnotics. Although hypnotics

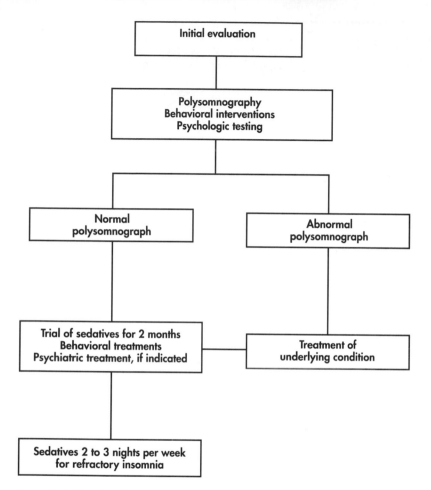

Figure 10-1 Flow chart for the evaluation and treatment of severe insomnia. (From Wooten V: *Psychiatr Ann* 20[8]:466, 1990.)

may be appropriately prescribed for long-term insomnia, a diligent evaluation is necessary before hypnotics are prescribed. As shown in Figure 10-1, drugs are most appropriately prescribed when clear evidence of disturbed sleep occurs without an apparent or direct cause. In contrast to cases involving long-term insomnia, other cases involve healthy individuals who wish to carry out their day-to-day activities free from the residual effects of insomnia. For these individuals, benzodiazepine or newer nonbenzodiazepine hypnotics, and to a lesser extent antidepressant or antihistamine medications, are appropriately prescribed. Other drug classes to be considered include phenothiazines, which may improve sleep in psychotic patients; phenytoin to treat the paroxysmal nightmares associated with psychomotor attacks; beta-adrenergic antagonists to treat disturbed sleep in association with hyperthyroidism; and H_2-receptor blockers or proton pump inhibitors for patients with peptic ulcer disease, nonulcer dyspepsia, or gastroesophageal reflux disorder. Many patients have "pseudoinsomnia"; that is, they complain of poor sleep, but polysomnograph studies are normal. These patients benefit best from no drug intervention.

Neurochemical Effects of Hypnotics

Psychotropics with a significant role in treating sleep disturbances are currently categorized as follows:

1. Neurotransmitter metabolism modifiers, including precursors such as L-tryptophan or levodopa
2. Enzyme inhibitors that affect the synthesis or catabolism of the neurotransmitter
3. Drugs that alter the distribution or utilization of the transmitter, for example, reserpine, alpha-methyldopa, or monoamine oxidase inhibitors (MAOIs)

Treatment is carried out with the recognition that many drugs have distinct or opposite actions on the CNS at different concentrations; that is, complex dose-response relationships exist. For example, some drugs have a stimulatory effect followed by a sedative effect. Feedback mechanisms that operate within the CNS may also be responsible for complex or paradoxic pharmacologic responses.

BENZODIAZEPINES

Considerable attention has been devoted to the pharmacology of the benzodiazepines. As discussed in Chapter 7, these agents modulate gamma-aminobutyric acid (GABA) transmission and interact with specific receptor sites in the brain. As discussed in Chapter 4, GABA is the most abundant inhibitory neurotransmitter in the CNS. Most neurons that release this neurotransmitter, however, are interneurons that modulate activity by presynaptic and postsynaptic inhibition. Many intrinsic neurons found within the dorsal raphe nuclei and their terminals form inhibitory synapses with serotonergic receptor sites or cells. Terminals are also identified within the locus ceruleus, but the cell bodies of origin are unknown. Although GABA inhibits the activity of the locus ceruleus, the exact mode of action is unclear. A minority of neurons, such as Purkinje's cells in the cerebellum or the GABA neurons of the nigrostriatal pathway, project distantly in the brain, probably having complex effects. Moreover, the classic benzodiazepines such as diazepam appear to bind without substantial regional differences. Benzodiazepine-1 receptors, located primarily on postsynaptic membranes, are distinguished from benzodiazepine-2 receptors, which are presynaptic. The anxiolytic and antiepileptic effects are thought to be related to the agonistic effect on benzodiazepine-1 receptors, whereas sedation may result from activation of the benzodiazepine-2 receptors.[16] There are also benzodiazepine omega receptors, which are discussed later.

The classic benzodiazepines used as hypnotics to treat sleep disturbances are outlined in Table 10-1. These include triazolam (Halcion), estazolam (ProSom), temazepam (Restoril), flurazepam (Dalmane), and quazepam (Doral). The chemical structures for selected benzodiazepine and nonbenzodiazepine hypnotics are presented in Figure 10-2.

Pharmacologic Effects

In general, benzodiazepines alter sleep by binding to the benzodiazepine receptor and the GABA receptor-chloride channel molecular complex. The classic benzodiazepines generally shorten sleep latency, reduce the number of awakenings and duration of wakefulness during the night, and increase total sleep time. The latency to REM sleep is prolonged by the benzodiazepines, but this effect may be caused by the suppression of the first episode of REM sleep rather than to a delay in its appearance. Non-REM sleep is changed considerably by the classic benzodiazepines. The duration of stage 1 is reduced, and that of stage 2 is increased. Moreover, EEGs

Table 10-1 Clinical Profile of Selected Hypnotic Drugs

Sedative	Adult dosages (mg)	Onset of effects (hr)	Elimination half-life (hr)	Active metabolite	Comments
Triazolam (Halcion)	0.125-0.5	1-2	1.5-5.5	No	Higher dosages may lead to residual effects and rebound insomnia. Most useful for sleep onset.
Temazepam (Restoril)	15-30	2-3	10-15	Yes	Soft-gel capsule 10-20 mg is free of residual effects; useful for sleep onset.
Flurazepam (Dalmane)	15-30	½-1	3-150*	Yes	Hypnotic effect related to metabolites; residual effect likely with accumulation with continuous use. Useful for nocturnal awakenings when daytime sedation is acceptable.
Zolpidem (Ambien)	5-10	½-1	2.6	No	Free of residual effects. Maintains stages 3 and 4 of sleep.
Oxazepam (Serax)	15-30 (in elderly 10-20)	2-3	5-20	No	Free of residual effects but rather slowly absorbed; used mainly as an anxiolytic but sustains sleep.
Zaleplon (Sonata)	5-10	½-1	1	No	Free of residual effects. Maintains stages 3 and 4 of sleep.

*With active metabolites.

show slowing of electrophysiologic activity, in particular, the emergence of delta waves, k-wave potentials, and theta activities that are less abundant. Perhaps the *most significant* effects of benzodiazepines are their effects on stage 4 (deep) sleep. Benzodiazepines may diminish the release of growth hormone that normally occurs during this stage. Stage 4 disruptions may also decrease REM sleep. Paradoxically, some insomniacs show an increase in REM sleep while others report having nightmares when taking benzodiazepines. After the withdrawal of benzodiazepines, sleep stages 2 and 4 remain altered much longer than do other sleep stages.

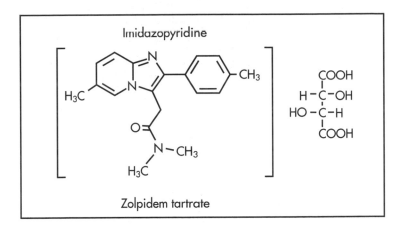

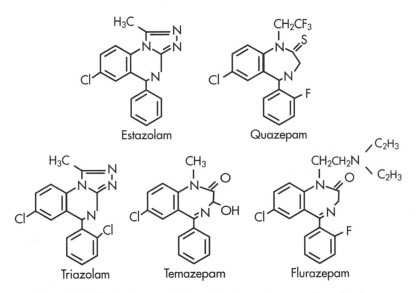

Figure 10-2 Chemical structures for benzodiazepines and newer nonbenzodiazepines.

Clonazepam. The nonclassic benzodiazepine clonazepam may modify sleep less markedly because it has only a few agonistic effects. Clonazepam is particularly useful as a hypnotic because it inhibits REM sleep, but stage 4 sleep is actually enhanced during the night of administration but decreased the following night. Clonazepam may be most beneficial in patients with sleep disturbance superimposed on another condition, for example, neurodegenerative disorders such as Alzheimer's disease or Parkinson's disease or nocturnal myoclonus with periodic leg movement (restless leg syndrome).

Similarities and differences of barbiturates. Although barbiturates may affect the chloride channels differently than the benzodiazepines, the neuropharmacologic effects of both classes of drugs are similar. For example, pentobarbital and phenobarbital exert hypnotic effects in patients by shortening sleep latency and reducing intermittent awakenings during the night. In contrast to benzodiazepines, barbiturates, when given for an extended period, may induce a rebound REM sleep when discontinued. This REM sleep is often accompanied by nightmares. Thus benzodiazepines have distinct advantages in this regard.

Pharmacokinetics

The absorption, metabolism, and elimination of benzodiazepines are nearly identical to each other, but distribution is not. Individual differences are characterized in the latter part of this section.

Absorption. The most important factors governing the choice of benzodiazepines to treat insomnia are the dose, the individual rate of absorption, the distribution (most relevant for single-dose effects), and the elimination half-life (most important in treating chronic insomnia). Sleep induction by means of benzodiazepines depends entirely on the rate of absorption from the gut because benzodiazepines penetrate the blood-brain barrier easily. Most benzodiazepines are rapidly absorbed, but absorption may be slowed by food and antacids. The more rapidly absorbed drugs have a faster onset of action, whereas those that are slowly absorbed may not have a desired effect at all. Of the currently marketed hypnotics, flurazepam is the most rapidly absorbed, followed by triazolam, which has an intermediate absorption rate, and temazepam, with a slow absorption rate. Thus the time at which the medication is given to the patient before he or she retires is very important.[14] Obviously, a drug with a slow absorption rate (e.g., oxazepam) may be most appropriate for treating anxiety when a sustained effect with minimal initial drowsiness is sought. Once absorbed, a hypnotic is distributed to the blood and to the highly vascular tissues, that is, the brain, heart, liver, and lungs, and then distributed peripherally to less vascular tissues. This rapid distribution results in an initial rise in the plasma concentration, but the subsequent fall in concentrations results mainly from elimination by metabolism and excretion. The absorption rate after intramuscular injection of many benzodiazepines, with the possible exception of lorazepam, is slower than with oral administration.

Distribution and accumulation. The duration of clinical action of benzodiazepines in single doses depends on distribution, whereas accumulation becomes important with multiple doses. This means that absorption rates and distribution to the CNS are mostly responsible for a single-dose effect. A long half-life does not necessarily imply a long duration of sedation, nor does a short half-life imply a short duration of action for a hypnotic. Accumulation of course is determined by metabolic clearance and elimination half-life.

Distribution versus elimination. Because a particular pharmacodynamic effect is related to a specific plasma concentration, knowledge of distribution versus elimination half-life can be of great clinical utility. The duration of activity is short when the plasma level is within the phase that predominantly represents distribution but longer when the plasma level is within the elimination phase. In other words, *plasma concentration decay* occurs more rapidly during the distribution phase than during the elimination phase. Thus both distribution and elimination influence duration of activity, that is, half-life. In practical terms, this means that a relatively short duration of action may be expected when giving a single dose of a hypnotic that is not rapidly eliminated but is rapidly distributed. Thus although half-life is a familiar concept and often touted as the most important feature of benzodiazepines, it does have limitations in defining the duration of activity of a single dose.

Metabolism. Benzodiazepine metabolism occurs primarily in two ways: conjugation (combining with glucuronic acid and becoming inert) and oxidation (via the hepatic microsomal enzyme system). Furthermore, most benzodiazepines are initially metabolized by conjugation, with their active metabolites then undergoing oxidation. Some short-acting benzodiazepine derivatives, for example, oxazepam and lorazepam, are almost completely inactivated by one-step conjugation in the liver and have few residual morning-after effects. Indeed, benzodiazepines eliminated as rapidly as these may even result in early-morning insomnia, whereas other benzodiazepines, for example, flurazepam (which initially undergoes conjugation), may produce persistent long-acting metabolites (which eventually undergo oxidation) that cause a lingering impairment in alertness, motor performance, and cognitive functioning. Benzodiazepine metabolism is largely age dependent; the elimination half-life of diazepam, for instance, may increase threefold to fourfold in persons 20 versus 80 years of age because of declining oxidative capabilities (age-related hepatic changes), thus increasing the bioavailability of the drug (see Table 10-1).

Benzodiazepines transformed in the liver by attachment of the benzodiazepine molecule to glucuronic acid (conjugation) are then excreted in the urine as pharmacologically inactive metabolites. However, some benzodiazepines form active metabolites, which complicates their pharmacologic properties. In addition, if the hepatic-detoxification system is compromised, as in viral hepatitis, benzodiazepine activity is prolonged, and the potential exists for physical complications.

Metabolic basis for categorizing benzodiazepines. Benzodiazepines are characterized on the basis of elimination half-life. Triazolam is the most rapidly excreted hypnotic, with an elimination half-life of 1.5 to 5.5 hours. Oxazepam has an elimination half-life of 5 to 20 hours, and the half-lives of lorazepam, temazepam, alprazolam, and chlordiazepoxide are between 10 and 30 hours and generally longer in geriatric patients. Triazolam may be useful when next-day sedation has occurred, but in some patients, rapid washout may provoke rebound insomnia, next-day anxiety, and anterograde amnesia.[11] Lorazepam also has a propensity for anterograde amnestic effects. The lack of active metabolites may make oxazepam preferable in patients with liver disease or other conditions in which liver function may be compromised.

Elimination versus distribution. As noted, the influence of distribution on plasma concentration decay is important. Although using the elimination half-life alone to predict duration of action is taught in most pharmacology courses, this guideline is misleading.[21] However, *with repeated ingestion*, the elimination half-life again becomes useful as a concept for predicting the rate and extent of metabolic accumulation. Furthermore, the prescriber must recognize that slow elimination of a parent compound or an active metabolite is most disadvantageous when drugs are being used nightly. To show how this information can be translated into clinical usefulness, the compound temazepam is used as an example. Temazepam has a distribution phase similar to that of its parent compound, diazepam, but it has an elimination half-life of only 8 hours and has insignificant amounts of other metabolites. Thus residual sequelae with temazepam are unlikely unless inappropriately high dosages are prescribed.

Clinical decision making based on pharmacokinetics. Benzodiazepines and the nonbenzodiazepine agents zolpidem and zaleplon (discussed later) are preferred as hypnotics because of their safety and lower potential for overdose. The more lipid-soluble agents readily enter the CNS. For instance, flurazepam enters within 10 minutes, whereas oxazepam enters within 18 to 35 minutes. Slowly excreted drugs with relatively long half-lives (e.g., flurazepam) may promote ease of sleep onset and reduce prolonged anxiety the following day. Long-acting agents are also less likely to provoke untoward reactions on abrupt withdrawal. On the other hand, long-acting benzodiazepines induce next-day levels of subjective sleepiness and may result in hangover effects. In short, the difference between the slowly and the rapidly excreted benzodiazepines provides a precarious guide for the individual patient, given large differences in tolerance and sensitivity.

The next-day performance and any side effects of a hypnotic agent are more often influenced by the dose of the drug than by its elimination half-life. Pulling together the variables mentioned is challenging, but based on these observations, one could surmise the following:

1. A first-choice drug for sleep-onset insomnia is triazolam.
2. A first-choice drug for sleep-maintenance insomnia is temazepam.
3. A first-choice drug for early-morning awakening is flurazepam, which induces sleep of long duration.

Patient implications. That persons with insomnia represent a heterogeneous group is implicit in this discussion. Thus selection of a drug, the prediction of its effects, and the long-range treatment of most types of insomnia must allow for drug variability among patients. The hazards of well-monitored treatment with hypnotic drugs are small, although true physiologic addiction nonetheless may occur. Persons who may be advised not to take hypnotic agents include pregnant women, alcoholics, those who must arise and function in the middle of the night, and those with symptomatic sleep apnea.

Side Effects

Benzodiazepines used as hypnotics are unlikely to have severe adverse effects. The most common side effects of benzodiazepines are related to mental alertness. The patient must be advised to be careful about driving or operating hazardous machinery. Fortunately, tolerance to most side effects quickly develops. The blood pressures of inpatients must be monitored routinely; a drop in pressure of 20 mm Hg (systolic) on standing warrants withholding the drug and notifying the prescriber.

As noted in Chapter 7, unnecessarily high dosages and unnecessarily long treatment periods are the main problems associated with benzodiazepine use. These problems often result in adverse effects, undoubtedly because of misuse. Impaired performance, anterograde amnesia, and other adverse effects of hypnotics are potentially troublesome.

A number of the adverse effects associated with benzodiazepines are discussed in Chapter 7. Also, insomnia on cessation of treatment may arise when rebound phenomena emerge, in particular, when short-acting drugs are withdrawn suddenly. Rebound insomnia occurs most often when a relatively large dose of a rapidly eliminated drug is prescribed and used nightly. Rebound insomnia is not observed when benzodiazepine sedatives are used in appropriate doses for a limited time. The potential for dependence is minimized by the intermittent use of low dosages, limited duration of ingestion, or gradual withdrawal when continuous treatment has been given for longer than a month.

Implications

Therapeutic versus toxic levels. Therapeutic levels of benzodiazepines have comfortable margins of safety compared with other sedative-hypnotic class agents. However, overdoses when taken with alcohol have led to death, and many deliberate overdoses seem to involve alcohol. Thus it is difficult to assess or determine what supply of benzodiazepines would be considered safe. The continued use of benzodiazepines for more than several weeks should be applied in the context of the critical appraisal of risks and benefits in individual cases. The near-total replacement of the 50 or more previously available barbiturates by the benzodiazepines has resulted in a lower incidence of toxicity and a similar but not superior hypnotic effect. These agents cause less respiratory and cardiac depression than do the barbiturates, although overdosage clearly results in respiratory depression. Tolerance of benzodiazepines, in contrast to the barbiturates, is less marked and is never complete.

Use in pregnancy. The safety of benzodiazepines use during pregnancy has not been established, and animal studies suggest that these drugs are not free of hazard. Prolonged administration of benzodiazepines at either low or high dosages in the last trimester of pregnancy is reported to produce arrhythmias, hypertonia, poor sucking, and hypothermia in neonates. Benzodiazepines cross the placenta and enter breast milk. Thus ingestion during pregnancy and lactation should be avoided.

Use in the elderly. Older adults are known to rely on sleeping pills much more often than do younger adults.[9] However, the metabolism and elimination of CNS depressant drugs (discussed in detail in Chapter 21) is decreased in many older adults with low renal glomerular filtration rates, possibly in those with reduced hepatic blood flow, and in those with decreased activity of hepatic drug-metabolizing enzymes. In general, starting dosages are initially cut in half, and daytime alertness is monitored to detect serious impairment. Ideally, a short-acting benzodiazepine or preferably nonbenzodiazepine given at a lower dosage is best prescribed. On the other hand, some older patients may respond poorly to short-acting drugs and may prefer longer-acting agents because of the potential to reduce generalized daytime anxiety. The overall choice for young and old alike depends on individual clinical features.

Interactions. Discussions of drug interactions with benzodiazepines found in Chapter 7 are relevant to those prescribed as hypnotics. The sedative effect of benzodiazepines is of course increased in combination with antipsychotics, sedating antidepressants, other hypnotics, analgesics, anesthetics, and alcohol. In healthy young adults, small doses of temazepam and moderate doses of alcohol may produce no significant additive effect and may not necessarily prolong the effects of benzodiazepines. They clearly do in elderly patients or in those who indeed have alcohol dependence. Antacids and anticholinergic drugs may decrease the absorption of benzodiazepines; cimetidine slows their metabolism to a minor degree. For other interactions, see Chapter 7.

Patient education. Benzodiazepines have great potential for abuse. Consequently, patients and families need education about the following points:
1. Benzodiazepines prescribed for insomnia should be taken as directed.
2. Over-the-counter drugs may potentiate the actions of benzodiazepines.
3. Driving should be avoided until tolerance develops.
4. Alcohol and other CNS depressants potentiate the effects of benzodiazepines.

5. Hypersensitivity to one benzodiazepine may indicate hypersensitivity to another.
6. Benzodiazepine treatment should not be stopped abruptly.

Specific Benzodiazepine Hypnotics

The choice of an individual hypnotic may depend on the drug's potential to do the following:
1. Shorten sleep onset when there is difficulty falling asleep
2. Reduce nocturnal wakefulness
3. Provide an anxiolytic effect the next day

The clinical profiles of selected compounds are provided in Table 10-1. Three specific compounds, designated short-acting (triazolam), intermediate-acting (temazepam), and long-acting (flurazepam), are discussed in detail.

Short-acting benzodiazepines: prototype drug, triazolam. Triazolam is metabolized principally by hepatic microsomal oxidation. Hepatic clearance occurs at a high rate, depending on blood flow in the liver and activity of hepatic microsomal enzymes. Significant drug interaction (as discussed in Chapter 6) occurs with nefazodone (Serzone), which inhibits these enzymes. Essentially, the dosage of triazolam should be reduced by 50% to 75% when coadministered with nefazodone. Triazolam is rapidly eliminated after the administration of single doses and does not accumulate. Advantages and disadvantages may occur as a consequence of the following properties:

- *Advantages:* The rapid elimination results in no hangover effect.
- *Disadvantages:* (1) The very short-acting agents compound early-morning rebound insomnia, and anxiety may occur; (2) the complete disappearance of triazolam and its metabolites from the blood within a day of discontinuing long-term treatment may result in severe rebound symptoms of drug withdrawal; and (3) abrupt withdrawal may cause confusion, toxic psychosis, convulsions, or a condition resembling delirium tremor including sweating and diarrhea.

Long-term treatment should therefore be stopped slowly.

Intermediate-acting benzodiazepines: prototype drug, temazepam. Among the hypnotics available in alternative formulations with differential rates of absorption is temazepam. This drug is available as a soft gelatin capsule and has a mean peak plasma concentration time of approximately 1 hour. In contrast, the typical hard gelatin capsule is absorbed relatively slowly and has a delay of approximately 2 hours. With temazepam, the major metabolite is an inert conjugate. Thus this compound has virtually no active metabolites to prolong its effect.

Because temazepam is metabolized by conjugation rather than by oxidation, its metabolic pathway is less likely to be influenced by factors such as age. Although this knowledge may imply a clinical advantage for temazepam over flurazepam or triazolam among older adults, such an advantage has not been clearly established. The effects of temazepam are thought to be restricted to the night of ingestion as a result of its relatively short half-life. However, with a mean half-life of 13 to 14 hours in some individuals, this drug should be characterized as an intermediate-acting benzodiazepine. Large doses may cause hangover effects.

Long-acting benzodiazepines: prototype drug, flurazepam. Flurazepam produces a complex mixture of short-acting and long-acting metabolites on repeated dosing. Steady-state levels are reached 2 to 3 weeks after ingestion. An accumulation may cause impairment of waking performance. Single doses generally cause a full night's sleep, with little residual impairment, and the 30-mg dose may result in an anxiolytic effect throughout the day.

NONBENZODIAZEPINE HYPNOTICS: ZOLPIDEM AND ZALEPLON

Zolpidem (Ambien) and zaleplon (Sonata) are new-generation nonbenzodiazepine hypnotics. Zolpidem of the imidazopyridine class has a unique mechanism of action, modulating the $GABA_A$ receptor chloride channel complex. This results in sedative, anxiolytic, anticonvulsant, and myorelaxant properties. The major effect occurs on the alpha subunit of the $GABA_A$ receptor complex, referred to as the *benzodiazepine omega receptor,* that is, the benzodiazepine-GABA receptor complex. Thus this agent shares some properties with the benzodiazepines.

The pharmacologic profile of zolpidem is characterized by rapid absorption and elimination, with an ultrashort half-life (see Table 10-1). Zolpidem has no active metabolites and is unlikely to accumulate during short-term use (i.e., several weeks). Daytime drowsiness or residual effects are minimal or lacking, and rebound effects (e.g., cognitive effects), as described with many benzodiazepine agents, do not occur. Zolpidem has been shown to have little unfavorable effect on stage 3 or 4 sleep or REM sleep; that is, the integrity of sleep and sleep architecture are maintained.[20] Zolpidem reduces time to sleep onset, increases total sleep time, and decreases the number of awakenings during the sleep period. The drug appears to be effective in transient, short-term, and chronic insomnia.

Zaleplon, approved by the U.S. Food and Drug Administration in 1999, shows great promise in the treatment of insomnia (Figure 10-3). Zaleplon is a nonbenzodiazepine hypnotic from the pyrazolopyrmidine class. This medication affects the brain similarly to zolpidem and also represents less risk of tolerance and dependence than benzodiazepines. Studies have demonstrated that zaleplon enables patients with insomnia to fall asleep quickly without producing many of the morning-after side effects associated with other hypnotic medications.

A 5- or 10-mg dose of both zolpidem and zaleplon results in significant effects on the median time to sleep onset compared with placebo. Compared with the benzodiazepines, zolpidem has a superior adverse effect profile with less residual sedation. Zaleplon's adverse effect profile is similar to that of zolpidem, but zaleplon

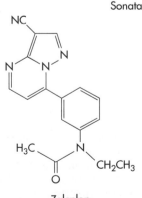

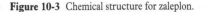

Figure 10-3 Chemical structure for zaleplon.

has no residual sedation, no tolerance, minimal rebound insomnia, and no resultant functional impairment. Generally, zaleplon has demonstrated a slightly lesser effect on the nervous system than zolpidem. For example, rebound insomnia occurs more often in elderly outpatients receiving zolpidem 5 mg (19%) in comparison to placebo (6.8%), zaleplon 5 mg (8.4%), or zaleplon 10 mg (8.8%).[6] Common side effects include drowsiness, dizziness, headache, and gastrointestinal upset, occurring in a small percentage of cases. Significant drug interactions do not occur except with alcohol, which potentiates the effect of zaleplon (and zolpidem).

Switching a patient from a benzodiazepine hypnotic to a nonbenzodiazepine hypnotic may carry the risk of rebound or symptoms of abrupt withdrawal, especially if continuous benzodiazepine therapy has occurred at higher dosages. Therefore the benzodiazepine should be withdrawn gradually, perhaps over 1 to 2 weeks. After a washout of 2 to 3 days, especially for benzodiazepines with longer half-lives, zolpidem or zaleplon may then be started at 10 mg for adults or 5 mg for older patients or patients with hepatic dysfunction.

Treatment Considerations

Hypnotics are sometimes introduced at unnecessarily high dosages because dose-ranging studies have occurred in patients with chronic insomnia. Such studies may provide information relevant to the use of hypnotics to treat chronic insomnia but are not relevant for treating "normal" insomnia. A further trend toward higher dosing is encouraged when an immediate first-night effect is sought and when high dosages of ultrarapidly eliminated drugs are prescribed for treating difficulties in sustaining sleep. Such philosophies and approaches initially resulted in significant problems with triazolam, resulting in the 0.5-mg tablet being withdrawn from the U.S. market and guidelines for short-term use (up to 21 days) being established. This agent has been totally withdrawn from some European countries because of safety concerns.

Dosage Strategies

When prescribing any of the hypnotics shown in Figure 10-1, the clinician should strive to use the lowest effective dosage by choosing the compound with the most suitable pharmacologic profile.

The *ideal dosage* preserves normal sleep architecture to the extent possible during ingestion and after withdrawal. The *ideal pharmacokinetic profile* should (1) meet the clinical requirement to shorten sleep onset, (2) reduce nocturnal wakefulness, or (3) provide the anxiolytic effect required during the next day. In every case, the goal is to be as free as possible from untoward effects on daytime functioning. The appropriate use of any hypnotic must depend more on whether the profile solves the clinical problems just mentioned and depend less on the particular individual characteristics of the hypnotic.

Effects on Electroencephalograms

A significant concern in patients evaluated for primary sleep disorder may be the effects of benzodiazepines on sleep physiology. As mentioned earlier, these compounds may cause striking electroencephalographic changes during sleep. An overall decrease in the number of sleep-stage shifts throughout the night may occur. In addition, alterations in normal sleep patterns may occur and may be manifested differently in different individuals. Clearly, benzodiazepines decrease non-REM sleep stages 1, 3, and 4 and increase sleep stage 2, increasing the latency to REM (stage 5) sleep and diminishing REM sleep for the most part. These effects are similar to but less marked than those of the barbiturates. The effects of zolpidem and zaleplon are less significant. REM episodes or bursts in REM latency may have considerable inherent variability in response to benzodiazepines or may be erratic, with either a decrease or an increase in latency during chronic treatment. REM rebound during drug withdrawal tends to be dose related and most obvious after discontinuance of high dosages of benzodiazepines.

Benzodiazepine Withdrawal

A discussion of withdrawal from regimens of benzodiazepines and other similar sedative hypnotic agents can be found in Chapter 7. Indeed, withdrawal of hypnotics after long-term use usually leads to resurfacing of the original symptoms, difficulties in sleeping, and anxiety. Although rebound insomnia may occur with the benzodiazepines, the frequency and severity vary. Withdrawal symptoms are minimized by tapering rather than stopping treatment abruptly, and tapering is strongly advised with drugs that are short acting; also, beta-adrenergic blocking drugs or clonidine may be useful to reduce rebound or withdrawal in difficult cases. Undesirable side effects such as impaired memory, anxiety, confusion, depersonalization, and hallucinations may be more related to the direct effect of the drug than to withdrawal itself.

Dependence

Dependence on the newer benzodiazepine and nonbenzodiazepine hypnotics has not proven to be a major clinical problem, although frequent review is prudent. Zolpidem and zaleplon have been reported to have much lower abuse liability when compared with the benzodiazepine hypnotic triazolam.[6,8] Dependence and addiction are more likely to occur in patients with coexisting psychiatric disturbances or histories of addictive disorders or in patients with personality or somatoform disorders.

OTHER DRUGS USED TO TREAT INSOMNIA
Antidepressants

Many conventional antidepressants are prescribed to enhance sleep because of their sedating properties. The sedative effects and half-lives of antidepressants are profiled in Table 10-2. Antidepressants commonly prescribed to enhance sleep include trazodone (Desyrel), nefazodone (Serzone), mirtazapine (Remeron), amitriptyline (Elavil), trimipramine (Surmontil), and doxepin (Sinequan). Although these antidepressant compounds are not specifically indicated for treating insomnia, they are often prescribed for that purpose, especially with coexisting depression or anxiety.

Hypnotics

Chloral hydrate, the first hypnotic, was developed in 1868 and is still useful today (Table 10-3). Chloral hydrate in doses of 0.5 to 1 g is widely used and has a rapid onset of action. Chloral hydrate is cross-tolerant with alcohol, is inexpensive, and is available in syrup form for those who have difficulty swallowing pills. Ethchlorvynol (Placidyl) is another hypnotic; compared with chloral hydrate, ethchlorvynol peaks later and is more slowly excreted. Glutethimide (Doriden) has a rapid onset of action, rapid metabolism, high mortality with overdosage, and great potential for abuse.

Table 10-2 Antidepressant Sedative Effect and Elimination Half-Life

Agent	Sedative effect	Half-life (hr)
Trazodone (Desyrel)	+++	4-9
Amitriptyline (Elavil)	+++	31-46
Doxepin (Adapin, Sinequan)	+++	8-24 (51)*
Maprotiline (Ludiomil)	++	21-25
Imipramine (Tofranil)	++	11-25
Nortriptyline (Aventyl, Pamelor)	++	18-44
Amoxapine (Asendin)	+	8-30
Protriptyline (Vivactil)	+	67-89
Desipramine (Norpramin)	+	12-24
Sertraline (Zoloft)	None to +	26-98†
Fluoxetine (Prozac)	None	48-216
Fluvoxamine (Luvox)	None to +	15-19
Paroxetine (Paxil)	None to +	21
Venlafaxine (Effexor)	+	3-11†
Nefazodone (Serzone)	+ to ++	2-4
Mirtazapine (Remeron)	+++	35

+++, Marked; ++, moderate; +, mild.

*Active metabolite, desmethyldoxepin, has a longer life than parent compound (51 hours ± 17 hours).

†Includes active metabolite.

Diphenhydramine and L-Tryptophan

Among the over-the-counter agents, diphenhydramine (Benadryl), a histamine blocker, possesses a mild sedative effect and is commonly prescribed to enhance sleep.[11] L-tryptophan, withdrawn from the U.S. market, exerts mild sedative properties at high dosages and is an amino acid precursor to CNS serotonin production. L-tryptophan has no significant side effects and results in maximum benefit at doses of approximately 2 to 3 g.

Melatonin

Melatonin has received much attention as an over-the-counter sleep aid. Changes in the melatonin secretion cycle area may be associated with sleep disturbances in older individuals. Melatonin is produced and secreted by the pineal gland at night and has a role in the regulation of the sleep-wake cycle. Among sleep-disturbed patients— even those who are generally healthy—the frequency of sleep disturbance is strongly associated with changes in the melatonin cycle.

The therapeutic effects of melatonin replacement therapy in melatonin-deficient patients with insomnia have been discussed by Haimov and others.[15] This report indicates that melatonin doses of 1 to 3 mg administered in a sustained-release or fast-release formulation improved initiation and maintenance of sleep. Sustained-release melatonin in doses of 2 or 3 mg may be especially effective for sleep maintenance, whereas fast-release melatonin primarily improves the initiation of sleep. A study by Garfinkel found treatment with nightly doses of 2 mg of controlled-release melatonin significantly improved sleep efficiency.[13] Objective measures

Table 10-3 Other Sedatives (Forerunners of Benzodiazepine Sedatives)

Generic name	Trade name	Comments
Alcohols, Aldehydes, and Propanediols		
Ethanol	Generic	Not recommended*
Ethchlorvynol	Placidyl	Not recommended*
Chloral hydrate	Generic	1-2 g to induce sleep
Paraldehyde	Generic	Not recommended*
Meprobamate	Equanil, Miltown, generic	Not recommended*
Tybamate	Tybatran, Solacen, generic	Not recommended*
Barbiturates		
Amobarbital	Amytal, generic	Administer 100-800 mg/hr intravenously in diagnosis or parenterally for emergency sedation
Methohexital	Brevital	Administer 10 mg/5 sec intravenously (average dose = 70 mg) for electroconvulsive therapy only
Pentobarbital	Nembutal, generic	Can be used for treatment of withdrawal from most sedative addictions†‡
Phenobarbital	Luminal, generic	30-90 mg/day†‡
Secobarbital	Seconal, generic	Not recommended†
Structural Relatives of Barbiturates (Nonbarbiturates)		
Glutethimide	Doriden	Not recommended*
Methyprylon	Noludar	Not recommended*
Methaqualone	Quaalude, generic	Not recommended*
Antihistamines		
Diphenhydramine	Benadryl	25-50 mg§
Hydroxyzine	Atarax, Vistaril	Not recommended*
Promethazine	Phenergan, generic	Not recommended*

Modified from reference 4.
*These agents are not recommended for routine use as sedatives.
†Short-acting barbiturates, although not generally recommended, are sometimes used to induce sleep because of their low cost; phenobarbital is an inexpensive sedative that is not often abused.
‡Pentobarbital and phenobarbital are often used to treat addiction to sedative-hypnotic drugs.
§Diphenhydramine and other antihistamines are sometimes used as sedatives in pediatric practice. These are not recommended for use in elderly individuals.

showed improvement in sleep parameters as early as 1 to 3 weeks after the onset of melatonin therapy. Sleep latency was decreased, although not significantly, and total sleep time was improved substantially. The only adverse effect in this study was pruritus, which resolved spontaneously.

Generally, the efficacy of melatonin has not been demonstrated among patients who are not melatonin deficient. Tolerance to melatonin does not develop, and sleep quality may deteriorate with the cessation of melatonin treatment. Benzodiazepines may suppress endogenous melatonin production. Thus melatonin replacement therapy may improve the sleep in older individuals who have received long-term treatment with benzodiazepines.[10] Melatonin may also augment the effect of benzodiazepines or enable dosage reduction or discontinuation of a benzodiazepine sedative-hypnotic, while maintaining good sleep quality with no apparent rebound insomnia.[12] Apart from a direct hypnotic effect, exogenous melatonin can affect sleep through its phase-resetting action on the biologic cycle. Evening melatonin administration may favorably affect the timing of sleep onset, may improve patients with advance sleep-phase syndrome, and has been reported to entrain sleep to day-night cycles in individuals with blindness.[10]

Presently, no melatonin formulation has gained approval from any regulatory authority. Clinical trials are needed to determine recommended dosages, timing, and duration of melatonin use and safety. Studies in animals have noted that melatonin may constrict coronary and cerebral arteries, which could place older patients taking melatonin at risk for heart attacks and strokes.[18] Possible drug-drug interactions with melatonin include conjugated estrogens. Because of a lack of sufficient data on melatonin's efficacy, safety, dose-response relationships, interactions, and purity, caution is advised for long-term use. For those who do use melatonin regularly, careful monitoring for adverse effects is advisable.

DISCUSSION

The pharmacotherapy of insomnia often occurs in the context of other pathophysiologic disturbances or psychiatric disorders. Hypnotics are useful when used in the absence of these conditions or as an adjunct treatment while patients are receiving behavioral therapy. Daytime residual effects, special problems of elderly patients, interactions with alcohol dependence, and effects on respiratory drive are just a few of the treatment issues associated with hypnotic agents; a full discussion of these is beyond the scope of this chapter.

Most prescriptions for hypnotics are written for 30 days or less. The vast majority of individuals with insomnia are not prescribed hypnotic medication; on the other hand, a significant portion of individuals with chronic insomnia self-medicate. Obviously, disparities exist in the pattern of hypnotic medication prescription, including the disproportionately high rate of prescription among geriatric patients. Older sedative hypnotic class agents, including barbiturates, chloral hydrate, methaqualone, and meprobamate, are discussed in Chapter 7. Other agents, such as antihistamines and heterocyclic antidepressants, prescribed because of their sedating effects, are compared with the benzodiazepines in Chapter 7. Generally, the older group of sedative hypnotic agents, with the exception of chloral hydrate, is not recommended. Ironically, some states require the triplicate form of prescription for benzodiazepines, which has discouraged their use and has resulted in an increase in the prescription of older sedative-hypnotic agents such as meprobamate and barbiturates for hypnotic and anxiolytic use.

Many so-called natural sleep aids and over-the-counter agents are ultimately quite harmful to patients, whereas benzodiazepines and nonbenzodiazepine hypnotics (zolpidem and zaleplon) are remarkably nontoxic and safe. The majority of drug-related suicide attempts involve the combination of several agents, including newer hypnotics combined with alcohol. Despite the overall safety and efficacy of the benzodiazepines and newer nonbenzodiazepine hypnotics, they may also produce unwanted effects in the elderly (see Chapter 21). Long-acting agents may result in daytime impairment, and ultrashort-acting agents may be associated with rebound insomnia and innocent dose escalating. Triazolam once received much attention in the popular press because of its alleged profile of severe side effects. However, data are conflicting, and *no data exist* regarding its ability to produce daytime anxiety or possible disinhibition resulting in rage, psychosis, or amnesia. For example, a 20% incidence of anterograde amnesia is associated with triazolam, but approximately 45% of untreated patients with insomnia also have memory problems, so it is difficult to determine the clinical significance of triazolam's effect on memory.[19]

NONPHARMACOLOGIC TREATMENT STRATEGIES FOR INSOMNIA

The use of behavioral techniques, including progressive relaxation, biofeedback, cognitive approaches, stimulus control instructions, sleep restriction therapy, and other attempts to normalize the sleep-wake cycle, are effective and ideally combined with a pharmacologic treatment for insomnia. In many cases, simply educating an individual about better sleep hygiene may produce significant benefit. For others, behavioral interventions may be necessary to return the individual to a normal sleeping pattern.

Sleep Hygiene Education

Many persons with difficulty sleeping can alleviate the problem by making some adjustments to their daily habits. Maintenance of a regular sleep schedule is advised; this includes awakening at the same time every day rather than sleeping late on weekends or after a late night. Proper sleep hygiene may also be maintained by physical and mental activity during the day and by exposure to bright sunlight or artificial bright light of 2000 to 3000 lux (an ordinary fluorescent light bulb is equivalent to 1000 lux). The sleeping environment needs to be adequately dark and quiet. Patients may be counseled to do something they find relaxing just before bedtime. Eating a light snack before bed may be helpful, but alcohol and caffeine must be avoided, even as much as several hours (up to 12 hours for caffeine) before bedtime. Finally, if patients experience anxiety about their sleeplessness, it may be useful for them to remove the clock from their bedroom so that they do not stare at it all night.

Relaxation. Relaxation training may be an effective intervention for those who are anxious as bedtime approaches. Some elderly persons experience this anxiety, although they may have nothing scheduled the next day. Biofeedback, abdominal breathing, and progressive muscle relaxation are potentially effective interventions. Patients require instruction in these methods, and they must be advised to practice and perfect their techniques before using these strategies at bedtime.

Stimulus control. Stimulus control instruction may be especially useful to patients who present with a shift in the sleep-wake cycle (Box 10-3). Stimulus control therapy instructions, which encourage the individual to lie down with the intention of going to sleep only when drowsy, may be more effective than prescribed hypnotics. In addition, individuals are encouraged not to use the bed for purposes other than sleep or sexual activity. Going to another room and later returning to bed to sleep, if unable to fall asleep, may be a potent intervention. Setting the alarm for the same time each morning, regardless of how much sleep is achieved the night before, and avoiding daytime napping are the other crucial factors among those listed in Box 10-3.

Box 10-3 Stimulus Control Therapy*

Retire only when sleepy.

Use bed and bedroom only for sleep (and sexual activity).

Go to another room if unable to sleep and return to bed only when
 sleepy.

Set alarm at same hour each day, irrespective of amount of sleep attained.

Avoid daytime napping.

Adhere to sleep hygiene guidelines.

Modified from Mendelson WB: *Human sleep*, New York, 1987, Plenum; and Wooten V:
Psychiatr Ann 20(8):466, 1990.

*Method may be repeated as often as needed, and therapy may be continued indefinitely.

Sleep restriction therapy. Sleep restriction therapy attempts to consolidate a patient's fragmented sleep. If a sleep log demonstrates, for example, that an individual is spending 10 hours in bed throughout the day, only 5 of which are actually spent asleep, the patient is instructed to spend only 5 hours in bed. The goal is to increase sleep efficiency by forcing sleep to occur during a defined period. This is accomplished by diminishing the opportunity for the patient to sleep at other, nondesired times. After a few days of decreased time spent in bed, patients generally begin to spend more of that limited time asleep. When sleep begins to occur for more than 85% of that time, an extra 15 minutes can be added to their time spent in bed by having them retire earlier. After a few weeks, many patients reach the point where they are in bed for 7 hours and asleep for more than 90% of that time.

Treating Refractory Insomnia

The sleep laboratory is a useful tool in the assessment of refractory cases; unsuspected findings of a general medical nature, such as paroxysmal nocturnal dystonias or sleep apnea, may be revealed in as many as 50% of cases.[10] The initial approach outlined in the opening sections of this chapter, combined with accurate history, sleep hygiene instruction, and judicious prescription of appropriate hypnotic agents, generally leads to successful patient outcome.

OTHER SLEEP DISORDERS
HYPERSOMNIA AND EXCESSIVE SLEEPINESS

Hypersomnia is a persistent need for excessive sleep. Any disease or drug state affecting the sleep-wake cycle may be responsible. Sleepiness resulting from neurologic, endocrinologic, or psychiatric problems may be accompanied by other stigmas of disease. Sleepiness is typically provoked by prolonged monotony such as watching television or attending meetings. Driving for long distances, particularly on interstate highways, may be a culprit. In this section, primary idiopathic hypersomnia is discussed; the therapeutic goal may simply be to ensure that persistent hypersomnia is assessed and addressed through a careful evaluation in a sleep physiology laboratory. Table 10-4 distinguishes some of the other pertinent clinical characteristics of insomnia, idiopathic hypersomnia, narcolepsy, and other disorders that may be characterized by excessive daytime sleepiness.

Idiopathic Hypersomnia

Idiopathic hypersomnia involves prolonged nocturnal sleep that is normal on polygraphic study with continuous daytime drowsiness. It commonly develops in young adults who poorly tolerate late-night activities. The onset of hypersomnia may be difficult to identify; a change of work requirement or social obligation may precipitate a complaint in an individual who had previously coped with an abnormally increased need for sleep. These individuals often manifest "sleep drunkenness," a period of incapacitating drowsiness on first awakening, sometimes lasting for more than an hour. These individuals often take naps, usually prolonged, unlike the shorter naps of individuals with narcolepsy. Sleep requirements often impede fulfilling daytime obligations. Family history of hypersomnia is often present, and hypersomnia may be complicated by depression or impaired daytime concentration.

The pharmacologic approach to idiopathic hypersomnia involves combining a systematic scheduling of sleep, a prescription of stimulants (discussed in Chapter 16), and the use of a sleep diary with a rigid sleep practice that includes sleep hygiene. Napping is scheduled according to social demands. Stimulants are used primarily as adjuncts in a systematic fashion and are generally prescribed to maintain rather than to restore wakefulness. Two to six 18.75-mg tablets of pemoline, a long-acting stimulant, are prescribed, to be taken in divided doses in the morning. Amphetamines, including dextroamphetamine, and methylphenidate have a short duration of action and are taken in periodic divided doses on arising and before arising for sleep drunkenness (see Chapter 16). Occasionally, heterocyclic antidepressants such as protriptyline; activating selective serotonin reuptake inhibitors such as fluoxetine; bupropion (Wellbutrin); or MAOIs, especially tranylcypromine (Parnate); are used, with modest clinical response. The selective norepinephrine reuptake inhibitors (SNRIs) (reboxetine and tomoxetene), *not yet available,* may have some benefit as well. SNRIs are in the late stages of development for other conditions, that is, depression and attention deficit disorder.

Sleep Apnea

Sleep apnea is a generic term for breathing disorders that occur during sleep. The clinical picture is often of an obese, middle-aged or older man who smokes, uses large amounts of caffeine, and/or drinks alcohol frequently. Mild hypertension or cardiac arrhythmias may be present. The cardinal symptom is snoring. However, this may be absent when CNS sleep apnea or dysregulation of breathing is present, rather than upper airway obstructive mechanisms. Daytime sleepiness may be mild or may be quite noticeable to others or to the patient. It is common for individuals with sleep apnea to be asymptomatic or to have a tendency to deny that their sleep-related problems exist.

Although antidepressant medications may be useful and indicated in cases of sleep apnea, the greatest clinical implication is to withhold benzodiazepines and other sedating hypnotic agents that may further depress respiratory drive. Sleep hygiene and surgical intervention or other methods to improve the airway (e.g., nasal continuous positive airway pressure) are generally the best approaches for treating sleep apnea.

Table 10-4 Sleep Disorders

Disorder	Sleep-laboratory findings	Psychologic evaluation	Management and treatment
Somnambulism	Incidents occur out of stage 4 sleep; critical skills reactivity is impaired during incident	Psychiatric disturbances uncommon in children and common in adults	Prophylactic measures; children often outgrow disorders, so parents should be reassured; psychiatry evaluation for adults
Enuresis	Occurs during all sleep stages; dreaming is a common causal factor	Psychiatric disturbances infrequent with primary enuresis; psychologic evaluation often indicated for secondary enuresis	Parental counseling and reassurance critical so that parental mishandling does not create psychiatric problems; pharmacologic treatment (imipramine) may be indicated in older children
Night terrors	Occur out of stage 4 sleep; characterized by extreme vocalizations, motility, and autonomic response; recall minimal or absent	Psychiatric disturbances uncommon in children and common in adults	Parents should be reassured that children often outgrow disorder; for adults, psychologic evaluation is often indicated; use of stage 4 suppressants is under investigation

Nightmares	Occur out of REM sleep; characterized by less motility and autonomic response than with night terrors; recall is frequent and elaborate	Frequent nightmares in children or adults may indicate psychopathology; rule out drug withdrawal as a possible cause of nightmares	Parents should be reassured that nightmares in children are often transient; if episodes are frequent in children or adults, psychologic evaluation is indicated
Narcolepsy	Sleep attacks of narcolepsy may be accompanied by three auxiliary symptoms: cataplexy, sleep paralysis, and hypnagogic hallucinations (cataplexy is accompanied by sleep-onset REM periods)	Sleep attacks may be misinterpreted as laziness, irresponsibility, or emotional instability	Establishing diagnosis is critical; stimulants are effective for treatment of sleep attacks; imipramine is effective for treatment of auxiliary symptoms; danger exists in using imipramine and amphetamines simultaneously
Hypersomnia	Sleep-stage patterns normal, but sleep is extended; associated with postdormital confusion and difficulty in awakening; autonomic response variables are increased	Often a symptom of psychologic disorder (e.g., depression)	Stimulant drugs are effective; neurologic and psychologic evaluations are important in establishing diagnosis
Insomnia	Complaints of patients have been verified in sleep laboratory; sleep is more aroused (i.e., heart rate and respiration are increased); most hypnotic drugs lose effectiveness within 2 weeks	Most often a symptom of psychologic disturbance and not a primary disorder; depression a common feature	When insomnia is secondary to medical conditions, pharmacologic treatment may be useful; if psychologic factors are primary, pharmacologic therapy should be combined with psychotherapy

Periodic Leg Movements (Restless Leg Syndrome) and Nocturnal Myoclonus

Periodic leg movements (restless leg syndrome) may disrupt sleep and cause an individual to complain of light, broken, or restless sleep. Restless leg syndrome is probably a familial disorder, and the incidence increases markedly in individuals older than 45. The uncomfortable "creepy crawly" leg sensations that occur while the patient is at rest are usually relieved by movement. Thus active patients are asymptomatic during the day but are unable to fall asleep at night because of the sleep-related periodic leg movements that further disrupt sleep. The causes of restless leg syndrome are diverse and include underlying conditions such as amyloidosis and iron deficiency anemia. Benzodiazepines may be useful only to relieve symptoms. Many clinicians prescribe dopaminergic agents such as carbidopa/levodopa, pergolide, or bromocriptine for this purpose. Opioids and some anticonvulsants are also effective, although it is important to make sure that a sufficiently large dose of anticonvulsant is given. Finally, supplementation with iron, folate, and magnesium, as well as vitamin B_{12}, C, and E, is recommended for the elderly who have this problem.

Nocturnal myoclonus entails repetitive, stereotypic leg muscle jerks. Although the disorder may be ameliorated by means of benzodiazepines, specifically clonazepam, it may worsen with the use of tricyclic antidepressants; this distinction is crucial because these agents may be helpful in treating other types of insomnia. Phototherapy is another method for treating this syndrome; patients are exposed to artificial bright light, up to 10,000 lux, either in the evening right before they go to bed or in the afternoon.[5] For some people, an afternoon walk is enough to correct their circadian rhythms. When afternoon exposure to sunlight is not an option, light boxes can be used before bedtime. It may also help for people to wear dark glasses when they wake up in the morning.

NARCOLEPSY

Narcolepsy is a sleep disorder with a clear genetic component that occurs in as many as 1 or 2 individuals per 1000. Narcolepsy involves features related to REM sleep that suddenly and abnormally intrude on wakefulness during the day. The individual has an irresistible urge to nap for short periods. The paralysis of REM sleep may appear during the daytime, with attacks of cataplexy characterized by brief bilateral paresis, which may be brought on by laughter, anger, or surprise. During these periods of cataplexy, patients are unable to move, talk, or ambulate. However, consciousness and memory for the event are preserved, thus distinguishing this event from a seizure episode. Sleep paralysis and hypnagogic hallucinations may also occur in persons with narcolepsy. These dreamlike visual experiences may be accompanied by apprehension that someone else is present in the room.

These clinical features may be present in a classic case of narcolepsy. Paradoxically, wakeful periods may occur during the night. This feature is typically not found in idiopathic hypersomnia. Troublesome dreams and depression are other features seen in association with narcolepsy. Social, familial, and occupational functioning are often impaired. Pharmacologic and clinical approaches to narcolepsy are similar to those for idiopathic hypersomnia. Protriptyline and other conventional antidepressants that suppress REM sleep, and therefore narcolepsy symptoms, may be especially beneficial. Stimulants such as methylphenidate, pemoline, or modafinil (Provigil) may also be warranted (see Chapter 16). Modafinil in doses of 100 to 200 mg is a wakefulness-promoting agent specifically approved for reducing excessive daytime sleepiness caused by narcolepsy. Narcolepsy may also be managed with the use of scheduled naps and small, measured doses of caffeine.

PARASOMNIAS

Parasomnias are unwanted automatisms or automatic behaviors that occur during deep sleep. These often occur when cortical suppression of fixed-action patterns is lessened compared with other sleep stages. Perhaps the most common type of adult parasomnia is adult enuresis, which may be associated with cystitis, diabetes, or other nonpsychiatric medical conditions. Sleepwalking is another relatively rare parasomnia that occurs during adulthood, although a childhood or family history of sleepwalking may be present. Sleepwalking movements are usually slow, poorly coordinated, without integrated purpose, and not recalled by the patient. Rarely do these individuals harm themselves or others.[10]

Other sleep automatisms that may be considerations for pharmacologic intervention include bruxism and repetitive movements of the head or extremities. Stereotypic behavior such as sitting, standing, stroking the wall, saluting, or punching can also occur. In addition, night terrors, which rarely occur in adults, are distressing. Night terrors arise during deep sleep, and like other parasomnias, the details of the event are not remembered. Unlike nocturnal panic attacks, night terrors are not associated with other symptoms of panic or prolapsed mitral valve syndrome. Night terrors are different from nightmares, which may involve upsetting content, occur during REM sleep, and may not cause the individual to awaken (see Table 10-4).

COMORBID CONDITIONS

Using psychotropic drugs to treat sleep disorders has been addressed by largely focusing on insomnia and, to a lesser extent, other disorders. Insomnia and other sleep disorders often reflect a serious psychiatric disorder or are found in association with a general medical condition. Resolution of insomnia may avert subsequent psychiatric morbidity; however, more often it may be necessary to place the treatment of insomnia in the context of treating associated conditions and comorbid disturbances.

Covert physiologic factors or general medical conditions are the basis for nearly 40% of the cases of insomnia; if these factors are not identified, the patient's condition may actually worsen, even with effective conventional treatment (Box 10-4). For example, obstructive sleep apnea, as previously characterized, may be associated with cerebral hypoxia and may lead to physical and psychiatric complications. Conventional hypnotic agents may only worsen the condition. Administering antidepressants or improving the airway, for example, by use of continuous positive airway pressure, may be extremely helpful.

Several disorders that affect biologic rhythms may result in problems with initiating or maintaining sleep. As described in the discussion of insomnia, sleep-phase syndromes may occur in which the individual is unable to fall asleep at the desired time and then sleeps substantially longer than desired. These syndromes are commonly encountered among adolescents, college students, and shift workers, including health care professionals. Attempting to compensate by sleeping late on weekends or days off work is not particularly effective. Elderly individuals may have an advanced sleep-phase syndrome, retiring quite early and awakening after a normal 7 or 8 hours of sleep, for example, at 3 AM. This sleep pattern creates problems in the home or in other settings such as long-term care facilities, and leads to inappropriate prescription of hypnotic medication.[10]

Other cases of insomnia may simply be associated with the use of over-the-counter agents, alcohol, or drugs prescribed for other medical conditions, for example, antibiotics, thyroid preparations, cancer chemotherapeutic agents, and many other medications that can and do affect the sleep-wake cycle (see Box 10-4).

Box 10-4 Medical Causes of Insomnia

**Medical conditions that
can induce insomnia**
Cardiovascular disorders
Chronic obstructive pulmonary disease
Conditions associated with pruritus
Endocrine and metabolic disorders
Febrile illnesses and infections
Illnesses associated with pain
Inflammatory bowel disease
Neoplastic disorders
Urinary frequency

Drugs that can induce insomnia
Antihypertensives
Angiotensin-converting enzyme inhibitors
Beta-adrenergic blockers
Diuretics
Methyldopa
Reserpine
Autonomic agents
Anticholinergics
Cholinergic agonists
Cimetidine
Central nervous system stimulants
Amphetamines
Caffeine

Methylphenidate
Nicotine
Sympathomimetics
*Central nervous system
depressants*
Alcohol
Anxiolytics
Hypnotics
Narcotics
Opiates
Hormones
Corticotropin
Cortisone
Oral contraceptives
Progesterone
Thyroid hormone
  preparations
Others
Anticancer medications
Antidepressants
Digoxin
Monoamine oxidase
  inhibitors
Theophylline
Levodopa

Data from References 7 and 10.

REFERENCES

1. Ancoli-Israel S, Ramsdell J, Doghramji K: New ideas for the management of sleep disorders. In American Geriatric Society, editors: *Sleep disorders, supplement to clinical geriatrics,* Plainsboro, NJ, 1999, Multimedia HealthCare/Freedom.

2. Ancoli-Israel S, Roth T: Characteristics of insomnia in the United States: results of the 1991 National Sleep Foundation Survey. I, *Sleep* 22:S347, 1999.

3. Aserinsky E, Kleitman N: Regularly occurring periods of eye motility and concomitant phenomena during sleep, *Science* 118:273, 1953.

4. Baldessarini RJ: *Chemotherapy in psychiatry,* Cambridge, Mass, 1985, Harvard University.

5. Campbell SS and others: Light treatment for sleep disorders: consensus report. V. Age-related disturbances, *J Biol Rhythms* 10:151, 1995.

6. Elie R and others: Sleep latency is shortened during 4 weeks of treatment with zaleplon, a novel nonbenzodiazepine hypnotic, *J Clin Psychiatry* 60(8):536, 1999.

7. Erman MK: Insomnia, *Psychiatr Clin North Am* 10:525, 1987.

8. Evans SM, Funderburk FR, Griffiths RR: Zolpidem and triazolam in humans: behavioral and subjective effects and abuse liability, *J Pharmacol Exp Ther* 255(3):1246, 1990.

9. Foley DJ and others: Sleep complaints among elderly persons: an epidemiologic study of three communities, *Sleep* 18:425, 1995.

10. Folks D: Management of insomnia in the long-term care setting, *Ann Long-Term Care* 7(1): 7, 1999.
11. Folks DG, Burke WJ: Sedative hypnotics and sleep, *Clin Geriatr Med* 14(1):67, 1998.
12. Folks DG, Fuller WC: Anxiety disorders and insomnia in geriatric patients, *Psychiatr Clin North Am* 20(1):137, 1997.
13. Garfinkel LD and others: Improvement of sleep quality in elderly people by controlled-release melatonin, *Lancet* 346(8974):541, 1995.
14. Greenblatt DJ and others: Benzodiazepine hypnotics: kinetics and therapeutic options, *Sleep* 5(suppl 1):S18, 1982.
15. Haimov I and others: Melatonin replacement therapy of elderly insomniacs, *Sleep* 18(7): 598, 1995.
16. Hirsch JD, Garrett KM, Beer B: Heterogeneity of benzodiazepine binding sites: a review of recent research, *Pharmacol Biochem Behav* 23(4):681, 1985.
17. Keltner NL and others: *Psychobiological foundations of psychiatric care,* St Louis, 1998, Mosby.
18. Lamberg L: Melatonin potentially useful but safety, efficacy remain uncertain, *JAMA* 276:1011, 1996.
19. Mendelson WB: Pharmacologic treatment of insomnia. In Pies R, editor: *Advances in psychiatric medicine, Psychiatric Times* (suppl), Santa Ana, Calif, 1992, CME.
20. Merlotti L and others: The dose effects of zolpidem on the sleep of healthy normals, *J Clin Psychopharmacol* 9(1):9, 1989.
21. Nicholson AN: Hypnotics: clinical pharmacology and therapeutics. In Kryger MH, Roth T, Dement W, editors: *Principles and practice of sleep medicine,* Philadelphia, 1989, WB Saunders.

CHAPTER 11

Acute Psychoses and the Violent Patient

SCOPE OF THE PROBLEM

Violence and aggressive behavior are endemic in the mental health treatment setting and constitute a bona fide occupational hazard. Physical assaults on mental health professionals have been reported in all clinical settings, including inpatient, outpatient, emergency, and institutional settings. Clinicians report a 14.2% rate of assault in all settings. The risk of violence in hospital settings is increasing.[7] The inpatient setting is often characterized as having the risk of violent behavior and assault (33%); however, the highest percentage of assaults occurs in an outpatient or a private practice setting (47%). In teaching hospital emergency departments (EDs) with more than 40,000 visits, 32% report one verbal threat per day, 18% report weapons displayed at least once per month, and 43% report a staff member being attacked at least monthly.[4] Depp reported that 12% of 379 documented assaults over an 8-month period in an institutional setting involved staff nurses.[2] Lion, Snyder, and Merrill reported 203 incidences of assault against nursing staff over a 1-year period in a Maryland state hospital; as many as five times that number were thought to be unreported to the administration.[6] Given these percentages of violent behavior among all clinical settings, clinicians must learn the basic skills for management of aggressive or violent patients.

THE CLINICAL APPROACH

Clinicians' predictions of aggressive behavior or violence have shown some reliability. Patients with personality disorder, neurologic disorder, psychosis, head trauma, or mental retardation are predisposed to violence, but the highest risk comes from patients with a substance use disorder.[3] Patients tend to become aggressive or violent when they feel helpless, passive, or trapped. Successful interventions often alleviate these feelings and diminish the chances of loss of behavioral control. Usually, a prodromal pattern of behavior precedes overt violence. Sudden, unexpected violence is rare, and most violence is a predictable culmination of a 30- to 60-minute period of escalation.

The patient's posture, speech, and motor activity are key indicators a violent episode is forthcoming. Most violence is preceded by a period of increasing restlessness and pacing. Thus hyperactivity may be a sign that immediate intervention is necessary. One study found confusion, irritability, boisterousness, physical threats, verbal threats, and attacks on objects were common before the onset of violence.[5]

POLICIES ON VIOLENCE

Because violent behavior and assault are occupational hazards in all mental health settings, including EDs, the staff of each facility should thoughtfully develop policies and procedures that are appropriate to meeting the problems of its own patient population. Policies for the care of violent patients who are agitated or acutely psychotic should be reviewed, approved, and supported at the highest level of clinical administration. Procedures for the clinical management of a violent or aggressive patient should be rehearsed regularly. This chapter focuses on the pharmacologic treatment of the aggressive or violent patient, including diagnostic assessment, diagnostic categories, short-term and long-term treatment, and the implications important for successful clinical management.

DIAGNOSTIC CONSIDERATIONS

Assessment and Clinical Approach

The initial clinical approach to the care of the aggressive or violent patient clearly differs from the customary process of clinical diagnosis and treatment. Rapid assessment and swift symptomatic relief through immediate intervention are often necessary. Treatment is directed toward the target symptoms of agitated or aggressive behavior, often with little time for diagnostic sophistication. The primary goal is to ensure the safety of the patient, the staff, and others who may be innocent bystanders. Once the violence is contained, controlled, or concluded, the staff may begin to work on delineating the origin and pathogenesis of violence.

The clinical approach to aggressive behavior uses a number of strategies (Box 11-1). Initially, a variety of nonpharmacologic interventions may be used. Patients who may be on the verge of losing control often respond to a well-timed verbal intervention or isolation. Because potentially violent patients are terrified of losing control, they welcome these therapeutic efforts and may actually respond to an empathic response that takes charge of the situation. Of course, the nature of the setting, the staff, and the security resources largely determine whether the patient can be safely managed and will dictate the level of immediate response. The more secure the setting and the more experienced the staff, the less aggressive and restrictive the preferred intervention is likely to be.

During an interview with a violent or potentially violent patient, the clinician should focus on the patient's underlying feelings. Rationalization and intellectualization are not generally therapeutic and may serve only to increase the patient's sense of frustration. Ventilating anger reduces agitation. By acknowledging the patient's emotional state, the clinician may elicit some degree of emotional catharsis from the patient, thereby diminishing the patient's need or desire for further aggression.

During the assessment and interview of an aggressive or violent patient, the interviewer should stay at arm's length. The patient should never be left alone. Police, security personnel, or family should be asked to remain nearby to help control the patient if necessary. During the verbal intervention, it may be helpful to offer the patient food or drink; hot liquids should be avoided for obvious reasons. Food symbolizes nurturance and caring and may alleviate an angry patient's disruptive

---

Box 11-1 Clinical Approach to Aggressive Behavior

1. Talk
2. Observation
3. Redirection
4. Isolation
5. Medication—PO
6. Medication—IM
7. Seclusion
8. Restraint

PO, Orally; *IM*, intramuscularly.

behavior. Also, the patient's agitated behavior may signal the degree of loss of control. For example, the patient who cooperates with the initial verbal intervention and postures himself or herself in a restrained or secure fashion is more likely to comply with treatment.

The experience and skill of the interviewer is clearly important in defusing the threat of violent behavior. However, staff may actually contribute to violent episodes, especially in an inpatient or emergency setting. Conflicts over issues of power, dependency, or self-esteem constitute the psychodynamic themes that respond to verbal and psychotherapeutic crisis intervention. Thus the agitated paranoid, the borderline, or the mildly psychotic patient, through clarifying his or her grievances and ventilating frustrations, may in fact be able to "talk it out."

The ultimate threat is posed by a patient with a weapon. Ideally, the clinician explores the fear that led the patient to arm himself or herself. A weapon may symbolize a defense against feelings of helplessness and passivity. An immediate request to give up the weapon may heighten these feelings and further exacerbate the threat. Nonthreatening expressions of a desire to help, coupled with an expression of fear, is the response most likely to avert physical harm.[3] Of similar concern is a threat that may be posed by the staff's potential use of weapons, especially guns carried by police officers and security personnel who may be involved in an intervention. Generally and preferably, these employees should disarm themselves when in an emergency setting.

Ultimately, the agitated or aggressive patient requires symptomatic relief followed by a thorough evaluation of the origin and pathogenesis of the aggressive behavior. A number of algorithms have appeared in the literature regarding the initial clinical approach to these patients. A standard set of interview techniques to be used with an agitated or aggressive patient is summarized in Box 11-2. In addition, several

---

Box 11-2 Interview Techniques Used with Aggressive or Potentially Violent Patients

1. Secure a private but safe interview environment.
2. Approach the patient respectfully, professionally, and politely.
3. Maintain a nonthreatening, passive clinical approach.
4. Clarify, reassure, and gather data without interpretation or confrontation.
5. Listen uncritically and empathically in an unhurried fashion.
6. Offer food and drink as a symbol of help, assurance, and nurturance.
7. Involve family or friends in the clinical dialog.
8. Communicate positive expectations for the patient but prepare for the worst.
9. Provide the patient with options and the opportunity for making choices for treatment.
10. Assist the patient in focusing anger and grievances; for example, the staff is not usually a legitimate target.
11. Offer medication to maintain control as appropriate.
12. Ask security officers to stand by or sit in as appropriate (show of force).

Modified from Dubin WR: Psychiatric emergencies: recognition and management. In Stoudemire A, editor: *Psychiatry for medical students*, ed 3, Philadelphia, 1998, Lippincott-Raven; and Soloff PH. In Hales RE, Frances AJ, editors: *American Psychiatric Association annual review*, vol 6, Washington, DC, 1987, The Association.

management guidelines for the initial assessment are outlined in Box 11-3. Many of these suggested techniques and guidelines are appropriately combined with medication or followed by seclusion or restraint of the patient.

Using drugs to treat aggressive or violent behavior in a patient may occur without clear identification of syndromal or diagnostic features. Common diagnostic features of these patients are summarized in Box 11-4. The specific drug prescribed varies

---

Box 11-3 Management Approach to Aggressive or Potentially Violent Patients

Do	**Do not**
Anticipate violence	Ignore gut feelings
Respond to personal fears and feelings	Respond hastily to angry, threatening individuals
Call security at the first sign of violence	Compromise ability to maintain safety and security
Be aware of possible weapons	Antagonize or challenge a patient with a weapon
Offer food, drink, or medication	Touch or startle the individual
Restrain with an organized format	Restrain without a plan or without sufficient personnel
Offer injectable medicines if oral medicines are refused	Neglect looking for general medical causes of violence
Observe patients who are restrained or sedated	Bargain about the need for restraint, medication, or psychiatric admission
Hospitalize patients who are violent or uncooperative or patients who are psychotic or cognitively impaired	Forget medical and legal concerns and appropriate documentation
Warn potential victims of threatened violence	Overlook the usefulness of family and friends
Evaluate thoroughly	"Carry the coffin" by yourself: Do get help

Modified from Dubin WR. Psychiatric emergencies: recognition and management. In Stoudemire A, editor: *Clinical psychiatry for medical students*, Philadelphia, 1998, Lippincott-Raven; Rabin PL, Folks DG, Hollender MH: *Southern Med J* 75:1369, 1982; and Weissberg MP: *Am J Psychiatry* 136:787, 1979.

Box 11-4 Diagnostic Features Commonly Associated with Violence

Symptoms of agitation, confusion, or anxiety
Syndromes of mixed anxiety-depression or psychosis
Disorders of mood, thought, cognition, or perception
Disorders of drug and alcohol use
Disorders of personality or interpersonal functioning
Cases involving malingering and noncompliance

with the clinical diagnostic problem and involves some consideration of short-term versus long-term treatment, as well as the use of seclusion or physical restraint. Drug treatment is directed toward acute affective or cognitive symptoms responsible for the imminent loss of behavioral control. Thus agitation, hostility, belligerence, suspiciousness, and conceptual disorganization are treated initially, regardless of the underlying processes. In some cases, drug treatment addresses symptoms of primitive or disruptive forms of personality disorders such as borderline, narcissistic, histrionic, antisocial, schizotypal, or paranoid disorders. In other cases, drug treatment relieves symptoms that reflect an acute exacerbation of schizophrenia, bipolar disorder, delusional disorder, or psychotic or agitated depression. Occasionally, medication may simply represent the "chemical restraint" for short-term treatment of violence in progress. Thus incidents of violence resulting from psychotic ideation, cognitive impairment or manic excitement, extreme anxiety, or irritability or explosive behavior may all represent cases in which drugs are required to manage the violent behavior.

DRUG TREATMENT
SHORT-TERM TREATMENT

The acute drug treatment of the agitated or aggressive patient generally involves one of the following classes of agents:

1. The sedative-hypnotic class, usually a benzodiazepine administered orally
2. The neuroleptic or antipsychotic class, appropriately reserved for patients who are severely agitated or psychotic

The pharmacologic characteristics of these drugs are described in Chapters 5 and 7.

Benzodiazepines

Benzodiazepines are clearly efficacious in treating acute situational anxiety, but their use in aggressive or agitated patients carries some risk. Anxiolytics may result in disinhibition or further loss of control over feelings and may contribute further to rage, hostility, or aggression. Patients with a history of outbursts, belligerence, or assaultive or impulsive behavior are best not given benzodiazepines except with extreme caution. An example would be the patient with borderline personality disorder who has shown marked disinhibition of self-directed and other-directed violence, including suicide attempts and self-mutilation, when given benzodiazepines. However, acceptance and familiarity with anxiolytics, as well as the usefulness of a pill "to take the edge off," may prevent the escalation of anxiety or agitation in a patient who is potentially violent and may facilitate interpersonal interaction. Some clinicians prefer the use of low-potency agents, for example, oxazepam or diazepam, in oral doses of 10 to 30 mg and 2 to 10 mg, respectively. Lorazepam, a high-potency agent, in doses of 0.5 to 2.0 mg, is often prescribed and has the advantages of an intramuscular route of administration and reliable absorption.

Neuroleptics

Neuroleptic or antipsychotic medication is often given in single doses to a potentially violent or agitated patient to facilitate an evaluation. Haloperidol 2 to 5 mg oral concentrate or intramuscular administration is often effective in achieving symptomatic improvement. Newer antipsychotics such as risperidone, olanzapine, and quetiapine may be given in oral doses of 0.25 to 1.0 mg, 2.5 to 5.0 mg, or 12.5 to 50 mg, respectively. Thus, as a patient becomes progressively agitated, an antipsychotic agent is prescribed alone or in combination with 1 to 2 mg of lorazepam.

The potentially violent or acutely psychotic patient's treatment at some point may no longer be entirely voluntary or lend itself to oral medication. Medication may be initially presented to the patient in a firm but kind manner that indicates to the patient that his or her behavior is slipping out of control. The medication is now needed to prevent further loss of control. The patient may initially be given a choice of oral or parenteral medication to preserve self-esteem. Therapeutic work or evaluation can then continue after administration of the medication. On the other hand, a lack of response on the patient's part may suggest the need for a "show of force" such as physical restraint and/or seclusion.

Rapid Neuroleptization

Although verbal intervention is the mainstay and preferred method of evaluating and treating an acutely agitated or aggressive patient, antipsychotic agents with or without lorazepam represents the more effective drug treatment of the acutely violent or psychotic patient. Carefully titrated, repeated dosing of high-potency antipsychotic drugs (rapid neuroleptization) may be necessary over a short time (6 to 48 hours). This therapeutic technique is carried out in acutely psychotic, agitated, or violent patients. The technique is both safe and efficacious as an emergency treatment. The technique requires varying doses of medication given at 30- to 60-minute intervals; patients often begin to respond within 1 to 2 hours.

The technique of rapid neuroleptization is outlined in Box 11-5. Medications and dosages are listed in Table 11-1. Target symptoms of tension, anxiety, restlessness, hyperactivity, and motor excitement, as well as psychotic symptoms such as hallucinations, delusions, and disorganized thought, are ultimately addressed. However, initial treatment with antipsychotic medication does not fully relieve psychotic symptoms until appropriate antipsychotic drug treatment has been given for at least 7 to 10 days. Thus the goal is to calm patients so that they may cooperate in the evaluations, treatments, and further dispositions of their cases. Similarly, sedation may not necessarily be a therapeutic end point, especially because

---

Box 11-5 Technique of Repeated Dosing of Antipsychotics: Rapid Neuroleptization

Use a high-potency antipsychotic.*
Medicate at 4-hour intervals for a low-dose strategy.
Medicate at 30- to 60-minute intervals for a high-dose strategy.
Note response 20 minutes after a dose.
Observe for nontherapeutic effects after each dose.
Document levels of consciousness and vital signs before each dose.
Maintain close observation for patients in seclusion or restraint,
   as appropriate.

From Dubin WR, Weiss KJ, Dorn JM: *J Clin Psychopharmacol* 6:210, 1986.
*Low-potency neuroleptics and sedative-hypnotics are sometimes used but are not recommended (see Table 11-1).

Table 11-1 Repeated Dosing Techniques of Antipsychotics and Sedative-Hypnotics: Medications and Doses*

Medication	Parenteral (mg)	Oral (mg)	Range of usual daily dose (mg)
High-potency antipsychotics			
Haloperidol (Haldol)	5	15-100	100
Thiothixene (Navane)	10	30-100	100
Trifluoperazine (Stelazine)	10	20	30-100
Loxapine (Loxitane)	10	25	30-200
Low-potency antipsychotics			
Chlorpromazine (Thorazine)	25	50	100-400
Mesoridazine (Serentil)	25	50	50-200
Benzodiazepines†			
Diazepam (Valium)	5-10 (IV or IM)	5-10	5-40
Chlordiazepoxide (Librium)	12.5-50	12.5-50	50-200
Lorazepam (Ativan)	0.5-2	0.5-2	1.5-8
Sedative-hypnotic‡			
Sodium amytal	1 ml/min (IV)	—	150-500
Atypical Antipsychotics			
Risperidone (Risperdal)	N/A	0.25-2	0.5-8
Olanzapine (Zyprexa)	N/A	2.5-5	5-15
Quetiapine (Seroquel)	N/A	12.5-5.0	50-400
Ziprasidone (Zeldox)	10-20	10-20	40-160

Modified from Soloff PH. Emergency management of violent patients. In Hales RE, Frances AJ, editors: *American Psychiatric Association annual review,* vol 6, Washington, DC, 1987, The Association.
*Doses are arbitrary and not recommended for routine use but have been found effective by the authors. Doses for elderly individuals should be half the recommended doses for adults. Adverse effect may occur and should be monitored.
†With the possible exception of lorazepam, benzodiazepines are absorbed erratically or incompletely when given intramuscularly.
‡Use of sodium amytal is reserved for extreme cases of violence-in-progress.

drowsiness may simply delay the patient's evaluation and disposition. Although repeated dosing of antipsychotic medication may indeed obscure the patient's mental status or result in sedation, withholding this effective intervention may only serve to prolong the risk of violence.

Clinical response to repeated dosing of antipsychotics may be dramatic, with symptoms of hostility and belligerence resolved within 20 minutes of an initial injection of haloperidol 5 to 10 mg, and some improvement of psychosis within 6 hours. Forty-eight-hour response rates of 50% to 95% were reported in the original studies of acutely psychotic patients and involved modest dosages in some cases.[1,10] The most important variables in this technique are the choice of agent, the loading dose, the frequency of injection, and the time frame for titration (see Box 11-5 and Table 11-1). Although low-potency agents such as chlorpromazine or mesoridazine have been used, these agents are not recommended because of the potential for adverse effects (see Chapter 5). The preference is given to high-potency, nonsedating

Table 11-2 Guidelines for the Use of Intravenous Haloperidol in Critical Care Settings*

Degree of agitation	Dose (mg)
Mild	0.5-2.0
Moderate	2-10
Severe	Boluses up to 40

Titration and maintenance

Start with a low dosage and titrate in increments of 25% to 100%.

Allow 30 minutes before repeating a dose.

If agitation is unchanged, double the initial dose every 30 minutes until the patient becomes calm.

If the patient calms down, repeat the effective dose at regular dosing intervals, for example, every 2 to 8 hours.

Adjust the dosage and interval to patient's clinical course. Gradually increase the interval between doses until the interval is every 8 hours.

Once the patient's condition is stable for 24 hours, administer doses on a regular schedule, with supplemental doses as needed.

Once the patient's condition is stable for 36 to 48 hours, attempt to taper the dosage gradually. If agitation is severe, high boluses (up to 40 mg) may be required.

Modified from Dubin WR. Psychiatric emergenices: recognition and management. In Stoudemire A, editor: *Clinical psychiatry for medical students,* Philadelphia, 1998, Lippincott-Raven.

*Haloperidol is not specifically approved by the U.S. Food and Drug Administration for the intravenous route; careful documentation of the necessity and rationale must be made.

neuroleptics that may be combined with lorazepam 1 to 2 mg. Thus haloperidol (or an equivalent dose of an alternative high-potency antipsychotic) in single doses of 5 to 10 mg every 30 to 60 minutes (total maximum daily doses of 100 mg) is standard (see Box 11-5 and Table 11-1). Optimal efficacy usually occurs in the lower range of 10 to 30 mg. Regarding the simultaneous use of parenteral lorazepam, a ratio of 2 to 5 mg of haloperidol to 0.5 or 2 mg of lorazepam is generally effective for the acute control of many disruptive and violent patients.

Substance Abuse Related to Behavioral Control

For cases involving substance use disorders, especially alcohol dependence and withdrawal, antipsychotic agents serve to treat loss of behavioral control or psychotic symptoms; cross-tolerant agents such as the benzodiazepines (e.g., lorazepam) are preferred for the actual treatment of the withdrawal syndrome.

The Agitated Patient in the Medical Unit

Patients receiving general medical or surgical intensive care (including the burn unit) may require an alternative treatment approach to violent, aggressive, or acutely psychotic symptoms. In some cases, the patient may require an intravenous route of administration; patients may simply benefit from the rapid intravenous effect. Intravenous haloperidol may possess a lower incidence of extrapyramidal symptoms than seen with oral medication (Table 11-2). However, the use of intravenous haloperidol has not been specifically approved by the U.S. Food and Drug Administration and carries the risk of adverse effects. Documentation of the rationale for this technique must be provided. Coadministration of intravenous lorazepam 0.5 to 2.0 mg may also result in a more favorable clinical response, as noted with rapid neuroleptization.

Side Effects from Drugs Used to Treat Acute Psychosis and Violent Behavior

Side effects resulting from repeated dosing of conventional antipsychotics are generally uncommon and reversible. Muscle rigidity, drooling, dystonia, akathisia, bradykinesia, and others may occur in the first 24 hours after treatment. Extrapyramidal side effects that are not dose related may occur early, as may dystonic reactions. The most serious form of dystonia is laryngospasm, which compromises the airway by contracting the muscles of the larynx, leading to severe respiratory distress. Newer, "atypical" antipsychotics may have reduced potential for side effects, as discussed in Chapter 5.

The sedative or anticholinergic effects of conventional antipsychotic agents may mask or aggravate certain delirious or toxic metabolic confusional states. In general, these adverse effects are more common with low-potency neuroleptics, whereas the extrapyramidal symptoms are more typical of conventional high-potency antipsychotic agents. Akathisia is a sometimes subtle or unrecognized side effect that is often misdiagnosed. A patient who is agitated or who is having psychotic decompensation may reach a point where he or she cannot sit still, is restless or anxious, and finds relief only through pacing. The patient is literally wound up like a spring; he or she is irritable and feels like "jumping out of his or her skin." This drug-induced phenomenon can literally worsen the patient's clinical outcome and has been reported to lead to acts of suicide, violence, or homicide. Thus the patient who has received repeated doses of antipsychotic drugs and appears to be worsening, the patient who responds initially to antipsychotic medication but becomes agitated subsequently, or the patient who complies with drug treatment but has an apparent relapse should be suspected of having developed akathisia. See Chapter 17 for a discussion of treatment of this side effect.

Neuroleptic malignant syndrome, the potential for tardive dyskinesia (not well defined in these patients) or other serious side effects, and the possibility of sudden death are more likely to develop with long-term neuroleptic use. A final concern with repeated doses of antipsychotic agents arises when low-potency drugs are used (e.g., chlorpromazine), requiring large volumes of injectable medication. For example, 25 mg/ml can result in local tissue irritation, requiring adequate nursing techniques and prohibiting the administration of individual volumes any larger than 3 ml per site. Again, a high-concentration, high-potency neuroleptic is preferred for this practical reason alone.

Treating Acute Agitation

Sedative-hypnotic agents may be useful in the less common situations involving violence in progress. Acutely violent patients under temporary physical control or restraint may benefit greatly from sedatives if the goal is immediate sedation. Sodium amytal in doses of 200 to 500 mg may be given by slow intravenous push as a 2.5% or 5% solution at the rate of 1 ml/min until sleep is induced. The advantage of this technique is rapid and total control of behavior through sedation. Complications include potentiation of excitement when insufficient doses are given, laryngeal spasm, or respiratory depression. Barbiturates may potentiate the effects of other central nervous system depressants, including alcohol or other sedative hypnotic agents, as discussed in Chapter 7. Another alternative is the use of intravenous lorazepam in 0.5- to 2-mg doses or diazepam in 2- to 10-mg doses.

Lorazepam. The sedative-hypnotic agent used to treat alcohol or sedative hypnotic withdrawal or acute agitation when neuroleptics are ineffective alone is lorazepam (see Table 11-1). The intramuscular use of lorazepam in 1- to 2-mg doses is discussed in Chapter 7. Side effects may include ataxia, nausea, vomiting, amnesia, and confusion. Aggression is usually well controlled by means of a regimen of 8 mg or less of lorazepam in a 24-hour period, but sedative-hypnotics may not be effective in patients with acute psychosis. Lorazepam or an equivalent dose of clonazepam may also be especially useful in managing acute mania, as discussed in Chapter 6.

Restraints and Seclusion

A comprehensive discussion of the use of restraints and seclusion is beyond the scope of this text. However, some general guidelines for the use of restraints with or without seclusion are provided in Table 11-3. When verbal intervention and voluntary

Table 11-3 Intensive Care of the Violent Patient: Guidelines for Restraint with or without Seclusion

Guideline	Comments
Personnel and approach	A team of four or five personnel approach the patient confidently and calmly, with a firm but kind "show of force"; an explanation is provided for the seclusion and restraint; reassurance and clarification are provided throughout the process.
Technique	Restraint is achieved by use of leather straps, with patient's legs "spread eagle," one arm to one side, and one arm above the head with the head slightly raised.
Monitoring	Restraints are checked every 5 to 15 minutes as appropriate; toileting occurs at least every 4 hours, and requests for food and beverage are promptly met; the attending physician is notified of the restraint within 1 to 3 hours and attends the patient, in keeping with established policies.
Treatment	Verbal or drug intervention ensues immediately, and rapid neuroleptization is carried out, if appropriate, per protocol; restraint and then seclusion are discontinued only after the patient is calm, communicative, and cooperative.
Removal	Restraints are removed one at a time, except for the last two, which are removed simultaneously; the patient is debriefed, that is, given a clear explanation for the seclusion and restraint.

Modified from Binder RL, McCoy SM: *Hosp Community Psychiatry* 34:1052, 1983; Dubin WR: Psychiatric emergencies: recognition and management. In Stoudemire A, editor: *Clinical psychiatry for medical students*, ed 3, Philadelphia, 1998, Lippincott-Raven; and Dubin WR, Weiss KJ. In Michels R, et al: *Psychiatry*, vol 2, Philadelphia, 1985, JB Lippincott.

medication are refused or fail to benefit the violent patient, seclusion and restraint may be necessary to ensure safety and to facilitate treatment. Seclusion or restraint may be needed in the following instances:

1. To prevent imminent harm to the patient or others
2. To prevent serious disruption of the treatment program
3. To prevent significant damage to the physical environment
4. To enhance treatment as part of an ongoing plan of behavior therapy
5. To decrease the stimulation that a patient is receiving
6. At the request of the patient

Thus "the containment of the violent impulse, the isolation from frightening or confusing external stimuli, and the definition of disrupted ego boundaries may result in a therapeutic response."[11] An emergency setting may include patients brought in handcuffs by the police; in such cases, restraint is necessary so that a further measure of security and control is provided while assessment is carried out or treatment is begun.

Physical control such as seclusion and restraint are used when the patient's behavior exceeds the tolerance of the setting, a tolerance that may be defined by staffing patterns, patient population, or philosophy of care. Mechanical restraint or seclusion is an involuntary treatment requiring the use of force and the suspension of the patient's right to refuse treatment. Documentation must clearly outline the behavior requiring restraint, efforts to address the patient's behavior before the use of restraints, and the use of all medication. Continuous documentation with monitoring and efforts to remove the restraints are obligatory (see Table 11-3). The clinician should be familiar with the legal and regulatory aspects of seclusion and restraint, as well as the clinical advantages and disadvantages of both.

LONG-TERM TREATMENT

Long-term treatment of the aggressive, psychotic, or violent patient may be carried out in more restrictive settings. However, shorter hospital stays have resulted in the frequent need to effectively intervene in crisis units and outpatient settings. Long-term management may occur within the community, for example, assertive community treatment or in a long-term care setting. Patients with psychoses, mental retardation, personality disorders, or disorders of cognitive impairment represent the majority of cases.

The long-term treatment of aggressive or violent behavior ideally combines medication with nonpharmacologic interventions. Psychotherapy or psychosocial approaches are especially helpful for patients with personality disorders, as well as for those who are cognitively impaired. Compliance with medical regimen or adherence to a treatment plan may also be a significant treatment issue. The motivation of the patient, the patient's ability to achieve self-control, issues regarding transference and countertransference, the development of "affective" awareness and insight, and the appreciation of the consequences of violence all represent essential psychotherapeutic tasks.

Generally, no one drug may be recommended for the long-term management of the violent or aggressive patient. Several medications or classes of medications have been suggested, depending on the underlying cause. Antipsychotics, mood stabilizers, antidepressants, and beta-blockers are depicted in Table 11-4. Most recently, newer-generation antidepressants, antiepileptic, and nonbenzodiazepine anxiolytic drugs have emerged as beneficial long-term medications. A more specific discussion of some of these categories and agents follows.

Antipsychotics

As outlined in Table 11-4, antipsychotics are especially useful for treating schizophrenia, mania, and other syndromes in which significant agitation or psychotic symptoms are present. Haloperidol or fluphenazine may be reasonable choices for the patient in whom depot administration is desirable in aftercare, for example, the patient with paranoid schizophrenia. The atypical antipsychotic agent Risperdal may become available in a depot formulation in the near future. Clozaril may be used for patients who are refractory to at least two other antipsychotic agents (preferably atypicals). Several reports have demonstrated decreases in violent episodes in patients receiving Clozaril. Of course, patients receiving long-term treatment are subject to the long-term side effects of antipsychotic agents, as outlined in Chapter 5.

Mood Stabilizer: Lithium

Lithium is an effective treatment for aggression and hypersexuality in patients with mania and for the prophylaxis of manic-depressive disorder. Lithium is also useful in decreasing agitation, aggression, and the potential for violence in many patients. Lithium has been successfully applied to treating children and adolescents with chronic aggressive behavior and conduct disorders. The advantages of lithium versus antipsychotic agents with respect to short-term and long-term side effects are obvious in these cases. Generally, lithium produces the best results in cases with a strong mood component related to the aggressive or violent behavior. Lithium is not currently approved for uses other than to treat bipolar disorder or mania.

Antiepileptics: valproate. Valproate has proven to be a useful agent for aggressive behavior and for acute agitation. It is commonly used as an alternative to lithium. This agent may be uniquely effective in rapid mood cycling and in geriatric patients.[8,13] Posttraumatic stress disorder, behavioral dyscontrol, agitated dementia, and psychosis secondary to trauma or medical conditions have been reported to respond to treatment with valproate at concentrations of 50 to 120 µg/ml.[14]

Carbamazepine. Carbamazepine is useful in the treatment of aggression in psychiatric patients with or without seizures. This drug is discussed in detail in relation to bipolar disorder (see Chapter 6) and epilepsy (see Chapter 9). Psychotic patients, predominantly patients with schizophrenia or cognitive impairment associated with aggression and excitability, benefit from carbamazepine with or without an antipsychotic as an adjunct. Carbamazepine may be especially useful in patients with temporal lobe abnormalities or in agitation, aggressiveness, and emotional lability in patients with episodic dyscontrol syndrome.

Gabapentin and lamotrigine. Gabapentin (Neurontin) and lamotrigine (Lamictal) have also been used in the treatment of aggressive behavior. Starting doses and dosage ranges for agitation and aggressive behavior are similar to those used in seizures as outlined in Chapter 9.[13]

Nonbenzodiazepine Anxiolytic

Buspirone (BuSpar) has been used successfully in patients with aggressive behavior syndromes with or without cognitive impairment. Aggressive or agitated patients with brain injury and mental retardation or developmental disorder also appear to respond to buspirone alone or when coadministered with another agent. Standard

Table 11-4 Long-Term Psychopharmacologic Treatment of Aggression

Agent	Indications	Approximate dose* (mg)	Special clinical considerations†
Antipsychotic: conventional, atypical	Aggression directly related to psychotic symptoms; management of violence or aggression by use of single dose or rapid neuroleptization	Standard antipsychotic doses	Oversedation; multiple side effects, including risk of tardive dyskinesia when used long term
Clozapine	Patients refractory to at least 2 conventional or atypical antipsychotics	75-600 mg in divided doses Requires baseline evaluation or monitoring of blood counts for toxicity	
Carbamazepine or valproate	Aggression related to mood cycling or seizures; aggression possibly related to general medical condition	Maintain serum levels at 6-12 µg/ml of carbamazepine and 50-120 µg/ml of valproate	Monitor for evidence of toxic effects; watch for microsomal induction and drop in serum level of carbamazepine
Gabapentin or lamotrigine	Aggression related to mood cycling, seizures, or general medical condition	Standard dosages used for seizures	Often used in combination with other agents
Lithium	Aggression and irritability related to manic excitement or cyclic mood	Maintain serum levels at 0.6-1.2 mEq/L	May augment effects of antidepressants, antipsychotics, or carbamazepine

Benzodiazepines	Nonpsychotic agitation or aggression; most useful for mood (mania) and anxiety (panic)	Standard anxiolytic doses; clonazepam especially useful	Possible induction of paradoxic rage; problems with oversedation
Buspirone	Long-term management of use of anti-anxiety and serotonergic properties	15-60 mg in divided doses	Onset of action up to 30 days at sufficient dose; may be used secondarily as an adjunct to another agent
Beta-blockers	Recurrent aggression in patients with cognitive impairment or irritability when aggression is not directly related to psychosis	50-400 mg/day of propranolol or equivalent agent in divided doses	Latency period before onset of action may be 4-6 weeks; metoprolol, atenolol, pindolol, and nadolol are alternative agents
SSRIs	Aggression associated with dysphoric mood, personality disorder, or cognitive impairment	Low dosages may be effective	Onset of action at 3-4 weeks
Trazodone	Agitation associated with mood or sleep disturbances	Low dosages, 25-50 mg during the day; higher dosages, up to 150 mg at night	Often used as an adjunct to another drug

Modified from Maletta GJ: *Psychiatr Ann* 20:454,1990.
SSRIs, Selective serotonin reuptake inhibitors.
*Doses for geriatric patients should be started at lower levels and individually titrated over time.
†Trazodone in 25- to 50-mg doses may also be useful alone or as an adjunct to another agent.

therapeutic doses of 15 to 60 mg have been effective.[9,12] Similarly, selective serotonin reuptake inhibitors (SSRIs), generally at low dosages (e.g., sertraline 25 to 50 mg or citalopram 10 to 30 mg), may also be useful. Trazodone at dosages of 25 to 50 mg two to four times a day and/or 150 mg at bedtime is a useful adjunct.

Beta-Blockers

Propranolol (or equivalent dosages of nadolol or pindolol) is useful in treating chronic or recurrent aggression, especially in patients with brain injury or psychiatric syndromes secondary to general medical conditions. Chronic or recurrent aggression or irritability in patients whose aggression is not directly related to psychotic ideation may also benefit, particularly from this class of drug. Aggression in patients with head trauma, seizures, Wilson's disease, mental retardation, minimal brain dysfunction, Korsakoff's psychosis, and other neuropsychiatric disorders responds to daily doses of 50 to 400 mg of propranolol; a response time of several days to 6 weeks is typical. Side effects include lowered blood pressure, decreased pulse rate, and rarely, respiratory difficulties, nightmares, ataxia, and lethargy. Most patients receive concomitant treatment with an antipsychotic, antidepressant, or mood-stabilizing medication. A careful medical examination should be performed to identify patients with relative contraindications to beta-blocking agents, such as those with cardiopulmonary distress, asthma, insulin-dependent diabetes mellitus, cardiac disease, severe renal disease, or hyperthyroidism.

The initial dosages of propranolol are 20 mg three times a day; dosages may be increased by 60 mg every 3 to 4 days to a maximum of 640 mg/day. Dizziness, wheezing, and ataxia are all indications for decreasing the dosage. The highest tolerated dosage should be given for at least 1 month before concluding that the patient is nonresponsive. Prospective studies and further use of propranolol and other, similar agents are needed. Ratey and others reported a significant decline in the frequency of nadolol-treated aggression when compared with controls.[9] Thus nadolol, metoprolol, or pindolol may also prove to be beneficial in treating aggression in psychiatric patients with chronic conditions.

IMPLICATIONS AND TREATMENT ISSUES

There are many special concerns about the treatment of aggression and violence in patients with psychiatric disorders, particularly in an ambulatory setting. Counter-transference issues, inappropriate response, safety concerns for staff and bystanders, the duty to protect potential victims, and other ongoing issues must be addressed. As patients become less violent, a risk of despondency ensues. Aggressive patients presumably value being aggressive. To relinquish such behaviors is to be confronted with passivity, dependence, and the helplessness inherent in being weak. Thus the therapeutic task in treating violence, both short term and long term, includes consideration of these aspects of management of patient care. These considerations, together with drug treatment, supportive interventions, seclusion, restraint, and maintenance medication, are intended to culminate in improved therapeutic outcome and to reduce the potential for harm.

REFERENCES

1. Anderson WH, Kuehnle JC: Strategies for the treatment of acute psychosis, *JAMA* 229: 1884, 1974.
2. Depp FC: Violent behavior patterns on psychiatric wards, *Aggressive Behavior* 2:295, 1976.

3. Dubin WR, Wilson S, Mercer C: Assaults against psychiatrists in outpatient settings, *J Clin Psychiatry* 49:338, 1988.
4. Lavoie FS and others: Emergency department violence in the United States teaching hospitals, *Ann Emerg Med* 17:1127, 1988.
5. Linaker OM, Busch-Iversen H: Predictors of imminent violence in psychiatric inpatients, *Acta Psychiatr Scand* 92:250, 1995.
6. Lion JR, Snyder W, Merrill GL: Underreporting of assaults on staff in state hospitals, *Hosp Community Psychiatry* 32:497, 1981.
7. Pane GA, Winiarski AM, Salness KA: Aggression directed toward emergency department staff at a university teaching hospital, *Ann Emerg Med* 20:283, 1991.
8. Pope HG and others: Valproate in the treatment of acute mania: a placebo-controlled study, *Arch Gen Psychiatry* 48:62, 1991.
9. Ratey JJ and others: Nadolol to treat aggression and psychiatric symptomology in chronic psychiatric inpatients: a double-blind, placebo-controlled study, *J Clin Psychiatry* 53:41, 1992.
10. Slotnick VB: Management of the acutely agitated psychotic patient with parenteral neuroleptics: a comparative symptoms effectiveness profile of haloperidol and chlorpromazine. Paper presented at the Fifth World Congress of Psychiatry, Mexico City, Nov 1971.
11. Soloff PH: Emergency management of violent patients. In Hales RE, Frances AJ, editors: *American Psychiatric Association annual review*, vol 6, Washington, DC, 1987, The Association.
12. Stanislav SW and others: Buspirone's efficacy in organic-induced aggression, *J Clin Psychopharmacol* 14(2):126, 1994.
13. Wengel SP, Folks DG: Mood stabilizers. In Klein DL, Hay DG, editors: *Treatment of agitation in dementia*, Washington, DC, American Psychiatric Press (in press).
14. Wilcox J: Divalproex sodium in the treatment of aggressive behavior, *Ann Clin Psychiatry* 6:1:17, 1994.

CHAPTER 12

Alcoholism and Other
Substance Use Disorders

This chapter focuses on pharmacologic agents used to ameliorate withdrawal syndromes, modify drug-seeking behavior, and treat psychiatric disorders in substance-dependent individuals. Chapter 15 examines drugs of abuse without reference to treatment considerations. Although there is some overlap in the content of these two chapters, there is little redundancy.

EPIDEMIOLOGY

Accurate assessment of the extent and character of substance abuse and dependence patterns is difficult because of several significant measurement problems. Because the use of most drugs is illicit or unacceptable, most surveys are likely to provide conservative estimates of prevalence as a result of underreporting by respondents. Because substance use patterns change, national survey data may be outdated by the time they are reported. Marked variation exists in patterns among persons from various cultural groups and geographic regions. Furthermore, data from emergency departments and other treatment facilities, as well as data from arrest records or reports of overdose deaths, measure only those individuals who are unsuccessful in their drug use patterns. Despite these limitations, it is possible to outline some of the trends in substance use disorders that are pertinent to pharmacologic interventions.

Historical Perspective

Before the 1960s, the abuse of all substances with the exception of alcohol was relatively rare and confined primarily to certain underprivileged inner-city populations, individuals within the entertainment world, or criminals. Marijuana use began to increase in the 1960s, particularly among urban men. This use increased with the emergence of a counterculture that rejected traditional values and sought to find meaning, truth, or escape in pharmacologically induced altered states of consciousness. Subsequently, the civil rights movement, the Vietnam War, birth control pills, and the development of a range of legitimate psychotropic medications were contributing factors in a sharp rise in substance use. For example, during the 1960s and 1970s, marijuana use spread to rural areas, increasing the incidence of use at least once in a lifetime (lifetime experience incidence) in 1979 to 31% in 12- to 17-year-olds and 68% in young adults.[13] During the 1980s, the use of marijuana and other hallucinogens declined. Also, the nonmedical use of sedative-hypnotic agents, in particular barbiturates, appeared to level off. Cocaine became more commonly abused, its use increasing in 1982 to a lifetime experience rate of 28.3% among young adults. Since the mid-1980s, cocaine use has remained stable or even decreased slightly. During the 1990s, heroin use has increased, although use now involves a greater cross-section of society, including more affluent populations and adolescents.

Methamphetamine and designer amphetamines are also used in much greater frequency. During the 1980s and 1990s, a major shift in the gender pattern of substance use took place. Traditionally, men were more likely to smoke tobacco, drink alcoholic beverages, or use illicit drugs, but more women have recently been noted to be drug users than in the past.[22]

National Surveys

Recent National Institute on Drug Abuse surveys suggest that 37% of the population reported the use of one or more illicit substance in their lifetime; 13% had used illicit substances in the past year, and 6% had used them in the month before the survey. More than two thirds of people aged 18 to 25 had used an illegal substance, and more than 15% of the U.S. population older than 18 have serious substance use problems. About two thirds of this group abuses primarily alcohol, the other one third primarily other substances. In the late 1990s, the substance use problem's total annual cost to society was estimated at almost $200 billion.[22]

A large recent survey showed that the lifetime prevalence of a U.S. diagnosis of substance abuse or dependence among the U.S. population older than 18 was 16.7%.[42] The lifetime prevalence for alcohol abuse or dependence was 13.8%; for nonalcohol substances, it was 6.2%. In 1995, 6.1% of the population age 12 years or older were current illicit drug users; that is, they used an illegal drug in the previous month. Alcohol and nicotine (tobacco) are the most commonly used substances, but marijuana, hashish, and cocaine are also commonly used. In general, for all four of these substances—alcohol, marijuana, nicotine (tobacco), and cocaine—a gradual but consistent decrease has occurred in the United States from around 1980. However, since 1993, substance abuse has been increasing among children and adolescents.

The comorbidity of substance dependence with psychiatric disorders is significant. Comorbidity, also known as *dual diagnosis*, is the diagnosis of two or more psychiatric disorders in a single patient. A recent large community survey reported that 76% of men and 65% of women with a diagnosis of substance abuse or dependence had an additional psychiatric diagnosis.[47] The most common comorbidity involves two substances of abuse, usually alcohol and another substance. Other psychiatric diagnoses commonly associated with substance abuse are antisocial personality disorder, phobias and other anxiety disorders, bipolar mood disorder, major depressive disorder, and dysthymic disorder. In general, the most potent and dangerous substances have the highest comorbidity rates. For example, comorbidity of psychiatric disorders is more common for opioid and cocaine use than for marijuana use. Substance abusers are at risk to develop psychiatric disturbances and anxiety, depression, and other psychiatric disorders are often associated with self-medication (primarily alcohol use). Substance-dependent patients with a comorbid psychiatric condition are much more likely to relapse and to have a significantly poorer prognosis (Table 12-1).[22]

Pregnancy Considerations

Drug abuse, particularly cocaine use, in pregnant women and its effects on the fetus and infant are epidemiologic concerns.[22] The consequences of cocaine use during pregnancy include complications both prenatally and during delivery. Toxic effects from cocaine and alcohol can result in congenital malformations and drug withdrawal symptoms in infants. These withdrawal symptoms may last for several weeks beyond birth.

Table 12-1 Estimated Prevalence of Extramedical Use and Dependence in Total Study Population and Lifetime Dependence Among Users

	Proportion with a history of dependence	Proportion with a history of extramedical use	Dependence among drug extramedical users
Tobacco*	24.1 ± 1.0	75.6 ± 0.6	31.9†
Alcohol	14.1 ± 0.7	91.5 ± 0.5	15.4 ± 0.7
Other drugs	7.5 ± 0.4	51.0 ± 1.0	14.7 ± 0.7
Cannabis	4.2 ± 0.3	46.3 ± 1.1	9.1 ± 0.7
Cocaine	2.7 ± 0.2	16.2 ± 0.6	16.7 ± 1.5
Stimulants	1.7 ± 0.3	15.3 ± 0.7	11.2 ± 1.6
Anxiolytics‡	1.2 ± 0.2	12.7 ± 0.5	9.2 ± 1.1
Analgesics	0.7 ± 0.1	9.7 ± 0.5	7.5 ± 1.0
Psychedelics	0.5 ± 0.1	10.6 ± 0.6	4.9 ± 0.7
Heroin	0.4 ± 0.1	1.5 ± 0.2	23.1 ± 5.6
Inhalants	0.3 ± 0.1	6.8 ± 0.4	3.7 ± 1.4

From Anthony JC, Arria AM, Johnson EO: Epidemiological and public health issues for tobacco, alcohol, and other drugs. In Oldham JM, Riba MB, editors: *Review of psychiatry,* vol 14, Washington, DC, 1995, American Psychiatric Press.
Note: Weighted estimates from National Comorbidity Survey data gathered in 1990 to 1992; N = 8098 persons ages 15 to 54. *Extramedical use* refers to the use of the drug listed without a physician prescription and supervision or in ways not intended by such a prescription if one was given.
*N = 4414.
†Not estimated.
‡Anxiolytics, sedatives, and hypnotic drugs, grouped.

Psychologic Considerations

Psychologic (and neurobiologic) alterations induced by drug use may have significant influences on the personalities of those exposed persistently to drugs.[29] Drug-related nonfatal emergencies, deaths, and emergency visits for the treatment of alcohol abuse are well-known phenomena. Thus there is the need to continue studying determinants of drug and alcohol abuse and to further develop pharmacologic agents that may be useful in treatment.

GENETIC, ENVIRONMENTAL, AND OTHER INFLUENCES
Genetic Influences

The study of genetic contributors to alcohol and substance abuse is just beginning. The lack of knowledge about the genetic aspects of drug addiction is marked, in contrast to the wealth of knowledge about the genetic aspects of alcoholism, for which a hereditary relationship has been well established. Adoption studies and twin studies focusing on drug abuse have begun to improve our understanding of genetic (and environmental) factors that contribute to substance use disorders.[22] Generally, abuse of substances is highly correlated with antisocial personality disorder, and antisocial personality disorder, in turn, is often predicted by the presence of antisocial personality behavior in a first-degree relative.[15] Alcohol problems among biologic relatives often predict increased drug or alcohol abuse or both in those without antisocial personality disorder who are adopted, but not in adoptees with the disorder.[3] Offspring of tobacco smokers are more likely to become tobacco smokers and to become tobacco dependent than are members of the general population.

A higher rate of opioid dependence is found among the siblings and relatives of opioid addicts than among the general population. Interestingly, one study measured a euphoric response to a single 1-mg oral dose of alprazolam in a sample of 12 nonalcoholic sons of alcoholics. Nine of the men with a family history of alcoholism experienced euphoria, whereas only 2 of the 12 control subjects without a family history of alcoholism had a euphoric response.[6]

Other studies of risk or possible genetic contributors to substance abuse include the longitudinal studies of Kandel, Simcha-Fagan, and Davis, who found that delinquency was highly predictive of drug abuse in adolescents and young adults.[21] Another study identified the influence of older brothers, peers, and parents on younger brothers' drug use.[2] The results showed that older brothers who did not use drugs could offset the effects of parental drug use on younger brothers. Also, younger brothers were least likely to use drugs if both older brothers and peers abstained.

Environmental Influences

Drug-taking patterns are apparently influenced by factors relating to the family constellation and psychosocial environment. Possibly the lack of realistic, rewarding alternatives and the paucity of legitimate role models may render drug-taking behaviors more attractive. Peer influence plays a central role in the initiation, development, and maintenance of drug abuse patterns. The media may also have a profound effect on substance abuse patterns. Alcohol, marijuana, and tobacco have been romanticized such that engaging in these behaviors sometimes may confer on the user a variety of attributes perceived to be positive. Although the dangers of cocaine, alcohol, and tobacco use receive attention in newspapers and magazines and on television, these drugs also are portrayed as an exciting province of the rich, the famous, and the popular. Moreover, young individuals growing up in families with parents or older siblings who are substance abusers tend to become substance abusers themselves. Parental attitudes or perceived parental attitudes influence the adolescent's decision to start drinking alcoholic beverages or taking drugs. Other familial factors possibly related to drug abuse include family instability, parental rejection, and divorce.

Psychologic Factors

Whether drug abuse or dependence results from specific personality factors or psychodynamics and whether drug-use patterns are associated with certain personality types remain controversial. Youthful drug abusers have been characterized as having external locus of control; in addition, lowered self-esteem and increased anxiety and depression have been noted among these abusers.[28] Psychodynamic conceptualizations have suggested that abuse of alcohol and drugs is an attempt to self-medicate a variety of dysphoric states. In addition, the muting and antiaggression properties of the opioids and other compounds may diminish painful psychic states, at least temporarily, and allow the narcotic-dependent individual to cope.

It is sometimes difficult to tell whether the psychopathologic features associated with alcohol or substance abuse are secondary or primary to the pharmacologic effect of the chronic use of the particular drug. Also, the adaptation to the experience of becoming and being a drug-dependent person in a society that stigmatizes and punishes such behavior must be appreciated. Most likely, substance abusers vary markedly in premorbid personality patterns and in psychopathologic features. Systematic studies of opioid addicts in methadone treatment have demonstrated the heterogeneity of psychiatric diagnoses in these populations. Perhaps the choice of drug may reflect personality patterns or psychopathology. Thus whether stimulants, narcotics, opioids, alcohol, or other sedative-hypnotic depressants are used may depend on the specific individual's makeup and may account for great heterogeneity among substance-abuse populations.[4,28] The use of marijuana, hallucinogens, or stimulants may be avoided because these substances weaken the connection to reality and amplify paranoid, psychotic, or anxiety states. In general, a careful drug-use history, with particular emphasis on which drugs are perceived as pleasant and beneficial and which have led to adverse reactions, may facilitate the clinical approach.

Drug-Related Influences

All too often the sense of control that derives from substance abuse is related to the effect of a rapid rate of change of consciousness or perception in almost any direction.[28] For example, cocaine is perceived to be more desirable than an oral amphetamine; a rapidly acting benzodiazepine may be more subject to abuse than are drugs that are slower in onset. Moreover, the conditioned learning important in maintaining drug abuse patterns and in initiating relapse may also be an important environmental influence. For example, the dysphoric symptoms that the drug-taking behavior allayed or controlled or certain situations that have come to be associated with drug-taking behaviors become in time the conditioned stimulus for the experience of drug cravings and drug-seeking behavior. Learning may be an important determinant of the subjective perception of the drug experience; for example, marijuana is used in some cultures as a work enhancer and an appetite suppressant, in contrast to its publicized effects in America as a drug that decreases motivation and stimulates the appetite for sweet food.

Neurobiologic Influences

Recent neurochemical research has focused on opioids and cocaine. Cocaine and other abusable stimulants have varied actions on multiple neurotransmitter systems. Essentially, these compounds exert their primary effects on dopaminergic systems, but they also affect noradrenergic, serotonergic, and cholinergic systems.[22] Cocaine increases dopamine concentration in the synaptic cleft, resulting in increased neurotransmission in brain reward systems. Chronic use of cocaine or other stimulants causes catecholamine receptor supersensitivity. Autoreceptor feedback systems may ultimately decrease dopaminergic transmission. This action may explain the anhedonia seen in chronic cocaine users. Cocaine may also impair the ability of neurons to use dopa. Also, the benzodiazepine receptor may be affected by cocaine through complex interactions. Studies of these receptors and their interactions with the gamma-aminobutyric acid (GABA) neurotransmitter systems may further explain some of the phenomena seen in both cocaine and benzodiazepine withdrawal. In addition to the opioids, a receptor specific for tetrahydrocannabinol (THC), the active ingredient in marijuana, has been identified in the human brain.[8] This discovery may lead to a better understanding of the effects of marijuana, both positive (e.g., appetite stimulation, nausea prevention) and negative (e.g., perceptual and memory disturbance). The toxic effects of marijuana may be caused by its effect on the cells of the hippocampus, which are known to be important in learning and memory.[22]

The availability of animal models that simulate drug addiction in humans has enabled identification of specific regions in the brain that are important in addictive disorders. The locus ceruleus plays an important role in physical dependence to opioids. The mesolimbic dopamine system is involved in clinically evident drug-seeking behavior. Molecular and cellular changes or adaptations occur in various brain regions responsible for behavioral features of addiction and dependence. Intracellular messengers, especially G-proteins and cyclic adenosine monophosphate (cAMP) systems, are involved. As pathophysiologic mechanisms are understood, pharmacologic interventions can be developed.[29]

DIAGNOSTIC CONSIDERATIONS

The appropriate treatment of an individual with substance use disorder relies on the characterization of the specific drug(s) and pattern of use, and an understanding of the psychologic set and social situations attendant to the behavioral patterns. The nature and degree of drug-induced effects, as well as the presence of abstinence phenomena, must be evaluated through history and physical assessment, including a complete history of substance use.

The recognition and treatment of alcoholism and other substance use disorders require knowledge of the pharmacokinetics and pharmacodynamics of specific substances of abuse. The presence of substance abuse or dependence must be considered with respect to known therapies for the acute management of intoxication and withdrawal, and options for long-term rehabilitation. Several aspects of substances more often abused are discussed in Chapter 15. However, some consideration of the diagnostic approach is necessary with respect to pharmacologic agents that are used specifically to treat alcohol and drug abuse and dependence.

Often, no clear delineation distinguishes the appropriate use of a psychoactive substance from misuse, abuse, or dependence. Although the scope of this problem has been considered with respect to epidemiologic, genetic, environmental, and neurobiologic contributors, most of the factors determining an individual's susceptibility to substance use are not well understood. Studies of populations at risk for developing substance abuse have identified factors that foster the development and continuance of substance abuse. However, the relative contribution of these factors varies among individuals, and no single factor appears to account entirely for the risk. Diagnosis and classification of substance abuse disorders reflect prevailing cultural attitudes and theoretic biases. In recent years, it has become recognized that these disorders may exist independent of other psychiatric conditions. Thus the current nomenclature permits the independent diagnosis of substance use and dependence apart from other psychiatric disorders.

American Psychiatric Association Considerations

The American Psychiatric Association (APA) has considered the problem of psychiatric substances to be a medical disorder when the use of "psychoactive substances" constitutes or meets established criteria.[1] From a pharmacologic perspective, *dependence* is a state in which a syndrome of specific withdrawal signs and symptoms follows reduction or cessation of drug use. *Tolerance* refers to a state in which the physiologic or behavioral effects of repeated doses of a psychoactive substance decrease over time, or a greater dose of drug is necessary to achieve the same effect. *Withdrawal* is a physiologic state that follows cessation or reduction in the amount of the drug used. *Abuse* is a residual category for patterns of drug use that do not meet the criteria for dependence. *Substance dependence* is therefore defined as a pattern of substance use of at least 1 month's duration that impairs social or occupational functioning and the presence of psychologic or physical problems or

Box 12-1 Criteria for Substance Dependence

At least three of the following persist for at least 1 month or have occurred repeatedly over a significant period of time:

- Substance taken in larger amounts or over a longer period than originally intended
- Substance used to relieve or avoid stress (may not apply to cannabis, hallucinogens, or PCP)
- One or more unsuccessful attempts to cut down or to control substance use or a persistent desire to do so
- Considerable time spent in activities necessary to obtain the substance, using the substance, or recovering from its effects
- Symptoms of intoxication or withdrawal occur when expected to fulfill major obligations at work, school, or home
- Important activities or obligations are reduced or unmet due to the substance use
- Continued substance use despite knowledge that a persistent or recurrent social, psychologic, or physical problem is related to use of the substance
- Marked tolerance with increased amount of the substance (at least 50%) to achieve intoxication or a desired effect: markedly diminished effect with use of the same amount of substance
- Characteristic withdrawal symptoms

Modified from *Diagnostic and statistical manual of mental disorders-TR*, ed 4, Washington, DC, 2000, The Association.

situations in which use of the substance is physically hazardous, for example, driving while intoxicated. *Addiction* is often used as a synonym of *dependence* but carries a more negative and pejorative connotation. Specific criteria for substance dependence are shown in Box 12-1. Box 12-2 lists the DSM-IV categories of "psychoactive substances."

Comorbidity

Much of the current treatment approach to alcoholism and other substance use disorders has focused on the association with other psychopathologic features. Dually diagnosed patients constitute 30% to 50% of psychiatric patients and up to 80% of substance abusers. The comorbid pathologic characteristics found consist of both axis I and axis II disorders within the nomenclature.[1] The most prevalent disorders include mood disorders, anxiety disorders, psychotic disorders, attention deficit and conduct disorders, and personality disorders, particularly those that fall within the cluster B disorders characterized as antisocial, histrionic, borderline, and narcissistic.[27,48]

Most substances of abuse will magnify psychiatric symptoms. Nicotine and opioids are the exception. Opioids may even suppress comorbid conditions. Whether symptoms are drug induced or not, they must be treated. Treatment involves a combination of drug-focused and psychiatric approaches that best utilizes a multidisciplinary team. Progress is usually shown when both conditions are treated. Psychotherapy or counseling is usually necessary in patients with comorbid psychiatric disturbance.

> **Box 12-2 Psychoactive Substance Categories According to the DSM-IV**
>
> | | |
> |---|---|
> | Alcohol | Inhalants |
> | Amphetamines | Nicotine |
> | Caffeine | Opioids |
> | Cannabis | Phencyclidine (arylcyclohexylamines) |
> | Cocaine | Sedative-hypnotics* or anxiolytics |
> | Hallucinogens | |
>
> From *Diagnostic and statistical manual of mental disorders-TR*, ed 4, Washington, DC, 2000, The Association.
> *These drugs may precipitate drug-drug interactions.

DRUG TREATMENT
OBJECTIVES

The pharmacologic approach to substance use disorders ideally combines psychotherapy, behavioral techniques, and adjunctive interventions that may serve to improve adherence to the medical regimen. To provide appropriate treatment, the psychosocial and cultural characteristics of the patient must be considered, as well as the pharmacology and pattern of abuse of the particular psychoactive substance. Drug treatment uses one, two, or all of the following strategies:
1. Administration of agents that produce some of the effects of the abused substance
2. Administration of agents that deliver some of the abused substance but with reduced toxicity
3. Administration of agents intended to block the reinforcing effects of the abused substance or to make the abused substance aversive

Treatment should be conceptualized for both initial and long-term phases.

Short-Term Treatment Objectives

During the initial phase, terminating drug use and establishing a stable, drug-free state must be the primary therapeutic goal. Identifying the substance use problem and helping the patient accept the proposed intervention may require some degree of confrontation in a family, occupational, social, or vocational setting. During the initial treatment phase, provisions must be made for long-term interventions. Whereas establishing a therapeutic alliance is essential to the treatment process, patients often resume abuse without informing the therapist. Thus intermittent or routine screens may be performed, and objective data on drug abuse status may actually facilitate an open and trusting therapeutic relationship. In the context of this relationship, objectives of short-term treatment include the following:
1. Relieving subjective symptoms of distress and discomfort resulting from intoxication or withdrawal
2. Preventing and treating serious complications of intoxication, withdrawal, or dependence
3. Achieving a drug- or alcohol-free state
4. Preparing for and referral to longer-term treatment or rehabilitation
5. Engaging the family in the treatment process

Long-Term Treatment Objectives

The objective of long-term treatment or rehabilitation is to maintain the alcohol- or drug-free state through ongoing psychologic, family, and vocational interventions. Long-term treatment involves behavioral, psychologic, and psychosocial interventions to maintain abstinence. Changes in lifestyle, work, or friendships may be necessary. Halfway houses, therapeutic communities, and other residential treatment situations may be useful treatment modalities. Treatment of underlying psychiatric or medical illnesses may reduce the impetus for self-medication. Self-help groups such as Alcoholics Anonymous (AA), Narcotics Anonymous (NA), and Cocaine Anonymous provide education, emotional support, and hope to substance abusers and their families. Many patients who come for treatment do so in the context of a dysfunctional family structure. For these individuals, involving the family, particularly spouses and children, may provide great benefit.

DRUGS USED TO TREAT ALCOHOLISM

An estimated 5% to 7% of Americans are dependent on alcohol in a given year; 13% have alcohol dependence at some time during their lives. Simply defined, *alcohol dependence* is a repetitive but inconsistent and sometimes unpredictable loss of control of drinking that produces symptoms of serious dysfunction or disability. There are marked gender differences in alcohol dependence and abuse; the prevalence is about 5% to 6% for men and 1% to 2% for women. The prevalence is highest among men ages 18 to 64 and women ages 18 to 24, with a gradual drop afterward.[35] Alcoholism is believed to account for 20% to 50% of all hospital admissions but is diagnosed in fewer than 5% of patients. Alcohol use is also highly correlated with suicide, homicide, and accidents.

Drug Treatment of Alcohol Intoxication or Withdrawal (Short Term)

Patients who come to medical attention for treatment of alcohol intoxication or withdrawal may show various types of impairment. Many patients present with profound social and financial problems that our health care system is ill equipped to handle. Particularly frustrating is the patient with profound social needs who does not require medical treatment or who refuses medical treatment. The acute alcohol withdrawal syndrome varies greatly in severity. Although severity of withdrawal is generally proportional to the level and duration of alcohol intake, many other factors, such as previous episodes of dependence and concurrent medical illness, influence the syndrome's severity. Most episodes are mild and require neither hospitalization nor pharmacologic intervention.

Although prescribing sedative-hypnotic agents to manage withdrawal on an ambulatory basis is taboo, these drugs are useful in more restrictive clinical settings. Generally, comprehensive nursing care, the routine use of nutritional supplements, and prompt attention to complicating illnesses are responsible for the present low rates of delirium tremens and mortality resulting from alcohol withdrawal. Although paraldehyde, chloral hydrate, barbiturates, and other sedative-hypnotic agents are effective in suppressing the alcohol withdrawal syndrome, the benzodiazepines are superior when given in adequate dosages for sufficient periods of time.

Use of benzodiazepines. The basic principle in using benzodiazepines to treat alcohol withdrawal is rapid substitution of a sufficient amount to suppress withdrawal, followed by a gradual tapering of the drug level over several days. Drugs with long-acting properties, such as chlordiazepoxide (Librium), diazepam (Valium), and clonazepam (Klonopin), are useful in that they self-taper. These long-acting agents enable once-daily dosing. However, lorazepam, with short-acting properties and ease of metabolism and elimination, is preferred in most cases at dosages of 1 to 2 mg orally on an as-needed basis. Parenteral administration must be considered for patients who cannot take drugs by mouth. Lorazepam is promptly and reliably absorbed from intramuscular sites. If suppression of withdrawal is delayed and hallucinosis develops, dopaminergic blockers such as haloperidol (Haldol) or risperidone (Risperdal) may be required in addition to benzodiazepines.

Symptoms of acute withdrawal may benefit from beta-blockers (e.g, atenolol) to decrease autonomic arousal. Coadministration with benzodiazepines facilitates detoxification. For milder withdrawal, clonidine may be as effective, and lofexidine can have similar efficacy with less hypotension and sedation.

Other agents. Barbiturates may be used for treating alcohol withdrawal; however, chloral hydrate and paraldehyde should be considered obsolete because of toxic effects. Phenytoin (Dilantin) is sometimes used as part of the treatment for alcohol withdrawal, but no evidence exists to support its use routinely except in patients who have a history of seizures unrelated to alcohol withdrawal. Unlike phenytoin, valproate (Depakene) suppresses alcohol withdrawal seizures in animals and may be useful in treating alcohol withdrawal in humans.

Thiamine should be administered to all alcohol users as soon as possible (and before the administration of glucose) to prevent the development of Wernicke's encephalopathy, which is characterized by ataxia, nystagmus, ophthalmoplegia, and changes in mental status. The encephalopathic symptoms tend to improve with thiamine repletion. Levels of magnesium and other electrolytes should be determined and deficits replaced. Other details of detoxification management are beyond the scope of this chapter. Korsakoff's psychosis (characterized by gait disturbances, memory loss, confabulation, and neuropathy) is also caused by thiamine deficiencies but is not reversed by thiamine repletion therapy.

Maintenance Treatment of Alcoholism (Abstinence)

The goal of long-term treatment of alcoholism is to maintain abstinence through a comprehensive treatment program that includes psychologic, family, and social interventions. Pharmacologic agents can deter alcohol consumption by making the ingestion of alcohol aversive (sensitizing agents) or by producing unpleasant effects that deliberately lengthen the metabolism of alcohol to create an aversion to alcohol (conditioning agents).

Disulfiram (Antabuse) has been widely used to treat alcoholism. This agent inhibits the enzyme aldehyde dehydrogenase, which metabolizes acetaldehyde to acetic acid. When this enzyme is inhibited, ingestion of alcohol causes a rise in the acetaldehyde level and brings on an unpleasant syndrome characterized by facial flushing, tachycardia, pounding in the chest, decreased blood pressure, nausea, vomiting, shortness of breath, sweating, dizziness, and confusion.[5] Deaths have occurred. Patients taking disulfiram must be informed about the danger of the drug's combination with even small amounts of alcohol. Alcohol present in foods, shaving lotion, mouthwashes, or over-the-counter medications may produce a reaction. The usual dose of disulfiram is 250 to 500 mg/day. Disulfiram may interact with other medications, notably anticoagulants and phenytoin. It should not be used in patients with liver disease. Other contraindications may include myocardial disease, severe pulmonary insufficiency, renal failure, disorders of cognitive impairment, neuropathy, psychosis, difficulty with impulse control, or suicidal ideation. Certain medications, such as vasodilators, beta-adrenergic agonists, monoamine oxidase inhibitors (MAOIs), or antipsychotic agents, may also represent relative contraindications.

More recently, two classes of agents have demonstrated efficacy in alcohol dependence: opioid antagonists (e.g., naltrexone) and serotonergic agents (e.g., selective serotonin reuptake inhibitors [SSRIs], buspirone [BuSpar]). Two carefully controlled trials have examined the opioid antagonist naltrexone (ReVia) in reducing relapse among chronic alcoholics.[33,46] Both trials showed that 50 mg/day significantly reduced relapse. Naltrexone is well tolerated and reduces consumption rates. Several components of the alcohol drinking sequence are affected, including lowered cravings, decreased reinforcement of drinking, and increased headache and nausea that further reduces quantity of intake.[9] Patients treated with naltrexone show increased ability to participate in therapy or counseling. Patients who received both naltrexone and coping skills training were the most successful at not relapsing. These studies suggest the potential utility of naltrexone, particularly when combined with other therapeutic approaches, in preventing relapse.

Nalmefene is a newer opioid antagonist that is structurally similar to naltrexone but with a number of pharmacologic advantages for the treatment of alcohol dependence. These advantages include no dose-dependent associated toxic effects to the liver, greater oral bioavailability, longer duration of antagonist action, and more competitive binding with opioid receptor subtypes thought to reinforce drinking.[25] The major side effect is nausea, with adverse effects occurring in fewer than 15% of patients who have participated in studies. Doses of 20 to 80 mg have been effective in preventing relapses to heavy drinking and reducing alcohol craving. This agent may become available for the practicing clinician in the near future as a first-line treatment of alcohol dependence.

Serotonergic agents have also shown modest efficacy in reducing alcohol relapse.[39,44] Recent studies with SSRIs (i.e., fluoxetine, sertraline, citalopram) have been effective in reducing alcohol use in nondepressed heavy drinkers.[37,44] Other agents that may reduce consumption include buspirone ($5HT_{1A}$ agonist), ritanserin ($5HT_2$ agonist), and ondansetron ($5HT_3$ agonist).[23]

Acamprosate (calcium acetol homotaurine) is a structural analog of GABA and has agonist effects at GABA receptors and inhibitory effects at NMDA receptors. In clinical trials, acamprosate reduced relapse drinking and craving for alcohol and had minimal side effects.[38] This medication has been approved in several European countries for the prevention of alcohol relapse and is currently under clinical testing in the United States. Acamprosate should be considered an adjunctive therapy to a comprehensive psychosocial treatment plan and not a sole treatment modality.

The use of lithium to treat patients with alcohol use disorders not comorbid with bipolar disorder was supported by some early anecdotal reports by small double-blind, placebo-controlled studies. However, a large Veterans Administration collaborative study showed no benefits of lithium over placebo for patients with or without depressive symptoms.[11]

DRUGS USED TO TREAT OPIOID DEPENDENCE AND ABUSE

Opioid dependence (addiction) is defined as a cluster of cognitive, behavioral, and physiologic symptoms in which the individual continues use of opioids despite significant opioid-induced problems. Opioid dependence is characterized by repeated self-administration that usually results in opioid tolerance, withdrawal symptoms, and compulsive drug taking. Dependence may occur with or without the physiologic

---

Heroin Use Is Increasing

Heroin use in the United States has begun to shift from a low-incidence endemic pattern to widely diffused and rapidly spreading epidemic proportions over the last 10 years. Data analyses from disparate sources confirm that heroin use is on the rise, most disturbingly among high school students. Although limited by survey methods that tend to underestimate the presence of "hard core" drugs (e.g., heroin), a statistically significant increase has been seen in the percentage of people in large metropolitan areas who report that heroin is "fairly or very easy" to obtain. The heroin addict at the turn of the 21st century is much more likely to be younger and less experienced with the drug and drug culture than the long-time users of the 1990s.

---

symptoms of tolerance and withdrawal. Usually, there is a long history of opioid self-administration, typically via intravenous injection in the arms or legs, although recently the intranasal route or smoking also is used. A history of drug-related crimes, drug overdoses, and family, psychologic, and employment problems is common. Physical problems, including skin infections, hepatitis, human immunodeficiency virus (HIV) infection, or irritation of the nasal and pulmonary mucosa, may develop. Physical examination usually reveals puncture marks along veins in the arms and legs and "tracks" secondary to sclerosis of veins.

Symptoms of opioid withdrawal include anxiety, restlessness, runny nose, tearing, nausea, and vomiting. Tests for opioids in saliva and urine can help support a diagnosis of dependence. The physiologic effects of opioids are caused by stimulation of receptors that modulate endogenous hormones, enkephalins, endorphins, and dynorphins. Mu, kappa, sigma, delta, and epsilon opioid receptors have been identified.[22] Morphine, heroin, and methadone act primarily through mu receptors and produce analgesia, euphoria, and respiratory depression. Drugs that appear to be mediated through the kappa receptors include the so-called mixed agonist antagonists butorphanol and pentazocine, which produce analgesia with less respiratory depression. The sigma receptor appears to imitate the receptor for the hallucinogen phencyclidine (PCP). The delta receptor binds endogenous opioid peptides. At high dosages, opioid drugs lose their receptor specificity and have agonist or antagonist properties at multiple receptor subtypes. The most common method of ending heroin dependence is simply to stop the drug and experience withdrawal without any pharmacologic support. Going "cold turkey," so named for the goose flesh produced by the heroin withdrawal, is a time-honored method for initiating abstinence. Narcotics Anonymous, a support group approach based on the 12 Steps of Alcoholics Anonymous and a commitment to abstinence, has been helpful to many who are able to take advantage of the practical advice, emotional support, and bonding offered during meetings.

Methadone hydrochloride is a highly effective agent in ameliorating the signs and symptoms of opioid withdrawal. Although the use of methadone (and LAAM [Levo-alpha-acetylmethadol]) to detoxify or maintain patients with opioid dependence requires special licensing; this regulation is waived for inpatients with life-threatening, general, or psychiatric conditions. The procedure for detoxification with methadone involves stabilizing the patient on a daily dose that is determined by the patient's response to a dose of 10 mg every 2 to 4 hours as needed. During the first 24 hours, 10 to 40 mg will stabilize most patients and control abstinence symptoms. Once the stabilization dose is determined, the drug can be slowly tapered by 5 mg/day. When the methadone dose drops below 20 to 30 mg/day, many patients begin to complain of renewed but milder abstinence symptoms. These may be ameliorated by the addition of clonidine.

The treatment of acute opioid withdrawal may benefit from the use of clonidine. Clonidine is a nonopioid antihypertensive drug that has been used successfully to reduce symptoms of opioid withdrawal. Clonidine acts by stimulating midbrain alpha-2 adrenergic receptors. Thus it reduces the noradrenergic hyperactivity that accounts for many symptoms of opioid withdrawal. Clonidine suppresses nausea, vomiting, diarrhea, cramps, and sweating but does little to reduce the muscle aches, insomnia, and drug craving that often accompanies opioid withdrawal. Protocols for clonidine detoxification are as follows: on the first day of treatment, clonidine-aided detoxification involves 0.1 to 0.3 mg in three divided doses, which is usually sufficient to suppress signs of opioid withdrawal. Higher dosages may be used in an inpatient setting with the availability of monitoring for hypertension and sedation, and the dosages are adjusted until withdrawal symptoms are reduced. If the patient's blood pressure falls below 90-60 mm Hg, the next dose should be withheld, after which tapering may be resumed while the patient is monitored for signs of withdrawal. Clonidine-aided withdrawal usually takes 4 to 6 days, whereas withdrawal from methadone alone usually takes 10 to 14 days. Clonidine's advantages over methadone are that it does not produce opioid-like tolerance or physical dependence, it prevents postmethadone rebound in withdrawal symptoms, and patients can be immediately given an opioid antagonist once they have completed the clonidine-assisted withdrawal process.

Administering naltrexone combined with clonidine can speed withdrawal and lessen withdrawal symptoms from opioids. For example, a dose of naltrexone 12.5 mg can be followed by clonidine, up to 0.6 mg with an average daily dose of approximately 0.3 mg.[31,45] Another technique is opioid detoxification with buprenorphine (Buprenex), a partial opioid agonist. Daily sublingual doses of 2 to 8 mg of buprenorphine have enabled the switch from methadone as well as detoxification of heroin. The coadministration technique with naltrexone, as with clonidine, has also been successful with buprenorphine.[40]

Rapid detoxification from opioids can be achieved if the patient is hospitalized, briefly anesthetized, and treated with naltrexone. Ideally, the patient can leave the hospital 12 hours after admission without feeling any withdrawal and safely start on maintenance naltrexone in a cohesive outpatient treatment program. The risks of general anesthesia combined with the lack of outcome studies over time make rapid anesthesia assisted detoxification an unproven method.

Maintenance Therapy: Methadone

Methadone (Dolophine) or LAAM (a long-acting congener of methadone) maintenance continues as the preferred modality for treating opioid dependence. Opioid replacement therapy alleviates drug hunger with high dosages of methadone, blocking the dependency by means of cross-tolerance. Methadone is typically administered orally. Because of its reliable absorption and delay in peak plasma levels of 2 to 6 hours after ingestion, patients are protected against sharp peaks in serum levels and continuation of tolerance. Methadone can ultimately be administered once daily, and opioid maintenance programs using methadone can be undertaken with confidence. Patient progress is monitored by means of counseling and urine drug testing.

No single dose of methadone is optimal for all patients. Some may benefit from maintenance on low dosages (10 to 20 mg/day), whereas others require more than 100 mg/day to achieve maximum benefit. Although 40 to 60 mg of methadone is usually sufficient to block opioid withdrawal symptoms, higher dosages may be needed during maintenance treatment to block cravings for opioids and associated drug use. In general, higher dosages (i.e., greater than 60 mg/day) are associated with better retention and outcomes.[7] If higher dosages are used, monitoring of plasma methadone concentrations may be helpful, with the aim of maintaining minimum levels of 150 to 200 ng/ml.

LAAM

LAAM (Levo-alpha-acetylmethadol or levomethadyl [Orlaam]) is a long-acting replacement therapy that reduces cravings for opioids.[32] LAAM is usually prescribed in doses of 20 to 140 mg with an average of 60 mg. Some patients prefer LAAM to daily methadone because dosing can be as infrequent as three times per week, thus allowing fewer clinic visits and expanded integration into work or other rehabilitative activities. Whereas treatment with LAAM has been shown to be comparable to methadone treatment with respect to reduction of opioid use, retention rates are reportedly higher for patients treated with methadone.[7] In general, longer duration of LAAM treatment is associated with better outcomes.

The criteria for withdrawing patients from long-term maintenance on methadone or LAAM include demonstrated progress toward a drug-free lifestyle, stability in personal and occupational adjustment, absence of other substance use disorders, and successful treatment and remission of any comorbid psychiatric disorder. Constipation and sweating are common side effects of methadone and LAAM that may persist.

A substantial number of pregnant women who are dependent on opioids also have HIV/AIDS. On the basis of preliminary data, women who receive methadone maintenance are more likely to be treated with zidovudine (AZT). It has been well established that administration of zidovudine to HIV-positive pregnant women reduces by two-thirds the rate of HIV transmission to their infants. Comprehensive methadone maintenance, along with sound prenatal care, has been shown to decrease obstetrical and fetal complications as well.

Opioid antagonists. The use of opioid antagonists in treating opioid dependence is based on the high relapse rate after detoxification. Naltrexone (ReVia) is a long-acting, orally effective agent that, when given either as 50 mg/day or 100 or 150 mg three times per week, produces substantial blockade of the effects of large doses of injected opioids.[36] Adverse effects may include dysphoria, anxiety, and gastrointestinal distress. Naltrexone is contraindicated in patients with acute hepatitis or liver failure. Patients must be free of opioid dependence for 1 week before naltrexone can be used.

Opioid overdose, a life-threatening emergency, should be suspected in any patient who comes to medical attention with coma and respiratory suppression. Treatment of suspected overdose includes emergency support of respiration and cardiovascular functions. Parenteral administration of the opioid antagonist naloxone (Narcan) 0.4 to 0.8 mg rapidly reverses the coma and respiratory suppression but does not result in the relief of depression caused by other sedatives such as alcohol or barbiturates. Naloxone can precipitate opioid withdrawal, causing the patient whose life has just been saved to be extremely ungrateful. Naloxone's short half-life makes its use impractical for treating opioid dependence.

STIMULANTS: COCAINE, AMPHETAMINES, AND OTHER STIMULANTS
Drugs Used to Treat Cocaine Abuse and Dependence

The use of cocaine and crack cocaine underwent an epidemic increase in the 1980s and early 1990s. Cocaine remains a major drug of abuse after a relatively long quiescent period during which its use was limited to a small subgroup of the population. The pure drug has been available for only approximately 100 years, but chewing coca leaves has been a practice for 2000 years. Cocaine is an alkaloid extracted from the leaves of the native South American plant. Cocaine is a local anesthetic that blocks the initiation and propagation of nerve impulses and is a potent sympathomimetic agent that potentiates the actions of catecholamines in the autonomic nervous system, causing tachycardia, hypertension, and vasoconstriction. Cocaine is also a central nervous system (CNS) stimulant, increasing arousal and producing mood elevation and psychomotor activation.

There has been a major shift from snorting cocaine to intravenous injection and smoking freebase cocaine. Freebase cocaine, known as *crack*, is inexpensive and widely available. Thus the dramatic increases in hospital admissions for treatment, emergency care, and deaths reflect not only the increased number of users but also new ways of ingesting this drug.

Cocaine intoxication is characterized by elation, euphoria, excitement, pressured speech, restlessness, stereotypic movements, and bruxism (grinding of the teeth). Sympathetic nervous system stimulation occurs, including tachycardia, mydriasis, and sweating. Paranoia, suspiciousness, and psychosis may occur with prolonged use. Overdosage produces hyperpyrexia, hyperreflexia, seizures, coma, and respiratory arrest.[44]

Cocaine produces effects in multiple neurotransmitter systems, including reuptake blockade of dopamine, norepinephrine, and serotonin.[22] Dopamine reuptake inhibition results in increased extracellular dopamine concentration in the mesolimbic and mesocortical reward pathways.

Cocaine has a short plasma half-life of 1 to 2 hours, which correlates with its behavioral effects. Along with the decline in plasma levels, most users experience a period of dysphoria, which often leads to additional cocaine use within a short period. The dysphoria of the "crash" is intensified and prolonged after repeated usage. Abusers uniformly report control over early stimulant use. As use continues, however, the individual binges until immediate supplies are exhausted. This compulsive use pattern and impairment of self-control are the best indicators of stimulant abuse and of the severity of abuse.

Clinical presentations involving cocaine abuse and dependence include a mixture of acute and chronic symptoms with different intensities. Cocaine intoxication, delirium, delusions, postuse dysphoria, and withdrawal may be present. Cocaine may cause severe drug intoxication or death through an extension of its sympathomimetic properties. Chronic medical complications may include malnutrition, anorexia, nutritional deficiencies, dehydration, endocrine abnormalities, and complications linked to the route of administration.

Effective pharmacologic treatment of cocaine abuse and dependence remains an open question. Strategies are based on the premise that altered neurochemistry underlies the chronic high-intensity use (binge) and crash that follows. No consensus exists regarding optimal treatment strategies. Clearly, accurate diagnostic assessment of the cocaine abuser is important because symptoms appearing during abstinence might provide guidance to what pharmacologic adjuncts are potentially useful. Treatment generally focuses on one of the following three areas: acute sequelae, craving, or withdrawal. Psychologic supports and behavioral therapy are generally applied when treating these patients. Hospitalization may be required for individuals who are chronic freebase or intravenous cocaine users or concurrent alcohol users. Furthermore, individuals who have significant psychiatric or medical comorbidity, psychosocial impairment, or lack of motivation, or who were not successfully treated as outpatients may also need inpatient care.[44]

Although no panacea exists for treating cocaine dependence, a wide range of psychotropic medications have been used, including stimulants, antidepressants, precursors to neurotransmitters, neuroleptics, and other agents that exert multiple effects on brain neurotransmission. Agents that are useful have a relatively rapid onset of action, including amantadine, bromocriptine, levodopa (L-dopa), carbidopa, methylphenidate, and carbamazepine.

Dopaminergic drugs. Amantadine (Symmetrel) may exert its therapeutic effect by releasing neuronal stores and delaying uptake of dopamine and norepinephrine, thereby increasing availability to the postsynaptic receptor sites. This drug theoretically could be given with L-dopa, carbidopa, or tyrosine to enhance the clinical effect. Dosages of 200 to 300 mg/day reduce cocaine craving for several days to a month. Although amantadine initially is effective without significant side effects, its usefulness appears to be limited to the acute withdrawal phase.[26]

Bromocriptine, a dopamine agonist, also appears to reduce the density of the inhibitory receptors or autoreceptors on dopamine neurons that exert a rapid anticraving effect. Dosages of 0.5 to 1.5 mg/day may be useful. Abstinent cocaine users report an antagonist effect of bromocriptine when using cocaine. Higher dosages are poorly tolerated because of the side effects. Oral craving is reduced in many cases. Thus bromocriptine may be useful in abstinent cocaine abusers as an antagonist, similar to the way disulfiram or naltrexone is used with alcoholics or opioid addicts, respectively.[26]

Methylphenidate (Ritalin) has been studied for treatment of cocaine abuse. Treated subjects report tolerance, diminished craving, and a mild sense of stimulation. Disadvantages include tolerance, abuse potential, and poor patient acceptance.

Mazindol, a catecholamine reuptake blocker, has been useful in Parkinson's disease and may significantly reduce cocaine-induced craving. Tolerance and abuse do not occur, nor does rebound depression.[10] Bupropion (Wellbutrin) has also been reported to be useful at dosages of 100 to 300 mg three times a day.[24]

Carbamazepine. Carbamazepine (Tegretol) has been used in cocaine dependence. Theoretically, carbamazepine, through its ability to reverse cocaine-induced kindling, reverses cocaine receptor supersensitivity that results from chronic cocaine use.[22] Patients receiving treatment in an open trial have shown significant reductions in cocaine craving with the use of this drug.

Antidepressants. The anhedonia, anergia, and consequences of chronic cocaine abuse can result in a syndrome known as *intracranial self-stimulation.* Desipramine, imipramine, and amitriptyline treatment have been used, and use in an animal model seems to reverse the changes that occur at catecholamine receptors as a result of repeated stimulant use. In essence, the tricyclic antidepressants (TCAs) restore hedonic capacity and decrease cocaine craving. Whether desipramine and possibly other antidepressants, for example, trazodone, nefazodone, or the SSRIs, have some ability to block the physiologic effects of cocaine has been the subject of speculation.[22] However, to determine conclusively whether antidepressants block cocaine's effects or have anticraving effects or both remains a subject of further study.

Other agents. Mood disorders and attention deficit disorder may be common in cocaine users. Resemblance of the cocaine withdrawal syndrome to depression may predict increased cocaine use in follow-up. Thus pharmacologic treatment of depression, as described in Chapter 6, may be an important pharmacologic strategy. Lithium and valproate may also diminish craving, particularly in persons who meet diagnostic criteria for cyclothymia or who have family histories of bipolar disorder. These agents are not generally considered blocking agents for cocaine euphoria and have not been established as particularly useful for these patients. Treatment of underlying attention deficit disorder may also be necessary to treat cocaine abuse successfully.

Cocaine overdose. Cocaine has no specific antagonist for the treatment of acute sequelae. Management of overdose is largely symptomatic and is aimed at reversing epileptogenic, cardiorespiratory, and metabolic effects. Lorazepam for transient agitation, together with a beta-blocking agent, may be useful for persistent symptoms. Suicidal ideation and depressive symptoms that occur during the postcocaine crash are transient and require no acute treatment other than close observation. Antipsychotic agents may be used briefly for severe psychotic symptoms. However, psychotic symptoms seem to be short-lived and usually remit after sleep normalization. Symptoms of depression or psychosis that do not remit within approximately 3 days may necessitate conventional treatment.

Nondrug approaches. Psychotherapy, group therapy, and behavioral techniques have all been found to be useful in treating cocaine users.[16] Self-help groups such as Cocaine Anonymous may also be useful as a primary treatment modality or as an adjunct to another treatment. Many cocaine-dependent patients use alcohol or other drugs, particularly sedatives and heroin, and may require treatment for abuse of these substances.

Amphetamine Dependence and Abuse

Although the subjective effects of amphetamines are similar to those of cocaine, important differences can be identified in their mechanisms of action. Cocaine epidemics stimulated many more attempts at pharmacologic intervention than did the amphetamine epidemic of the 1960s and the more recent methamphetamine epidemic of the 1990s. Thus little is known about the pharmacologic treatment of amphetamine dependence or its complications.

As a group, amphetamines are structurally related to the catecholamine neurotransmitters norepinephrine, epinephrine, and dopamine. These drugs release endogenous catecholamines from nerve endings and are catecholamine agonists at receptors in the peripheral, autonomic, and central nervous systems. One of the primary effects of amphetamines and related compounds is CNS stimulation, which results in characteristic activation of behavior. Amphetamines are potent anorexics and have been used extensively as appetite suppressants. Thus intoxication with stimulants such as amphetamines, methylphenidate, or other sympathomimetics produces a clinical picture similar to that of cocaine intoxication. Chronic users of amphetamines engage in a pattern similar to that of chronic cocaine abusers, escalating doses for several days, then abstaining. Paranoid psychosis similar on diagnosis to schizophrenia may result (i.e., amphetamine psychosis). Underlying psychiatric illnesses such as mood disorder or attention deficit disorder may also be present, as in cocaine dependence.[12,43]

Designer amphetamines such as MDMA, MDEA, MMDA, and STP cause the release of catecholamines and serotonin. Serotonin is implicated as the major neurochemical pathway involved in the effects of hallucinogens. Therefore the clinical effects of designer amphetamines are a cross between classic amphetamines and hallucinogens. The pharmacology of MDMA (3,4-methylenedioxymethamphetamine) is the best understood among the designer amphetamines. Once in the neuron, MDMA can cause a rapid release of serotonin and inhibits the activity of serotonin-producing enzymes. Individuals taking SSRIs such as fluoxetine do not experience the effects of MDMA because they prevent MDMA from being taken up into the serotonergic neurons.

The clinical management of amphetamine-related disorders includes physical examination, general support, identification and treatment of associated psychiatric disorders, and use of the support mechanisms described with alcohol. Dopaminergic blockers such as haloperidol are generally preferred for treating amphetamine-induced paranoid and psychotic states that do not subside spontaneously within a few days. Lithium may be useful to blunt or block the euphoric effects of amphetamines.

Over-the-counter sympathomimetics. Over-the-counter sympathomimetic amines may be abused. Use of these medications, sold as appetite suppressants, decongestants, or bronchodilators, may become evident with signs of intoxication similar to those present with amphetamine intoxication. However, a greater tendency for autonomic effects is present with use of these over-the-counter sympathomimetic amines and may result in a hypertensive crisis.

Caffeine. The use of caffeine and related compounds such as theophylline is ubiquitous in the United States. Caffeine is present in chocolate and a variety of prescription and over-the-counter agents that are used as stimulants, appetite suppressants, analgesics, and cold and sinus preparations. The physiologic effects of these agents include cardiac stimulation, diuresis, bronchodilation, and CNS stimulation. These compounds may augment the actions of neurotransmitters such as norepinephrine and may have a direct stimulatory effect on nerve endings. CNS effects of caffeine include psychomotor stimulation, increased attention and concentration, and suppression of the need for sleep. Caffeine may exacerbate the symptoms of anxiety disorders and increase requirements for neuroleptic or sedative medications. In moderate to heavy users, a withdrawal syndrome characterized by lethargy, hypersomnia, irritability, and severe headache may ensue. Treatment of caffeine dependence consists of limiting consumption and substituting decaffeinated forms of beverages such as coffee or cola. No other definitive treatments are available.

DRUGS USED TO TREAT NICOTINE DEPENDENCE

Heavy or persistent smokers who abruptly stop smoking typically experience nicotine withdrawal syndrome that consists of craving, irritability, impatience, hostility, restlessness, anxiety, depression, difficulty in concentrating, confusion, disturbed sleep patterns, increased appetite, decreased heart rate, and increased slow waves on the electroencephalogram (EEG). Pharmacologic treatments for nicotine dependence are divided into the following groups: (1) agents that produce some of the effects produced by nicotine, (2) agents that deliver nicotine but with reduced toxicity, and (3) agents intended to block the reinforcing effects of smoking or to make smoking aversive.

Nicotine is an alkaloid drug present in the leaves of the tobacco plant. Nicotine addiction and tobacco use are legally sanctioned forms of substance abuse. Tobacco is clearly the most lethal substance in our society. The percentage of Americans who smoke has declined; however, the number of young women who smoke tobacco products has increased because tobacco companies continue to market tobacco as a chic product.

Nicotine has several effects on the somatic, autonomic, and central nervous systems. It agonizes the nicotinic cholinergic receptor sites and stimulates autonomic ganglia in the parasympathetic and sympathetic nervous systems, producing salivation, increased gastric motility and acid secretion, and increased catecholamine release. Tobacco is a mild psychostimulant, producing increased alertness, increased attention and concentration, and appetite suppression. Tobacco can be used to prevent weight gain, which makes this drug attractive, particularly to some individuals concerned about weight control. Repeated use of nicotine produces tolerance and dependence. The degree of dependence is considerable; 70% of those who quit using tobacco relapse within 1 year.

The treatment of nicotine-dependent patients follows the general principles common to treatment of dependence on all addictive substances. Short-term goals consist of reducing or stopping the tobacco use, followed by treatment designed to support and encourage abstinence. Few patients can reduce tobacco use on their own; most require a smoking cessation program.[14] The most successful treatment combines pharmacologic and behavioral therapies.

Generally, attempts to produce stimulation, appetite suppression, or other amphetamine-like effects in smokers do not reduce tobacco use. Using sedatives, tranquilizers, or propranolol has not been of substantial aid in smoking cessation. Lobeline, an alkaloid that is structurally similar to nicotine, has been proposed as a treatment for tobacco dependence and withdrawal. Although this compound has some cross-tolerance with nicotine and is marketed as an over-the-counter preparation, it is not significantly superior to placebo in helping smokers stop smoking.[19]

Nicotine Gum

Nicotine in the form of chewing gum (nicotine polacrilex [Nicorette]) can suppress important components of tobacco withdrawal and can be particularly useful in achieving long-term success. Symptoms that are relieved include irritability and impatience, with some reduction in restlessness, anxiety, hunger, insomnia, and changes in heart rate. The gum is a sweet-flavored resin containing 2 or 4 mg of nicotine, which is released slowly when the gum is chewed.[17] Proper use of the gum can reduce the craving for tobacco and decrease discomfort during the withdrawal period. Nicotine ingested through the gastrointestinal tract is extensively metabolized on the first past through the liver. Nicotine gum (nicotine polacrilex) prevents this problem via buccal absorption. The original recommendation was to use one piece of 2-mg gum every 15 to 30 minutes as needed for craving. More recent works suggest scheduled dosing, for example, one piece of 2-mg gum per hour, or higher, or 4 mg for heavy smokers. Also, the original recommendation of 3 months may be too short. Many experts now believe that longer treatment is required, but no definitive recommendation for time interval is given. Nicotine absorption from gum peaks 30 minutes after beginning to use the gum. Venous nicotine levels from 2- and 4-mg gum are about one third and two thirds, respectively, of the steady-state levels of nicotine achieved with cigarette smoking. Nicotine gum is available as an over-the-counter medication.

Nicotine Nasal Spray

Nicotine nasal spray is a nicotine solution in a nasal spray bottle, similar to those used with antihistamines. This treatment produces droplets that average about 1 mg per administration. The formulation produces a more rapid rise in nicotine levels than docs nicotine gum. Peak nicotine levels occur within 10 minutes, and venous nicotine levels are about two thirds that of between-cigarette levels. Smokers use this product ad lib up to 30 times per day for 12 weeks including a tapering period.

Nicotine Inhalers

Nicotine inhalers are plugs of nicotine placed inside a hollow cigarette-like rod. The plugs produce a nicotine vapor when warm air is paced through them. Absorption from the nicotine inhaler is primarily buccal rather than respiratory. These inhalers produce venous nicotine levels that rise more quickly than with gum but less quickly than with nicotine nasal spray. Blood levels are about one third that of cigarette levels. As with the nasal spray, the inhalers may be used ad lib for about 12 weeks. The failure to relieve all symptoms of tobacco withdrawal is likely related to the dose or route of administration.

Nicotine Patches

Another means of delivery of nicotine is the nicotine skin patch. Currently, four types of transdermal nicotine patches are available (Table 12-2).[41] Three of the patches are for 24-hour use, and one is for 15-hour (waking) use. Patches applied each morning significantly increase abstinence rates when combined with a behavioral or a smoking cessation program. Their use significantly reduces cravings for cigarettes or other tobacco products. They maintain a steady blood level of nicotine that declines no more than 25% to 40% from peak to trough over the course of the day, allowing simple, convenient, once-daily therapy.[34]

Nicotine patches are generally prescribed beginning with the highest dosing system, except for individuals weighing less than 100 pounds. Two of the patches are available over the counter. Regardless of the product choice, Prostep, Habitrol, Nicoderm, or Nicotrol, each is prescribed for 4 to 6 weeks, with subsequent weaning to the next lower dose for 2 to 4 weeks. Generally, the weaning process takes from a minimum of 6 weeks to a maximum of 12 weeks. Again, these treatments are best combined with a behavioral or a smoking cessation program. Box 12-3 presents guidelines for nicotine patch use.

The use of nicotine patches requires absolute motivation and abstinence during the treatment phase. Adjustments in the dosages of concomitant medications may be necessary, for example, decreases in benzodiazepines, TCAs, beta-blockers,

Table 12-2 Nicotine Transdermal Systems

Agents (trade name)	Dosages (delivery rate in vivo)	Comments (apply to all three systems)
Nicoderm	21 mg/day	Rotate skin sites; consider nonthera-
	14 mg/day	peutic effects (i.e., nicotine excess
	7 mg/day	versus withdrawal symptoms);
Habitrol	21 mg/day	topical reactions are most common
Prostep	14 mg/day	side effect; other side effects, in
	7 mg/day	descending order of frequency, are
	22 mg/day	diarrhea, dyspepsia, muscle ache,
	11 mg/day	abnormal dreams, and insomnia.
Nicotrol	15 mg/day	

Box 12-3 Guidelines for Use of the Nicotine Patch (Nicotine Transdermal Systems)

The goal of the program is complete abstinence.

Patients must read instructions and have questions answered for appropriate use.

Quality, frequency, and intensity of support and a formal smoking cessation program are recommended.

Patients who fail to quit using nicotine should be given a "therapy holiday" before another attempt.

Symptoms of withdrawal and excess overlap and should be considered assiduously.*

Nicotine transdermal systems should not be used for longer than 3 months.

Patches should be applied to a nonhairy, clean, dry site.

Skin sites should be alternated and should not be reused for 1 week.

*Excess nicotine causes abnormal dreams, insomnia, and gastrointestinal symptoms. Withdrawal from nicotine causes anxiety, somnolence, and depression, including somatic symptoms.

---

theophylline, insulin, or beta-adrenergic antagonists. In contrast, an increase in the dosage of adrenergic agonists such as phenylephrine may be necessary when the patient ceases to smoke.

Nontherapeutic effects such as allergic reactions and topical effects may occur as a result of the nicotine patch itself. The regimen for patients with cardiovascular and peripheral vascular diseases should be started carefully, and the benefits of nicotine replacement should be considered in the context of the cardiovascular disease. Patients with ischemic heart disease, severe cardiac arrhythmia, and vasospastic diseases should be screened and evaluated carefully before nicotine replacement is prescribed. Nicotine patches should be used with caution in patients with hyperthyroidism, pheochromocytoma, or insulin-dependent diabetes because nicotine causes the release of catecholamines by the adrenal medulla. Nicotine may delay the healing of peptic ulcers and accelerate hypertension. Because dependence on nicotine chewing gum has been reported, the use of a patch system beyond 3 months should be discouraged.

To minimize the risk of dependence, the patient should be encouraged to gradually withdraw from the nicotine replacement therapy after 4 to 6 weeks, progressively decreasing the dosage every 2 to 4 weeks. The most successful treatment of nicotine dependence combines both pharmacologic and behavioral approaches.

Bupropion (Zyban)

Several clinical studies have shown a high incidence of major depression occurring within days to weeks following smoking cessation and nicotine withdrawal.[22] Patients with personal or family histories of mood disturbances appear to be at great risk for depression following smoking cessation. Antidepressants have been shown to reduce the prevalence of depression and to improve the chances of remaining abstinent from nicotine. Antidepressants reported to be effective include desipramine, doxepin, and bupropion. A sustained-release formulation of bupropion (Zyban) was approved by the U.S. Food and Drug Administration as an adjunct in smoking cessation. The dose of antidepressant is similar to that used for depression. Essentially, 100 to 150 mg of bupropion begun approximately 1 to 2 weeks before the target quit date is advisable, along with brief counseling and education. Clinical trials have shown that sustained-release bupropion in doses of 100 to 300 mg is effective for smoking cessation and is accompanied by reduced weight gain and minimal side effects.[18] An additional study with sustained-release bupropion alone versus combination with a nicotine patch demonstrated significantly higher long-term rates of smoking cessation than those achieved with the use of either the nicotine patch alone or placebo.[20]

Other Forms of Nicotine

Many former smokers have adopted the use of oral tobacco in the form of snuff or chewing tobacco. This practice may reduce the hazards associated with smoke inhalation but does not qualify as a pharmacologic treatment of tobacco dependence.

Teratogenic Effects

Data regarding the teratogenic effects of nicotine in humans are inconclusive. Nicotine has been shown to produce skeletal abnormalities in the offspring of mice and therefore is not recommended for use during pregnancy.

DRUGS USED TO TREAT CANNABIS (MARIJUANA) DEPENDENCE

Some individuals use cannabis daily or almost daily. In many of these individuals, the capacity to function normally is seriously impaired. A withdrawal syndrome that is not life-threatening but that resembles mild sedative withdrawal has been reported. The relationship of this syndrome to marijuana-seeking behavior remains unclear. There are no specific therapeutic agents for cannabis withdrawal or dependence.

DRUGS USED TO TREAT ABUSE OF PHENCYCLIDINE AND SIMILAR AGENTS

Phencyclidine (PCP) is used as an anesthetic in veterinary medicine. The mechanism of action is not well understood, although recently this drug has been shown to bind the so-called sigma opioid receptor in the brain.

PCP intoxication has several definitive features based on empirical data. PCP and other similar agents produce amnestic, euphoric, hallucinatory states, and their effects may be unpredictable, resulting in a prolonged agitated psychosis with impulsive violence directed at self and others. The general approach to detoxification includes isolation in a quiet environment, supportive measures to prevent patients from harming themselves, maintenance of cardiorespiratory functions, and drug treatment that ameliorates psychotic symptoms. The removal of PCP, which is sequestered in acidic gastric fluids, can be aided by judicious use of gastric drainage.

Dopamine blockers such as haloperidol appear to be of value in treating PCP-induced acute psychotic states. Opioids such as meperidine and morphine may be valuable in certain cases but are not conventionally prescribed. In addition to haloperidol, benzodiazepines have been described as useful in decreasing agitation. Psychiatric hospitalization may be necessary in individuals with prolonged psychosis.

DRUGS USED TO TREAT SEDATIVE-HYPNOTIC AND ANXIOLYTIC ABUSE AND DEPENDENCE

Sedative-hypnotic class agents, unlike heroin, cocaine, amphetamines, marijuana, and other abusable substances, are produced almost entirely by pharmaceutical companies. Thus the diversion of these substances originates primarily from pharmaceutical and medical sources. Many adverse effects of sedative abuse may result, including acute drug effects and bodily damage resulting from accidents or overdoses. Discussion of the chronic effects of sedative-hypnotics is beyond the scope of this chapter. The treatment of sedative abuse or dependence usually occurs in two stages: detoxification and long-term treatment. The primary goal of treatment is abstinence.

The type of detoxification recommended is determined by evaluation of the patient's medical condition and social and personal circumstances. If no physical dependence exists, individuals may be treated as outpatients. However, hospitalization may be necessary for successful detoxification. Abrupt withdrawal from sedatives can lead to seizures or to toxic psychosis; death has been reported as a consequence to withdrawal.[30]

Several detoxification techniques are used for sedative-hypnotic class agents; each method involves substituting a prescribed sedative for one that has been abused. Once the patient's condition has been stabilized on a substitute drug regimen, the drug is reduced by approximately 10% per day, a generally acceptable rate of detoxification. The pentobarbital challenge test, presented in Table 12-3, involves the oral administration of 200 mg of pentobarbital followed by close observation to assess the degree of tolerance. Based on the patient's condition after the test dose, an estimated 24-hour pentobarbital requirement is determined; similarly, a phenobarbital substitution technique may be carried out, with the oral substitution of 30 mg of phenobarbital for each 100 mg of the estimated pentobarbital requirement. Medication is administered every 6 hours for approximately 24 hours. If a stabilization dose is reached, the substituted agent may then be reduced as previously described. Phenobarbital is generally preferred because it is longer acting and has better anticonvulsant activity than pentobarbital.

The conditions of patients who are addicted to both sedatives and narcotics must be stabilized on regimens of both types of drugs before detoxification can occur. It is important to remember that patients are restless and anxious and often have insomnia during and after detoxification. Given the significant heterogeneity of sedative abusers, it is essential to attempt to categorize the social and psychologic correlates of drug use in each patient so that a long-term treatment plan can be formulated.

Table 12-3 Pentobarbital Challenge Test: Initial Response to 200 mg of Pentobarbital

Response	Degree of tolerance requirement* (mg)	Patient's condition
Asleep and sedate	None	None
Drowsy; marked intoxication	400-600	Mild
Comfortable; minimal intoxication	600-1000	Marked
No effect	1000	Extreme

*Phenobarbital may be preferred and substituted at a dose of 30 mg for pentobarbital, 100 mg.

Long-term treatment of sedative abuse is customized and may include residential drug-free programs or self-help groups using 12-step counseling techniques. Some patients may be found to have comorbid psychiatric disorders. If pharmacologic treatment is deemed necessary for anxiety, the use of an antidepressant or a nondependence-producing anxiolytic such as buspirone should be considered.

REFERENCES

1. American Psychiatric Association: *Diagnostic and statistical manual of mental disorders-TR*, ed 4, revised, Washington, DC, 2000, The Association.
2. Brook JS and others: The role of older brothers in younger brothers' drug use viewed in context of parent and peer influences, *J Genet Psychol* 151:59, 1990.
3. Brooner RK and others: Antisocial behavior of intravenous drug abusers: implications for diagnosis of antisocial personality disorder, *Am J Psychiatry* 149:482, 1992.
4. Brown RA and others: Cognitive-behavioral treatment for depression in alcoholism, *J Consult Clin Psychol* 65(5):715, 1997.
5. Chick J, Gough K, Falkowski W: Disulfiram treatment of alcoholism, *Br J Psychiatry* 161: 84, 1992.
6. Ciraulo DA and others: Parental alcoholism as a risk factor in benzodiazepine abuse: a pilot study, *Am J Psychiatry* 146:1333, 1989.
7. Cooper JR: Establishing a methadone quality assurance system: rationale and objectives. In *Improving drug abuse treatment. National Institute on Drug Abuse Research Monograph Series #106*, Washington, DC, 1991, DHHS, p. 358.
8. Culhane C: Marijuana's brain receptor found, *US Journal*, Dec 11, 1990:11.
9. Davidson D and others: Effects of naltrexone on alcohol self-administration in heavy drinkers, *Alcohol Clin Exp Res* 23(2):195, 1999.
10. Diakogiannis IA, Steinberg M, Kosten TR: Mazindol treatment of cocaine abuse: a double-blind investigation, *NIDA Res Mongr Ser* 105:514, 1990.
11. Dorus W and others: Lithium treatment of depressed and nondepressed alcoholics, *JAMA* 262:1646, 1989.
12. Ellinwood EH: Amphetamine psychosis: a multidimensional process, *Semin Psychol* 1: 208, 1969.
13. Fishburne PM, Abelson HI, Cisin I: National survey on drug abuse. Main finding: 1979, *Department of Health and Human Services Pub No. ADM-80-976*, Washington, DC, 1980, US Government Printing Office.
14. Greene HL, Goldberg R, Ockene JK: Cigarette smoking: the physician's role in cessation and maintenance, *J Gen Intern Med* 3:75, 1988.
15. Grove WM and others: Heritability of substance abuse and antisocial behavior: a study of monozygotic twins reared apart, *Biol Psychiatry* 27:1293, 1990.
16. Higgins ST, Budney AJ, Bickel WK: Applying behavioral concepts and principles to the treatment of cocaine dependence, *Drug Alcohol Depend* 34:87, 1994.
17. Hughes JR: Treatment of nicotine dependence. In Schuster CR, Gust SW, Kuhar MJ, editors: *Pharmacological aspects of drug dependence: toward an integrative neurobehavioral approach: handbook of experimental psychology series*, vol 11, New York, 1996, Springer-Verlag.
18. Hurt RD and others: A comparison of sustained-release bupropion and placebo for smoking cessation, *N Engl J Med* 337(17):1195, 1997.
19. Jaffe JH: Pharmacological agents in treatment of drug dependence. In Meltzer HY, editor: *The third generation of progress*, New York, 1987, Raven.
20. Jorenby DE and others: A controlled trial of sustained-release bupropion, a nicotine patch, or both for smoking cessation, *N Engl J Med* 340(9):685, 1999.
21. Kandel D, Simcha-Fagan O, Davis M: Risk factors for delinquency and illicit drug use from adolescence to young adulthood, *J Drug Iss* 16:67, 1986.
22. Keltner NL and others: *Psychobiological foundations of psychiatric care*, St Louis, 1998, Mosby.
23. Kosten TR, McCance-Katz E: New pharmacotherapies. In Oldham JM, Riba MB, editors: *Review of psychiatry*, vol 14, Washington, DC, 1995, American Psychiatric Press.

24. Margolin CH and others: Bupropion reduces cocaine abuse in methadone-maintained patients, *Arch Gen Psychiatry* 48:87, 1991.

25. Mason BJ and others: A double-blind placebo-controlled study of oral nalmefene for alcohol dependence, *Arch Gen Psychiatry* 56:719, 1999.

26. Meyer RE: New pharmacotherapies for cocaine dependence . . . revisited, *Arch Gen Psychiatry* 49:900, 1992.

27. Meyer RE: The disease called addiction: emerging evidence in a 200-year debate, *Lancet* 347:162, 1996.

28. Millman RB: General principles of diagnosis and treatment. In Frances AJ, Hales RE, editors: *American Psychiatric Association annual review,* vol 5, Washington, DC, 1986, The Association.

29. Nestler EJ, Fitzgerald LW, Self DW: Neurobiology. In Oldham JM, Riba MB, editors: *Review of psychiatry,* vol 14, Washington, DC, 1995, American Psychiatric Press.

30. O'Brien CP, Woody GE: Sedative-hypnotics and antianxiety agents. In Frances AJ, Hales RE, editors: *American Psychiatric Association annual review,* vol 5, Washington, DC, 1986, The Association.

31. O'Connor PG and others: Ambulatory opiate detoxification and primary care: a role for the primary care physician, *J Gen Intern Med* 7:532, 1992.

32. Olivetto and others: Effect of LAAM dose on opiate use in opioid-dependent patients: a pilot study, *Am J Addict* 7:272, 1998.

33. O'Malley SS and others: Naltrexone and coping skills therapy for alcohol dependence: a controlled study, *Arch Gen Psychiatry* 49:894, 1992.

34. Palmer KJ, Faulds D: Transdermal nicotine: a review of its pharmacodynamic and pharmacokinetic properties, and therapeutic use as an aid to smoking cessation, *Drugs* 44:498, 1992.

35. Regier DA and others: One-month prevalence of mental disorders in the United States, *Arch Gen Psychiatry* 45:977, 1988.

36. Resnick RB, Schuyten-Resnick E, Washton AM: Assessment of narcotic antagonists in the treatment of opioid dependence, *Annu Rev Pharmacol Toxicol* 20:463, 1980.

37. Schuckit MA: Genetic and clinical implications of alcoholism and affective disorder, *Am J Psychiatry* 143:140, 1986.

38. Sass RB, Schuyten-Resnick E, Washton AM: Assessment of narcotic antagonists in the treatment of opioid dependence, *Annu Rev Pharmacol Toxicol* 20:463, 1996.

39. Sellers EM, Higgins GA, Sobell MB: 5-HT and alcohol abuse, *Trends Pharmacol Sci* 13:69, 1992.

40. Shi JM and others: Three methods of ambulatory opiate detoxification, *NIDA Res Monogr Ser No. 132, NIH Publ No. 93-3505,* Washington, DC, 1993, US Government Printing Office.

41. Silagy C and others: Meta-analysis on efficacy of nicotine replacement therapies in smoking cessation, *Lancet* 343:139, 1994.

42. Substance Abuse and Mental Health Services Administration Office of Applied Studies: *Preliminary Estimates from the 1995 National Household Survey on Drug Abuse,* Washington, DC, 1995, U.S. Government Printing Office.

43. Swift RM: Alcoholism and substance abuse. In Stoudemire A, editor: *Clinical psychiatry for medical students,* Philadelphia, 1990, JB Lippincott.

44. Swift RM: Pharmacologic treatments for drug and alcohol dependence: experimental and standard therapies, *Psychiatr Ann* 28(12):697, 1998.

45. Vining E, Kosten TR, Kleber HD: Clinical utility of rapid clonidine-naltrexone detoxification or opioid abuse, *Br J Addict* 83:567, 1988.

46. Volpicelli J and others: Naltrexone in the treatment of alcohol dependence, *Arch Gen Psychiatry* 49:867, 1992.

47. Warner LA and others: Prevalence and correlates of drug use and dependency in the United States. Results from the National Comorbidity Survey, *Arch Gen Psychiatry* 52:219, 1995.

48. Woody GE, McLellan AT, Bedrick J: Dual diagnosis. In Oldham JM, Riba MB, editors: *Review of psychiatry,* vol 14, Washington, DC, 1995.

CHAPTER 13

Sexual Dysfunction

LUIS BENCOMO AND DAVID G. FOLKS

Human sexuality may be affected by biologic, psychologic, or cultural factors. Most of these factors play a role independently or together cause sexual dysfunction. Adequate sexual functioning plays a significant role in a person's ability to form an intimate and loving relationship. Estimates of sexual disorders are variable, but some studies indicate that up to 30% of the population are affected.[31] Multiple factors account for this variability, including the individual's unwillingness to report certain problems. A clinician may also not adequately perform a thorough sexual history of a patient; moreover, bias in sample populations tends to overrepresent sexual dysfunction among the female gender. In some cultures, sexual disorders, whether transitory or enduring, may affect up to 50% of marital or intimate relationships.[21]

The most adequate demographic survey of the incidence and prevalence of sexual dysfunction in the general adult population (18 to 59 years of age) in the United States is the National Health and Social Life Survey (Table 13-1).[18] Among those with medical illnesses or postsurgical conditions, the prevalence of sexual dysfunction resulting from contributing psychologic factors has been difficult to establish because of the covarying effects of the general medical illness. Increased orgasmic and erectile dysfunction occurs among the medically ill, whereas a decrease in the incidence of premature ejaculation occurs in those patients.[31] In about 30% of sexually dysfunctional individuals who have axis I psychiatric disorders (e.g., major depression), the disorder is not a primary etiologic agent in the sexual dysfunction.[14]

Sexual dysfunctions have been traditionally understood as deviations from the normal human sexual response cycle (Box 13-1).[21] Since the 1960s, this model has been the dominant paradigm of sexual response in western cultures. Of course the meaning of sexual behavior and functioning, that is, what makes it unnatural, dysfunctional, or pathologic, must be constructed with a clear understanding of dominant cultural beliefs. Nonetheless, the human sexual response provides clinicians with a relative norm with which they can obtain a clear phenomenology of the specific nature of the sexual dysfunction. The clinician who assesses for sexual dysfunction should consider quantifying both time intervals (e.g., in foreplay) and physiologic responses (e.g., vaginal lubrication). These data are then compared with the human sexual response cycle and further elaborated on in DSM-IV.[3]

Human sexual behavior is motivated behavior in which physiologic drives are expressed bodily, are experienced by a sentient person, and if only in fantasy, nearly always involve an erotic relationship with another person (or object surrogate such as a fetish). When sexual behavior fails despite efforts that are appropriate for the desired end, then sexual dysfunction has occurred. The cause of the dysfunction may be biologic or psychologic or a combination of the two.

Biologic or general medical causes of sexual dysfunction are determined by a careful review of systems as well as a general physical examination. History of an

Table 13-1 Percentage of Sexual Problems in the General Population of Adults (18-59 Years) by Gender

Sexual problem	Men	Women
Lack of interest in having sex	15.7	33.4
Unable to climax	8.2	24.1
Climax too quickly	28.5	10.3
Physical pain during intercourse	3.0	14.4
Sex not pleasurable	8.1	21.2
Anxious about performance	17.0	11.5
Arousal (erection/lubrication) problems	10.4	18.8

From Reference 18.

Box 13-1 Human Sexual Response Cycle

Sexual behavior is characterized by four distinct phases:

1. *Desire phase (appetitive phase):* consists of fantasies of sexual activity and the desire to have sexual activity and involves physical, cognitive, and behavioral components
2. *Excitement phase:* characterized by a subjective sense of sexual excitement and pleasure with accompanying physiologic changes, including penile tumescence in the male and pelvic engorgement and vaginal lubrication and swelling of the external genitalia in the female
3. *Orgasmic phase:* characterized in both sexes by the peaking of sexual pleasure with release of sexual tension and rhythmic contractions of the perineal muscles and pelvic reproductive organs
4. *Resolution phase:* characterized by a sense of general relaxation and well-being, and muscle relaxation (For the man, there is a refractory period to orgasm; however, women can have multiple orgasms without a refractory period.)

An abnormality in any one of the first three phases is usually associated with a DSM-IV diagnosable sexual dysfunction, the exception being the resolution phase, in which there can be postcoital dysphoria and postcoital headaches but no DSM-IV diagnostic sexual dysfunction.

---

endocrine, vascular, or neurologic disorder deserves special attention; other more common medical and surgical causes of sexual dysfunction in men and women are shown in Box 13-2. Drugs are often a precipitant or perpetuator of sexual dysfunction and often contribute to the disorder in patients who are already compromised by disease. Table 13-2 shows many drugs reported to adversely affect sexual response. Alcohol and drug abuse, beta-adrenergic blockers, centrally acting antihypertensives, antiandrogens, and psychotropic agents, especially selective serotonin reuptake inhibitors (SSRIs), are known to cause sexual dysfunction. SSRIs have their primary effect in the orgasmic/ejaculation phases. This topic is discussed in greater detail later in this chapter.

To ascertain the psychologic causes of sexual dysfunction, a complete psychosocial and psychosexual history should be taken. Box 13-3 lists the data

Box 13-2 Medical and Surgical Causes of Sexual Dysfunction

Medical illnesses associated with sexual dysfunction
Cardiovascular
  Atherosclerotic disease
  Hypertension
  Myocardial infarction
  Cardiac failure and angina
Renal
  Chronic renal failure
Genitourinary
  Pelvic-genital infection
  Atrophic vaginitis
  Endometriosis
  Peyronie's disease
  Testicular disease
  Genital trauma
Endocrine
  Diabetes mellitus
  Hypogonadal states

Hyperprolactinemia
Pituitary dysfunction
Thyroid dysfunction
Adrenal disease
Neurologic
  Multiple sclerosis
  Peripheral neuropathy
  Central nervous system tumors
  Stroke
  Spinal chord diseases

Surgical procedures associated with sexual dysfunction
Prostatectomy
Mastectomy
Vaginal surgeries
Episiotomy
Lumbar sympathectomy

important for the assessment of an individual's sexual development and behavior. To obtain sexual data, the clinician should establish an atmosphere of candor and relative comfort. The clinician may then ask any question relevant to the diagnosis and treatment of the sexual dysfunction. If the clinician is confident that the information being obtained is important, then that attitude will be conveyed to the patient and a condition of relative comfort will exist between them. If the sexual history follows the line of questioning and developmental stages suggested in Box 13-3, the patient has a schema of what to expect. This format reduces anxiety and generates a certain degree of structure so that the patient can anticipate what will be asked regarding his or her sexual behavior. Questions will focus on an individual's mental, emotional, and physiologic responses to his or her sexual experience. The human sexual response cycle serves as a framework for appreciating the physiologic response of the patient.

The multiple determinants of sexual dysfunction may not become apparent until the person or couple is in therapy for several sessions. The etiology of cognitions and emotions that cause sexual dysfunction may be understood using a variety of theoretical frameworks. These include psychodynamic, behavioral, cognitive, and social learning theories. Many cases of sexual dysfunction that are psychologic in origin are not directly or universally related to any one specific etiologic event or psychodynamic structure. Thus a careful history elaborating the patient's psychologic constitution is necessary to confirm the pertinent psychologic factors for a given patient.

DIAGNOSTIC CONSIDERATIONS

Sexual disorders are characterized by a disturbance or disruption in the processes that define the human sexual response cycle (see Box 13-1). In addition, pain associated with sexual intercourse may result in a sexual disorder. Sexual dysfunction

Table 13-2 Classes of Medications That May Affect Sexual Response

Drug	Sexual response
Antihypertensives	
Diuretics	Libido, erectile, ejaculation problems
Timolol (ocular)	Libido, erectile, low ejaculate problems
Central-acting adrenergic inhibitors	Libido, erectile, ejaculation problems
Peripheral-acting adrenergic inhibitors	Libido, erectile, ejaculation problems
Alpha-adrenergic blockers	Low incidence of sexual dysfunction
Combined alpha- and beta-adrenergic blockers	Erection, ejaculation, delayed detumescence problems
Vasodilators	No sexual dysfunction
Angiotensin-converting enzyme inhibitors	19% had worsening of sexual dysfunction
Slow channel calcium-entry blocking agents	No reports when used alone
Psychotherapeutic agents	
Antidepressants	Libido, arousal, and orgasm problems with tricyclic antidepressants, monoamine oxidase inhibitors, and selective serotonin reuptake inhibitors, including venlafaxine; no reports of sexual dysfunction with nefazodone and bupropion
	Breast pain, impotence with mirtazapine
	Priapism
	Libido, arousal, and orgasm problems
Lithium	Libido and erectile problems
Carbamazepine	Decreased libido or erectile problems (13%)
Conventional antipsychotics	Libido, erectile, ejaculation problems
Anxiolytics	Libido, erectile, ejaculation problems
Benzodiazepines	Anorgasmia
Buspirone	No reported sexual dysfunction
Stimulants	Impotence, changes in libido
	Exogenous hormones
Hormones	
Androgens	Libido decreased, impotence, testicular atrophy
Anabolic steroids	Azoospermia
Testosterone	No negative effect on sexual function
Estrogens	Decreased vaginal atrophy; decreased libido in males
Cancer agents	
Alkylating chemotherapy agents	Gonadal dysfunction in males and females
Other chemotherapeutic agents	Gonadal dysfunction in males and females with procarbazine and vinblastine
	Suppressed testicular and adrenal androgen synthesis with ketoconazole
Carbonic anhydrase inhibitors	Libido, erectile problems
Antiepileptic drugs	
Carbamazepine, phenytoin	Decreased libido or erectile problems

Adapted from Reference 8.

Box 13-3 Data Gathering in Taking a Comprehensive Sexual History

Childhood
First sex play with peers
Family sleeping arrangements
Sex play with siblings
Sexual abuse, incest, or molestation
Parental attitudes toward sex
Sources of sexual knowledge

Pubertal
Menarche or first ejaculation:
   subjective reaction
Secondary sex characteristics:
   subjective reaction
Body image
Masturbation fantasies and behavior
Homoerotic fantasies and behavior
Dating experiences (physical
   intimacies)
Intercourse
Age at first occurrence
Reaction to first intercourse

Young adult
Lengthy or live-in relationships
Pattern of sexual activities with others
Paraphilic behaviors
Previous marriages
Courtship
Parental attitudes toward spouse
Sexual activity (dysfunction?)
Reasons for termination of marriage
Venereal diseases, including HIV exposure

Adult
Present primary sexual relationship
Development of relationship
Significant nonsexual problems
   (e.g., money, alcohol, in-laws)
Infertility; contraceptive practices
Children (problems?)

Sexual behaviors
Extramarital affairs
Intercourse frequency during
   relationship
Variety of sexual behaviors
   (e.g., oral-genital, masturbation)
Previous dysfunction (in either
   partner)
Elaboration of onset and history of
   present problem (without
   partner present)
Perception of partner's reaction to
   problem
Homosexual activity
Possible exposure to HIV

HIV, Human immunodeficiency virus.

may also result in consistent impairments of the normal patterns of sexual interest or response. A disturbance in the subjective sense of pleasure or desire or in the objective performance of sexual functioning may also result in dysfunction. Sexual dysfunction may be subtyped as being lifelong when the disorder has been present since the onset of sexual functioning. Acquired sexual dysfunction is designated when the sexual dysfunction develops only after an initial period of normal functioning. Acquired sexual disorders may be generalized in cases in which sexual dysfunction is not limited to certain situations, partners, or stimulation. A situationally bound sexual disorder is limited to certain types of stimulation, situations, or partners. Of course, normative sexual functioning and norms of sexual dysfunction are difficult to determine. Sexual functioning varies widely among individuals, based on differing cultural, religious, and other influences.[21]

GENERAL EVALUATION AND TREATMENT PRINCIPLES

Because a patient may have difficulty discussing sexual problems, the presentation of the chief sexual complaint and the history of the present illness may be imprecise. Thus significant time may be required to consider the problem; more than one session may be necessary to complete this task. A patient whose sexual dysfunction involves a partner or spouse should ideally include the partner's view of the problem. Finally, asking patients about their notions concerning the etiology of the sexual disorder and their expectations for treatment is helpful in determining important patient cognitions.

The eventual development of a treatment plan depends on the specifics of each case and requires the consideration of several favorable prognostic factors (Box 13-4). The evaluation will often reveal that sexual dysfunctions are secondary to marital or relationship problems; the sexual complaint is the ticket of entry into the care system, and treatment should initially be based on the presenting complaint. Once treatment has begun, relationship issues may be given priority, and the goals of treatment can be redirected.

FEMALE SEXUAL DISORDERS
Female Hypoactive Sexual Desire Disorder

Female hypoactive sexual desire disorder is characterized by a deficiency or absence of sexual fantasies coupled with a lack of desire for sexual activity. This disturbance affects up to 35% of women.[3,28] Specific causes may include the following: (1) psychologic conflict, (2) problems in the relationship, (3) sexual inhibition, (4) previous unsatisfactory sexual experiences, or (5) history of sexual abuse. Female hypoactive sexual desire disorder may also occur secondary to ongoing depression, anxiety, or situational stress.[14] The disorder may occur in part or wholly due to general medical problems involving hypogonadal states.[13] The diagnosis of hypoactive sexual desire disorder may be difficult to make because it is mainly subjective and there are no specific "norms."

The treatment of hypoactive sexual desire disorder includes sexual therapy, marital and cognitive therapy, and medications, including hormonal intervention. Drugs that have been used successfully include bupropion, testosterone, and

---

Box 13-4 Sexual Dysfunction: More Favorable Prognostic Factors

- Recent onset of symptoms
- Mild to moderate severity of dysfunction
- History of good sexual function
- Identifiable situational stress factors
- Good mental health
- Absence of paraphilia
- A cooperative spouse or partner who is willing to participate in treatment

yohimbine.[29] The use of a testosterone patch, however, may result in virilizing effects. Yohimbine (Yocon), an alpha-2 presynaptic adrenergic antagonist, decreases sympathetic adrenergic activity and increases parasympathetic cholinergic activity. Several clinical reports from uncontrolled trials of yohimbine show varying degrees of efficacy. Because of the potential for side effects, yohimbine's use is not recommended in geriatric, pediatric, female, or psychiatric patients treated with mood-stabilizing drugs or antidepressants. Yohimbine has also been reported to induce panic attacks and may increase the risk of panic attacks in individuals with prior histories of panic attacks.

Female Sexual Aversion Disorder

Sexual aversion disorder is characterized by persistent and recurrent aversion to and avoidance of almost all genital or sexual contact with a sexual partner. This is a rare disorder that often involves a history of sexual abuse or trauma (e.g., incest, rape). Patients may provide a history of a rigid or puritanical background. Marital discord or infidelity by a partner may also contribute to the development of sexual aversion disorder, with or without dyspareunia (painful sexual intercourse).

The treatment of sexual aversion disorder includes cognitive-behavioral therapy, marital therapy, and generally, an attempt to remove any underlying cause. If the aversion is the result of a phobic disorder, benzodiazepines or serotonergic antidepressants such as the SSRIs or $5HT_2$ antagonists (e.g., nefazodone) may be useful in decreasing anxiety and tension.[14,15] For individuals who meet the clinical criteria for traumatic anxiety (acute or posttraumatic), treatments that are generally effective for traumatic anxiety (e.g., SSRIs, monoamine oxidase inhibitors [MAOIs], or $5HT_2$ antagonists) may also improve the symptoms of sexual aversion disorder.

Female Sexual Arousal Disorder

Female sexual arousal disorder is characterized by a persistent or recurrent inability to obtain or maintain adequate lubrication throughout the sexual act. Female sexual arousal disorder occurs in approximately 5% to 30% of women.[31] This disorder is usually associated with decreased libido. The perimenopause or hormonal fluctuations (patterns) in premenopausal women may influence the onset or course of sexual arousal disorder. Medications or other general medical problems may also have an etiologic relationship to the disorder. Psychologic factors or other psychosocial influences may also be responsible for the onset or development of sexual arousal disorder. Guilt, fear, history of sexual trauma, negative attitudes toward sex, or inadequate stimulation may also produce the disturbance.

The treatment of sexual arousal disorder may include hormonal therapy, with the use of estrogen replacement therapy or estrogen creams in menopausal women.[35] The application of lubricating gels has also been successful. Treatment should be preceded by a general medical and psychosocial history to determine the possibility of other underlying causes. Cognitive-behavioral therapy and psychoeducational approaches have also been effective modalities in the treatment of sexual arousal disorder.

Female Orgasmic Disorder

Female orgasmic disorder is characterized by delayed or absent orgasm following a normal phase of sexual excitement. This disorder is common and affects up to 25% of women.[31] Inhibited orgasms may be lifelong or acquired. However, most cases involve individuals who have experienced this orgasmic disorder over the course of their lives.

Orgasmic disorder may be generalized or situational. For example, the patient may be able to obtain orgasm through self-masturbatory practices but not with her partner. Multiple factors may contribute to the disturbance. These factors include adequacy (or inadequacy) of sexual stimulation, conflict in the interpersonal relationship with a sexual partner, medications, and other biologic problems that may contribute to the disorder. A thorough psychosexual and general medical history may serve to delineate the cause(s) of this dysfunction.

The treatment for inhibited orgasm (anorgasmia) is a program of directed masturbation that may be effectively used together with individual or couples therapy. Sildenafil (Viagra) has also been used for this purpose in clinical practice; however, this agent does not currently have a U.S. Food and Drug Administration (FDA) indication for treatment of inhibited orgasm disorder or drug-induced anorgasmia in women.[5] Moreover, medication-induced orgasmic disorders can be effectively treated.

Dyspareunia

Dyspareunia is characterized by recurrent and consistent genital pain associated with sexual intercourse. This disorder often is associated with vaginismus or is secondary to surgical procedures or a history of salpingitis or endometriosis. Patients often complain of chronic pelvic pain. Multiple psychosocial or psychologic factors may contribute to dyspareunia. Misconceptions about sexual intercourse, fear, and anxiety may also contribute to the disturbance. A history of rape or childhood sexual abuse may be found in some cases of dyspareunia. In these cases, the patient may meet clinical criteria for posttraumatic stress disorder, and antidepressant or anxiolytic medications may be useful.

Treatment generally begins with a thorough general medical examination with a focus on gynecologic and neurologic examinations to rule out underlying general medical disorders. Direct treatment may include psychoeducational approaches or formal psychotherapy focused on the issues of sexual trauma, using cognitive-behavioral (exposure) techniques as well as anxiety management techniques such as stress inoculation and relaxation. Treatment may also include the use of marital or couples therapy when the focus of treatment is on relationship difficulties.

Vaginismus

Vaginismus is characterized by interference with sexual intercourse as a result of recurrent or persistent involuntary spasm of the musculature of the outer third of the vagina. General medical causes may be responsible for vaginismus.

Vaginismus is most commonly found in individuals who have experienced a sexual trauma or abuse with subsequent psychosexual conflicts. A strict or puritanical religious upbringing may sometimes be responsible for the development of vaginismus in adulthood. Treatment generally includes a thorough psychosexual evaluation to rule out underlying causes that may benefit from treatment. Psychotherapeutic approaches focus on anxiety management techniques using relaxation and desensitization. Other treatments include the systematic insertion of dilators of graduated sizes to decrease the spasm that occurs with this disorder. Individuals with underlying syndromes of anxiety or depression are best treated with antidepressant or anxiolytic medications, as discussed in Chapters 6 and 7.

MALE SEXUAL DYSFUNCTION

Male sexual dysfunction has more often been recognized by clinicians and patients since the introduction of sildenafil (Viagra). A significant number of male sexual dysfunction continue to go unreported.[25,31] As with female sexual disorders, the estimates for specific male sexual disorders are variable. Contributing factors include the patient's unwillingness to report sexual dysfunction, the clinicians' inadequate evaluation of sexual functioning, and bias in sample populations. Thus the rates for male sexual dysfunction vary widely, with the most frequently reported condition being premature ejaculation (at rates of 30% to 40%), followed by male erectile disorder (occurring at a rate of approximately 20% to 30%). Incidentally, the prevalence of male erectile disorder has been "increasing" because of increased clinician and patient awareness of the problem. Male orgasmic disorder is less frequently reported and is estimated to occur in approximately 5% to 10% of the male population. Dyspareunia is rarely reported in the male population.

Similar to female sexual disorders, male sexual disorders are categorized as sexual desire disorders, sexual arousal disorders, orgasmic disorders, and sexual pain disorders. Sexual dysfunction in men may be secondary to general medical conditions, including systemic illnesses or consequences of surgical procedures. Substance-induced sexual dysfunction may be related to a specific substance of abuse, including alcohol and prescribed medications. These disorders may be further subtyped into lifelong, acquired, generalized, or situational disorders.

Male Hypoactive Sexual Desire

Male hypoactive sexual desire is characterized by a general deficiency or absence of sexual desire. The diagnosis may be difficult to confirm because the condition is based on a subjective feeling with no norms.[18] A wide variability of sexual desire is reported among various patient populations. The estimated prevalence of hypoactive sexual desire in men is 15%. A lack of self-reporting of hypoactive sexual desire suggests that the condition is more common. This disorder often coexists in patients who experience erectile dysfunction.[9]

The evaluation and treatment of hypoactive sexual disorder includes a general medical evaluation to ascertain the presence of substance use disorder or general medical conditions or to identify an etiologic relationship with prescribed medications. This screening also includes a laboratory assessment to evaluate testosterone levels.[10] A psychosexual history is performed to rule out the presence of marital discord, conflict in a relationship, or other psychologic factors that may contribute to the disturbance.

Treatment options for hypoactive sexual desire disorder include cognitive-behavioral therapy, couples therapy, and medication. If testosterone levels are found to be low, supplementation with hormonal treatment is indicated. Medications such as yohimbine, an alpha antagonist, at 5.4 to 10.8 mg/day in divided doses, and bupropion (Wellbutrin) at 100 to 300 mg/day in divided doses, have been reported to improve sexual desire in men.[19,29] Of course, depression, including subsyndromal depression, or anxiety disorders may contribute to the disorder and must be treated accordingly.

Male Sexual Aversion Disorder

Sexual aversion disorder is characterized by persistent or extreme aversion or avoidance of genital sexual contact with a partner. This disorder is rare and requires general medical assessment and psychosexual evaluation to consider an underlying cause. Causative factors include a history of childhood sexual abuse, physical trauma, marital discord, and extreme anger or resentment toward the partner. Treatment includes cognitive-behavioral therapy, marital therapy, and counseling to assist the patient in processing past abuse issues and conflicts.

Male Erectile Disorder

Male erectile disorder is characterized by a persistent or recurrent inability to attain or maintain an adequate erection to complete the sexual act. Male erectile disorder occurs in approximately 20% to 25% of men.[6] The incidence and prevalence is higher among individuals 50 years of age and older. Risk factors for erectile dysfunction include aging, chronic illness, surgery, trauma of any kind, and various medications (Boxes 13-5 and 13-6). Psychologic factors may serve to cause inhibition of erectile mechanisms without the presence of a general medical problem or structural lesion.[36] For most patients, both psychologic and biologic etiologies are involved.

Erectile dysfunction is associated with a high incidence of depressive symptoms, regardless of age, marital status, or comorbidity.[30] Patients with erectile dysfunction have decreased libidos compared with control subjects. In addition, patients with depressive symptoms have lower libidos than patients without depressive symptoms. Patients with erectile dysfunction and depressive symptoms are more likely to discontinue treatment than are other patients with erectile dysfunction alone. These data emphasize the importance of multidisciplinary approaches to the treatment of erectile dysfunction.

A comprehensive sexual history, including the number of erections, time intervals, and quality of erections, are of utmost importance. In addition, the masturbatory capacity of the individual must be assessed to rule out situational causes of erectile dysfunction. A thorough general medical history and physical examination are performed to determine whether the erectile dysfunction may be caused by an illness

---

Box 13-5 Risk Factors and Illnesses Associated with Erectile Dysfunction

Cardiovascular
Hypertension
Myocardial failure

Neurologic
Multiple sclerosis
Sympathectomy
Central nervous system tumors
Neuropathy

Endocrinologic
Diabetes mellitus
Hypogonadism
Hyperthyroidism/hypothyroidism

Genitourinary
Peyronie's disease

Psychiatric disorders
Depression and anxiety

Surgery and trauma
Spinal cord injury
Abdominal perineal resection
Prostatectomy
Sympathectomy
Irradiation

or medication. A thorough psychosocial history serves to assess whether conflict in a relationship or other psychologic conflicts may be responsible for the erectile dysfunction. Laboratory assessment includes the evaluation of testosterone and prolactin levels as well as a comprehensive metabolic panel and testing of thyroid function. Other tests that may be performed include penile tumescence studies and prostate-specific antigen (PSA) levels.

The treatment of erectile dysfunction may include the use of surgical, mechanical, and pharmacologic interventions. Surgical or mechanical interventions may use vacuum constriction devices.[33] These devices generate negative pressure and cause tumescence, which is maintained by a constriction band at the penile base. Some reports indicate that vacuum constriction devices are effective in up to 90% of patients. Disadvantages include a lack of spontaneity, penile irritation, decreased penile sensation, and decreased ejaculation. Other devices used in the treatment of erectile dysfunction are penile implants and prosthetic devices. These devices are usually considered second- or third-line choices when other treatments have failed.

Box 13-6 Medications Associated with Erectile Dysfunction

Diuretics
Thiazides
Spironolactone

Antihypertensives
Methyldopa
Clonidine
Reserpine
Beta-blockers
Guanethidine
Verapamil

Cardiac
Clofibrate
Gemfibrozil
Digoxin

Tranquilizers
Phenothiazines
Butyrophenones

Antidepressants
Tricyclic antidepressants
Monoamine oxidase inhibitors
Lithium
Selective serotonin reuptake inhibitors

H$_2$ Antagonists
Cimetidine
Ranitidine

Hormones
Estrogens
Progesterone
Corticosteroids
Cyproterone acetate
Eulexin
Proscar
Gonadotropin-releasing hormone
    agonists

Cytotoxic agents
Cyclophosphamide
Methotrexate
Roferon-A

Anticholinergics
Disopyramide
Anticonvulsants

Miscellaneous
Metoclopramide
Baclofen
Carbonic anhydrase inhibitors
Nonsteroidal antiinflammatory
    drugs
Tobacco
Alcohol
Amphetamines
Opioids

They can cause poor sensation and are associated with a high risk of infection at the site of the prosthesis.

Erectile dysfunction has been pharmacologically treated since the early 1980s. Papaverine and phentolamine have been used alone or in combination.[1] These agents are injected into the corpus cavernosa. Papaverine is a medication that increases intracellular cyclic adenosine monophosphate (cAMP). Phentolamine is a competitive alpha-1 and alpha-2 antagonist and is a direct relaxant of smooth muscle. Disadvantages of using these medications include pain at the injection site and a lack of spontaneity. These medications are also contraindicated in patients who take MAOIs. The urethral suppository alprostadil, a PGE_1 smooth muscle relaxant, has been used and carries a success rate of approximately 50%.[23] Side effects of alprostadil include pain and hypotension.

Oral pharmacologic agents in the treatment of erectile dysfunction include yohimbine, apomorphine, and sildenafil. Yohimbine has been prescribed in dosages of 5.4 to 10.8 mg with variable results.[24] Yohimbine is an alpha-2 antagonist that causes vasodilation. Adverse effects include nausea, anxiety, tremor, and palpitations. Apomorphine is a direct central D_2 receptor agonist; one tablet is typically taken sublingually, resulting in variable receptor agonist effects.[27] As with yohimbine, apomorphine has been studied only in small numbers of individuals; open-label clinical reports have yielded variable results.

Sildenafil is effective in a broad range of patients and has been reported to improve erections in numerous placebo-controlled trials.[7] Sildenafil is usually dosed initially at 50 mg and should be taken approximately 1 hour before sexual activity. The maximum dose of sildenafil is 100 mg, to be used no more than once daily. The effect of sildenafil lasts for approximately 4 hours.

Sildenafil is a selective inhibitor of cyclic guanosine monophosphate (cGMP) phosphodiesterase. This medication prevents the breakdown of cGMP and results in enhanced calcium efflux from cells. The precise mechanism of action of sildenafil is based on the physiologic mechanisms of erection of the penis, which involves the release of nitric oxide (NO) in the corpus cavernosum during sexual stimulation. NO then activates the enzyme guanylate cyclase, which results in increased levels of cGMP, producing smooth muscle relaxation in the corpus cavernosum and allowing the inflow of blood. Sildenafil has no direct relaxant effect on isolated human corpus cavernosum but enhances the effect of NO by inhibiting phosphodiesterase type 5 (PDE5), which is responsible for the degradation of cGMP in the corpus cavernosum. When sexual stimulation causes local release of NO, inhibition of PDE5 by sildenafil increases levels of cGMP in the corpus cavernosum, resulting in smooth muscle relaxation and the inflow of blood.

Clinical trials of sildenafil involved more than 3000 patients, 19 to 87 years of age, with erectile dysfunction of varying causes (biologic, psychologic, and mixed), with a mean duration of 5 years. Twenty-one studies were completed, and all resulted in statistical improvement compared with placebo. The greatest improvements were noted at doses of 50 and 100 mg, respectively. Regardless of baseline severity, cause, race, and age, sildenafil was effective in a broad range of patients, including those with histories of coronary artery disease, hypertension, other cardiac disease, peripheral vascular disease, diabetes mellitus, depression, coronary artery bypass graft, radical prostatectomy, transurethral resection of the prostate, and spinal cord injury, as well as in patients taking antidepressant, antipsychotic, or antihypertensive medications. Patients less likely to benefit were those with atherosclerotic disease restricting blood flow.

Sildenafil potentiates the hypotensive effects of nitrates and therefore is contraindicated in patients who are concurrently using organic nitrates (Box 13-7).

Box 13-7 Nitrates Contraindicated in Combination with Sildenafil

Generic name	Trade name
Isosorbide dinitrate	Isordil and Sorbitrate
Isosorbide mononitrate	Ismo, Monoket, and Imdur
Nitroglycerin IV	Tridil and Nitro-Bid
Nitroglycerin ointment 2%	Nitro-Bid and Nitrol
Nitroglycerin spray	Nitrolingual
Nitroglycerin sublingual	Nitrostat
Nitroglycerin SR	Nitro-Bid
Nitroglycerin, transdermal	Deponit, Minitran, Nitro-Dur, Nitrodisc, and Transderm-Nitro

---

Use of sildenafil may not be advisable with anatomic deformation of the penis or in patients who have conditions that may predispose them to priapism (e.g., sickle cell anemia, multiple myeloma, leukemia). Sildenafil metabolism is principally mediated by cytochrome P-450 isoenzyme 3A4. Drugs that inhibit this isoenzyme have been shown to increase levels of sildenafil plasma concentrations, and include cimetidine, erythromycin, clarithromycin, ketoconazole, and other drugs that inhibit the metabolism of P-450 3A4.

In clinical trials, sildenafil exhibited adverse effects, which most commonly included headache (16%), flushing (10%), dyspepsia (7%), nasal congestion (4%), and abnormal vision (3%). The abnormal vision was mild and transient, predominantly resulting in a color tinge to vision, increased sensitivity to light, or blurred vision. More than a 100-mg dose produced significant dyspepsia in 17% of the patients. The recommended dose is 50 mg orally as needed, 1 hour before sexual activity, with a range of 30 minutes to 4 hours before sexual activity. Based on effectiveness and tolerability, the dose may be increased to a maximum of 100 mg or decreased to 25 mg. The maximum recommended dosing frequency is once per day. The cost of the drug is approximately $7 per tablet. The 25-, 50-, and 100-mg strengths are all the same cost, and insurance coverage varies, with some companies providing limitations of 6 to 10 tablets per month.

The understanding of erectile dysfunction has increased in the past few years.[26] The introduction of sildenafil together with a better understanding of the underlying disorders has resulted in more frequent diagnosis as well as increased awareness by the public and by clinicians. Oral agents such as sildenafil enable clinicians to treat this disorder more readily. Media attention and direct consumer marketing have also increased the number of patient inquiries about erectile dysfunction.

Male Disorders of Orgasm

Male orgasmic disorder is characterized by a persistent delay in or the absence of orgasm following a normal phase of sexual excitement. This disturbance is uncommon in men, affecting approximately 1% to 2% of the general population.[25,29] Orgasmic disorders are generally associated with negative attitudes toward sex, most often in individuals who come from strict religious or puritanical backgrounds.[18] This reflects a cultural perspective in which sex has negative connotations, or is taboo or sinful. Another cause of this disorder is marital discord or distress or other relationship problems.

The treatment of male orgasmic disorder includes a thorough evaluation to rule out underlying general medical problems, substance use disorder, or medications that may contribute to the disorder. If psychologic or psychosocial factors are identified, sexual therapy may be efficacious in treating this disorder.

Premature ejaculation is an orgasmic disorder characterized by persistent or recurrent ejaculation that occurs with minimal sexual stimulation. The ejaculation occurs before or soon after penetration and before the individual wishes ejaculation to occur. This disorder is the most common problem among men with sexual dysfunction.[25] It occurs in approximately 30% to 40% of adult men. Some of the factors etiologically related to premature ejaculation include severe psychosocial stress, anxiety or depressive disorders, or significant levels of anger.[32] Premature ejaculation tends to occur in individuals of a younger age.

The nonpharmacologic approach to the treatment of premature ejaculation includes individual counseling or couples therapy. Successful interventions include the "start/stop" technique, or another successful procedure, the "squeeze" technique, developed by Masters and Johnson.[20] These behavioral treatments have a success rate of approximately 60% to 95%. However, many individuals will relapse, with only 25% successfully treated at 3 years.

The pharmacologic treatment of premature ejaculation includes use of SSRIs or clomipramine, which have been successfully and paradoxically used in these cases. The SSRIs are known to increase the intravaginal ejaculatory latency time; various reports of treatment of premature ejaculation have described the utility of the SSRIs. Controlled studies as well as open-label trials of SSRIs in the treatment of medication suggest that paroxetine (Paxil) is associated with the longest delay in ejaculatory latency time.[34] Fluoxetine (Prozac) and sertraline (Zoloft) have also been reported as being effective.[4,22] Clomipramine (Anafranil), an SRI, has also been reported to be effective in these cases.[2] The usual doses for SSRIs in the treatment of premature ejaculation are the same as the usual starting doses for depression. SSRIs may be used intermittently (i.e., with pulse dosing) or routinely (i.e., scheduled). Studies in which SSRIs were prescribed on a scheduled basis have shown superior efficacy in treating premature ejaculation.

SEXUAL DYSFUNCTION CAUSED BY MEDICATION AND MEDICAL DISORDERS

Sexual disorders secondary to chronic illnesses, chronic pain, or the side effects of medications may be reversed by general medical interventions. Improvement in the patient's overall physical condition and relief of pain may restore sexual function. Drug holidays, a change of medication, or discontinuation of medication may sometimes reverse medication-induced sexual dysfunction.

Sexual dysfunction secondary to acute effects of substance abuse or alcoholism often remits once the abuse is controlled. Prolactin-secreting tumors may be treated by surgical resection or administration of bromocriptine. Inhibited desire in men or male arousal disorders may be treated with the use of exogenous testosterone, provided there is no evidence of prostate cancer. Sexual dysfunction caused by trauma, disease, or the sequelae of surgery may be treated by using the general principles of rehabilitation medicine. Those with irreversible damage may be taught sexual techniques that enable them to maintain sexual relationships and referred to self-help associations such as multiple sclerosis, ostomy, and cardiac support groups.

Sexual dysfunction secondary to estrogen deficiency may be responsive to estrogen replacement therapy (provided no medical contraindications exist), which improves the patient's sense of well-being and increases the ability to lubricate vaginally. Postmenopausal women for whom hormonal replacement therapy is contraindicated should be informed about over-the-counter vaginal lubricants.

Multiple psychotropic medications can induce sexual dysfunction. Antidepressants, antipsychotics, and anxiolytics are the medications most often described in the literature.[11,16,29] The current literature focuses on the SSRIs because they are the most widely prescribed antidepressant and psychotropic agents.[12,17] Initial data for the SSRIs reported the incidence of sexual dysfunction at 3% to 10%; however, newer data indicate that rates up to 60% occur, compared with rates of 96% occurring with the tricyclic antidepressant (TCA) clomipramine. The clinical criteria for substance-induced sexual dysfunction are outlined in Box 13-8.

Specific neurotransmitter systems may be involved in the pathophysiology of drug-induced sexual dysfunction. Dopamine has a key role in facilitating desire and sexual arousal. Norepinephrine may also facilitate sexual desire. Serotonin has an inhibitory effect, although some studies have suggested that $5HT_{1A}$ receptors have a role in increasing sexual behavior. Prolactin, as previously mentioned, has also been implicated as having a negative influence on sexual arousal. Some antipsychotics and SSRIs increase the release of prolactin from the hypothalamus and may cause hyperprolactinemia, which in turn may cause sexual dysfunction. Examples include risperidone and citalopram.

Antidepressant-induced sexual dysfunction may include decreased libido or desire, disorders of arousal, and disorders of orgasm. Clinicians need to screen patients for other possible causes of sexual dysfunction before attributing sexual dysfunction to a specific antidepressant medication. General medical conditions or coexisting psychiatric disorders (e.g., depression) may cause sexual dysfunction. A thorough sexual history may also help determine whether psychosocial factors or psychologic causes account for the sexual dysfunction.

SSRIs have been reported to cause sexual dysfunction across the sexual response cycle except in the resolution phase. Decreased sexual desire has been reported with the SSRIs in various reports with the incidence ranging from 40% to 60%. SSRIs have not been associated with, or implicated in, sexual aversion disorder.[27] Sexual arousal disorders are an uncommon side effect of SSRIs in women. However, a few reports have paradoxically implicated SSRIs in increasing sexual arousal in women. SSRIs have been associated with erectile disorder in men, however, much less often

---

Box 13-8 Criteria for Substance-Induced Sexual Dysfunction

- Clinically significant sexual dysfunction that results in marked distress or interpersonal difficulty predominates in the clinical picture
- Evidence from the history, physical examination, or laboratory findings that the sexual dysfunction is fully explained by a substance use or medication
- The disturbance is not better accounted for by sexual dysfunction that is not substance or medication induced

Specify: With Impaired Desire, With Impaired Arousal, With Impaired Orgasm, With Sexual Pain

Modified from American Psychiatric Association: *Diagnostic and statistical manual-TR*, ed 4, Washington, DC, 2000, The Association.

than with TCAs or MAOIs. Paroxetine is the SSRI most often associated with erectile dysfunction, probably because of its significant anticholinergic effect.

Delay in orgasm and absence of orgasm are often encountered as adverse effects of SSRIs in both men and women.[28] This is probably a result of the central serotonergic inhibitory effects of these agents. Reports that both men and women experience spontaneous orgasms while taking SSRIs have also emerged. However, no cases of premature ejaculation caused by SSRIs have been documented. No reports of dyspareunia or vaginismus caused by SSRIs have been published. Nor have reports of painful ejaculation occurred, except in the TCAs clomipramine and imipramine.

The treatment of SSRI-induced sexual dysfunction requires a thorough evaluation of other possible causes of the sexual dysfunction. These include underlying general medical conditions, substance use disorders, comorbid psychiatric disturbances, or a primary sexual disorder. After a thorough evaluation, SSRI-induced sexual dysfunction may be treated with the antidotes shown in Table 13-3.

Table 13-3 Drugs Used to Treat Antidepressant-Induced Sexual Dysfunction

Drug	Symptom/indicator	Dosage
Bethanecol	Erectile dysfunction	10-40 mg prn
Amantadine	Anorgasmia	100 mg prn; 1 hr before sexual activity
	Erectile dysfunction	100 mg bid
	Hypoactive desire	100 mg bid
Bupropion	Anorgasmia	75-150 mg prn; 1-2 hr before sexual activity
	Hypoactive desire	75-150 mg bid
	Arousal	75-150 mg bid
Buspirone	Anorgasmia	20-60 mg/day
	Hypoactive desire	20-60 mg/day
	Erectile dysfunction	20-60 mg/day
Cyproheptadine	Anorgasmia	4-16 mg prn; 1 hr before sexual activity
	Hypoactive desire	4-16 mg/day
Dextroamphetamine	Anorgasmia	5-20 mg prn
	Hypoactive desire	2.5-5 mg bid
Granisetron	Anorgasmia	1 mg prn; 1 hr before sexual activity
Gingko biloba	Hypoactive desire	60 mg bid-qid
Methylphenidate	Anorgasmia	5-20 mg prn
	Hypoactive desire	5-20 mg/day
	Arousal	5-20 mg/day
Pemoline	Anorgasmia	18.75 mg prn
	Hypoactive desire	18.75-75 mg/day
	Arousal	18.75-75 mg/day
Sildenafil	Erectile dysfunction	50-100 mg/day; 4 hr-1/2 hr before sexual activity
Yohimbine	Anorgasmia	5.4-10.8 mg prn
	Hypoactive desire	5.4 mg/day to 5.4 mg tid
	Arousal	5.4 mg/day to 5.4 mg tid

REFERENCES

1. Althof SE and others: Sexual, psychological and marital impact of self-injection of papaverine and phentolamine: a long-term prospective study, *J Sex Marital Ther* 17:101, 1991.

2. Althof SE and others: A double-blind crossover trial of clomipramine for rapid ejaculation in 15 couples, *J Clin Psychiatry* 56:402, 1995.

3. American Psychiatric Association: *Diagnostic and statistical manual-TR,* ed 4, Washington DC, 2000, The Association.

4. Balon R: Antidepressants in the treatment of premature ejaculation, *J Sex Marital Ther* 22:85, 1996.

5. Bartlik B and others: Medications with the potential to enhance sexual responsivity in women, *Psychiatr Ann* 29:46, 1999.

6. Benet AE, Melman A: The epidemiology of erectile dysfunction, *Urol Clin North Am* 22(4):699, 1995.

7. Bootell M, Gepi-Attee S, Gingell JC, Allen MMJ: Sildenafil, a novel effective oral therapy for male erectile dysfunction, *Br J Urol* 78:257, 1996.

8. Buffum J: Prescription drugs and sexual function, *Psychiatr Med* 10:181, 1992.

9. Buvat J and others: Recent developments in the clinical assessment and diagnosis of erectile dysfunction, *Ann Sex Res* 1:265, 1990.

10. Carani C and others: Effects of androgen treatment in impotent men with normal and low levels of free testosterone, *Arch Sex Behav* 19:223, 1990.

11. Crenshaw TL, Goldberg JP: *Sexual pharmacology: drugs that affect sexual function,* New York, 1996, WW Norton.

12. Ellison JM: Antidepressant-induced sexual dysfunction: review, classification, and suggestions for treatment, *Harvard Rev Psychiatry* 6:177, 1998.

13. Fagan PJ, Schmidt CW Jr: Sexual dysfunction in the medically ill. In Stoudemire A, Fogel BS, editors: *Psychiatric care of the medical patient,* ed 2, New York, 2000, Oxford University Press.

14. Fagan PJ and others: Sexual dysfunction and dual psychiatric diagnoses, *Compr Psychiatry* 29:278, 1988.

15. Gitlin MJ: Psychotropic medications and their effects on sexual function: diagnosis, biology, and treatment approaches, *J Clin Psychiatry* 55:406, 1994.

16. Gitlin MJ: Sexual side effects of psychotropic medications, *Psychiatr Clin North Am Annu Drug Ther* 4:61, 1997.

17. Labbate LA: Sex and serotonin reuptake inhibitor antidepressants, *Psychiatr Ann* 29:571, 1999.

18. Laughman E, Gagnon J, Michael R, Michaels S: *Sex in America,* Chicago, 1994, University of Chicago Press.

19. Mann K and others: Effects of yohimbine on sexual experiences and nocturnal penile tumescence and rigidity in erectile dysfunction, *Arch Sex Behav* 25:1, 1996.

20. Masters WH, Johnson VE: *Human sexual inadequacy,* Boston, 1970, Little, Brown.

21. Masters WH, Johnson VE: *Human sexual response,* Boston, 1970, Little, Brown.

22. Mendels J, Camera A, Sikes C: Sertraline treatment for premature ejaculation, *J Clin Psychopharmacol* 15:341, 1995.

23. Padma-Nathan H and others: Treatment of men with erectile dysfunction with transurethral alprostadil, *N Engl J Med* 336:107, 1997.

24. Pittler EE: Yohimbine for erectile dysfunction: a systematic review and meta-analysis of randomized clinical trials, *J Urol* 159(2):433, 1998.

25. Sadock VA: Normal human sexuality and sexual and gender identity disorders. In Sadock BJ, Sadock VA, editors: *Comprehensive textbook of psychiatry,* ed 7, Philadelphia, 2000, Lippincott Williams & Wilkins.

26. Schiavi RC, Segraves RT: The biology of sexual function, *Psychiatr Clin North Am* 18:7, 1995.

27. Segraves RT: Effects of psychotropic drugs on human erection and ejaculation, *Arch Gen Psychiatry* 46:275, 1989.

28. Segraves RT: Antidepressant-induced orgasm disorder, *J Sex Marital Ther* 21:192, 1995.

29. Segraves RT: Effects of antipsychotic, antianxiety, and mood-stabilizing agents on sexual functioning, *Primary Psychiatry* 6:37, 1999.

30. Shabsigh R and others: Increased incidence of depressive symptoms in men with erectile dysfunction, *Urology* 52:848, 1998.
31. Spector HP, Carey MP: Incidence and prevalence of the sexual dysfunctions: a critical review of the empirical literature *Arch Sex Behav* 19:389, 1990.
32. Strassberg DS and others: The role of anxiety in premature ejaculation: a psychophysiological model, *Arch Sex Behav* 19:251, 1990.
33. Turner LA and others: External vacuum devices in the treatment of erectile dysfunction: a one-year study of sexual and psychosocial impact, *J Sex Marital Ther* 17:81, 1991.
34. Waldinger MD, Hengeveld MW, Zinderman AH: Paroxetine treatment of premature ejaculation: a double-blind, randomized, placebo-controlled study, *Am J Psychiatry* 151: 1377, 1994.
35. Walling M, Andersen BL, Johnson SR: Hormonal replacement therapy for postmenopausal women: a review of sexual outcomes and related gynecologic effects, *Arch Sex Behav* 19: 119, 1990.
36. Weiss HD: The physiology of human erection *Ann Intern Med* 76:793, 1972.

UNIT III

Drug Issues Related to Psychopharmacology

CHAPTER 14

Drugs Used
for Electroconvulsive Therapy

*"In 1959, I vividly remember visiting a psychiatric hospital in Indonesia
where ECT was administered without the use of any special apparatus. In
this hospital, they used only the cord from the electric outlet connected to two
electrodes strapped to the patient's temples. At the time of the treatment, a
nurse was stationed at the electrical outlet holding the plug in her hand.
At a nod from the doctor, the nurse inserted the plug into the outlet and
an immediate grand mal seizure ensued. With the next nod, the plug was
withdrawn, and the patient had his convulsion and recovered uneventfully."*

Memoirs of Zimund M. Lebensohn (1999).

Electroconvulsive therapy (ECT) is an effective and predictable treatment option for
individuals with severe or refractory depression.[42,47,64] Although this treatment form
has undergone considerable scrutiny, it remains a major psychiatric intervention. In
1995, approximately 60,000 people in the United States underwent ECT, translating
into 1 million individual treatments.[54] Between 6% and 8% of psychiatrists provide
this treatment.[29,50] This once reviled and supposedly barbaric treatment has
recaptured a strong endorsement from clinicians and a renewed interest from the
media. A book titled *Undercurrents: A Therapist's Reckoning With Her Own Depression*
tells the story of Dr. Martha Manning, a clinical psychologist, whose depression
became so debilitating she agreed to ECT. In a television appearance, Dr. Manning
convincingly recommended ECT for those not helped by antidepressants. Like most
patients who benefit from ECT, her attitude toward this treatment is favorable.[34,46]

HISTORY OF ECT

ECT is a somatic, or physical, therapy. Somatic therapies are basically a European
contribution and have led to Nobel Prizes for two individuals. The first recognized
somatic therapy was developed by von Jauregg of Vienna in 1918.[35] He used malarial
therapy to treat general paresis, winning the Nobel Prize in 1927 for his efforts. Four
more somatic therapies were developed in the 1930s. In 1933, insulin shock
(convulsive) therapy was developed by Sakel in Vienna. In 1934, Metrazol convulsive
therapy was developed by von Meduna in Hungary. In 1935, psychosurgery was
developed by Muniz in Portugal, and in 1938, ECT was developed by Drs. Ugo
Cerletti and Luciano Bini in Rome. Insulin and Metrazol convulsive therapies were
abandoned more than 50 years ago because of unpredictability, relative ineffective-
ness, and a propensity to instill doom. Psychosurgery, although the source of a Nobel
Prize for Dr. Muniz in 1949, is rarely used today. Only ECT remains a mainstream
treatment option.

ECT, available for more than half a century, has proved to be remarkably safe and
effective.[4,27] During those 50 years, critics emerged and affected both public and

professional perceptions of this treatment. ECT has weathered these concerns and misperceptions and continues in use today.

As noted, ECT emerged as a treatment form in 1938. Within 2 years, ECT was being administered to patients in the United States. Its adoption was swift and far-ranging as clinicians responsible for large numbers of patients in overcrowded and underfunded public hospitals looked for answers. Lebensohn captures the essence of the new treatment's acceptance when he writes, "Most treatment methods in medicine that are relatively easy to administer are often overused at first."[35] It was.

Although ECT proved to be effective, its theoretical underpinning was faulty. Early 20th century psychiatrists such as von Meduna believed schizophrenia and epilepsy were incompatible.[58] Although not true, this false belief led to an effective treatment form.

The early advocates of ECT envisioned dramatic relief from severe mental illness in an era in which the only psychopharmacologic weapons were barbiturates, bromides, paraldehyde, and chloral hydrate. Over time, inappropriate use, overuse, and disappointing results, coupled with growing distrust of psychiatric hospitals, created a climate of hostility toward ECT. The emergence of antipsychotics and other psychopharmacologic agents in the 1950s foreshadowed the decline of ECT.

By the 1960s and early 1970s, ECT came under harsh criticism, and legislation was passed to limit its use.[60] ECT use came to a near standstill. During the 1980s, ECT reemerged as a viable treatment alternative when more conventional treatment approaches failed. With the application of rigid treatment criteria and careful pretreatment evaluation, many psychiatric patients, particularly those with depression, have responded to ECT. Currently, ECT is recognized as an effective treatment for a variety of affective and other disorders.

Historical Perspective on the Negative View of ECT

To appreciate the safety and efficacy of modern ECT, it is important to understand why the "old" ECT procedure caused such great distress (Box 14-1). The old ECT was literally applied as an electrical current passed through the brain, causing an epileptic, or grand mal, seizure. It was given without benefit of anesthesia or muscle relaxant. The convulsion was accompanied by various complications, including muscle soreness, fractures, dislocations, sprains, and tongue lacerations. As barbaric as this may sound, it was significantly more humane and scientific than the approach used in some Third World countries. Rereading the excerpt from Lebensohn's memoirs at the beginning of this chapter will reinforce this assertion.

Box 14-1 Consequences of "Old" Electroconvulsive Therapy

Full grand mal seizure
Problems associated with full seizure
- Muscle soreness
- Fractures
- Dislocations
- Sprains
- Tongue lacerations
- 1 in 1000 patients died
- 40% of patients were injured

MODERN ELECTROCONVULSIVE THERAPY

During ECT, an electrical current is passed through the brain. The seizure resulting from ECT should be at least 25 seconds in duration (typical range is 25 to 60 seconds with up to 120 seconds being acceptable).[25] Recent evidence suggests the duration of the seizure may not be as important to ECT's antidepressive effect as the intensity of the seizure.[20,32,64] Seizures longer than 180 seconds should be interrupted by administration of an intravenous benzodiazepine or barbiturate.[30] Collectively, between 220 and 250 seconds is thought necessary for a therapeutic series of ECT. As the treatment series progresses, the seizure threshold can increase as much as 200%, necessitating a stronger stimulus.[56] Subconvulsive stimulation, on the other hand, can cause bradycardia (to the point of asystole) and either restimulation or atropine is needed to counter this unopposed parasympathetic surge.[7]

The events performed before, during, and after treatment, including primarily nursing, medical, or shared responsibilities, follow in roughly sequential order and are outlined in Box 14-2. Electrodes are typically placed bilaterally, but unilateral placement is not uncommon and is correlated with less memory impairment.

Seizure activity is monitored by electroencephalography (EEG). Blood pressure and heart rate are also monitored. Oxygen is administered immediately before and after the treatment because of the interruption of breathing caused by succinylcholine (Anectine) and the seizure. Typically, patients receive ECT two to three times per week up to a total of 6 to 12 treatments (or until the patient improves or is obviously not going to improve).

Indications

"Failure to respond to adequate pharmacological treatment for major depression is now the most common indication for use of electroconvulsive therapy (ECT)."[18]

Approximately 65% of depressed patients will have a full recovery, 20% to 25% will have a partial recovery, and 5% to 10% will exhibit significant symptoms after 2 years of treatment.[10] Individuals prescribed ECT usually come from the latter group. ECT has a very important role in psychiatric treatment because it offers hope when patients and families have lost hope. ECT is particularly helpful when a patient is drug resistant or when speed of action is desirable (e.g., with suicidal ideation). Approximately 85% to 90% of patients receiving ECT have severe depression or bipolar disorder.[29,47,59] Patients with depression respond better and faster to ECT than to other treatments.[9,14] Specifically, patients with melancholic depression (psychomotor changes), psychotic depression (hallucinations and delusions), suicidal tendencies, acute mania, catatonia, and prominently affective schizophrenia are significantly helped by ECT.[3,27,41,48,64] Conditions such as Parkinson's disease, neuroleptic malignant syndrome, and Huntington's disorder also respond to ECT.[1,6,39,40] Box 14-3 lists indicators for ECT, Box 14-4 lists the disorders, depressive symptoms, and conditions responsive to ECT, and Box 14-5 (p. 372) lists situations in which ECT can be prescribed as a first-line agent.

ECT seems particularly suited to the elderly patient because there are no drug side effects, it is safe, and it is effective.* Administering ECT to children and adolescents is more controversial, but both clinicians and parents advocate its use, when needed, in this population.[13,16,33,62] ECT is not useful for treating mild depressions, behavior disorders, phobias, anxiety, somatoform disorders, or personality disturbances (Box 14-6, p. 372).

*References 2, 17, 22, 23, 26, 27, 51, and 66.

Box 14-2 Electroconvulsive Therapy Administration

Preparation
Medical

The patient must have a pretreatment evaluation, including physical examination, electrocardiogram, laboratory work (blood cell count, blood chemistry studies, and urinalysis), and baseline mental status examination that includes a formal assessment of cognition. A computed tomography scan or magnetic resonance imaging of the head may also be indicated and performed.

Nursing

A consent form must be signed. Because ECT is often given as a treatment of last resort, some patients are so profoundly depressed by the time ECT is ordered that obtaining their "informed consent" is not possible. In such cases, involving family members and requesting assistance from the facility's legal staff may be necessary.

Medical

1. Eliminate the routine use of benzodiazepines or barbiturates for nighttime sedation because of their ability to raise the seizure threshold and cause shorter seizures (less than 25 to 30 seconds in duration).[a] Chloral hydrate may be used as an alternative drug regimen. A subconvulsive stimulus may be harmful to the patient.[b] Discontinue antidepressant and lithium regimens to prevent adverse effects or the potential for neurotoxicity.[c,d]

2. Obtain the services of a trained electrotherapist and an anesthesiologist/nurse anesthetist. Whether an anesthesiologist/nurse anesthetist provides care significantly different from that of a psychiatrist is a subject of debate. Pearlman and others[b] found no deaths attributable to ECT in surveying 9 years of psychiatrist-administered anesthesia.[b]

Before treatment
Nursing

1. The patient should receive nothing by mouth from the midnight preceding treatment until after the treatment.

2. Give anticholinergic as ordered. Atropine can be given 1 hour before treatment or be given by intravenous (IV) administration immediately before treatment. Atropine reduces the risk of aspiration and prevents parasympathetic surge (see Box 14-8). Glycopyrrolate (Robinul) may be given as an alternative agent.

3. Ask the patient to urinate before treatment. (Seizure-induced incontinence is common.)

4. Remove the patient's hairpins and dentures.

[a]Fink M: *Am J Psychiatry* 144:1995, 1987.
[b]Reference 45.
[c]Reference 14.
[d]Reference 3.

Continued

Box 14-2 Electroconvulsive Therapy Administration—cont'd

Before treatment
Nursing—cont'd
5. Take the patient's vital signs.
6. Be positive about the treatment and attempt to reduce the patient's pretreatment anxiety.

During treatment
Medical or nursing
1. Insert an IV line.
2. Attach electrodes to the proper place on the head. Electrodes are typically held in place with a rubber strap.
Nursing
   Insert bite-block.
Medical
1. Give methohexital (Brevital) 0.75 to 1.5 mg/kg body weight or another IV anesthetic for anesthesia. The barbiturate causes immediate anesthesia, preempting the anxiety associated with waiting for the "jolt to hit" and the anxiety caused by succinylcholine (Anectine). (Succinylcholine causes paralysis but not sedation, thereby leaving the patient conscious but unable to breathe.)
2. Place blood pressure cuff on one arm to monitor seizure duration (typically shorter than seizure recorded on electroencephalograph). Inflate the cuff before administering succinylcholine.
3. Give IV succinylcholine. Fasciculations should occur in all muscles except those below the blood pressure cuff. Stimulate with nerve stimulator to ascertain paralysis.[e] Succinylcholine prevents the external manifestations of a grand mal seizure, thus minimizing the risk of fractures, dislocations, and other problems while not affecting the "brain seizure."
4. The anesthesiologist/nurse anesthetist mechanically ventilates the patient with 100% oxygen immediately before the treatment.
5. Give the electrical impulse.
6. Observe the length of the seizure. The seizure should be longer than 25 seconds in duration to be of therapeutic value. If the seizure is shorter than 25 seconds long, a decision must be made whether to stimulate another seizure. Up to four attempts may be made. Coffey and others[f] augmented ECT with the administration of caffeine, 242 mg IV push, pretreatment to maintain or increase seizure duration.
Medical or nursing
1. Monitor the patient's heart rate, heart rhythm, and blood pressure; electroencephalography is also used.
2. Ventilation and monitoring should continue until the patient recovers.

[e]Reference 28.
[f]Reference 15.

Box 14-2 Electroconvulsive Therapy Administration—cont'd

After treatment
Medical

The anesthesiologist mechanically ventilates the patient with 100% oxygen until the patient can breathe on his or her own.

Nursing
1. Monitor for respiratory problems.
2. Because ECT causes confusion and disorientation, it is important to help reorient the patient to time, place, and person as he or she emerges from this groggy state.
3. Observe the patient until he or she is oriented and is steady on his or her feet.

Medical and Nursing

Carefully document all aspects of the treatment for the patient record.

Box 14-3 Indications for ECT

- *Major depression:* ECT is appropriate treatment when associated with the following:
    1. Nonresponse to an adequate trial of antidepressants
    2. High suicide potential
    3. Dehydration
    4. Depressive stupor
    5. Catatonia
    6. Delusions
- Prophylaxis of recurrent major depression, (i.e., "maintenance ECT")
- Severe mania—not controlled by medications
- Postpartum psychosis after nonresponse to antidepressants
- Schizophrenia-catatonic type when nonresponsive to medications
- Movement disorders refractory to treatment (e.g., Parkinson's disease, neuroleptic malignant syndrome, tardive dyskinesia)

Adapted from Reference 7.
ECT, Electroconvulsive therapy.

Box 14-4 Disorders, Depressive Symptoms, and Conditions That Respond to Electroconvulsive Therapy

Disorders	Depressive symptoms	Conditions
Severe depression	Anhedonia	Tardive dystonia
Treatment-refractory depression	Anorexia	Tardive dyskinesia
	Delusions	Akathisia
Catatonia	Insomnia	Parkinsonian symptoms
Mania	Muteness	Neuroleptic malignant syndrome
Some types of schizophrenia	Psychomotor retardation	
	Suicidal ideations	

From Reference 57.

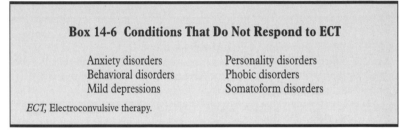

Box 14-5 Situations in Which ECT Can Be a First-Line Treatment

ECT is typically prescribed after antidepressants have failed but can be considered a first-line treatment in these situations:
1. When immediate intervention is warranted (e.g., catatonia, suicide, malnutrition)
2. When the risks of other treatments are greater than the risk of ECT
3. When a history of successful response from ECT exists
4. When the patient prefers ECT

Adapted from Reference 5.
ECT, Electroconvulsive therapy.

Box 14-6 Conditions That Do Not Respond to ECT

Anxiety disorders	Personality disorders
Behavioral disorders	Phobic disorders
Mild depressions	Somatoform disorders

ECT, Electroconvulsive therapy.

Contraindications

The American Psychiatric Association (APA) takes the position that only brain tumor with increased intracranial pressure is an absolute contraindication to ECT. Relative contraindications include other intracranial tumors, intracerebral hemorrhage, recent myocardial infarction, cerebrovascular accident, osteoporosis, unstable vascular aneurysm, chronic obstructive pulmonary disease (COPD), pulmonary disease, retinal detachment, coronary heart disease, and pheochromocytoma.[30] Ziring likens ECT to lifesaving surgery; if a patient's life is in jeopardy, use of lifesaving procedures outweighs almost all potential risks.[65] Box 14-7 presents conditions known to be high risk for ECT, and physiologic effects associated with ECT are presented in Box 14-8.

Safety of ECT (Mortality Rates)

ECT is a safe procedure. Death as a result of ECT is rare.[22,53,64] The mortality rate for an individual treatment is about 1 per 50,000, with approximately 1 death per 10,000 patients occurring. This mortality rate (0.002% to 0.004% per treatment) approximates that for uncomplicated anesthesia and is lower than mortality rates for childbirth (0.01%).[14,21] Mortality is most often associated with cardiovascular complications (Box 14-9); however, even these complications are less problematic with ECT than with antidepressants. When contrasted to the death by suicide of those diagnosed with major depression (15 per 100), the use of ECT is easily justified. ECT is not only safe but also equieffective if not superior to antidepressants, and because ECT works faster, it provides an economic advantage as well.[18,36,47,64] Finally, ECT has proved safe for elderly patients, even in the so-called old-old (older age 85).[22,61]

Box 14-7 Conditions Resulting in Increased Risk from Electroconvulsive Therapy

Absolute contraindication	Brain tumor with increased intracranial pressure
Very high risk	Recent myocardial infarction
	Recent cerebrovascular accident
	Intracranial mass lesion
High risk	Angina pectoris
	Congestive heart failure
	Severe pulmonary disease
	Severe osteoporosis
	Major bone fractures
	Glaucoma
	Retinal detachment
	Thrombophlebitis
	Pregnancy

Modified from Reference 65.

Box 14-8 Physiologic Effects of Electroconvulsive Therapy

Aspiration: during anesthesia induction; right after ECT
Cardiovascular complications (see Box 14-9)
Changes in cerebrovascular dynamic
Increased oxygen consumption
Hyponatremia
Migraine headaches
Memory impairment (typically transient)
Drowsiness (transient)
Confusion (transient)
Headache
Uncommon effects (~0.4% of treatments)
  Muscle aches
  Oral lacerations
  Bone fractures
  Dislocations
  Compression fractures of lumbar spine

From References 24, 30, 63, and 65.

Disadvantages of ECT

The major disadvantage of ECT is that it provides only temporary relief. About 20% of those treated relapse within 6 months, and 50% to 60% relapse within 1 year. Most of these individuals will need another series of treatments. Some psychiatrists order maintenance or continuation ECT (once per month for 6 to 12 months or longer). Maintenance ECT has been found safe, efficacious, well tolerated, and cost-effective, while reducing relapse, recurrence, and rehospitalization.[49,55]

**Box 14-9 Cardiovascular Complications
of Electroconvulsive Therapy**

Arrhythmias
Myocardial infarction
Congestive heart disease
Cardiac arrest
Parasympathetic surge with decreased cardiac output (at moment of
    electrical stimulus):
    Bradycardia
    Hypotension
    Asystole
Sympathetic surge with increased cardiac output (during seizure):
    Tachycardia
    Hypertension
    Arrhythmia

Memory impairment, both retrograde (memory before treatment) and antero-grade (ability to learn new things and memory after treatment), has been frequently cited as a side effect of ECT. Anterograde amnesia is typically transient, whereas retrograde memory loss is more problematic, taking longer to return.[13] Memory of events closest in time to ECT is most commonly affected. Memory is impaired for events occurring before and after each treatment, and confusion occurs immediately after each treatment. However, there seems to be no substantial loss of mental function once the treatment series is completed. By 6 months, almost all patients have recovered their full memory. Furthermore, because depression can cause memory loss, it is not always clear whether memory impairment is related to ECT or to depression. Confusion, no matter how severe, clears within days to weeks.[53]

Although bilateral ECT (bECT) is thought by some to be more effective, unilateral ECT (uECT) reduces anterograde memory loss and disorientation related to treatment.[5,64] Frances, Weiner, and Coffey reported memory actually improved after nondominant-hemisphere uECT.[19] When uECT is used, both electrodes are placed on the nondominant hemisphere (usually the right hemisphere), and electrical impulses are delivered at 2.5 times the seizure threshold. uECT is a recommended method for administering ECT.[30,42]

HOW ELECTROCONVULSIVE THERAPY WORKS

More than 100 theories have been proposed to explain the efficacy of ECT.[52] Although ECT's efficacy is established, the mechanism of effectiveness is not well understood. Most likely, ECT's efficacy is associated with complex changes in the monoaminergic systems, including changes in second messenger systems, downregu-lation of postsynaptic beta-receptors, decreased functioning of 5HT autoreceptors, and increased sensitivity of $5HT_{1A}$ and $5HT_3$ receptors.[31,44]

Charlton moves away from antidepressant explanations of efficacy and suggests that ECT causes an antidelirium effect.[12] Charlton believes that serial seizures act as a "deep and restorative sleep," allowing the brain to "reset" after a period of sleep deprivation and sleep-related symptoms (e.g., hallucinations, delusions, psychomo-tor retardation).

DRUGS USED IN ELECTROCONVULSIVE THERAPY

Three major drug classes are used to enhance ECT: anticholinergics, anesthetics, and muscle relaxants. Typically, the anticholinergic is atropine or glycopyrrolate, the anesthetic is methohexital (Brevital), and the muscle relaxant is succinylcholine (Anectine). Before treatment, the anticholinergic is given to reduce secretions and to minimize aspiration. Once the patient is ready for the treatment, the anesthetic is given intravenously. Methohexital induces anesthesia and is an amnesic. Together these properties reduce treatment-associated anxiety. One can easily imagine the fear associated with waiting for the "jolt" to hit that patients in the premodern ECT era experienced. A second rationale for the use of methohexital is that it induces anesthesia before the third category of drug, the muscle relaxant, is given. Succinylcholine is given intravenously to prevent the musculoskeletal aspects of seizure activity, but it does not affect consciousness. Without the addition of methohexital, the suffocating effect of succinylcholine would terrify the patient.

ANTICHOLINERGICS: ATROPINE AND GLYCOPYRROLATE
Atropine

Atropine, derived from a common plant, *Atropa belladonna*, is the prototypical anticholingeric agent. It inhibits the effects of acetylcholine (ACh) on the parasympathetic system and crosses the blood-brain barrier to cause central effects as well. Atropine is given before ECT for two reasons (1) to inhibit salivation and respiratory tract secretions to prevent aspiration-associated respiratory problems and (2) to prevent the parasympathetic surge outlined in Box 14-8. Some question the need for anticholinergic premedication for ECT.[37]

Pharmacokinetics. Atropine is well absorbed from the gut. It can be given orally (onset 30 minutes) or intramuscularly/subcutaneously (onset 15 minutes) 1 hour before ECT. Most often it is given intravenously (onset 1 minute) just before delivery of ECT. Atropine readily crosses the blood-brain barrier, is metabolized in the liver, and is excreted in the urine. It has a duration of action of 4 hours and a half-life of 2 to 3 hours. A typical dose ranges from 0.4 to 0.6 mg.

Side effects. The most common side effects associated with atropine are dry mouth, blurred vision, constipation, urinary hesitancy, and possibly urinary retention. (See Chapter 17 for an explanation of muscarinic cholinergic receptors.) More serious reactions include paralytic ileus and anaphylactic reactions. Central nervous system (CNS) effects reported include confusion, memory deficits, agitation, restlessness, and disorientation. Occasional adverse responses include nervousness, flushing, fever, tremor, bradycardia, palpitations, nausea and vomiting, photophobia, and skin rashes. Atropine is used cautiously when a patient is known to have a history of glaucoma, prostatic hypertrophy, cardiac arrhythmias, current fever, or obstructive uropathy. Because atropine has been reported to cause or increase confusion in elderly patients, its use has declined to some degree.

Interactions. When atropine is given concurrently with other anticholinergic drugs, an additive effect occurs. Particularly common drug-drug interactions are found between atropine and the following drugs with anticholinergic properties: antihistamines, antipsychotics, antiparkinson agents, tricyclic antidepressants (TCAs), amantadine, benzodiazepines, and monoamine oxidase inhibitors (MAOIs). Caution should also be used when atropine is given concurrently with sympathomimetics (an increased sympathomimetic response), cholinesterase inhibitors (decreased cholinesterase effect), digitalis, slow-release digoxin, and neostigmine (an increased potential for side effects).

Glycopyrrolate

Glycopyrrolate (Robinul) is an anticholinergic drug with the advantage of not crossing the blood-brain barrier. This property prevents the CNS-related anticholinergic effects associated with atropine (e.g., confusion, memory deficits). It has the same peripheral nervous system side effects as atropine, including dry mouth, depression of bronchial secretions, bronchial dilation, mydriasis, vagal inhibition, and gastrointestinal and urinary tract relaxation. Glycopyrrolate has a half-life of 2.5 hours. A typical pretreatment dose of glycopyrrolate is 0.2 mg intravenously. Onset of action occurs 1 minute after intravenous dosage.

ANESTHETICS: METHOHEXITAL AND PROPOFOL

The following are the four objectives for ECT anesthesia[30]:
1. Rapid induction
2. Attenuation of the physiologic effects of ECT
3. Rapid recovery from ECT
4. Minimization of antagonistic effects of anesthetic drugs on seizure duration

Methohexital

Methohexital (Brevital) is an ultrashort-acting barbiturate used to induce anesthesia and is the preferred agent for inducing a light coma preceding delivery of ECT. Less often, propofol (Diprivan) is used for this purpose. The primary efforts in modern ECT have been directed at eliminating the overt manifestations of seizure activity. Induction of anesthesia is the first step in that process. Succinylcholine provides the sought-after muscle relaxation needed to reduce observable convulsions, but it does not induce anesthesia. Consequently, if only succinylcholine were to be given to the patient, the patient would experience muscle paralysis, including respiratory paralysis, while conscious. The emotional reaction to suffocation would be panic; therefore anesthesia induction with methohexital is required.

Pharmacokinetics. Methohexital is given intravenously just before the intravenous administration of succinylcholine. Methohexital rapidly crosses the blood-brain barrier and quickly depresses the CNS, causing unconsciousness within 10 to 15 seconds. The duration of effect is relatively short (5 to 7 minutes) as a result of a natural redistribution to adipose tissue and other less vascular sites. Methohexital is metabolized by the liver, is excreted in the urine, and has a half-life of 3 to 8 hours.

The amount of methohexital used for ECT is typically 40 to 120 mg given intravenously (or 0.75 to 1.5 mg/kg) for adults.[30,46]

Side effects. The major side effects of methohexital are respiratory depression, hypotension, myocardial depression, and decreased cardiac output. Consequently, methohexital is used cautiously in persons with asthma, hypotension, and severe cardiovascular disease. Other potentially life-threatening reactions include anaphylactic reactions, cardiac arrhythmias, peripheral vascular disease, apnea, laryngospasm, and bronchospasm. Bothersome and occasionally serious side effects include prolonged unconsciousness, headache, restlessness and anxiety, nausea and vomiting, dyspnea, hiccups, and a variety of skin rashes.

Interactions. Methohexital has several potentially serious drug interactions. Most notably, other CNS depressants increase CNS and respiratory depression. Furosemide (Lasix), a commonly prescribed drug in older patients, interacts with methohexital to cause substantial orthostatic hypotension. In addition, a number of drugs have decreased effectiveness when given concurrently with methohexital.

Propofol

Propofol (Diprivan) is an alternative to methohexital and produces hypnosis within 40 seconds of intravenous administration. It is highly lipid soluble and has a long half-life as a result of its extensive distribution. The appropriate dosage for propofol-anesthesia induction is 2 to 2.5 mg/kg for adults younger than 55. Propofol is associated with a better side effect profile than methohexital but is also known to reduce seizure length.[8] Propofol is associated with smaller blood pressure changes and faster resolution of anesthesia than other anesthetics.[30]

MUSCLE RELAXANT: SUCCINYLCHOLINE
Succinylcholine

Succinylcholine (Anectine) is an ultrashort-acting (30 to 60 seconds), noncompetitive, depolarizing neuromuscular blocker used for several short-duration procedures, including ECT. Competitive nondepolarizing agents (e.g., tubocurarine) block nicotinic-M receptors on the motor end-plate, thus preventing muscle activation by ACh. Depolarizing agents such as succinylcholine are ACh agonists that mimic ACh but are longer acting. Initially, the muscle is highly stimulated, but because succinylcholine remains connected to the receptor, the motor end-plate is prevented from repolarizing. In other words, the muscle is in a state of constant depolarization. The resulting paralysis prevents musculoskeletal seizures. The initial stimulation caused by succinylcholine lasts about 30 seconds and produces strong muscle contractions (fasciculations) in a roughly rostrocaudal (head to toe) direction (Table 14-1). Recovery of muscle tone occurs in reverse order. Succinylcholine has no effect on the CNS, so it causes paralysis without altering consciousness or the ability to feel pain.

Pharmacokinetics and dosage. Succinylcholine is given intravenously about 1 minute after methohexital administration and is metabolized rapidly by plasma and liver pseudocholinesterases. It should be noted that a number of situations and conditions can prolong the effects of succinylcholine, including reduced amounts of pseudocholinesterase, liver disease, pregnancy, cancer, and atypical pseudocholinesterase. The last is because of an inherited abnormal gene and occurs in almost 4% of the population.

Table 14-1 Rostrocaudal Order of Paralysis by Succinylcholine*

Levator muscles of the eyelids	Muscles of the glottis
Muscles of mastication	Intercostals
Limb muscles	Diaphragm
Abdominal muscles	All other skeletal muscles

Adapted from Reference 43.
*Read down.

Whereas competitive nondepolarizing neuromuscular blockers can be reversed with cholinesterase inhibitors, succinylcholine effects are intensified by these agents. (See the following section for an explanation.) Complete paralysis from succinylcholine occurs within 30 to 60 seconds. Succinylcholine has the shortest duration—about 5 minutes or so—of all neuromuscular blockers. For ECT, an intravenous dose of succinylcholine 0.4 to 1 mg/kg body weight is given.

Interactions. Several drugs prolong the effect of succinylcholine. Perhaps the most important are the cholinesterase inhibitors (e.g., neostigmine). The discussion of this interaction also serves to clarify the difference between nondepolarizing and depolarizing muscle relaxants. Whereas cholinesterase inhibitors are used as antidotes for competitive nondepolarizing neuromuscular blockers, they have the opposite effect if given to reverse succinylcholine effects. This seeming paradoxical result is caused by a profound difference in mechanisms of action between succinylcholine and nondepolarizing agents. The nondepolarizing drugs paralyze by blocking nicotinic-M receptors (i.e., receptor antagonists). Succinylcholine, an agonist, works by depolarizing the muscle and lingering on the receptor until broken down by pseudocholinesterases, thus preventing subsequent depolarizations. Substances that would inhibit these enzymes retard the breakdown of succinylcholine. In other words, the antidote for nondepolarizing paralysis will actually potentiate the paralysis caused by succinylcholine. An exception to this principle occurs when succinylcholine neuromuscular blockade evolves to a phase II block. Discussion of phase I versus phase II blockade is beyond the scope of this text. Other interactions are found in Table 14-2.

Side effects. A major adverse effect associated with succinylcholine is malignant hyperthermia. It is a relatively rare hypermetabolic condition brought on by accelerated muscle metabolism. There is an inherited tendency to develop malignant hyperthermia, and those individuals with a family history should be given another muscle relaxant such as a nondepolarizing agent. Other concerns include histamine release (causing hypotension and bronchoconstriction), cardiovascular changes (including cardiac arrest and arrhythmias), respiratory depression and apnea, hyperkalemia, myoglobinemia, myoglobinuria, and postoperative muscle pain.

Table 14-2 Drug Interactions with Succinylcholine

Benzodiazepines	Reduce the duration of neuromuscular blockade
Phenelzine, promazine, oxytocin, some nonpenicillin antibiotics, quinidine, beta-adrenergic blockers, procainamide, lidocaine, trimethaphan, lithium, furosemide, magnesium sulfate, acetylcholine, anticholinesterases	Enhance the duration of neuromuscular blockade
Nondepolarizing muscle relaxants	Synergistic or antagonistic effect
Digitalis glycosides	Toxicity of both drugs causing cardiac arrhythmias?
Narcotic analgesics	Increased incidence of bradycardia, sinus arrest

Adapted from Reference 43.

Other Agents: Esmolol and Labetalol

Box 14-9 includes the results of the sympathetic surge that occurs during seizure. The addition of sympatholytic agents reduces these autonomic changes but also may shorten seizure duration.[38] Esmolol (Brevibloc) 1.3 to 4.4 mg/kg or labetalol (Normodyne) 0.13 to 0.44 mg/kg is effective in reducing cardiovascular responses to ECT.[11] Esmolol is a beta-1 blocker that decreases sympathetic influence on the heart, thereby reducing cardiac excitability and output. This lowers the blood pressure. After intravenous injection, onset of action occurs in fewer than 5 minutes, with a duration of action between 10 and 30 minutes. The serum half-life is 9 minutes. Labetalol is both an alpha-1 blocker and a nonspecific beta-blocker. It lowers blood pressure and prevents reflex tachycardia. It has an immediate onset of action after intravenous infusion and a duration of action of about 5 hours. The serum half-life is between 6 and 8 hours. Patients with hypertension or cardiovascular disease or those who are frail or medically ill can usually be safely treated with ECT.

REFERENCES

1. Aarsland D and others: Maintenance electroconvulsive therapy for Parkinson's disease, *Convulsive Ther* 13(4):274, 1997.
2. Alexopoulos G and others: ECT in the high-risk geriatric patient, *J Am Geriatr Soc* 32: 651, 1989.
3. American Psychiatric Association: *APA task force on electroconvulsive therapy*, Task Force No. 14, Washington, DC, 1978, The Association.
4. American Psychiatric Association: *The practice of electroconvulsive therapy, recommendations for treatment, training, and privileging: a task force report of the American Psychiatric Association*, Washington, DC, 1990, The Association.
5. Beale MD and others: Recent developments in electroconvulsive therapy, *J S C Med Assoc* 91(3):93, 1995.
6. Beale MD and others: ECT for the treatment of Huntington's disease: a case study, *Convulsive Ther* 13(2):108, 1997.
7. Bezchlibnyk-Butler KZ, Jeffries JJ: *Clinical handbook of psychotropic drugs*, Seattle, 1997, Hogrefe & Huber.
8. Borgeat A: Propofol: pro- or anticonvulsant? *Eur J Anesth* 15(suppl):17, 1997 (abstract).
9. Bowden CL: Current treatment of depression, *Hosp Comm Psychiatry* 36:1192, 1985.
10. Broquet KE: Status of treatment of depression, *South Med J*, 92(9):846, 1999.
11. Castelli I and others: Comparative effects of esmolol and labetalol to attenuate hyperdynamic states after electroconvulsive therapy, *Anesth Analg* 80(3):557, 1995.
12. Charlton BG: The 'anti-delirium' theory of electroconvulsive therapy action, *Med Hypotheses* 52(6):609, 1999.
13. Chatterjee A: Electroconvulsive therapy, *Lancet* 345(8948):518, 1995 (letter).
14. Coffey CE, Weiner RD: Electroconvulsive therapy: an update, *Hosp Community Psychiatry* 41:515, 1990.
15. Coffey CE and others: Caffeine augmentation of ECT, *Am J Psychiatry* 147:579, 1990.
16. Fink M: Electroconvulsive therapy, *Lancet* 345(8948):519, 1995 (letter).
17. Fogel B: Electroconvulsive therapy in the elderly: a clinical research agenda, *Int J Geriatr Psychiatry* 3:181, 1988.
18. Folkerts HW and others: Electroconvulsive therapy vs. paroxetine in treatment-resistant depression: a randomized study, *Acta Psychiatr Scand* 96(5):334, 1997.
19. Frances A and others: ECT for an elderly man with psychotic depression and concurrent dementia, *Hosp Community Psychiatry* 40:237, 1989.
20. Geretsegger C and others: Propofol and methohexital as anesthetic agents for electroconvulsive therapy (ECT): a comparison of seizure-quality measures and vital signs, *J ECT* 14(1): 28, 1998.
21. Gitlin MC and others: Splenic rupture after electroconvulsive therapy, *Anesth Analg* 76: 1363, 1993.

22. Gromley N and others: The safety and efficacy of electroconvulsive therapy in patients over age 75, *Intern J Geriatr Psychiatry* 13(12):871, 1998.

23. Greenberg L, Fink M: Use of electroconvulsive therapy in geriatric patients, *Clin Geriatr Med* 8(2):349, 1992.

24. Greer R, Stewart R: Hyponatremia and ECT, *Am J Psychiatry* 150(8):1272, 1993.

25. Hass S and others: ECT-induced seizure durations, *J Kentucky Med Assoc* 94(6):223, 1996.

26. Hay DP: Electroconvulsive therapy in the medically ill elderly, *Convuls Ther* 5(1):8, 1989.

27. Hay DP: Electroconvulsive therapy. In Sadavoy J, Lazarus LW, Jarvik LF, editors: *Comprehensive review of geriatric psychiatry*, Washington, DC, 1991, American Psychiatric Association.

28. Henneman EA and others: Peripheral nerve stimulators in the critical care setting, *Crit Care Nurs* 15(6):82, 1995.

29. Hermann RC and others: Diagnoses of patients treated with ECT: a comparison of evidence-based standards with reported use, *Psychiatr Serv* 50(8):1059, 1999.

30. Hick EM, Black JL: AANA journal course: update for nurse anesthetists-anesthetic management during electroconvulsive therapy—effects on seizure duration and antidepressant efficacy, *AANA* 67(1):8792, 1999.

31. Ishihara K, Sasa M: Mechanisms underlying the therapeutic effects of electroconvulsive therapy (ECT) on depression, *Jpn J Pharmacol* 80(3):185, 1999 (abstract).

32. Kales H and others: Relationship of seizure duration to antidepressant efficacy in electroconvulsive therapy, *Psychol Med* 27(6):1373, 1997.

33. Kellett JM: Electroconvulsive therapy, *Lancet* 345(8948):518, 1995 (letter).

34. Krahn LE: Childhood-onset schizophrenia associated with parkinsonism in a patient with a microdeletion of chromosome 22, *Mayo Clin Proc* 73(10):956, 1998.

35. Lebensohn ZM: The history of electroconvulsive therapy in the United States and its place in American psychiatry. A personal memoir, *Comprehens Psychiatry* 40(3):173, 1999.

36. Markowitz J and others: Reduced length and cost of hospital stay for major depression in patients treated with ECT, *Am J Psychiatry* 144:1025, 1987.

37. Mayur PM and others: Atropine premedication and the cardiovascular response to electroconvulsive therapy, *Br J Anesth* 81(3):466, 1998.

38. McCall WV and others: Effect of esmolol pretreatment on EEG seizure morphology in RUL ECT, *Convuls Ther* 13(3):175, 1997.

39. McKinney P, Kellner C: Multiple ECT late in the course of neuroleptic malignant syndrome, *Convuls Ther* 13(4):269, 1997.

40. Moellentine C and others: Effectiveness of ECT in patients with parkinsonism, *J Neuropsychiatry Clin Neurosci* 10(2):187, 1998.

41. Mukherjee S and others: Electroconvulsive therapy of acute manic episodes: a review of 50 years' experience, *Am J Psychiatry* 151(2):169, 1994.

42. Murugesan G: Electrode placement, stimulus dosing and seizure monitoring during ECT, *Aust NZ J Psychiatry* 28(4):675, 1994.

43. Olin BR: *Drug facts and comparisons.* St Louis, 1995, Wolters Kluwer.

44. Owens MJ: Molecular and cellular mechanisms of antidepressant drugs, *Depression Anxiety* 4(4):153, 1996-1997 (abstract).

45. Pearlman T and others: Should psychiatrists administer anesthesia for ECT? *Am J Psychiatry* 147:1553, 1990.

46. Pettinati HM and others: Evidence of less improvement in depression in patients taking benzodiazepines during unilateral ECT, *Am J Psychiatry* 147(8):1029, 1990.

47. Potter W, Rudorfer M: Electroconvulsive therapy: a modern medical procedure, *N Engl J Med* 328(12):882, 1993.

48. Prudic J, Sackeim HA: Electroconvulsive therapy and suicide risk, *J Clin Psychiatry* 60(suppl 2):104, 1999.

49. Rabheru K, Persad E: A review of continuation and maintenance electroconvulsive therapy, *Can J Psychiatry* 42(5):476, 1997.

50. Reid WH and others: ECT in Texas: 19 months of mandatory reporting, *J Clin Psychiatry* 59(1):8, 1998.

51. Rice EH and others: Cardiovascular morbidity in high-risk patients during ECT, *Am J Psychiatry* 151(11):1637, 1994.

52. Sackeim HA: Central issues regarding the mechanisms of action of electroconvulsive therapy: directions for future research, *Psychopharmacol Bull* 30(3):281, 1994.

53. Sackeim HA and others: Effects of stimulus intensity and electrode placement on the efficacy and cognitive effects of electroconvulsive therapy, *N Engl J Med* 328(12):839, 1993.

54. Shulins N: Reviled electroshock therapy improved and effective, *Las Vegas Sun* March 19, 1995:11b.

55. Stiebel VG: Maintenance electroconvulsive therapy for chronic mentally ill patients: a case series, *Hosp Community Psychiatry* 46(3):265, 1995.

56. Swartz CM: ECT or programmed seizures? *Am J Psychiatry* 150(8):1274, 1993.

57. Swartz CM: Seizure benefit: grand mal or grand bene? *Neurol Clin* 11(1):151, 1993.

58. Swayze VW II: Frontal leukotomy and related psychosurgical procedures in the era before antipsychotics (1935-1954): a historical overview, *Am J Psychiatry* 152(4):505, 1995.

59. Tancer ME and others: Use of electroconvulsive therapy at a university hospital: 1970 and 1980-1981, *Hosp Community Psychiatry* 40(1):64, 1989.

60. Thompson JW, Blaine JD: Use of ECT in the United States in 1975 and 1980, *Am J Psychiatry* 144:557, 1987.

61. Tomac TA and others: Safety and efficacy of electroconvulsive therapy in patients over age 85, *Am J Geriatr Psychiatry* 5(2):126, 1997.

62. Walter G and others: Views about treatment among parents of adolescents who received electroconvulsive therapy, *Psychiatric Serv,* 50(3):701, 1999.

63. Weinstein MD: Migraine occurring as sequela of electroconvulsive therapy, *Headache* 33(1):45, 1993.

64. Wijeratne C and others: The present status of electroconvulsive therapy: a systematic review, *Med J Austr (MJA)* 171:250, 1999.

65. Ziring B: Issues in the perioperative care of the patient with psychiatric illness, *Med Clin North Am* 77(2):443, 1993.

66. Zwil AS, Pelchat RJ: ECT in the treatment of patients with neurological and somatic disease, *Int J Psychiatry Med* 24(1):1, 1994.

CHAPTER 15

Drugs of Abuse

Leland Allen

Substance abuse has been labeled by many as the greatest problem facing American society today, but the roots of substance abuse can be traced back for centuries. Many substances viewed today as drugs of abuse at one time had legitimate roles in society: Native Americans used (and still use) peyote as part of religious rituals; Sigmund Freud was both a user and advocate of cocaine; Sir Arthur Conan Doyle's famous character, Sherlock Holmes, was a frequent user of opium; and until 1903, the secret ingredient (at 60 mg per 8-ounce bottle) in the original formula of Coca-Cola was cocaine. Today, use and abuse of illicit substances is pervasive and is associated with frequent comorbidities such as human immunodeficiency virus (HIV) infection and other sexually transmitted diseases, teenage pregnancy, rape, assault, and murder. According to the National Household Survey on Drug Abuse for 1996, 13 million Americans admitted to using illicit substances, a number that was stable from the previous year. Nicotine, alcohol, and caffeine, all legal drugs, are used and abused by a far larger segment of the population. Table 15-1 provides a month-at-a-glance view of psychoactive substance use in the United States.

Treatment and diagnosis of alcoholism and other substance abuse disorders are reviewed elsewhere in this text (also see Table 15-2). The focus of this chapter is the epidemiology and psychopharmacology of commonly abused substances. The approach centers on major classes of drugs and representative drugs from each class, as identified in the DSM-IV (Box 15-1).

ALCOHOL

Alcohol abuse is the number one problem in North America, both economically and in terms of the number of people directly affected. It has been estimated that in 1995, alcohol abuse costs exceeded $166 billion.[14] These economic data reflect health care expenditures, or direct costs, and the indirect costs related to crime, premature death, loss of productivity, and social welfare. An estimated 13.7 million Americans either abuse alcohol or are addicted to its use; after cardiovascular disease and cancer, alcoholism ranks third among the causes of death and disability in the United States.[4,22] Alcoholics have a death rate two to four times higher than that of nonalcoholics and die on average 20 years earlier than their nondrinking counterparts.[16] Approximately 100,000 deaths each year are directly related to alcohol.[7] About 30% of all traffic fatalities involve a drunken driver (representing a decrease from previous years). Other causes of alcohol-related mortality are suicide, liver disease, heart disease, homicide, and cancer.

The effects of alcoholism are commonly found among medical and psychiatric patients. It is estimated that among general hospital inpatients, 25% of the men and 4% to 35% of the women are alcoholics.[9,20]

Table 15-1 The Numbers Game

Substance	Number who used in past month
Heroin	200,000
Amphetamines	800,000
Cocaine/crack	1,500,000
Marijuana	10,000,000
Alcohol	11,000,000 (abusers)
Nicotine	61,000,000
Caffeine	130,000,000

Adapted from Nash JM: Addicted: why do people get hooked? *Time* May 5:68, 1997.

Table 15-2 12-Month Prevalence Rate of Mental Disorders in the United States

Diagnosis	Percentage of population older than 17 years of age	Number of persons
Anxiety disorders	12.6	20,034,000
Phobia disorders*	10.9	17,331,000
Mood disorders	9.5	15,143,000
Alcohol disorders	**7.4**	**11,766,000**
Major depression†	5.0	7,950,000
Drug disorders	**3.1**	**4,929,000**
Cognitive impairment	2.7	4,293,000
Obsessive-compulsive disorder	2.1	3,339,000
Antisocial disorder	1.5	2,385,000
Panic disorders*	1.3	2,067,000
Bipolar disorder†	1.2	1,908,000
Schizophrenia	1.1	1,749,000
Somatization	0.2	365,000

From Regier DA and others: The de facto US mental and addictive disorders service system: epidemiologic catchment area prospective 1-year prevalence rates of disorders and services, *Arch Gen Psychiatry* 50:85, 1993.
Note: Bold denotes mental disorders related to content of this chapter specifically.
*Also calculated in anxiety statistics.
†Also calculated in mood disorders statistics.

Pharmacokinetics

The chemical name for beverage alcohol is ethanol (CH_3CH_2OH). It is primarily metabolized in the liver; however, a significant amount of alcohol is metabolized in the stomach as well. The oxidation process can be described chemically as follows:

$$CH_3CH_2OH \longrightarrow CH_3CHO + H_2 \longrightarrow CH_3COOH \longrightarrow CO_2 \text{ \& } H_2O$$
$$\text{[alcohol dehydrogenase]} \quad \text{[aldehyde dehydrogenase]}$$

At each step of the metabolizing process, an enzyme breaks down the chemical. Ethanol is broken down by alcohol dehydrogenase to acetaldehyde and hydrogen.

Box 15-1 DSM-IV Criteria for Substance Dependence and Substance Abuse

Substance dependence

Maladaptive use of a substance that leads to impairment or distress as manifested by any three of the following occurring in a single year:

1. Tolerance to the effect of the substance
2. Withdrawal symptoms when use is stopped
3. Increasing frequency or quantity of use
4. Unsuccessful efforts to cut down or quit
5. Time devoted to getting or using the substance
6. Ordinary activities curtailed in favor of the substance
7. Continued substance use despite knowledge of adverse effects

Substance abuse

Maladaptive use of a substance leading to impairment or distress as manifested by one of the following occurring in a single year, but not having met the criteria for dependence:

1. Major role obligations at work, school, or home curtailed in favor of or because of substance abuse
2. Use of a substance when it is hazardous
3. Substance-related legal problems
4. Continued use despite adverse social/interpersonal effects

Modified from American Psychiatric Association: *Diagnostic and statistical manual of mental disorders-TR*, ed 4, Washington, DC, 2000, The Association.

The hydrogen molecule from alcohol metabolism causes the liver to bypass normal energy sources, that is, the hydrogen from glucose metabolism, and to use the hydrogen from ethanol. This excess of hydrogen production erroneously signals the liver that the body is in a "fed" state, causing the liver to cease producing glucose. This can lead to profound, life-threatening hypoglycemia. Aldehyde dehydrogenase breaks down acetaldehyde to acetic acid, which is an innocuous substance. When enzymatic action on acetaldehyde is blocked by the aldehyde dehydrogenase blocker disulfiram (Antabuse) or by loss of normal hepatic function, acetaldehyde can accumulate, causing an unpleasant illness consisting of malaise, nausea, and flushing. Large concentrations of acetaldehyde in the liver can cause hepatocyte (liver cell) necrosis, leading to cirrhosis and ultimately death. Acetaldehyde also interferes with vitamin activation. The alcohol dehydrogenase in gastrointestinal tissue of nonalcoholic men oxidizes a significant amount of the alcohol in the gut before it enters the bloodstream. However, Frezza and others have discovered that the gastrointestinal tissue of women and of alcoholic men contains little alcohol dehydrogenase.[2] The inability of women's bodies to make this first-pass metabolism accounts for their enhanced vulnerability to the effects of alcohol and confirms an age-old suspicion that women become intoxicated more easily than men, even considering differences in body mass and composition.

The mechanism of action of ethanol is unclear. Certainly, complex interactions with neurons occur and include effects on the actual lipids in neuron cell membranes, as well as specific interactions with ligand-gated and voltage-gated ion channels in neurons. Ligand-gated ion channels include gamma-aminobutyric acid (GABA), glycine, glutamate, and N-methyl-D-aspartate (NMDA) receptors. Voltage-gated channels include Ca^{++} and Na^{+}-K^{+} cotransporters. Ethanol exerts both acute and chronic effects on these neurons, which probably explains withdrawal symptoms after chronic use.

Alcohol is absorbed partially from the stomach (20%) but mostly from the small intestine (80%). If a person with an empty stomach ingests alcohol, it is in the bloodstream within 20 minutes. The type of beverage consumed affects the rate of absorption. Beer contains 4% to 6% ethanol; wine, 12% ethanol; and whiskey, 40% to 50% ethanol. Ethanol in beer and wine is absorbed more slowly than that in liquor, but the alcohol content does not account completely for its absorption rate. Food slows alcohol absorption in the stomach but has less effect on small intestine absorption.

Ethanol is distributed equally in all body tissue, including the brain, according to water content. Large persons or persons with great amounts of body water can ingest more alcohol than small persons or persons with less body water. Alcohol affects the cerebrum and cerebellum before it affects the spinal cord and the vital centers because the former areas contain more water.

The rate of absorption largely determines how quickly a person will become intoxicated and is affected by the gastric emptying time. The metabolic rate, which is relatively constant (nonlinear kinetics), largely determines how long alcohol will affect the body. The body can metabolize 15 ml of alcohol (1 ounce of whiskey or 1 glass of beer) every 60 minutes. In persons who drink alcohol frequently for years, hepatic drug-metabolizing levels are increased to hasten alcohol metabolism. Hot coffee, "sweating it out," and other home remedies do not increase alcohol metabolism, nor do they speed the "sobering-up" process. Scientists have attempted unsuccessfully to develop a drug to prevent or decrease intoxication. In late-stage alcoholism, the metabolism rate decreases because the damaged liver can no longer adequately metabolize the alcohol.

Tolerance to alcohol occurs and is probably related to elevated hepatic enzyme levels (pharmacokinetic tolerance) or to cellular adaptations (pharmacodynamic tolerance). The naive drinker may be noticeably intoxicated after two to three drinks, whereas the "practiced" drinker may be able to handle a six-pack or two (both pharmacokinetic tolerance) and the long-term drinker may walk around almost unaffected even though having a very high blood alcohol level (pharmacodynamic tolerance). Tolerance does not tend to develop to any degree for respiratory depression. Blood alcohol levels slightly above those in which the chronic alcoholic was functioning have caused death.

Physiologic Effects

Central nervous system. Central nervous system (CNS) effects are related to sedation and toxicity (Table 15-3). Initially, alcohol exerts an anxiolytic effect. It stimulates dopamine in the reward pathway at first, but then these levels eventually decrease to normal when drinking. When not drinking, dopamine levels drop, so the chronic drinker persists in consuming alcohol just to feel "normal."

As alcohol concentrations increase, cognitive and motor skills diminish. At high concentrations, the vital centers of the brain become depressed, and a slower, stuporous-to-unconscious mental state develops. Large amounts of alcohol can cause progressive depression of brainstem functions to the point that reflexes such as the gag reflex or automatic functions such as respiratory drive are impaired. Death can

Table 15-3 Drugs of Abuse: Effects, Overdose, and Withdrawal

Drugs	Effects	Overdose	Withdrawal
Narcotics	Euphoria, respiratory depression, constricted pupils, nausea, constipation	Slow, shallow breaths; clammy skin; coma; convulsions, respiratory arrest; death	Watery eyes, runny nose, yawning, loss of appetite, irritability, tremors, panic, cramps, nausea, chills, sweating
Depressants	Slurred speech, disorientation, drunken behavior without evidence of alcohol	Shallow respirations, clammy skin, dilated pupils, weak and rapid pulse, coma, death	Anxiety, insomnia, tremor, delerium, convulsions, death
Stimulants	Increased alertness, excitation, euphoria, rapid pulse, hypertension, insomnia, anorexia	Agitation, hyperthermia, hallucinations, convulsions, death	Apathy, sleep, irritability, depression, disorientation
Hallucinogens	Illusions and hallucinations, poor time and distance perception	Longer and more intense "trips," psychosis, death	No withdrawal syndrome reported
Cannabinoids	Euphoria, disorientation, relaxed inhibitions, increased appetite	Fatigue, paranoia, psychosis	Insomnia, hyperactivity, anorexia

From *Federal Register* 55(159):33590, Washington, DC, Aug 16, 1990.

occur from respiratory depression or aspiration of stomach contents. Symptoms of alcohol intoxication can be predicted based on alcohol blood levels (Table 15-4). Ingestion of ethanol often leads to amnesia for the period of intoxication.

Historically, the brain damage associated with chronic alcohol use was thought to be caused by nutritional deficiencies. Persons with alcoholism eat poorly, which leads to pathologic change. It is now known, however, that brain damage occurs even when a nutritious diet is maintained. In fact, all persons with alcoholism have some brain cell loss, and atrophy of the brain can be seen on computed tomograms (CT) of the brain.[6,18]

Wernicke's encephalopathy and Korsakoff's psychosis are caused by thiamine deficiency in the diet. Patients for whom alcohol comprises a significant percentage of their caloric intake are likely to be thiamine deficient. In addition, thiamine absorption is blocked directly by alcohol, further exacerbating the deficiency. Wernicke's encephalopathy, expressed by confusion, nystagmus, and ophthalmoplegia or loss of control of eye movements, can be reversed by thiamine intake.[10] Korsakoff's psychosis is not reversed by thiamine intake. It is characterized by gait disturbances, memory loss, confabulation, and neuropathy.

Peripheral nervous system

Neuropathy. Neuropathy is a general term used to indicate loss of function of a nerve. Alcohol causes peripheral neuropathy primarily through nutritional deficiencies, and neuropathies may be either motor or sensory. Sensory neuropathy is usually the initial manifestation, with patients complaining of vague pain, burning, or

Table 15-4 Clinical Effects of Alcohol

Blood alcohol level	Physiologic effect
0.05	Euphoria, decreased inhibitions
0.10-0.15	Labile mood, loquaciousness, impaired judgment, tremors, poor attention
0.15-0.20	Decreased motor skills, slurred speech, diplopia
0.25	Altered perceptions
0.30	Alterations in equilibrium
0.35	Apathy
0.40	Stupor, coma
0.40-0.50	Severe respiratory depression, death

numbness in extremities. Untreated, patients can lose all sensation in their extremities. This can predispose the patient to pressure sores identical to those found in people with diabetes. Sensory neuropathy can be objectively demonstrated by a loss of deep-tendon reflexes or a loss of pinprick sensation or of heat-cold discrimination in the legs or arms. Motor neuropathy presents as weakness, typically affecting distal muscle groups more than proximal ones. Distal muscles will atrophy because of the loss of motor input, and patients with motor neuropathy will have loss of the interosseus muscles of the hand, leading to a wasted, bony appearance. No specific treatment for neuropathy exists, and abstinence from alcohol and nutritional replacement frequently fails to resolve the condition.

Liver. Cirrhosis and other diseases of the liver are the physical health problems most commonly associated with alcohol abuse. Cirrhosis is the fifth leading cause of death in the United States and occurs in up to 20% of chronic alcoholics. In cirrhosis, normal hepatocytes are replaced with fibrous, nonfunctioning scar tissue that obstructs blood flow, leading to portal hypertension, ascites, and esophageal varices. As the functioning liver is replaced by scar tissue, symptoms and signs of liver failure become evident. The patient with liver dysfunction has low serum protein levels, high serum ammonia and bilirubin levels, and blood clotting problems. The reduction in normal hepatocytes decreases the liver's ability to metabolize drugs and toxins, leading to an increased sensitivity of the patient to the side effects or toxic effects of common medications. Alcohol metabolism is also reduced in the cirrhotic liver, leading to a loss of tolerance to the effects of alcohol. Alcohol may also cause an acute hepatitis, or inflammation of the liver. This is clinically characterized by abdominal pain, fever, nausea, vomiting, malaise, jaundice, and occasionally, overt liver failure and death.

Gastrointestinal tract. Alcohol is a chemical irritant. It burns the mouth and throat and prompts the stomach to secrete more hydrochloric acid. Gastric ulcers and gastritis are caused and then worsened by alcohol. People with alcoholism experience ulcers, gastritis, bleeding, and hemorrhage in the stomach. Ulcers can eventually perforate, creating a life-threatening situation. Likewise, esophageal varices caused by cirrhosis can rupture, leading to fatal hemorrhage. A malabsorption syndrome is caused by irritation of the intestinal lining. This seems to affect B vitamins generally and to lead to a deficiency of vitamin B_1 (thiamine) in particular.

Pancreas. The pancreas is both directly and indirectly affected by alcohol. Acute and chronic pancreatitis are common in chronic drinkers (about 5%) and may lead to diabetes.[5]

Other organs. Alcohol directly affects muscle tissue, a condition known as *alcohol myopathy,* leading to skeletal muscle death or weakness. Other organs affected by alcohol include the eyes (loss of peripheral and night vision), the heart (hypertension, enlarged left ventricle, disturbances in the normal cardiac rhythm, and a reduction in systolic function), and reproductive organs (as a depressant, alcohol can cause impotence). Paradoxically, while the disinhibiting effects of alcohol can increase libido, the aforementioned mentioned physiologic effects can thwart the physical component of sex.

Drug Interactions

In general, acute alcohol ingestion decreases metabolism of other drugs by competing for hepatic enzymes. Chronic drinking, on the other hand, tends to increase metabolism of other drugs related to hepatic enzyme induction. When chronic drinking causes cirrhosis, however, any drug metabolized by the liver will have a prolonged half-life, so health care professionals must be cognizant of potential drug toxicities in alcoholics. A few examples of important interactions follow.

Disulfiram. Disulfiram (Antabuse) inhibits the breakdown of acetaldehyde by the enzyme aldehyde dehydrogenase (see Chapter 12). Because acetaldehyde is toxic, the person who drinks alcohol while taking disulfiram becomes ill (sweating, flushing of the neck and face, a throbbing headache, nausea and vomiting, palpitations, dyspnea, tremor, and weakness). This combination can also cause arrhythmias, myocardial infarction, cardiac failure, seizures, coma, and death. The unpleasant response to alcohol reinforces the efforts of the person with alcoholism to stop drinking.

Naltrexone. Naltrexone (ReVia), an opiate receptor antagonist, reduces the urge to drink while also diminishing the alcoholic high and is used to treat alcoholism.[12,15,19]

CNS depressants. Alcohol taken with other CNS depressants causes profound CNS depression, often leading to death. For instance, diazepam, which is not lethal when taken alone (even in large doses), can lead to death when it is combined with alcohol. Individuals taking barbiturates, antipsychotic drugs, antidepressants, benzodiazepines, and other CNS depressants should avoid alcohol. Chloral hydrate and lorazepam (Ativan) have been associated with intentional sedating of unsuspecting persons in bars. A combination of chloral hydrate and alcohol (the legendary "knockout drops") was used years ago to "recruit" men for ship duty or for robbery. Lorazepam and alcohol have been used by prostitutes to debilitate their clients in order to rob them.

Other interactions include the following:

Interactant	Effect
Acetaminophen	Can lead to acetaminophen-induced liver toxicity
Cephalosporins	Possible disulfiram-like responses
Antidepressants	Additive CNS effects
Ascorbic acid	Increased alcohol clearance
Cimetidine	Possible increased peak alcohol blood levels
Verapamil	Inhibited alcohol metabolism
Warfarin	Acute alcohol use: increased warfarin levels
	Chronic alcohol use: decreased warfarin levels

Withdrawal and Detoxification

Ethanol suppresses glutamate, which enhances cortisol. When the long-time drinker withdraws from alcohol, glutamate is free to increase serum cortisol. Increased levels of cortisol cause anxiety, insomnia, anorexia, and decreased libido. Furthermore, dopamine depletion in the reward pathway occurs, leaving the abstinent ethanol-dependent person anhedonic.

Increased psychomotor activity as a consequence of alcohol withdrawal is called the *alcohol-withdrawal syndrome*. Sedation is the predominant effect of alcohol, but as sedation wears off, psychomotor activity increases. This is referred to as a *rebound phenomenon*. As the CNS becomes more irritated, the normal drinker feels sick and irritable (a hangover) but lives through it. People who drink heavily or who have alcoholism have to drink again to resedate the psychomotor system. Eventually, people with alcoholism have to drink large amounts of alcohol just to feel normal. Some reach the point at which they cannot drink enough, and CNS irritability is not sedatable. Alcoholic tremors, sweating, palpitations, and agitation then occur. Most often, these symptoms occur after alcohol ingestion has stopped, but in some cases, they occur while the person with alcoholism is drinking.

Alcoholic hallucinosis, a state of auditory hallucinations, is a phenomenon that alcoholics sometimes experience. The brain begins to invent sensory input. Alcoholic hallucinations typically begin 48 hours or so after drinking has stopped. Frightening voices or sounds are heard, usually within the context of a clear sensorium.

The ultimate level of CNS irritability is delirium tremens (DTs), which typically develop 72 hours after drinking cessation. During DTs, the body not only invents sensory input but also has extreme motor agitation. Hallucinations become visual (e.g., the proverbial pink elephants), and the sufferer is tremulous and terrified. Tonic-clonic (grand mal) seizures can occur. Hypertensive crises can result in death if not treated. Treatment for DTs involves administration of a short course of benzodiazepines.

AMPHETAMINES

Amphetamines were developed in 1887 (see Chapter 16). They have medicinal uses, such as in the attention-deficit hyperactivity disorder in childhood (see Chapters 20 and 21) and narcolepsy (see Chapter 10). They are seldom prescribed for obesity today. Amphetamine and methamphetamine are known as *speed, crank, ice, bennies, dexies,* and other names. Derivatives of amphetamines include MDMA (Ecstasy), MDA (love drug), and other designer drugs that are created to bypass legal definitions of controlled substances.

Pharmacokinetics

Amphetamines are indirect-acting catecholamine agonists that cause the release of norepinephrine and dopamine from nerve endings (see Chapter 16). Amphetamines also block norepinephrine reuptake in presynaptic nerve endings. Amphetamines are well absorbed from the gastrointestinal tract. They are usually given orally but may also be administered intravenously or smoked. They are eliminated from kidneys mostly unchanged; hence, conditions that slow their excretion (e.g., kidney disease, alkaline urine) result in an intensification of effect.

Physiologic Effects

CNS effects of amphetamine use include wakefulness, alertness, heightened concentration, energy, improved mood to euphoria, insomnia, anorexia, and amnesia. Non-CNS effects include hypertension, hyperthermia, and occasionally, cardiac conduction abnormalities. Toxic levels of amphetamines cause severe hypertension, cerebral hemorrhage, seizures, and coma. Patients may become acutely psychotic and may be prone to violent outbursts, even committing murder. See Chapter 16 for a more complete discussion.

Withdrawal and Detoxification

Although amphetamines are highly addictive, physical withdrawal is relatively mild. Psychologic withdrawal is severe, however, because the drugs are so pleasurable. The process is gradual and safe for persons withdrawing from amphetamines under medical supervision. Cold turkey withdrawal without medical supervision causes agitation, irritability, and severe depression. In general, the low of withdrawal will be inversely proportional to the high experienced. A number of approaches are used, all aiming to restore depleted neurotransmitters. Monoamine precursors such as phenylalanine and tyrosine, tricyclic antidepressants, and the dopamine agonist bromocriptine are three approaches for increasing the availability of depleted catecholamines.

CANNABIS

Marijuana is the most commonly used illicit drug in the United States. In 1995, it was estimated that 2.4 million people smoked their first joint. Marijuana use is especially prevalent among youth and young adults. Marijuana is made from the chopped leaves and flowers of the *Cannabis* plant and is usually smoked. In some countries, the resin of the plant is used to make a drink that is more potent. The active ingredient is tetrahydrocannabinol (THC), although several other cannabinoids are known to be present in marijuana.

Mechanism of Action

The precise mechanism of action of THC is not known, but there appear to be specific receptors in the brain for THC, and endogenously occurring cannabinoids have been recovered.

Physiologic Effects

THC produces a calm, mildly euphoric state. Sensations are said to be heightened, and in some instances, hallucinations occur. Psychomotor retardation occurs, so persons under the influence of THC should not operate heavy machinery or automobiles. Time perception is said to be distorted. Users often experience increased appetite.

Data regarding long-term effects of THC use are conflicting. Some evidence exists indicating that neurologic function may deteriorate with chronic use, but other studies show no such effect. Perhaps the most pressing long-term health issue is the effect of marijuana smoke on the lungs and the development of emphysema and other chronic sequelae of smoke inhalation. Chronic use does not seem to produce physiologic dependence.

COCAINE

Coca leaves have been used as stimulants for thousands of years. Coca plants grow high in the Andes, and the Inca Indians chewed coca leaves long before the Spanish explorers arrived. Cocaine is extracted from the coca plant and is a fine, white, odorless substance with a bitter taste. It was introduced to Western medicine as an anesthetic in 1858. Freud was known to use cocaine and believed it to be a remedy for morphine addiction. Cocaine and its offspring crack are the most costly illicit drugs to society with respect to crime, morbidity, and mortality. It has been reported that 1.75 million people were active users in 1996. The problems associated with these drugs extend to every level of society. If viewed as a separate category, cocaine-related deaths would rank as the fifth leading cause of death among young men in New York City.[11]

Cocaine is available in several forms for different routes of administration. White powder is available for intranasal use (snorting), or it can be dissolved and injected intravenously. Rocks of cocaine base called *crack* have replaced powdered cocaine as the most commonly used form of the drug. Crack is smoked, as is freebase cocaine. Any of these forms can be ingested orally as well. The intravenous route is the most efficient way to use cocaine in terms of bioavailability of the dose. Smoking crack or freebase is almost as efficient as intravenous use and can cause an immediate high. Intranasal and ingested cocaine are not nearly as well absorbed, and the onset of action is slower with these two routes.

Pharmacokinetics

Cocaine passes the blood-brain barrier quickly, causing an instantaneous high, but it is rapidly metabolized by the liver, so the "rush," although exhilarating, does not last long. Cocaine affects both the CNS and the peripheral nervous system (PNS) by blocking norepinephrine and dopamine reuptake into neurons, thereby depleting these neurotransmitters. Tolerance to CNS and PNS effects develops quickly with crack use because neuronal norepinephrine stores are depleted (and decreased norepinephrine levels is one explanation for the depression associated with cocaine use), causing a need to increase drug amounts to achieve the desired effect. Tolerance develops to otherwise lethal amounts.

Physiologic Effects

Cocaine and its derivatives are addictive stimulants. Although physical dependence is less severe than with opioid abuse, psychologic dependence is intense. Euphoria, increased mental alertness, increased strength, anorexia, and supposed increased sexual stimulation are major desired effects of cocaine and its derivatives. CNS effects include stimulation of the medulla, resulting in deeper respirations, euphoria, increased mental alertness, dilated pupils, anorexia, and increased strength. Less common reactions are specific hallucinations and delusions. Some persons taking cocaine report "bugs" crawling beneath the skin (formication) and foul smells. The primary effect is a dopaminergic stimulation of mesolimbic and mesocortical reward pathways.[8]

Chronic cocaine use leads to catecholamine receptor supersensitivity and probably the eventual destruction of dopaminergic neurons. This result may account for the anhedonia found in some chronic cocaine users.[8] Increased motor activity, tachycardia, and high blood pressure are other effects. Cocaine can also provoke cardiac arrest. In a survey of unexpected, nontraumatic deaths of men between ages 20 and 40, Shen and others found a full third between 1980 and 1989 were cocaine related.[17] Cocaine is a potent vasoconstrictor that can cause spasm of any blood vessel. This is most striking when the vessels are the coronary arteries, causing acute myocardial infarction. Patients have also died from ingestion of cocaine and the subsequent necrosis of the bowel. Necrosis of the nasal septum is seen in chronic snorters of cocaine, related to vasoconstriction. Other complications of cocaine use include headache and chronic cough.[21] Cocaine use during pregnancy leads to prematurity, stillbirth, small gestational size, and CNS damage in the newborn.[1]

HALLUCINOGENS

Hallucinogens, also referred to as *psychotomimetics* or *psychedelics*, alter perception. There are two basic groups of hallucinogens: natural hallucinogens and manufactured hallucinogens (synthetic). Natural hallucinogenic substances include mescaline (peyote [from cactus]), psilocybin (psilocin [from mushrooms]), and perhaps marijuana *(Cannabis sativa)*. Synthetic or semisynthetic substances include lysergic acid diethylamide (LSD), 2,5-dimethoxy-4-methylamphetamine (STP), phencyclidine (PCP), dimethyltryptamine (DMT), and methylenedioxyamphetamine (MDA).

Hallucinogens can heighten awareness of reality or can cause a terrifying psychosis-like reaction. Users report distortions in body image and a sense of depersonalization. Particularly frightful is a loss of the sense of reality. Hallucinations and illusions depicting grotesque creatures such as a "dog with a snake for a tongue" can be extremely frightening. Emotional consequences of such effects are panic, anxiety, confusion, and paranoid reactions. Some people have had frank psychotic reactions after minimal use. In the jargon of the hallucinogens, such an experience is a "bad trip."

Pharmacokinetics

LSD is taken orally and is quickly absorbed. Other hallucinogens may be smoked, snorted, or ingested. The sites and mechanisms of action are unclear, but almost certainly, serotonin is the key neurotransmitter involved in the effects of hallucinogens.

Physiologic Effects

LSD and other hallucinogens are relatively safe drugs, at least in terms of their physiologic effects. Sympathetic stimulation of the autonomic nervous system can produce hyperthermia, hypertension, pupillary dilation, tremor, and tachycardia, but these effects are rarely fatal. Nausea and vomiting can occur and are most often associated with mescaline or peyote. Tolerance quickly develops to the psychologic effects of hallucinogens, but there is no physiologic or psychologic dependence.

INHALANTS

A broad range of volatile substances can be and are inhaled. These include glues, solvents, gases (e.g., nitrous oxide), and aerosol propellants. Many of these are organic, petroleum-based products. They typically produce CNS depression, although they can cause excitability. Chronic use can lead to cerebral or cerebellar dysfunction, and death can occur as a result of asphyxiation or arrhythmia. Table 15-5 lists chemicals commonly found in inhalants.

OPIOIDS

Narcotics, or opioids, are widely abused and include heroin, morphine, codeine, meperidine (Demerol), methadone (Dolophine), and fentanyl (Sublimaze). Heroin use, after a period of dormancy, is regaining its appeal among drug abusers. Users find heroin less expensive than cocaine. Narcotics can be swallowed, smoked,

Table 15-5 Chemicals Commonly Found in Inhalants

Adhesives	
Airplane glue	Toluene, ethyl acetate
Rubber cement	Hexane: toluene; methyl chloride; acetone; methyl ethyl ketone; methyl butyl ketone
PVC cement	Trichloroethylene
Aerosols	
Paint sprays	Butane; propane (U.S.); fluorocarbons; toluene; hydrocarbons ("Texas Shoe Shine," a spray paint containing toluene)
Hair sprays	Butane; propane (U.S.); fluorocarbons
Deodorants; air fresheners	Butane; propane (U.S.); fluorocarbons
Analgesic spray	Fluorocarbons
Asthma spray	Fluorocarbons
Anesthetics	
Gaseous	Nitrous oxide
Liquid	Halothane; enflurane
Local	Ethyl chloride
Cleaning agents	
Dry cleaning	Tetrachloroethylene; trichloroethane
Spot removers	Tetrachloroethylene; trichloroethane; trichloroethylene
Degreasers	Tetrachloroethylene; trichloroethane; trichloroethylene
Solvents	
Polish remover	Acetone, ethyl acetate, toluene
Paint remover	Toluene; methylene chloride; methanol
Paint thinners	Toluene, methylene chloride; methanol
Correction fluid thinners	Trichloroethylene; trichloroethane
Fuel gas	Butane
Lighter	Butane; isopropane
Fire extinguisher	Bromochlorodifluoromethane
Food products	
Whipped cream	Nitrous oxide
Whippets	Nitrous oxide
"Room odorizers" (Locker room; Rush; Poppers)	(Iso)amyl nitrite; (iso)butyl nitrite; isopropyl nitrite; butyl nitrite, cyclohexylnitrite

From Lowinson JH, Ruiz P, Hillman RB, Langrod JG: *Substance abuse: a comprehensive textbook,* Baltimore, 1992, Williams & Wilkins.

snorted, injected into soft tissue (skin-popping), and mainlined (injected intravenously). Initially, veins in the antecubital space are used, but as veins scar and sclerosis ("tracks") develops, other veins are used, requiring the abuser to inject less accessible vascular structures such as the femoral vein or artery, the dorsal vein of the penis, or even directly into the heart. The needle is often passed from one user to another. Infections, including acquired immunodeficiency syndrome (AIDS) and hepatitis, are known to spread by shared needles and have prompted controversial needle exchange programs.

Pharmacokinetics

Opioids are metabolized in the liver and excreted by the kidneys. They are not absorbed as well from the gut and are readily metabolized there and in the liver. A much more potent effect is achieved with parenteral administration. Drugs that compete for liver metabolism increase the effect of opioids.

Physiologic Effects

Opioids relieve pain by increasing the pain threshold and by reducing anxiety and fear. Naturally occurring neurotransmitters, the endorphins, mediate pain and regulate mood. The opioids are endorphin agonists. It is their effect on mood (a feeling of euphoria) that attracts people who abuse these drugs. Such individuals often refer to the euphoric mood created by heroin as "better than sex." In addition to the euphoria, an overall CNS depression occurs. Drowsiness, or "nodding," and sleep are common effects. When heroin is combined with cocaine (speedballing), abusers can become poetic in describing the effect—euphoria and analgesia.

Heroin is a prodrug of morphine and more readily passes the blood-brain barrier. Once heroin enters the brain, it is metabolized to morphine, so it becomes trapped in the brain.[3] This property of heroin (reduction to morphine) causes a more sustained high than that of regular morphine because higher levels are achieved in the CNS.

CNS effects of opioids include respiratory depression related to decreased sensitivity to hypercarbia as a stimulus for respiration at the medullary center. Respiratory depression is the primary cause of death among people who abuse opioids. Peripheral effects include reduced gastrointestinal mobility, causing nausea, vomiting, and constipation; decreased gastric, biliary, and pancreatic secretions; urinary retention; hypotension; and reduced pupil size. Pinpoint pupils are a sign of opioid overdose.

Narcotic Antagonists

Opioids are the only class of commonly abused drugs that have a specific antidote. Naloxone (Narcan), a narcotic antagonist, is the drug of choice when opioid overdose is suspected. Naloxone blocks the neuroreceptors affected by opioids, so patients respond in a few minutes to an intravenous injection. Respirations improve, and the patient consciously responds. However, because most opioids have a longer-lasting effect than naloxone, the antagonist must often be repeated to maintain adequate respirations. The nurse administering naloxone must carefully observe the patient to determine whether additional antagonist will be needed. Naltrexone (ReVia) is also a narcotic antagonist used to treat alcohol dependence. Narcotic antagonists do not interrupt the effects of nonnarcotics. The treatment strategy with these agents is further discussed in Chapter 12.

Interactions

The effects of opioids are increased when they are combined with other CNS depressants. Because substance abusers commonly use multiple drugs, the potential for deadly combinations is real. If it is known that heroin has been taken and naloxone does not reverse CNS depression, it can be safely assumed that other depressants were also taken. In such cases, supportive care is indicated.

Withdrawal and Detoxification

The unassisted withdrawal from alcohol or barbiturates can be fatal, but the unassisted withdrawal from opioids is rarely fatal. Withdrawal symptoms are related to the degree of dependence and the abruptness of discontinuance. Maximum intensity is reached within 36 to 72 hours and subsides in 5 to 10 days. Withdrawal symptoms can be categorized as early, intermediate, and late appearing. Early symptoms of withdrawal include yawning, tearing, rhinorrhea, and sweating. Intermediate symptoms include flushing, piloerection, tachycardia, tremor, restlessness, and irritability. Symptoms that are late appearing include muscle spasm, fever, nausea, diarrhea, vomiting, repetitive sneezing, abdominal cramps, and backache. Treatment is primarily symptomatic and supportive.

Specific Drugs

Morphine is the prototype opioid and is useful in alleviating pain. Oral administration has a variable onset, but intravenous morphine provides almost immediate effect. It is metabolized in the liver, excreted in the urine, and has a half-life of 2.5 to 3 hours.

Drugs related to morphine include hydromorphone (Dilaudid), levorphanol (Levo-Dromoran), and meperidine (Demerol). Hydromorphone is a derivative of morphine and more potent; levorphanol is a drug whose action is identical to that of morphine but used for less severe pain; and meperidine, a synthetic narcotic analgesic, is commonly abused.

Several narcotics have both agonist and antagonist activity. Because of the antagonist activity, their abuse potential is less severe. They include pentazocine (Talwin), oxymorphone (Numorphan), alphaprodine (Nisentil), butorphanol (Stadol), and nalbuphine (Nubain). Fentanyl (Sublimaze), an anesthetic commonly used in surgical anesthesia, is similar to but 100 times stronger than morphine and 20 to 40 times stronger than heroin. It is said to produce an "unbelievable" high.

Methadone (Dolophine), although an opioid similar to morphine, is used to prevent withdrawal symptoms. Methadone is given orally and is poorly metabolized in the liver. Accordingly, it has a much longer half-life (15 to 30 hours) than morphine. Because of the long half-life, once-a-day dosage is effective for treatment of chronic pain and has led to the founding of methadone clinics where people who abuse opioids receive tapering doses of methadone so that they can be gradually weaned from narcotics.

Heroin is derived from morphine and is referred to as a *semisynthetic drug*. It was originally thought to be a cure for morphine addiction but proved to be far more addictive than morphine. Heroin is injected, and deaths have occurred because the concentration of heroin in the street drug is variable.

Codeine is used primarily as a cough suppressant. Its abuse preceded the general drug abuse of the mid to late 1960s because codeine was easily available in over-the-counter cough syrups. Ease of access was eliminated at about the same time that drug abuse became recognized as an emerging national problem. Codeine is not a drug choice for many substance abusers today because it causes a significant degree of nausea in many who use it, even at therapeutic doses for legitimate purposes. Derivatives of codeine such as hydrocodone and oxycodone are commonly used for legitimate medical reasons and are popular drugs for abuse because the purity of a commercially manufactured tablet is attractive to potential buyers.

PHENCYCLIDINE

Phencyclidine (PCP), a synthetic drug, traditionally was used as an animal tranquilizer. The mechanism of action is not well understood, but recently, this drug has been shown to bind sigma opioid receptors in the brain. Emergency room personnel are familiar with this drug because PCP-intoxicated persons are often brought to the emergency room; they literally change from coma to violent behavior and back. Caution must be exercised when caring for these patients because of their unpredictable behavior. Ketamine (Special K, vitamin K) is related to PCP and has risen in popularity as a "club drug" with youth. It is a general anesthetic used in day surgery. Euphoria, hallucinations, and disorientation are primary effects. Bad trips are referred to as a *K-hole*. Flashbacks are known to occur.

Pharmacokinetics

PCP is taken orally or intravenously and is smoked and snorted. Oral PCP takes effect in 5 minutes. Phencyclidine is well absorbed by all routes. Its high lipid solubility causes it to reach the brain soon after dosing. Effects last for 6 to 8 hours. PCP can be found in the blood and urine for up to 10 days after intake.

Ketamine can be injected, snorted, ingested, or smoked. Recently, users have combined it with marijuana or tobacco, sometimes selling to or sharing with unsuspecting victims.

Physiologic Effects

The user experiences a high with PCP or ketamine. Euphoria and a peaceful, easy feeling can occur and are sought. Perceptual distortions are common. Memory and attention are impaired.

The undesired effects of PCP are many and serious. Blood pressure and heart rate are elevated. Other effects include ataxia, salivation, and vomiting. Psychologic symptoms include hostile, bizarre behavior; a blank stare; and agitation. Catatonia with muscular rigidity alternating with violent outbursts is particularly frightening to bystanders. PCP is toxic to neurons in both the cortex and cerebellum.[13]

SEDATIVE-HYPNOTICS

Several types of drugs fall into the sedative-hypnotic class, and their abuse potential is staggering. The original type of drug in this class was barbiturates, such as phenobarbital or pentobarbital. Benzodiazepines are commonly prescribed and abused drugs. More recently, newer drugs such as gamma-hydroxybutyrate (GHB) have gained popularity with youth as club drugs.

Barbiturates and benzodiazepines are used to relieve anxiety or to produce sleep (see Chapter 10). Barbiturates have a narrow therapeutic index, the lethal dose being only slightly higher than the therapeutic dose, whereas benzodiazepines have a much wider therapeutic index and are not lethal when used alone. These drugs produce both physical and psychologic dependence.

Currently, barbiturates are categorized as ultrashort acting (e.g., thiopental), short to intermediate acting (e.g., secobarbital), and long acting (e.g., phenobarbital). Abused barbiturates tend to come from the short- to intermediate-acting group. Barbiturates are used in some headache preparations (Fiorinal, Fioricet, and Esgic Plus). Benzodiazepines are used for treatment of anxiety disorders and for sleep disturbances. GHB is manufactured from products available at health-food stores and is used as a performance-enhancing drug in competitive athletics, in addition to being used as a depressant.

Pharmacokinetics

Barbiturates, when abused, are usually taken orally, as are benzodiazepines and GHB. They are metabolized by the liver and excreted by the kidneys. When these drugs are combined with alcohol, dangerous levels of CNS depression can occur.

Physiologic Effects

Sedative-hypnotics depress the CNS, thus decreasing awareness of external stimuli, shortening the attention span, and decreasing intellectual ability. These effects are mediated through actions at the GABA receptor. Regular sleep patterns are changed, with loss of rapid eye movement sleep. These drugs are used to treat insomnia, to soften withdrawal from heroin, and as anticonvulsants. People who abuse drugs take barbiturates and benzodiazepines to maintain a state of relatively anxiety-free living. These drugs are also taken to counteract the effects of amphetamines, to "come down," or to replace heroin when it is not available. The acutely intoxicated person has an unsteady gait, slurred speech, and sustained nystagmus. Chronic users have mental symptoms that include confusion, irritability, and insomnia. As previously stated, tolerance develops rapidly, and important physiologic dependence occurs. Barbiturates also induce hepatic microsomal enzymes and by doing so can increase the metabolism and shorten the half-life of important drugs such as oral anticoagulants, steroids, and some antibiotics. Interactions with these drugs must be monitored closely.

Overdose

Whereas barbiturates can be lethal in overdose, benzodiazepines are not. Both barbiturates and benzodiazepines affect GABA receptors, but benzodiazepines simply enhance the effect of existing GABA on these receptors. The effect of benzodiazepines does not transcend the level of endogenous GABA. On the other hand, in larger doses, barbiturates not only enhance GABA but also mimic GABA. Thus the effect of barbiturates is significantly greater than that of benzodiazepines. These two apparently contradictory effects are mediated through different subunits on the GABA receptor.

The toxic dose of barbiturates varies; in general, an oral dose of 1 g results in serious poisoning, and doses of 2 to 10 g can be fatal. Acute overdose is manifested by CNS and respiratory depression. Although tolerance for the anxiolytic properties of barbiturates can be rather steep, tolerance to respiratory depression is more gradual. Eventually, the abuser reaches a point where the amount of drug needed to feel good is not much less than the amount needed to kill. Treatment for severe overdose is supportive. Overdose of benzodiazepines likewise produces CNS depression, but as noted, it is not lethal unless combined with ethanol or some other depressant. Acute intoxication with benzodiazepines can be reversed with flumazenil, but this must be done with caution to avoid producing acute withdrawal seizures.

Withdrawal and Detoxification

Symptoms of withdrawal from barbiturates are severe and can cause death. Symptoms usually begin 8 to 12 hours after the last dose is taken. Minor withdrawal symptoms include anxiety, muscle twitching, tremor, progressive weakness, dizziness, distorted visual perception, nausea and vomiting, insomnia, and orthostatic hypotension. More serious withdrawal symptoms include seizures and delirium, beginning approximately 16 hours after the last dose and lasting up to 5 days. Untreated, withdrawal symptoms may not decline in intensity for some time. Detoxification requires a cautious and gradual reduction of these drugs. One approach is to reduce the patient's regular dose by 10% each day. Barbiturates can be detected in the urine for up to 3 weeks, as can benzodiazepines.

REMARKS

This chapter is in no way an exhaustive reference. Instead, it is written so that the reader will have a backbone of information about drugs of abuse that are commonly encountered in mental health and medical settings. In the information age, perhaps the greatest accomplishment is the proliferation of information available on the Internet. The following sites are recommended:

www.nida.nih.gov
www.ncadd.org
www.drug-abuse.com
www.health.yahoo.com/health/Diseases_and_Conditions/Mental_Health/
    Addiction_and_Recovery
www.nasadad.org

REFERENCES

1. Buehler BA: Cocaine: how dangerous is it during pregnancy? *Nebr Med J* 80(5):116, 1995.
2. Frezza M and others: High blood alcohol levels in women: the role of decreased gastric alcohol dehydrogenase activity and first-pass metabolism, *N Engl J Med* 322(2):95, 1990.
3. Goldstein GW, Betz AL: The blood-brain barrier, *Sci Am* 255: 74, 1986.
4. Grant B and others: Epidemiologic Bulletin No. 35: Prevalence of DSM-IV alcohol abuse and dependence, United States 1992, *Alcohol Health Res World* 18(3):243, 1994.
5. Gupta PK, al-Kawas FH: Acute pancreatitis: diagnosis and management, *Am Fam Physician* 52(2):435, 1995.
6. Ibañez J and others: Chronic alcoholism decreases neuronal nuclear size in the human entorhinal cortex, *Neurosci Lett* 183(1-2):71, 1995.
7. Institute of Medicine: Prevention and treatment of alcohol-related problems: research opportunities, *J Stud Alcohol* 53(1):5, 1992.
8. Kaufman E, McNaul JP: Recent developments in understanding and treating drug abuse and dependence, *Hosp Community Psychiatry* 43(3):223, 1992.
9. Lewis DC, Gordon AJ: Alcoholism and the general hospital: the Roger Williams Intervention Program, *Bull NY Acad Med* 59:181, 1983.
10. Manzo L and others: Nutrition and alcohol neurotoxicity, *Neurotoxicology* 15(3):555, 1994.
11. Marzuk PM and others: Fatal injuries after cocaine use as a leading cause of death among young adults in New York City, *N Engl J Med* 332(26):1753, 1995.
12. Miller NS: Pharmacotherapy in alcoholism, *J Addict Dis* 14(1):23, 1995.
13. Nakki R and others: Cerebellar toxicity of phencyclidine, *J Neurosci* 15(3 Pt 2):2097, 1995.
14. The National Institute on Drug Abuse: *The economic costs of alcohol and drug abuse in the United States—1992,* Washington, DC, 2000, National Institute on Drug Abuse.
15. O'Brien CP: Treatment of alcoholism as a chronic disorder, *Alcohol* 11(6):433, 1994.
16. Poldrugo F and others: Mortality studies in the long-term evaluation of treatment of alcoholics, *Alcohol* 2 (suppl):1551, 1993.
17. Shen WK and others: Sudden unexpected nontraumatic death in 54 young adults: a 30-year population-based study, *Am J Cardiol* 76(3):148, 1995.
18. Sullivan EV and others: Anterior hippocampal volume deficits in nonamnesic, aging chronic alcoholics, *Alcohol Clin Exp Res* 19(1):110, 1995.
19. Volpicelli JR and others: Effect of naltrexone on alcohol "high" in alcoholics, *Am J Psychiatry* 152(4):613,1995.
20. Wallerstedt S and others: The prevalence of alcoholism and its relation to cause of hospitalization and long-term mortality in male somatic inpatients, *J Intern Med* 237(3):339, 1995.
21. Warner EA: Is your patient using cocaine? Clinical signs that should raise suspicion, *Postgrad Med* 98(2):173, 1995.
22. Whitfield C, Davis J, Barker L: Alcoholism. In Barker LR, Burton JR, Zieve PD, editors: *Principles of ambulatory medicine,* Baltimore, 1986, Williams & Wilkins.

CHAPTER 16

Drugs Used to Stimulate
the Central Nervous System*

STIMULANTS

Humans have been in search of stimulation for thousands of years. The ubiquitous caffeine molecule was repeatedly "discovered" in many forms and in many places, for example, as coffee in Arabia, as tea in China, as the kola nut in Africa, and as cocoa in Mexico.[11] The search continues today as scientists seek safer stimulants for attention-deficit hyperactivity disorder (ADHD), etc., while backstreet alchemists look for molecular configurations that will push stimulation to newer and greater heights.

There are two broad categories of stimulants: those stimulating the respiratory centers in the medullary brainstem (analeptics) and those stimulating the cortex (cerebral stimulants). Analeptic drugs are not discussed in this chapter, but more information can be found in a basic pharmacology text.

The drugs discussed in this chapter are the cerebral stimulants, commonly referred to as *psychostimulants* or just *stimulants*. These agents affect the cerebral cortex and have beneficial psychopharmacologic effects. The therapeutic potential of cerebral stimulants is compromised by their abuse potential.

The amphetamines (and chemical derivatives called *amphetamine congeners*) represent the major classes of cerebral stimulants and are treated as prototype stimulants in this chapter. Drugs such as methylphenidate (Ritalin) and pemoline (Cylert), caffeine, phenylpropanolamine, and other related compounds found in many over-the-counter preparations are examples of other cerebral stimulants.

AMPHETAMINES
Evolution of Amphetamine Use

1933	1937	WWII	1950s	1970
Bronchodilation	Narcolepsy	Battle fatigue	Depression	Use restricted by law

The amphetamines were first synthesized in 1887, but their stimulant effects were not reported in the literature until 1933.[40,44,48] First marketed in the United States in 1932 as bronchodilators, amphetamines were later used as respiratory stimulants, and by 1937, they had gained acceptance for the treatment of narcolepsy.[40,52] Once their mood-altering effects became widely known, these drugs became yet another

---

*The discussion of stimulants is unique in this text because stimulants are used therapeutically in several distinct disorders (e.g., ADHD, narcolepsy, depression) and in special populations (e.g., children, adolescents, the elderly). Furthermore, stimulants are often abused. Hence deciding how and where to discuss stimulants is not as straightforward as say the discussion of antidepressants might be. This chapter has been developed as a basic overview of stimulants, and more specialized discussions have been deferred to other chapters. For example, stimulants are also presented in Chapters 10, 20, 21, and 22. Specific abuses are discussed in Chapters 12 and 15.

option for individuals seeking arousal. By 1970, their use was severely restricted by the Controlled Substance Act, and they were classified as Schedule II drugs. A list of the sought-after effects of stimulants are found in Box 16-1.

Amphetamines gained popularity during World War II as a defense against battle fatigue. Close to 200 million amphetamine tablets were issued to American soldiers stationed in Britain during the war.[56] By the 1950s, stimulants were being used to treat depression.[5] By 1970, 10 billion stimulants were being manufactured legally in the United States.[56] These drugs came to be used by certain groups of individuals, for example, long-distance truck drivers, students, and night-shift workers, who valued the alertness stimulants provided.[48] Others, valuing the euphorigenic properties of amphetamines, made these drugs their drug of choice for abuse.

Today, stimulants are approved by the U.S. Food and Drug Administration (FDA) to treat ADHD, narcolepsy, and Parkinson's disease.[7] Non–FDA-approved indications are found in Box 16-2. At one time, amphetamines were a preferred treatment for obesity. However, because of the previously described propensity for abuse coupled with a tendency for pronounced tolerance and tachyphylaxis (unusually rapid tolerance), amphetamines are seldom prescribed for that use today.

Pharmacologic Effect

Four amphetamines are used clinically: dextroamphetamine (or D-amphetamine [Dexedrine]), amphetamine (a 50/50 combination of D-amphetamine and L-amphetamine [referred to as *racemic amphetamine*]), methamphetamine (Desoxyn), and an amphetamine mixture (Adderall). As noted, *amphetamine* is really two forms

---

Box 16-1 Sought-After Effects of Stimulants

Feelings of euphoria   Appetite suppression
Relief from fatigue   Wakefulness
Improved performance on selected tasks   Increased concentration
Increased activity   Inhibition of sleep

Box 16-2 Nonapproved Uses for Stimulants

Treatment-resistant depression
Major depression in medically or surgically ill patients
Augmentation of tricyclics, SSRIs, RIMA antidepressants
Obsessional disorder
Diagnostic test for tricyclic antidepressants
Negative schizophrenia
Cognitive symptoms of AIDS dementia
Adjuvants in pain management

Data from Reference 7.
SSRIs, Selective serotonin reuptake inhibitors; *RIMA,* reversible inhibitor of MAO-A; *AIDS,* acquired immunodeficiency syndrome.

of amphetamine combined in a 50/50 ratio.[35] These amphetamines are molecular mirror images and are designated as D-form (dextroamphetamine) and L-form (levamphetamine). These forms are more correctly referred to as *optical isomers*. This identical yet opposite molecular configuration accounts for the difference in effect. For example, dextroamphetamine is three to four times more potent as a central nervous system (CNS) stimulant than the L-isomer amphetamine.[52] The L-isomer is a more effective cardiovascular system stimulator. This differential affinity, known as *stereospecificity*, seems to primarily affect norepinephrine release and uptake.[31] Most amphetamine effects are related to increased availability of norepinephrine.[35]

Amphetamines are indirect catecholamine agonists that achieve pharmacologic effect by releasing *newly* synthesized norepinephrine and dopamine.[22,31,33] This is an important distinction and is supported by two important observations: (1) Reserpine, which is known to deplete existing stores of catecholamines (but does not influence the synthesis of catecholamines), *does not* hinder the effect of amphetamine. (2) Alpha-methyltyrosine, which blocks the synthesis of catecholamines, *does* hinder the effect of amphetamine.[31] Amphetamine mechanism of action is in contrast to stimulants such as cocaine and methylphenidate, which act on stored pools of catecholamines.[31] Amphetamines also increase catecholamine intrasynaptic availability by interfering with the presynaptic reuptake and by preventing enzymatic breakdown by monoamine oxidase. Other neurotransmitter systems affected include serotonin and various neuropeptide systems. Amphetamines have both CNS and peripheral nervous system (PNS) effects.

Central Nervous System Effects

Amphetamines stimulate the cerebral cortex, the brainstem, and the reticular activating system (RAS). The RAS is a group of ill-defined, interconnected nuclei located in the medulla, pons, and midbrain. These nuclei receive sensory input from the major sensory pathways and relay it to the cerebral cortex via the thalamus, the sensory relay center for the nervous system.[38] When the RAS is not stimulated, sleep can occur. When the RAS is stimulated, one awakens. Individuals already awake experience greater alertness when the RAS is stimulated.[38] Amphetamine's cortical effects accounting for its abuse potential include wakefulness, alertness, increased concentration, increased motor activity, improved physical performance, decreased fatigue, improved mood, inhibited sleep, and an anorexigenic effect. As noted earlier, an exaggeration of these pharmacologic effects is precisely the element of amphetamine use associated with adverse outcomes.

Amphetamines stimulate the reward center of the brain; this stimulation accounts for the great appeal of these drugs. The nucleus accumbens, a small subdivision of the basal ganglia, is a major component of the reward center.[15,24] By stimulating the reward center, amphetamines produce a sense of well-being usually reserved for accomplishment, love, or some other rewarding external source of gratification. J. Madeleine Nash states, "At a purely chemical level, every experience humans find enjoyable—whether listening to music, embracing a lover or savoring chocolate—amounts to little more than an explosion of dopamine in the nucleus accumbens, as exhilarating and ephemeral as a firecracker."[45] Although Nash's statement may seem overly reductionistic, amphetamines and other stimulants enhance or perpetuate a sense of well-being, and that is why they are abused. These sought-after effects of amphetamines begin to reverse themselves as the drugs wear off. A sense of well-being gives way to despair, concentration turns to irritation and distractibility, and improved physical performance and alertness become fatigue. That is, enhancement is followed by rebound depression approximately proportional to the previously experienced high. Some have likened it to a roller coaster ride. For many beginning users, such swings in emotion discourage further experimentation, but others find the highs irresistible and endure the lows. It should be noted that the "bottom" of the ride also leads to abuse. In other words, abuse of stimulants is motivated by both a desire to get high and by a desire to avoid anguish. This so-called rebound phenomenon is linked to dopaminergic stimulation of presynaptic autoreceptors (a negative feedback system).[23] Because presynaptic autoreceptors have a higher affinity for dopamine than do postsynaptic receptors, lowering dopamine levels cause the few molecules available to be attracted to presynaptic neurons (slowing the release of dopamine), reducing postsynaptic dopamine-receptor coupling even further.

Research indicates that the euphoric properties of amphetamines are more closely related to effects on dopaminergic rather than noradrenergic systems. This hypothesis stems from and is supported by observations that dopamine antagonists (e.g., haloperidol) block euphoria, whereas noradrenergic antagonists have little effect. Amphetamine's anorectic effect probably results from the stimulation of the lateral hypothalamic satiety center.

Because they stimulate the medulla, stimulants increase respirations. Such an effect serves to underscore the well-known fact that drugs have many intersystem and intrasystem effects; that is, although amphetamines produce primarily a cortical effect, they also stimulate subcortical areas.

Amphetamines in small doses may depress the CNS. Occasionally, individuals report a sedative effect after taking a small dose; CNS activity is a balancing of opposing actions between excitatory and inhibitory neurons, and small doses of amphetamines show a preference for inhibitory neurons. Small doses can cause a shift in the norm toward an overall inhibitory response, or CNS depression. This paradox is particularly beneficial in normalizing hyperkinetic motor activity and behavior.

Small doses of amphetamines and related drugs such as methylphenidate apparently stimulate the immature RAS in children with ADHD, thus improving function. Normalization of this system presumably enables the ADHD patient to sit and listen, to tune out extraneous stimuli, and to control bothersome motor activity. The mechanism of action for amphetamines and other stimulants used to treat ADHD in this population is discussed in Chapters 20 and 21.

Peripheral Nervous System Effects

The PNS effects with the greatest potential for harm involve the cardiovascular system and are related to the release of norepinephrine from sympathetic nerves. Amphetamines may increase blood pressure and heart rate. Tachycardia and tachyarrhythmias can also have serious implications in individuals with preexisting conditions. Paradoxically, amphetamines can decrease heart rate through the activation of the baroreceptor reflex as a result of increased blood pressure. This baroreceptor reflex increases parasympathetic input to the heart, thus causing bradycardia. Peripheral hyperthermia is triggered by the sympathoadrenal system.[18] Amphetamines also dilate the pupils and cause decongestion of the mucous membranes. Finally, stimulant use has been associated with sexual dysfunction and movement disorders.[27,29] Other effects related to abuse are outlined in Chapter 15.

Pharmacokinetics

Amphetamines given orally are well absorbed from the gut, have a high volume of distribution, have low protein binding, and are highly lipophilic, crossing the blood-brain barrier readily.[10] When given orally (the only legally approved route in the United States), they exert both CNS and PNS effects within 30 to 60 minutes. Amphetamines are available in several oral forms, including timed-release capsules, immediate-acting tablets, and an elixir. Other amphetamines come in a chewable, slow-release form.

Amphetamines are eliminated from the body in two distinct ways: by renal excretion of the unchanged amphetamine molecule and by metabolism. In some instances, most of a dose is unchanged and continues to produce an effect until excreted in the urine. Because amphetamine is a basic drug, urine pH influences excretion. Renal excretion of amphetamine is expedited by an acidic urine. For instance, at a pH of less than 5.6, amphetamine has a half-life of 7 hours, whereas alkalinizing the urine can increase the half-life up to 30 hours. (The average half-life of an amphetamine is 12 hours.)[52] Urinary alkalinization extends half-life because molecules are not ionized and are readily reabsorbed into the bloodstream. An average 7-hour increase in amphetamine half-life results from every 1-unit increase in pH.[47] Thus acidifying the urine (e.g., with cranberry juice) can hasten elimination of amphetamine, and alkalinization of the urine (e.g., with sodium bicarbonate) will slow elimination.

Amphetamines are metabolized by three metabolic pathways: aromatic hydroxylation producing an active metabolite, beta-hydroxylation by the enzyme dopamine beta-hydroxylase, or by oxidation. The distinctions among these metabolic routes are quite complex and beyond the scope of this text. Nonetheless, recognizing that the majority of an amphetamine dose often is excreted unchanged can help the clinician produce better outcomes through management of urine pH.

Side Effects

Amphetamine side effects are largely extensions of the effects noted in Table 16-1. Through the CNS, these drugs suppress appetite, resulting in weight loss (sometimes desired), cause insomnia (sometimes desired), produce overly anxious behavior and moodiness, and ignite euphoric feelings that can lead to inappropriate or overly ambitious decisions. Growth retardation is a concern in children who are given these drugs for ADHD. Other CNS effects include restlessness, irritability, dysphoria, dizziness, tremor, hyperpyrexia, talkativeness, aggressive behavior, confusion, panic, and increased libido.

A toxic paranoid psychosis, toxic delirium, or both can develop. Traditionally, the toxic psychosis caused by amphetamine's dopamine-potentiating properties has been viewed as a schizophrenia-like manifestation. Indeed, the use of dopamine antagonists (i.e., antipsychotic drugs) is effective in arresting these symptoms. Amphetamine psychosis follows a predictable course, initially manifesting as paranoid thinking and evolving to a rigid, persecutory, confused, and panic-stricken state. The latter can lead to violent outbursts. Because amphetamines increase norepinephrine, psychotic symptoms arising from amphetamine intoxication should be attributed partly to increased norepinephrine bioavailability.[8] Although cocaine can trigger psychotic symptoms, this phenomenon is much less common because of cocaine's much shorter duration of action.

Cardiovascular effects (most likely attributable to norepinephrine release by levamphetamine in racemic amphetamine) include elevated blood pressure, chilling, palpitations, and less often, tachycardia and tachyarrhythmias. Some patients have died from cardiovascular stimulation. Headaches, pallor, facial flushing, mucous membrane decongestion, mydriasis and photophobia, diarrhea, cramps, vomiting, dry mouth, and abdominal pain are also potential side effects of amphetamines.

Table 16-1 Side Effects/Overdose of CNS Stimulants

Side effect	Intervention/treatment/patient
CNS	
Anorexia (see Ketosis)	Pt: Take after meals.
Restlessness, insomnia	Pt: Take last dose at least 6 hours before bed. Decrease dose.
	Clin: Insomnia and restlessness associated with overdose can be treated with lorazepam 1-2 mg or diazepam 5-10 mg every 1-2 hr.
Restlessness, euphoria, panic, agitation	Clin: Decrease dose until the desired effects are achieved and the undesired side effects are minimized.
PNS	
Eye	
Mydriasis, photophobia	Pt: Wear sunglasses. Use artificial tears (use ointment at night).
Metabolic	
Ketosis, hyperglycemia, worsening of diabetic symptoms	Clin: Monitor glucose levels. Adjust insulin.
Cardiovascular	
Palpitations, tachycardia, hypertension, angina, arrhythmias	Clin: Monitor blood pressure and vital signs. Monitor caffeine intake and other sympathomimetics.
Severe hypertension/ tachyarrhythmias	Clin: Give IV propranolol 1 mg every 5-10 min prn to a total of 8 mg.
Gastrointestinal	
Dry mouth, constipation, diarrhea, anorexia, vomiting	Pt: Chew sugarless gum, eat hard candy, take frequent sips of water, use artificial saliva. Take with meals.

Overdose	Intervention/treatment/patient
Hypertension, tachycardia, hyperthermia, grand mal seizures	Clin: Give adrenergic blockers like phentalomine to decrease blood pressure and heart rate. Give activated charcoal 1 g/kg body weight. Acidify the urine. Give ammonium chloride to increase excretion.
Unconsciousness	Clin: Provide airway support.
Seizures	Clin: Give IV benzodiazapines: Lorazepam (Ativan) 1-2 mg Diazepam (Valium) 5-10 mg Clin: Give fluids until urine reaches 3-6 ml/kg/hr.
Toxic psychosis, delirum	Clin: Give chlorpromazine (Thorazine) 50 mg qid IM or haloperidol (Haldol) 5 mg bid IM

Note: Patient and clinician actions are denoted by *Pt* and *Clin*, respectively.
CNS, Central nervous system; *PNS,* peripheral nervous system.

Implications

Therapeutic versus toxic levels. Toxic effects generally reflect autonomic overstimulation and cause an extreme exaggeration of side effects. For example, acute toxicity produces dizziness, confusion, psychosis (i.e., hallucinations, paranoid delusions, grandiosity), arrhythmias, and hypertension. Therapeutic blood levels of amphetamines range from 5 to 10 μg/dl.[47] Some individuals can ingest much more than the recommended levels of amphetamines (about 5 mg to 40 mg/day for adults) without serious effects because of tolerance and tachyphylaxis. According to Lehne, some highly tolerant individuals need 1000 mg intravenously every few hours to sustain a euphoric state.[35]

Animal models suggest chronic use of amphetamine leads to long-term changes in dopaminergic, noradrenergic, and serotonergic systems. This thinking would support clinical observations that suggest a certain level of anhedonia lingers for some time among stimulant abusers after discontinuance of the drug(s).

Tolerance is an important consideration when treating with amphetamines. Tolerance occurs in two ways. The more significant mechanism depletes norepinephrine from nerve endings. As norepinephrine stores are reduced, more and more amphetamine is required to maintain a consistent response. Tolerance can occur after one or two doses. The second mechanism of amphetamine tolerance is ketosis, a byproduct of amphetamine-caused anorexia. As the individual stops eating, an alteration in metabolism occurs, resulting in ketosis that in turn leads to acidic urine. As noted previously, acidic urine hastens the excretion of amphetamine: anorexia → ketosis → acidic urine → increased urinary elimination of amphetamine.

Tolerance to almost all of the CNS and PNS effects can occur, including tolerance to appetite suppression, cardiovascular effects, and euphoria. However, no tolerance is observed for the psychotic effects of amphetamines. What this means is that abusers can take doses of amphetamines hundreds of times greater than therapeutic doses without harmful physical effects but remain vulnerable to amphetamine psychosis. These same high levels of amphetamine ingestion would kill someone who has not developed amphetamine tolerance.

Overdose results in sympathetic hyperactivity, that is, hypertension, tachycardia, and hyperthermia accompanied by delirium and toxic psychosis.[5] Grand mal seizures can occur as a physiologic response to an overdose of amphetamine. Deaths, although relatively rare, have been reported when tachycardias, tachyarrhythmias, hyperthermia, and seizures have converged to compromise body systems.[5]

Acute overdose treatment includes emptying the stomach of its contents, the administration of activated charcoal 1 g/kg body weight, and urine acidification. Strategies to treat overdose of amphetamines should also include using alpha-adrenergic blockers such as phentolamine to reduce blood pressure and lower pulse rate and the antipsychotic chlorpromazine (Thorazine) to counter psychotic manifestations. Chlorpromazine is also a relatively potent alpha-adrenergic antagonist and may contribute to hypertensive states. Other measures for overdose are supportive. Airway support is critical for patients who are unconscious, and external cooling approaches, including the use of cooling blankets, are required for hyperthermia. Seizures can be controlled with intravenous (IV) benzodiazepine, for example, lorazepam (Ativan) 1 to 2 mg or diazepam (Valium) 5 to 10 mg.[5] Fluids should be administered until urine flow reaches 3 to 6 ml/kg/hr.[47]

Use in pregnancy. Amphetamines are highly lipophilic and cross the placental barrier. Dextroamphetamine has a federal pregnancy category C rating (potential risk to the fetus) and racemic amphetamine is in category X (an absolute prohibition against use during pregnancy). Other cautions are listed in Box 16-3.

Box 16-3   Cautious Use, Precautions, and Contraindications for the Use of Stimulants

Cautious use
Patients suffering from anxiety, tension, agitation, restlessness
Patients suffering from cardiovascular problems (e.g., hypertension, arrhythmias)
Patients with seizure disorders (can lower seizure threshold)
Patients suffering from hyperthyroidism
Patients with history of drug abuse

Precautions
Abruptly withdrawing these agents after prolonged use can result in dysphoria and/or rebound insomnia.
Using psychostimulants in patients with attention-deficit hyperactivity disorder can unmask tics or tardive dyskinesia
Tourette's patients may worsen initially

Contraindications
Possibly patients recently known to abuse drugs or alcohol (must be used with extreme caution)
Patients with a history of psychosis
Patients with liver disease
Patients with anorexia nervosa
Patients with a diagnosis of anxiety
Patients with thyroid disease
Patients with glaucoma
Patients with severe hypertension, severe angina pectoris

Adapted from Reference 7.

Interactions. The more common drug interactions with amphetamines are found in Table 16-2.

METHYLPHENIDATE

Methylphenidate, a Schedule II agent, is the most commonly prescribed drug for ADHD and is structurally related to amphetamine (Figure 16-1). It is a milder cortical stimulant than amphetamine, being about half as potent, and appears to have a greater effect on mental activities than on motor activities.[10] Its mechanism of action is not fully understood; however, tolerance to the effects of this drug does occur to some extent. Methylphenidate is well absorbed from the gastrointestinal (GI) tract and reaches peak blood levels within 1 to 3 hours. Its half-life ranges from 1 to 7 hours, with a duration of effect after one dose of up to 6 hours. Methylphenidate is metabolized in the liver to inactive products (unlike the amphetamines), so urinary acidification or alkalinization does not affect its stimulatory abilities. It inhibits the cytochrome P-450 2D6 isoenzyme. Side effects are similar to those of the amphetamines already discussed (e.g., insomnia, restlessness, nervousness). In a few individuals, anemia and other blood dyscrasias

Table 16-2 Drug Interactions with Amphetamine and/or Methylphenidate

Interactant	Effect	Result
Acidifying agent (urinary) (e.g., ascorbic acid, fruit juices)	Decreased half-life and effect of amphetamine	Decreased CNS and PNS effects; may need to increase dosage
Alkalinizing agents (urinary) (sodium bicarbonate)—used for antidepressant overdose and for heartburn; acetazolamide; antacids, ammonium chloride, phenothiazines; haloperidol	Increased half-life and effect of amphetamine	Increased CNS and PNS effects; may need lower dosage
Anticholinergics	Additive cholinergic effect	
Anticonvulsants		
Phenytoin	Methylphenidate: increased phenytoin serum levels related to decreased metabolism	
Antidepressants		
MAOIs	Methylphenidate: hypertensive reaction	
TCAs	Methylphenidate: antidepressant serum levels rise; increased cardiovascular effects	
Moclobemide	Methylphenidate: increased blood pressure, enhanced effect over a long time	
	Methylphenidate and amphetamine: additive effects	
SSRIs	Amphetamine: hypertensive crisis, risk of stroke	
MAOIs	Amphetamine: slightly enhanced over a long period	
RIMA	Amphetamine: enhanced antidepressant effect; amphet-	
TCAs	amine plasma level elevated related to inhibited metabolism	

Continued

Table 16-2 Drug Interactions with Amphetamine and/or Methylphenidate—cont'd

Interactant	Effect	Result
Antihypertensives (guanethidine, clonidine)	Decreased antihypertensive affect of drug	
Antipsychotics	Antagonizes the effects of amphetamine	Decreased cerebral stimulant effect
		Decreased peripheral stimulant effect
Caffeine (cola, tea, coffee, chocolate)	Potentiates effect of amphetamine	
CNS depressants (alcohol)	Antagonism of desired stimulant effect	
Barbiturates	Amphetamine: effects of amphetamine antagonized	
Guanethidine	Amphetamine: reversal of hypotensive effect	
Hypoglycemic drugs (insulin, oral hypoglycemics)	Increased or decreased blood glucose levels	Poor diabetes control
Ketosis (starvation, diabetes)	Acidifies urine	Hastens elimination of amphetamine
Lithium	Decreased effect of one or both interactant	Poor control of psychotic disorder
MAOIs	Floods peripheral synapses with norepinephrine	Hypertensive crisis, stroke
OTC stimulants with caffeine (see Table 16-3)	Increased effect of amphetamine	
Phenylpropanalamine (Accutrim, Appedrine, Dexatrim capsules)	Increased sympathomimetic effect	Increased side effects of both drugs

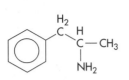

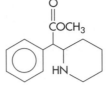

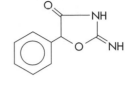

Amphetamine   Methylphenidate   Pemoline

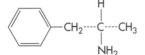

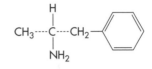

Dextroamphetamine   Levamphetamine

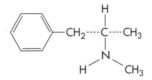

Methamphetamine

Figure 16-1 Chemical structures of amphetamine, methylphenidate, pemoline, dextroamphetamine, levamphetamine, and methamphetamine.

have been linked to methylphenidate treatment. Periodic complete blood cell counts can help the clinician monitor for these hematologic effects.

An overdose of methylphenidate manifests as CNS overstimulation similar to that found in amphetamine overdose. The side effects of methylphenidate are similar to those of amphetamine, and interventions discussed for amphetamines are appropriate for methylphenidate.

Implications

Use in pregnancy. There have been no reports of adverse effects on fetal development resulting from the use of this drug.

Interactions. Most of the interactions associated with amphetamines are also of concern with methylphenidate (see Table 16-2). Notable exceptions include the methylphenidate-mediated decrease in phenytoin metabolism and the lack of sensitivity to urinary acidifiers/alkalinizers.

PEMOLINE

Pemoline (Cylert) is an FDA-approved drug for the treatment of ADHD. It is only remotely similar to amphetamine and has minimal sympathomimetic activity.[56] Pemoline is well absorbed from the stomach, and peak serum levels occur within 2 to

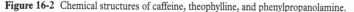

4 hours. The half-life is 12 hours in adults and approximately 7 hours in children. Once-per-day dosing is permitted. About half of each dose is excreted unchanged in the urine; the rest is metabolized before excretion.

Pemoline apparently acts by increasing the storage or synthesis of dopamine. A beneficial effect typically does not occur for 3 to 4 weeks. Pemoline causes less cerebral stimulation than do amphetamines or methylphenidate, and it is less effective. Pemoline also causes fewer peripheral sympathomimetic effects. Side effects, adverse responses, toxic effects, and appropriate interventions are similar to those for amphetamines. Exceptions include rarely occurring acute liver failure and significantly less intense cardiovascular side effects. Safety during pregnancy and breast-feeding has not been established. The abuse potential for pemoline is less than that for amphetamines or methylphenidate; hence, it is classified as a category IV drug.

OTHER STIMULANTS: CAFFEINE AND AMPHETAMINE-LIKE ANORECTICS

Many other drugs with stimulant qualities are available for stimulant seekers. Ma-huang, for instance, has been used since at least 3000 BC in China and is still a major ingredient in many "natural" herb products found in health stores. Most of these drugs are sold as anorectics, which are used for weight loss. Other stimulants can be found in foodstuff (e.g., caffeine), headache tablets, hay fever and cold remedies, and decongestants. Although some anorectics require a prescription, many can be purchased over the counter. (See Figure 16-2 for the chemical structures of the stimulants discussed in this section.)

CAFFEINE

Caffeine is the most widely used stimulant in the world. Coffee was discovered around 850 AD by Khaldi, a goat herder in northern Eygpt.[11] Technically, it was Khaldi's wayward goats that first sampled berries from the coffee bush, and noting the goats' euphoric state, Khaldi partook and was stimulated as well.[11]

Caffeine is found in coffee, cola, chocolate, and tea. It is an ingredient in more

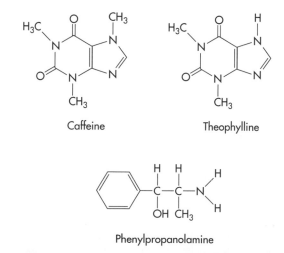

Caffeine   Theophylline

Phenylpropanolamine

Figure 16-2 Chemical structures of caffeine, theophylline, and phenylpropanolamine.

than 1000 over-the-counter medications.[34] More than half of the people in the United States could not start their days without their eye-opening cups of coffee. In fact, 80% of Americans ingest some form of caffeine daily, with an average adult consumption of 200 to 280 mg/day (about 2 cups of coffee).[53,54] It is coffee's CNS-stimulating potential with the accompanying mini-euphoria that makes it so popular.[25,26] Caffeine users often have the characteristics associated with substance abusers: tolerance, a withdrawal syndrome (lethargy, irritability, headache), persistent desire, and unsuccessful attempts to reduce or stop consumption despite physical and psychologic consequences.[19,50] Habitual coffee drinkers also refer to coffee's (caffeine's) relaxing effect. This "relaxation" is most likely related to relief from the withdrawal syndrome noted previously. Table 16-3 provides an interesting glimpse of the caffeine content of various beverages, pills, and foods.

The psychiatric significance of caffeine is related to its ability to produce a sustained anxiety-like syndrome in individuals hypersensitive to its sympathomimetic effects. The *Diagnostic and Statistical Manual of Mental Disorders,* fourth edition (DSM-IV), identifies this disorder as caffeine intoxication (305.90). Essential symptoms of this disorder include restlessness, nervousness, excitement, insomnia, flushed face, diuresis, and GI disturbance.[2] These symptoms can occur with dosages less than 250 mg/day (in caffeine-sensitive individuals), but in individuals diagnosed with caffeinism, higher dosages are usually required.[46] When dosages have exceeded 10 g/day, deaths have been reported.[47] Because 10 g of caffeine are equivalent to 89 to 100 cups of coffee, overdose occurs most often with tablets.

Coffee ingestion accounts for about 75% of all caffeine consumed.[11] The DSM-IV notes that coffee contains 80 to 180 mg of caffeine per cup, tea about half that amount, and colas about one third.[2] Caffeine-containing headache powders have one third to half the amount of caffeine found in a cup of coffee. Chocolate and cocoa typically contain less caffeine. From 20% to 30% of persons in the United States ingest between 500 and 600 mg of caffeine per day, and about 10% consume more than 1000 mg a day, the defining point for overuse.[28,51] As many as 10% of persons in the United States could be described as having caffeinism. However, caffeine "abuse" is significantly different from what is popularly called *drug abuse.*[20] Caffeine users do not need incrementally larger doses (hence no tolerance), and antisocial behaviors are not associated with caffeine use.[1]

Side Effects

Caffeine stimulates the CNS, producing alertness and focused concentration. At higher levels of consumption, caffeine produces insomnia and nervousness. Caffeine's recognized ability to relieve headache is thought to be related to its central vasoconstricting properties. On the other hand, caffeine causes vasodilation in the periphery. Caffeine's effects on the heart are well known—from increased rate to palpitations and arrhythmia. It relaxes smooth muscle in the bronchi, enabling respirations, and related drugs (e.g., theophylline) are prescribed for asthma. A faster heart rate coupled with vasodilation leads to increased urine output. Gastric acid and other secretions are also increased, leading to a variety of GI tract ailments. Not all the GI tract disorders associated with coffee are caffeine related. For instance, oils found in coffee are irritating to the stomach. The basal metabolic rate of regular coffee drinkers is increased by about 10%.[25]

Pharmacokinetics

Caffeine is easily absorbed from the GI tract. It reaches peak levels within 1 hour and has a half-life of 3 to 7 hours. It is metabolized by the P-450 1A2 isoenzyme.[4] Drugs

Table 16-3 Sources of Caffeine

Source	Caffeine content (approximate)
Beverages	
Coffee, brewed (drip)	60-180 mg/cup
Coffee, brewed (percolator)	40-170 mg/cup
Coffee, instant	30-120 mg/cup
Coffee, decaffeinated, brewed	2-5 mg/cup
Coffee, decaffeinated, instant	1-5 mg/cup
Tea, brewed, major U.S. brands	20-90 mg/cup
Tea, instant	25-50 mg/cup
Tea, iced	67-76 mg/12 oz
Cocoa	2-50 mg/cup
Chocolate milk	2-7 mg/cup
Milk chocolate	1-15 mg/oz
Baker's chocolate	25-35 mg/oz
Soft drinks*	
Jolt	100 mg/12 oz
Sugar-free Mr. Pibb	59 mg/12 oz
Mountain Dew	54 mg/12 oz
Tab	47 mg/12 oz
Coca-Cola	46 mg/12 oz
Diet Coke	46 mg/12 oz
Mr. Pibb	41 mg/12 oz
Dr. Pepper	40 mg/12 oz
Big Red	38 mg/12 oz
Pepsi-Cola	38 mg/12 oz
Diet Pepsi	36 mg/12 oz
RC Cola	36 mg/12 oz
7-Up, ginger ale, most root beers	0 mg/12 oz
Over-the-counter analgesics*	
Anacin, Midol, Vanquish	32 mg/tablet
Excedrin Extra Strength	65 mg/tablet or capsule
Over-the-counter cold preparations*	
Dristan	16 mg/tablet
Triaminicin†	32 mg/tablet
Over-the-counter stimulants*	
No Doz	100 mg/tablet
Vivarin	200 mg/tablet
Prescription medications*	
Darvon compound	32 mg/capsule
Fiorina	140 mg/tablet or capsule
Cafergot	100 mg/tablet

From Keltner NL: Central nervous system stimulants. In Schlafer M, editor: *The nurse, pharmacology, and drug therapy,* Redwood City, Calif, 1989, Addison-Wesley. Data for beverages; over-the-counter analgesics, cold preparations, and stimulants; and prescription medications adapted from References 11, 34, and 35.
*A representative sampling of the caffeine-containing preparations in these categories.
†This products also contain phenylpropanolamine.

Table 16-4 Interactions with Caffeine

Interactant	Result of interaction
Selective serotonin reuptake inhibitors (SSRIs)	Increased half-life of caffeine related to inhibition of P-450 1A2 isoenzyme
Electroconvulsive therapy (ECT)	Caffeine increases the duration of the seizure and is used to augment the effect of ECT
Clozapine	Increased plasma level of clozapine related to caffeine inhibition of P-450 1A2
Benzodiazepines/hypnotics and sedatives	Can interfere with sedation and cause insomnia instead
Disulfiram	Reduced clearance of caffeine by up to 30%
Lithium	Increases renal excretion of lithium; may increase lithium tremor

Data from References 4 and 7.

that inhibit this enzyme system (e.g., the selective serotonin reuptake inhibitors [SSRIs]) extend the half-life of caffeine. For instance, fluvoxamine (Luvox), a potent inhibitor of this enzyme, extends the half-life of caffeine to 31 hours.[7] Interactions with caffeine are found in Table 16-4.

Mechanism of Action

Caffeine apparently inhibits the breakdown of cyclic adenosine monophosphate (cAMP), a second messenger in the norepinephrine and dopamine neurotransmitter systems. The increase in cAMP bioavailability intensifies other CNS and PNS sympathomimetic effects.[47] An alternative explanation of caffeine's mechanism of action suggests it is related to the enhancement of calcium permeability in the sarcoplasmic reticulum.[35]

Implications

Caffeine withdrawal. Caffeine withdrawal is accompanied by headache (and occasionally vomiting), decreased arousal, and fatigue. Withdrawal effects are reversible with readministration of caffeine.

Use in pregnancy. Because caffeine is known to cross the placental barrier (with the potential to induce fetal malformation), some clinicians recommend cautious use of caffeine during pregnancy.[14]

PHENYLPROPANOLAMINE

Phenylpropanolamine is an ingredient in more than 100 prescription and over-the-counter anorectics, nasal decongestants, psychostimulants, and treatments for premenstrual syndrome.[13] Table 16-5 and Box 16-4 list several well-known compounds that are sold as anorectics. Phenylpropanolamine is often combined with caffeine. The amount of phenylpropanolamine ranges from 25 to 75 mg per tablet and should be used only by adults. At somewhat lower dosages (e.g., 12.5 mg) it is used in allergy, cough suppressant, and cold medications.

Psychiatrically, phenylpropanolamine is important because it intensifies stimulant properties of other sympathomimetics or antagonizes the effects of other psychotropic agents. Phenylpropanolamine is molecularly similar to amphetamine; however, it is a direct-acting sympathomimetic, whereas amphetamine is indirect acting. It acts as a pressor agent because of a strong alpha-1 effect and a relatively weak beta effect. Subsequent hypertension associated with phenylpropanolamine is often accompanied by a reflex bradycardia.[13] Signs and symptoms associated with phenylpropanolamine use in descending order (most common to least common) include hypertension, throbbing bilateral headache, nausea and vomiting, anxiety, palpitations, seizures, stroke, tremor, hallucinations, and tachycardia.[13]

Phenylpropanolamine is rapidly absorbed, has an onset of action within 3 hours, a

Table 16-5 Representative Over-the-Counter Weight Loss Products Containing Phenylpropanolamine

Product	Phenylpropanolamine content (mg)
Acutrim	75 (tablet)
Appedrine*	25 (tablet)
Dexatrim capsules*	25, 75 (capsule)
Grapefruit diet plan with Diadax	12.5, 30, 75 (capsule)
Phenoxine	25 (tablet)
Unitrol	75 (capsule)

*Also contains caffeine.

Box 16-4 Anorectic Drugs with and without Stimulation Effects

Nonamphetamine catecholamine stimulants
Schedule II
  Phenmetrazine (Preludin)
Schedule III
  Benzphetamine (Didrex)
  Phendimetrazine (Bontril, Prelu-2, Plegine)
Schedule IV
  Diethylpropion (Tenuate, Tepanil)
  Mazindol (Mazanor, Sanorex)
  Phentermine* (Adipex-2, Fastin, Obenix, Oby-Trim, Zantryl)
Nonregulated drugs
  Phenylpropanolamine (e.g., Acutrim, Dexatrim; see Table 16-4)

Serotonergic agents (non-CNS stimulating)
  Dexfenfluramine (Redux)
  Fenfluramine* (Pondimin)

CNS, Central nervous system.
*The combination of phentermine and fenfluramine (Fen-Phen) was used for weight loss until cases of valvular heart disease mandated that it be taken off the market. An increase in serotonin (i.e., fenfluramine) or an increase in catecholamines (i.e., phentermine) will result in an anorectic effect. Theoretically, the sedative effect of fenfluramine offsets the stimulating effect of phentermine.

half-life of 3 to 4 hours, and 80% to 90% is excreted in the urine unchanged. It has a low therapeutic index, and a number of deaths have been reported in patients taking phenylpropanolamine.

OTHER ANORECTICS

Other anorectics include catecholamine-enhancing drugs such as benzphetamine, diethylpropion, mazindol, phendimetrazine, phenmetrazine, and phentermine and serotonin-enhancing agents such as dexfenfluramine and fenfluramine (see Box 16-4). Dexfenfluramine and fenfluramine increase intrasynaptic serotonin through several mechanisms. Enhanced serotonin preferentially inhibits the ingestion of carbohydrates over fat or protein.[36] The combination of phentermine and fenfluramine (Fen-Phen) was used for weight loss until cases of valvular heart disease mandated it be taken off the market. An increase in serotonin (with fenfluramine) or an increase in catecholamines (with phentermine) results in an anorectic effect, and the use of these different but complimentary chemicals had great promise theoretically. Furthermore, it was thought the sedative effect of a serotonin enhancer would counterbalance the stimulating effect of a catecholamine enhancer. Although effective for many people, the aforementioned cardiovascular events prevent further marketing of this drug combination. These drugs have effects, precautions, and abuse potential similar to amphetamines.[55]

TREATMENT CONSIDERATIONS

Amphetamines, methylphenidate, and pemoline are used primarily to treat ADHD and narcolepsy (Table 16-6). Of children with ADHD, 60% to 70% remain symptomatic as adults, and drug dosages given in Chapter 21 may be applicable.[17] Information on the pharmacologic treatment of ADHD is found in Chapters 19 and 20.

Treatment of Depression

Stimulants have been used to treat depression and are also known to cause depression.[32,37,41] Although anecdotal reports of their antidepressive properties are encouraging, an extensive review of the literature does not support treating

Table 16-6 Adult Dosages of Major Central Nervous System Stimulants

Drug	Indications	Usual adult dose
Dextroamphetamine (Dexedrine), Schedule I	ADHD	5-40 mg/day
	Narcolepsy	5-60 mg/day in divided doses
	Depression	5-60 mg/day
Methylphenidate (Ritalin), Schedule II	ADHD	5-40 mg/day
	Narcolepsy	20-60 mg/day in divided doses
	Depression	10-30 mg/day
Pemoline (Cylert), Schedule IV	ADHD	37.5-112.5 mg/day

Data from References 5 and 7.
ADHD, Attention-deficit hyperactivity disorder.

depression with stimulants.[10] However, a number of other studies support the augmentation role of stimulants in depression.[42,56]

Treatment of Medically Ill and Geriatric Patients Who Are Depressed

Ayd and Zohar found a positive response to stimulants in medically ill and poststroke patients who were depressed.[6] Myers and Stewart reported promising results from methylphenidate with or without tricyclic antidepressants (TCAs) to treat depressed medically ill patients.[43] In a review of the literature, Roccaforte and Burke have found evidence to support stimulant use among elderly persons who have amotivational syndrome and depression.[52] Effects on cognition were less remarkable; however, this treatment alternative continues to be explored.[16] Other studies have found methylphenidate and dextroamphetamine helpful in treating apathetic and withdrawn elderly patients.[30,41,49] This topic is further discussed in Chapter 21.

Use as a Challenge Test for Predicting a Response to Antidepressants

Goff and Jenike suggested that a positive response (a euphoric response) to a dose of amphetamine might indicate a particular patient will respond positively to noradrenergic TCAs (e.g., amoxapine, desipramine, nortriptyline, protriptyline).[21] Patients who have a dysphoric response may respond more favorably to serotonergic antidepressants (SSRIs, amitriptyline, imipramine, clomipramine, nefazodone, venlafaxine). However, research on this topic is not conclusive. Little and Gay, for example, found stimulant responders fared better when undergoing chronic antidepressant treatment than did nonresponders.[39]

Caffeine Augmentation of Electroconvulsive Therapy

Giving pretreatment caffeine can help lengthen electroconvulsive therapy (ECT)-induced seizure time without increasing electrical stimulus.[3,12,46] Clinical efficacy does not appear to be compromised; furthermore, Coffey and others reported a higher response rate in the pretreatment caffeine group (95%) than in the control group (80%).[12]

Treatment of Schizophrenia

Goldberg and others sought to improve mood and cognition by coadministering dextroamphetamine and haloperidol.[22] Although the theoretic underpinning of their effort seems reasonable (i.e., amphetamine would selectively stimulate D_1 receptors in the frontal cortex), patients in the study did not improve. Chiarello and Cole reviewed 10 studies of stimulant-treated schizophrenia ($N = 430$).[10] Ninety-six patients improved, and 162 patients were either unaffected or worsened. It is hoped that a role exists for stimulants in the treatment of schizophrenia. Another study found no benefit when methylphenidate augmentation therapy was used in this population.[9]

Miscellaneous Uses

CNS stimulants have been used to treat mania, neurasthenia, pathologic fatigue, and obsessive-compulsive disorder. Further studies may reveal a more important role for this group of psychotropic drugs than is now realized.

PATIENT EDUCATION FOR INDIVIDUALS PRESCRIBED STIMULANTS

Safe and effective use of stimulants is facilitated when the patient and family are taught and understand the following:

- To take these drugs early in the day to prevent insomnia
- To decrease caffeine consumption related to its additive effect
- To take with meals or directly after eating to minimize anorectic effects
- To avoid over-the-counter preparations, as described in Table 16-3
- To avoid alcohol consumption
- To observe for rest deficits because these agents tend to cause patients to avoid rest behaviors
- To use with caution when driving because these drugs can mask fatigue
- To avoid chewing sustained-released forms of the drug because it will result in earlier and higher plasma levels
- To increase dosage only on the advice of the prescriber
- To observe caution when undertaking potentially hazardous tasks because amphetamines can mask extreme fatigue
- To notify the prescriber when experiencing nervousness, restlessness, insomnia, dizziness, anorexia, and GI disturbances because measures may be developed that can modify these effects

REFERENCES

1. Adamson RH, Roberts HR: Caffeine dependence syndrome, *JAMA* 27(18):1418, 1995.
2. American Psychiatric Association: *Diagnostic and statistical manual of mental disorders-TR,* ed 4, Washington, DC, 2000, The Association.
3. Ancill MB, Carlyle W: Oral caffeine augmentation of ECT, *Am J Psychiatry* 149(1): 137, 1992.
4. Applegate M: Cytochrome P450 isoenzymes: nursing considerations, *APNA* 5(1):15, 1999.
5. Arana GW, Hyman SE: *Handbook of psychiatric drug therapy,* Boston, 1991, Little, Brown.
6. Ayd FJ, Zohar J: Psychostimulant (amphetamine or methylphenidate) therapy for chronic and treatment-resistant depression. In Zohar J, Belmaker RH, editors: *Treating resistant depression,* New York, 1987, PMA.
7. Bezchlibnyk KZ, Jeffries JJ: *Clinical handbook of psychotropic drugs,* ed 10, Seattle, 2000, Hogrefe & Huber.
8. Breier A and others: Plasma norepinephrine in chronic schizophrenia, *Am J Psychiatry* 147(11):1467, 1990.
9. Carpenter MD and others: Methylphenidate augmentation therapy in schizophrenia, *J Clin Psychopharmacol* 12(4):273, 1992.
10. Chiarello RJ, Cole JO: The use of psychostimulants in general psychiatry, *Arch Gen Psychiatry* 44:286, 1987.
11. Chou T: Wake up and smell the coffee: caffeine, coffee, and the medical consequences, *West J Med* 157:544, 1992.
12. Coffey CE and others: Caffeine augmentation of ECT, *Am J Psychiatry* 147(5): 579, 1990.
13. Dilsaver SC, Votolato NA, Alessi NE: Complications of phenylpropanolamine, *Am Fam Physician* 39(4):201, 1989.
14. Eteng MU and others: Recent advances in caffeine and theobromine toxicities: a review, *Plant Foods Human Nutr* 51(3):231, 1997.
15. Fischbach GD: Mind and brain, *Sci Am* 267(3):48, 1992.
16. Flitman SS: Tranquilizers, stimulants, and enhancers of cognition, *Phys Med Rehab Clin North Am* 10(2):463, 1999.
17. Garfinkel BD, Amrami KK: A perspective on the attention-deficit disorders, *Hosp Comm Psychiatry* 43(5):445, 1992.
18. Gessa GL and others: Evidence that hyperthermia produced by d-amphetamine is caused by peripheral action of the drug, *Life Sci* 8:135-141, 1969.

19. Glass RM: Caffeine dependence: what are the implications? *JAMA* 272:1065, 1994.

20. Glass RM: Caffeine dependence syndrome, *JAMA* 273:1419, 1995.

21. Goff DC, Jenike MA: Treatment-resistant depression in the elderly, *J Am Geriatr Soc* 34: 63, 1986.

22. Goldberg TE and others: Cognitive and behavioral effects of coadministration of dextroamphetamine and haloperidol in schizophrenia, *Am J Psychiatry* 148(1):78, 1991.

23. Grace AA: The tonic/phasic model of dopamine system regulation: its relevance for understanding how stimulant abuse can alter basal ganglia function, *Drug Alcohol Depend* 37(2):111, 1995.

24. Graybiel AM: The basal ganglia, *Trends Pharmacol Sci* 18:60, 1995.

25. Greden JF: Anxiety or caffeinism, *Am J Psychiatry* 131(10):1089, 1974.

26. Greden JF and others: Anxiety and depression associated with caffeinism among psychiatric inpatients, *Am J Psychiatry* 135(8):963, 1978.

27. Hirschfeld RM: Management of sexual side effects of antidepressant therapy, *J Clin Psychiatry* 60(suppl 14):27, 1999.

28. Hughes JR and others: Should caffeine abuse, dependence, or withdrawal be added to DSM-IV and ICD-10? *Am J Psychiatry* 149(1):3340, 1992.

29. Jimenez-Jimenez FJ and others: Drug-induced movement disorders, *Drug Safety* 16(3): 180, 1997.

30. Kaplitz SE: Withdrawn apathetic geriatric patients responsive to methylphenidate, *J Am Geriatr Soc* 23:271, 1975.

31. King GR, Ellinwood EH: Amphetamines and other stimulants. In Lowinson JH, Ruiz P, Millman RB, Langrod JG, editors: *Substance abuse: a comprehensive textbook,* Baltimore, 1992, Williams & Wilkins.

32. Kosten TR and others: Depression and stimulant dependence: neurobiology and pharmacotherapy, *J Nerv Ment Dis* 186(12):737, 1998.

33. Kuczenski R: Biochemical actions of amphetamines and other stimulants. In Creese I, editor: *Stimulants: neurochemical, behavioral, and clinical perspectives,* New York, 1983, Raven.

34. Lecos C: The latest caffeine scorecard, *FDA Consumer* 18:14, 1984.

35. Lehne RA: *Pharmacology for nursing care,* ed 3, Philadelphia, 1998, Saunders.

36. Leibowitz SF, Alexander JT: Hypothalamic serotonin in control of eating behavior, meal size, and body weight, *Biol Psychiatry* 44(9):851, 1998.

37. Levin R: Psychostimulants for depression, *Am Fam Physician* 44(3):758, 1991 (letter).

38. Liebman M: *Neuroanatomy made easy and understandable,* ed 4, Gaithersburg, Md, 1991, Aspen.

39. Little KY, Gay TL: Acute stimulant response prediction of chronic trazodone effects. *Prog Neuropsychopharm Biol Psychiatry* 20(5):815, 1996.

40. Lovgren K: Amphetamines, *Emergency* 17(6):10, 1985.

41. Masand P and others: Psychostimulants for secondary depression in medical illness, *Psychosomatics* 32(2):203, 1991.

42. Metz A, Shader RI: Combination of fluoxetine with pemoline in the treatment of major depressive disorder, *Int Clin Psychopharmacol* 6(2):93, 1991.

43. Myers WC, Stewart JT: Use of methylphenidate, *Hosp Comm Psychiatry* 40(7):754, 1989.

44. Myerson A: The effect of benzedrine sulfate on mood and fatigue in normal and neurotic persons, *Arch Neurol Psychiatry* 36:816, 1936.

45. Nash JM: Addicted, *Time* 149(18):68, 1997.

46. Nehlig A and others: Caffeine and the central nervous system: mechanisms of action, biochemical, metabolic and psychostimulant effects, *Brain Res Rev* 17:139, 1992.

47. Olin BR: *Facts and comparisons,* St Louis, 1995, Wolters Kluwer.

48. Pickering H, Stimson GV: Prevalence and demographic factors of stimulant use, *Addiction* 89:1385, 1994.

49. Pickett P and others: Psychostimulant treatment of geriatric depressive disorders secondary to medical illness, *J Geriatr Psychiatry Neurol* 3(3):146, 1990.

50. Pickworth WB: Caffeine dependence, *Lancet* 345:1066, 1995.

51. Pilette WL: Caffeine: psychiatric grounds for concern, *J Psychosoc Nurs Ment Health Serv* 21: 19, 1983.

52. Roccaforte WH, Burke WJ: Use of psychostimulants for the elderly, *Hosp Comm Psychiatry* 41(12):1330, 1990.

53. Schreiber GB and others: Measurement of coffee and caffeine intake: implications for epidemiologic research, *Prev Med* 17:280, 1988.

54. Strain EC and others: Caffeine dependence syndrome: evidence from case histories and experimental evaluations, *JAMA* 272(13):1043, 1994.

55. Tinsley JA, Watkins DD: Over-the-counter stimulants: abuse and addiction, *Mayo Clin Proc* 73(10):977, 1998.

56. Warneke L: Psychostimulants in psychiatry, *Can J Psychiatry* 35:3, 1990.

CHAPTER 17

Drugs Used to Treat
Extrapyramidal Side Effects*

NORMAN L. KELTNER AND ELIZABETH WOODMAN TAYLOR

In general, understanding the drugs presented in this chapter informs and supports our conceptualizations of the pharmacologic effects caused by neuroleptic agents, effects both desired and undesired. Antipsychotic drugs cause somatic (motor) side effects ostensibly by reducing dopamine availability to the basal ganglia. High-potency antipsychotic drugs are much more likely to do this than are the low-potency or atypical agents. These undesired somatic effects are referred to as *extrapyramidal side effects* (EPSEs) and include dystonia, akathisia, akinesia, parkinsonism (tremor, rigidity, bradykinesia), tardive dyskinesia, and neuroleptic malignant syndrome. These reactions are covered extensively in Chapter 5 and are repeated in this chapter for reader convenience. Box 17-1 provides a summary of this information. To better understand EPSEs, a review of biochemical mechanisms associated with Parkinson's disease (PD) is presented, and based on an extension of that discussion, the phenomena of EPSEs are traced.

REVIEW OF PARKINSON'S DISEASE

PD, or idiopathic parkinsonism, is a chronic and progressive neurodegenerative disorder. This diagnostic term *(PD)* is reserved for conditions in which the cause of degeneration is unknown (idiopathic). *Parkinsonism,* a broader diagnostic term, identifies those motor impairments with PD symptoms for which a cause is known or suspected. Degeneration in PD occurs in pigmented brainstem nuclei. The substantia nigra, a major dopamine-generating site in the midbrain, is the primary target, but cell loss in the pigmented locus ceruleus also occurs. About 1% of substantia nigra neurons are lost per year, and total cell loss can approach 90% in severely impaired patients with PD.[1,45] A certain cell depletion threshold of about 50% to 60% of the neurons in the substantia nigra and perhaps 70% to 80% of the dopaminergic tracts and receptors in the basal ganglia must occur before symptoms become evident.[1] Increased activity by remaining healthy cells and hypersensitivity of dopaminergic receptors account for the lack of symptoms in individuals with significant dopaminergic cell loss below this threshold. Figure 17-1 compares a normal substantia nigra with an age-matched one from a patient with PD. It should be noted that the pigmentation is a product of dopamine synthesis. As less dopamine is synthesized, pigmentation is reduced and results in a paler midbrain. Figure 17-2 presents a schematic of basal ganglia dysfunction such as occurs in PD.

---

*Most patients taking neuroleptics experience extrapyramidal side effects (EPSEs). Accordingly, it could be argued this chapter should be a part of the primary chapter on antipsychotics (Chapter 5). Although this argument has merit, the best understanding of these drugs can be gained from a dedicated chapter such as this.

Box 17-1 Extrapyramidal Side Effects (EPSEs)

Akathisia	Subjective feeling of restlessness, restless legs, jittery feeling, nervous energy. It is the most common EPSE and responds poorly to treatment. Approximately 20%-25% of patients will develop akathisia. Most will develop within the first 10 days. If treatment with anticholinergics does not help, noncholinergics such as clonidine or a benzodiazepine may help. Dosage reduction from the neuroleptic typically works. **Diagnostic dilemmas: anxiety, psychosis, cocaine intoxication, alcohol withdrawal.**
Akinesia	Refers to absence of movement, but a slowed movement (bradykinesia) is more likely. Symptoms include weakness (hypotonia), fatigue, painful muscles, and anergy. Akinesia is treated effectively with most anticholinergics. Approximately 33% of patients will develop akinesia, most by the third week. **Diagnostic dilemmas: negative symptoms of schizophrenia, depression.**
Dystonias	These EPSEs manifest as abnormal postures that are caused by involuntary muscle spasms. About 10% of patients taking antipsychotics will develop dystonias. Dystonias tend to appear early in neuroleptic treatment (90% within the first 3 days). They include oculogyric crises, tongue protrusion, torticollis, and laryngeal-pharyngeal constriction, which can be life-threatening. Younger males are more likely to develop dystonias. These EPSEs are relatively rare among elderly individuals. **Diagnostic dilemmas: bizarre somatic symptoms of schizophrenia.**
Drug-induced parkinsonism	Parkinsonian symptoms, including tremor, bradykinesia, rigidity, and associated movements of dysphagia, dysarthria, loss of facial expression, sialorrhea, festinating gait, and increased muscle tone. Approximately 20% of patients develop this, most often within a few weeks to months. Incidence increases with age. **Diagnostic dilemma: Parkinson's disease.**
Tardive dyskinesia	*Tardive* means "late appearing." This disorder seldom occurs before 6 months of neuroleptic use. It is not related to dopamine-acetylcholine imbalance but is thought to be caused by hypersensitization of dopamine receptors. About 20%-35% of patients receiving chronic neuroleptic therapy eventually develop this EPSE. It affects muscles of the mouth and face and causes lip smacking, grinding of teeth, rolling or protrusion of the tongue, tics, and diaphragmatic movements that may impair breathing. Its severity fluctuates, and it disappears with sleep. It is most severe in young men and most common in elderly women. There are no drugs that cure tardive dyskinesia; anticholinergics worsen the condition. **Diagnostic dilemma: tremor.**

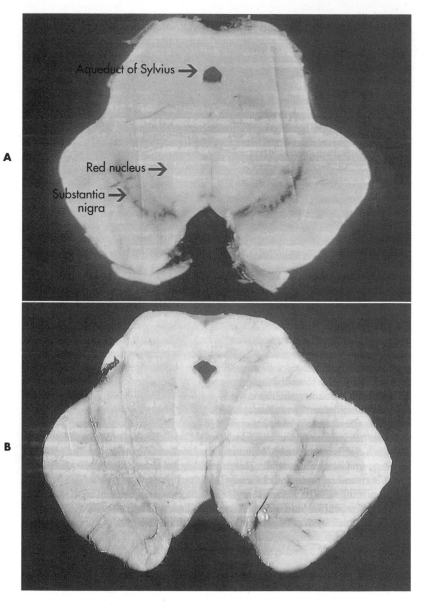

Figure 17-1 A, Brain slice illustrating a normal substantia nigra with adequate pigmentation. The substantia nigra is located in the zona compacta area of the midbrain. **B,** This midbrain is from a patient who suffered from Parkinson's disease. Note the loss of pigmentation. (**A,** Courtesy Dr. Cheryl Palmer, Department of Neuropathology, University of Alabama at Birmingham Brain Resource Program.)

The substantia nigra is part of a larger system, the *extrapyramidal system.* Anatomically, the extrapyramidal system lies rostral to (in front of) the motor strip in what is called the *premotor area* and projects to the basal ganglia. The extrapyramidal system differs from the pyramidal system both functionally and anatomically. The extrapyramidal system coordinates involuntary movement, which supports voluntary

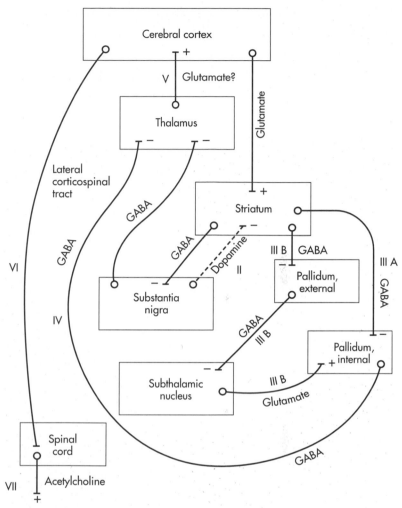

Figure 17-2 Diagram of the basal ganglia and movement pathways illustrating the feedback loop for voluntary movement and its relationship to involuntary supportive movement. *I*, The impulse from the cerebral cortex to the voluntary motor system is also signaled to the striatum. *II*, It is modulated by dopamine from the substantia nigra. *III*, Striatal output to the globus pallidus (there are two pathways: one directly to the globus pallidus internal *[III A]* and an indirect pathway from the globus pallidus external-subthalamic nuclei-globus pallidus internal *[III B]*). *IV*, Output from the globus pallidus internal to the thalamus. (Surgical destruction of the globus pallidus [i.e., pallidotomy] is successful in reducing symptoms of Parkinson's disease.) *V*, Thalamus to cerebral cortex. *VI*, Cerebral cortex to spinal cord nuclei (i.e., the corticospinal tract). *VII*, Spinal cord to specific motor nuclei. When disruption occurs in II, tremors, rigidity, and bradykinesia develop at VII (i.e., Parkinson's disease or extrapyramidal side effects).

movement. For example, when a person walks, a host of involuntary muscle activities support and facilitate those voluntary movements associated with walking. The extra-pyramidal system coordinates or fine tunes those involuntary actions. Another example is the simple act of sitting in a chair. Involuntary muscle tone and muscle support are required to sit successfully in a chair without falling over, slipping down, or slumping.

The *pyramidal system* is responsible for voluntary movement such as walking. Anatomically, the pyramidal system begins in the motor strip, extends down through the brain to the lower medulla, crosses over (decussates), and continues down the spinal cord, emerging at various points along the way to synapse with neurons innervating voluntary muscle throughout the body. Several terms arc used to describe all or part of this system anatomically (motor strip, precentral gyrus, corticospinal tract) and functionally (the voluntary system, the motor system, the pyramidal system). The motor strip of a normal brain, an intact motor strip in the brain of a patient with Alzheimer's disease, and the abnormal motor strip of a patient with amyotrophic lateral sclerosis are shown in Figures 17-3 to 17-5.

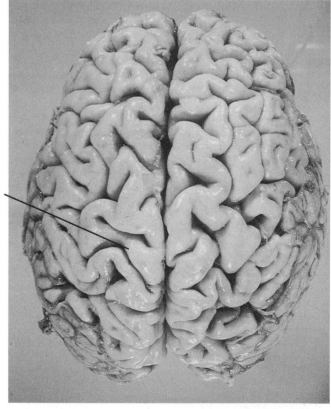

Normal
motor strip

Figure 17-3 Normal brain and precentral gyrus (motor strip). (Courtesy Dr. Richard Powers, Director, University of Alabama at Birmingham Brain Resource Program.)

The major cause of involuntary motor system disruption is a decrease in the availability of dopamine and a subsequent decrease in dopamine transmission (see Figure 17-2). Reductions in dopamine cause a profound effect on posture, walking, balance, and other muscle-dependent activities. For an individual to successfully negotiate everyday movement, two neurotransmitters, dopamine (inhibitory) and acetylcholine (ACh [excitatory]), must be in balance. In PD, there is too little dopamine and a relative excess of ACh. However, the role of acetylcholine seems to be secondary. For example, although drugs that deplete dopamine (e.g., antipsychotics) will cause parkinsonism, drugs that enhance acetylcholine (e.g., choline, physostigmine) do not cause parkinsonism.[12]

Dopamine deficiency can occur in the following three ways:

1. The brain produces less dopamine because of loss of dopamine-generating cells and dopaminergic tracts (i.e., PD).
2. Neuronal dopamine is depleted chemically, such as occurs with reserpine.
3. Dopamine is blocked at the postsynaptic receptor, such as occurs with antipsychotic drugs.

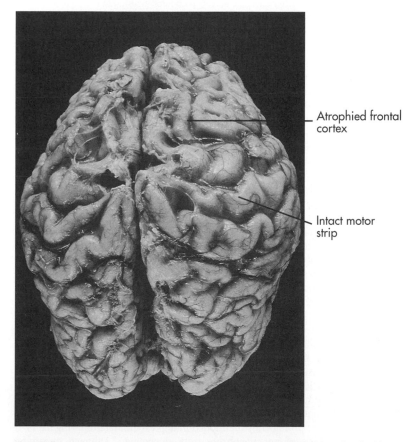

Atrophied frontal cortex

Intact motor strip

Figure 17-4 Brain of a patient with Alzheimer's disease. Note the atrophied frontal gyri, with the relative sparing of the motor strip. This pattern of pathology is consistent with the clinical observation that patients with Alzheimer's disease have cognitive impairment but adequate motor function. (Courtesy Dr. Richard Powers, Director, University of Alabama at Birmingham Brain Resource Program.)

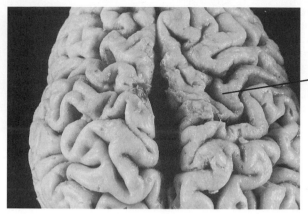

Focal atrophy of motor strip

Figure 17-5 Brain of a patient with amyotrophic lateral sclerosis. Note the obvious focal atrophy of the motor strip (and to a lesser extent the sensory postcentral gyrus), with sparing of frontal areas. These patients experience severe motor impairment. (Courtesy Dr. Richard Powers, Director, University of Alabama at Birmingham Brain Resource Program.)

The primary symptoms of PD—tremor, bradykinesia, and rigidity—are caused by massive destruction of nigrostriatal dopaminergic neurons in the zona compacta (or pars compacta) of the substantia nigra.[1,35] Many secondary symptoms are also present. Tremors are common, affecting about 75% of all patients with PD. Tremors can usually be detected in at least one arm or hand when the person is at rest. These resting tremors are in contrast to the "movement" tremors associated with long-term alcohol abuse. The latter are caused by lesions in the cerebellum. Whereas the basal ganglia fine tune involuntary movement in the extrapyramidal system, the cerebellum fine tunes voluntary movement in the pyramidal system.

Tremors are typically more amenable to treatment than are the other symptoms of PD. Bradykinesia, a generalized motor slowing, gives rise to yet other symptoms associated with PD. For example, masked facies (the slowing down of face movements); slowed arm swing; and difficulty initiating, maintaining, and stopping movement are all extensions of bradykinesia. Rigidity, sometimes referred to as *lead pipe* or *cogwheel rigidity,* impairs movement and makes the simple acts of getting out of a chair or gripping a pen so difficult that patients sometimes defer rather than attempt them. Tremor responds best to anticholinergic drugs, whereas rigidity and bradykinesia respond better to dopaminergic agents.[12]

Other important symptoms related to PD include postural difficulties, a gait disorder characterized by shuffling steps, and orthostatic hypotension. Falls can result from any or all of these and are a major source of injury. Gait and postural disturbances are the most treatment-resistant symptoms and are probably caused by nondopaminergic lesions downstream from the dopaminergic nerve terminals. Both dementia (15% to 20% incidence) and depression (approximately 40% incidence) occur in patients with PD.[18] Depression can be partially explained by the PD-related decrease in dopamine and a consequent decrease in its metabolite norepinephrine. Both deficiencies are prominently mentioned in depression literature. (Figure 17-6 depicts the synthesis of norepinephrine from dopamine.) Although dopamine deficiency constitutes the bulk of PD neurochemical abnormalities, other neuronal systems are also involved. Adrenergic, serotonergic, and cholinergic systems are disrupted and contribute to symptoms of depression and disturbed cognition.

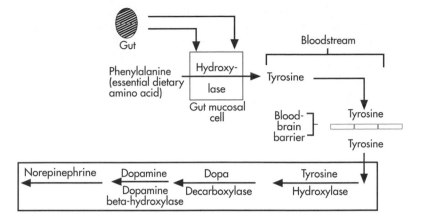

Figure 17-6 The dietary amino acid phenylalanine diffuses through mucosal cells in the gastro-intestinal tract and is metabolized to tyrosine. Tyrosine crosses the blood-brain barrier and enters brain neurons. In dopamine neurons, it is metabolized to levodopa and then to dopamine. In noradrenergic neurons, dopamine is converted further to norepinephrine and, in adrenergic neurons, is converted to epinephrine. In Parkinson's disease, dopaminergic neurons degenerate, creating an imbalance with opposing effects of acetylcholine that is released from nearby neurons (not shown). In drug-induced parkinsonism, dopaminergic neurons may be intact, but postsynaptic dopamine receptors are blocked.

Secondary symptoms found in PD include dysphagia, which makes eating difficult and causes excessive accumulation of saliva leading to drool (sialorrhea). Weight loss and choking are two more important consequences of dysphagia. The combined effect of bradykinesia and rigidity impair respirations (rigid, immobile respiratory muscles), bladder emptying (rigidity and retarded initiation of stream), and bowel evacuation (a rigid and immobile bowel), leading to constipation or incontinence.

REVIEW OF EXTRAPYRAMIDAL SIDE EFFECTS

EPSEs develop in up to 60% to 90% of patients receiving antipsychotic medications, and up to 50% of readmissions are related to these side effects.[2,9] Nonneuroleptic medications can also cause EPSEs. EPSEs can be roughly grouped into acute and chronic categories. Acute EPSEs occur early on in treatment (in the first month of treatment), with chronic forms developing later. It should be noted that some clinicians believe a minimal level of EPSEs (at least with traditional antipsychotics) indicates sufficient serum levels to support a therapeutic response.[8] The likely order of development, definition, and incidence of specific EPSEs are summarized next and then are followed by a more detailed explanation of each.[2,6,23,44,53]

1. Dystonic reaction (a spastic contraction of muscle groups) occurs in 10% of patients, most within the first 3 days.
2. Akathisia (restlessness, an irresistible need to move manifested objectively and subjectively) occurs in 20% to 25% of patients, usually within the first 10 days.
3. Akinesia (difficulty with or absence of movement) occurs in 33% of patients, with most cases developing by the third week of treatment.
4. Parkinsonism (tremor, rigidity, bradykinesia) occurs in 20% of patients, usually developing after weeks to months.

5. Tardive dyskinesia (abnormal, involuntary skeletal muscle movements of the face, tongue, trunk, and extremities) occurs at an annual cumulative rate of 5% and eventually affects 20% to 35%. It develops after months of continuous use.
6. Neuroleptic malignant syndrome (two cardinal symptoms are fevers and rigidity) occurs in fewer than 1% of patients taking neuroleptics, with an estimated 5% to 20% of untreated cases resulting in death. It develops within minutes to months after drug initiation.

Abnormal involuntary movement disorders develop because of a drug-induced imbalance between two major neurotransmitters, dopamine and ACh. As dopamine D_2 receptors are antagonized or occupied at levels between 60% and 75%, an optimal antipsychotic clinical effect occurs. At blockade levels not much higher (greater than 75% occupancy), EPSEs develop.[46,47] This imbalance is caused more readily by high-potency antipsychotic drugs; however, all antipsychotics can cause EPSEs.

Dystonia

Dystonic reactions occur very early in treatment and are characterized by involuntary contractions of muscles controlling posture, gait, or ocular movement. Positions become frozen and although frightening are not typically dangerous. Dystonias occur early in treatment, often appear suddenly, and can recur. Risk factors include young age, male gender, use of high-potency agents, use of high dosages, and intramuscular route of administration. About 10% of patients starting antipsychotic therapy develop dystonias. Three specific dystonic reactions bear special mention:

1. *Oculogyric crisis* is a dystonic reaction in which the eyes roll upward. This is a frightening experience.
2. *Torticollis* is a contracted state of the cervical muscle that produces torsion on the neck.
3. *Laryngeal-pharyngeal dystonia* is associated with gagging, cyanosis, respiratory distress, and asphyxia (particularly in young men). It is life-threatening and requires immediate intervention.

All dystonic conditions respond to intramuscular anticholinergic drugs.

Akathisia

Akathisia manifests as subjective and objective restlessness. It is the most common EPSE, occurs within the first 10 days of treatment, is less responsive to treatment than dystonia and parkinsonism, and probably accounts for more noncompliant behavior than do other EPSEs. Akathisia was first described in 1911, long before antipsychotic drugs were available, suggesting other variables may contribute to its occurrence (e.g., iron deficiency is suspected by some investigators). Subjectively, the patient often feels jittery or uneasy. He or she may report "nervous energy." Objectively, the patient is restless and literally cannot sit still. Planasky and Johnston discovered that 79% of suicidal schizophrenic patients were suffering with akathisia.[42]

Unfortunately, restlessness and verbal reflections of subjective anguish can be misinterpreted as a worsening of psychosis. Because akathisia can present as agitation, the clinician should not mistake the two because of their different treatment protocols.[25] If additional antipsychotic medication is given, the akathisia will worsen. Akathisia may respond to anticholinergic drugs such as trihexyphenidyl (Artane) or benztropine (Cogentin) but can also be resistant to this intervention. Benzodiazepines (e.g., lorazepam) may also be useful. However, Keepers and Casey pointed out that other approaches, including waiting for tolerance to develop and decreasing the dosage of the antipsychotic agent, might be the best ways to treat akathisia.[29]

Akinesia

Akinesia refers to an absence of or impairment of movement. More often, a state of bradykinesia, a slowing of movement, exists. Akinesia is experienced by about 33% of patients taking antipsychotic drugs.[53] Movement is difficult to initiate and difficult to maintain. The patient lacks spontaneity in movement and speech. Paradoxically, these same symptoms (for different reasons) are common in schizophrenia. If a manifestation of schizophrenia is occurring, more medication may be indicated; if it is akinesia, more medication will worsen the symptoms.

Parkinsonism

Parkinsonism occurs in approximately 20% of patients taking antipsychotics and develops within weeks to months. Symptoms mimic those of PD: tremors, rigidity, and bradykinesia. As would be expected, antipsychotic drugs intensify the symptoms of PD and should be avoided if possible for persons with this condition. Parkinsonian symptoms must be differentiated from the negative symptoms of schizophrenia because treatment approaches are different. Anticholinergic agents are effective and are used most for the treatment of drug-induced parkinsonism. Use of dopaminergic drugs such as levodopa is not indicated because of their inherent potential to increase psychotic symptoms. Amantadine (Symmetrel), possessing both anticholinergic and dopaminergic properties, is the exception and is ordered in the treatment of drug-induced parkinsonism for some individuals.

Tardive Dyskinesia

Tardive dyskinesia (TD) manifests as abnormal, involuntary movements of the face, tongue, trunk, and extremities. It is the most dreaded EPSE and was once thought to be irreversible. The term *tardive* means "late appearing," and TD typically appears after months of continuous use. Traditional antipsychotic drugs are the major culprits, but all antipsychotics, with perhaps the exception of clozapine, can cause TD. Although the other EPSEs are hypokinetic disorders caused by dopamine deficiency, TD is a hyperdopaminergic (and hyperkinetic) disorder related to dopamine receptor hypersensitivity. Because striatal dopaminergic receptors can become supersensitive, TD also develops as antipsychotic dosage reductions or withdrawal is instituted. Cholinergic deficits are also suspected. Although anticholinergic antiparkinsonism drugs are beneficial for most other EPSEs, they can exacerbate TD, no doubt related to cholinergic irregularities. TD has an annual prevalence rate of 5%, and a mean prevalence of 20% to 35% of continuous users develop it.[5] Most patients have mild symptoms, but about 10% will develop a debilitating form of TD.[2] Sometimes, TD appears as psychotropic agents are being withdrawn or reduced in dosage. This phenomenon, referred to as *withdrawal dyskinesia*, is reversible and subsides with time.

TD usually affects the muscles of the mouth and face and can also occur in the trunk and extremities. Signs of TD include lip smacking, grinding of the teeth, rolling or protrusion of the tongue, tics, and diaphragmatic movements, which may impair breathing. These involuntary movements fluctuate in severity and disappear during sleep. They can be controlled with great effort, but most individuals cannot sustain the effort for long. TD is most severe in young men and most common in women older than 70.[3] High dosages of antipsychotics and concurrent EPSEs increase the risk of TD.[54]

TD can be irreversible. If caught during the early stages, symptoms can be reversed or decreased in severity. Early detection and gradual dosage reductions (to 50%) have proven capable of mitigating the impact of TD.[2] Patient and family education should emphasize early detection by careful monitoring. The Abnormal Involuntary Movement Scale (AIMS) provides a mechanism for assessing TD. The dopamine agonist bromocriptine (Parlodel) has been used to treat this side effect, as has clonazepam (Klonopin) and vitamin E (which apparently works by neutralizing free radicals). Another approach involves the use of clozapine.[5,16,22,51] Numerous clinical trials have substantiated the efficacy of low dosages of clozapine in the treatment of TD.

Neuroleptic Malignant Syndrome

Neuroleptic malignant syndrome (NMS) is a potentially lethal hypodopaminergic side effect of antipsychotic drugs. Traditionally, a morbidity rate of 1% with a mortality rate of up to 30% was widely reported in the literature. Increased vigilance by physicians, nurses, and others has significantly reduced both the morbidity and mortality of the syndrome. Current thinking indicates an incidence of less than 1%. Before 1984, apparently 25% of patients developing NMS died, and since 1984, that percentage has declined to less than 12%. The American Psychiatric Association estimates 5% to 20% of untreated cases (some misdiagnosed) result in death.[2] NMS is most often associated with high-potency antipsychotic drugs, especially when prescribed with a large loading dose. NMS is not related to toxic drug levels and may occur after only a few doses.[34] Onset can occur within minutes or take months after drug initiation.

Important symptoms associated with NMS include hyperthermia, Parkinson-like symptoms of muscular rigidity and tremors, altered consciousness, increase in some laboratory values, and autonomic disturbances. Perhaps the two cardinal symptoms are elevated body temperature (up to 108° F with temperatures of 101° to 103° F more likely) and rigidity. Rigidity can range from muscle hypertonicity to severe lead pipe rigidity.[39] Altered consciousness includes confusion and even unresponsiveness. The muteness found in some patients may be related to state of consciousness also. Patients with NMS typically show a spike in creatinine phosphokinase (CPK) levels and an increase in white blood cell (WBC) count. CPK levels may reach 100,000 U/L, while WBC counts range to 40,000/mm^3.[39] The increase in CPK is caused by muscle rigidity and the subsequent rhabdomyolysis. Autonomic dysfunction includes hypotension, tachycardia, sialorrhea, sweating, and urinary incontinence.

Historically, risk factors associated with NMS have been dehydration, young adulthood, male sex, nonschizophrenic illness, and use of high-potency drugs. Because many patients do not associate these symptoms (e.g., fever, tachycardia, rigidity) with their antipsychotic medication, emergency room and primary care providers may be contacted first. These health care professionals should always rule out NMS in patients taking antipsychotics who develop high temperatures. Other risk factors include prolonged use of restraints; coadministration of lithium; poorly controlled EPSEs; withdrawal from anticholinergic medications; diagnosis of alcoholism, organic brain syndrome, or previous brain injury; extrapyramidal disorder (e.g., PD); iron deficiency; and catatonia.[39] Pharmacologic treatment has included bromocriptine (Parlodel), a dopamine agonist; dantrolene (Dantrium), a skeletal muscle relaxant via suppression of calcium release from the sarcoplasmic reticulum;

and amantadine (Symmetrel), another dopaminergic. Dursun and others found vitamins E and B$_6$ effective for a 74-year-old woman thought to be a poor candidate for the more conventional medications just mentioned.[21]

DRUGS USED TO TREAT PARKINSON'S DISEASE

The proposed model of PD found in Figure 17-7 suggests that this disease can be treated in one or two ways. The obvious approach would be to increase dopamine availability. Theoretically, an equally effective approach would aim at decreasing the availability of ACh (Figure 17-8). The two tactics basically capture the existing approaches to treating PD. Consequently, two classes of antiparkinsonism drugs exist for treating these patients: dopaminergic agents (those that increase dopamine) and anticholinergic agents (those that block ACh). Neuroleptic drug-induced parkinsonism is treated most often with the latter; however, dopaminergic drugs have a role and are discussed as well. Dopaminergic agents are discussed first.

Dopaminergic Agents

Because PD is caused by a deficiency in dopamine, the most direct approach to treating the disorder is to give the patient a dopaminergic drug. Although it would seem reasonable to give dopamine itself, such an approach does not work because dopamine is neither lipid soluble nor does it have a dedicated transport system to ferry it across the blood-brain barrier. Of course, the peripheral effects of dopamine are well known and include vascular constriction and positive inotropic effects on heart muscle. Therefore dopaminergic agents, which can cross the blood-brain barrier and increase dopamine levels in the brain, have been developed to treat PD. They fall into the following categories:

1. *Dopamine precursors*, for example, levodopa and carbidopa-levodopa (Sinemet): These drugs remain the gold standard for PD but are not prescribed for drug-induced parkinsonism. They interact with most psychotropic medications. In fact, in keeping with the dopamine model of schizophrenia, a central nervous system (CNS) side effect associated with these agents is psychotic-like

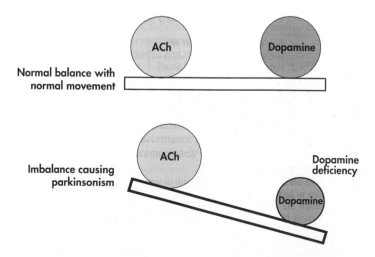

Figure 17-7 Normal and imbalanced states of acetylcholine *(ACh)* and dopamine.

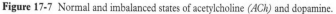

Schizophrenia hyperdopaminergic theory

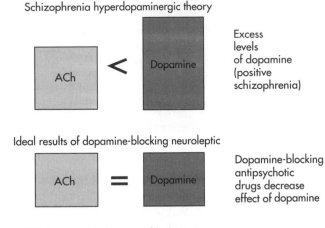

Excess
levels
of dopamine
(positive
schizophrenia)

Ideal results of dopamine-blocking neuroleptic

Dopamine-blocking
antipsychotic
drugs decrease
effect of dopamine

EPSEs caused by dopamine-blocking agent

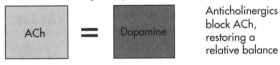

Antipsychotic drugs
block too much
dopamine, creating
a pseudoparkinsonism

Balanced state after anticholinergic antiparkinsonism drug given

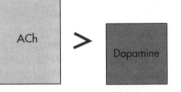

Anticholinergics
block ACh,
restoring a
relative balance

Figure 17-8 Theoretic neurochemical model of schizophrenia and chemical treatment.

symptoms such as hallucinations. COMT-inhibitors, which spare levodopa from enzymatic reduction by the enzyme catechol-*O*-methyltransferase, could be included here as well.

2. *Dopamine releaser:* Amantadine (Symmetrel) more effectively releases the dopamine remaining in the dopaminergic neurons in the brain and is thought to block neuronal dopamine reuptake. Amantadine is used to treat drug-induced parkinsonism.

3. *Dopamine agonists:* Bromocriptine (Parlodel) and pergolide (Permax) directly stimulate dopamine receptors. These drugs are inferior to levodopa but superior to amantadine and anticholinergics in the treatment of PD. Bromocriptine is used to treat NMS.

4. *Dopamine metabolism inhibitor:* Selegiline (Eldepryl) blocks the metabolism of dopamine by inhibiting MAO-B, an enzyme that breaks down dopamine. Selegiline is typically given with levodopa to extend the life of the dopamine derived from levodopa administration. MAO-A breaks down serotonin and norepinephrine. The monoamine oxidase inhibitors (MAOIs) used in the treatment of depression (see Chapter 6) inhibit both A and B subtypes. Selegiline is not used to treat drug-induced parkinsonism.

Because of this book's focus, only the dopaminergic drugs used in the treatment of EPSEs are discussed.

Amantadine. Amantadine increases the intrasynaptic availability of dopamine by enhancing its release from otherwise depleted dopaminergic neurons and is thought to inhibit dopamine reuptake as well. Amantadine has a relatively strong anticholinergic effect (although milder than that of the other anticholinergics), making it unique among the dopaminergic antiparkinsonism drugs. Unlike levodopa, amantadine can be used to treat drug-induced parkinsonism, no doubt related to its anticholinergic properties. Amantadine is less effective than levodopa but more effective than the anticholinergics in treatment of PD.[38] Amantadine appears most effective in relieving akinesia and less effective in modifying dystonic symptoms.[6] Amantadine has a unique role among the anticholinergic antiparkinsonism drugs in the treatment of sexual disorders induced by neuroleptics and selective serotonin reuptake inhibitors (SSRIs).

Amantadine is well absorbed from the gastrointestinal (GI) tract, with peak plasma levels occurring in about 4 hours. The mean half-life is 15 hours. Amantadine is excreted unchanged by the kidneys; therefore impaired renal function can lead to an extended half-life and amantadine intoxication. Amantadine's excretion is hastened by acidifying the urine.

Amantadine, first used as an antiviral drug, is one of the drugs given for treatment of early PD because its effectiveness depends on availability of residual dopamine. In more advanced stages in which dopamine levels are depleted, greater efficacy occurs when combining amantadine with levodopa or some other antiparkinsonism drug. A major drug interaction can occur when administering amantadine with other anticholinergic drugs. Theoretically, amantadine is less likely to interact with high-potency than with the low-potency antipsychotic drugs.

Common side effects (5% to 10% of patients) of amantadine are nausea, dizziness, light-headedness, and insomnia.[38] Slightly less common side effects include depression, anxiety, irritability, hallucinations, confusion, anorexia, dry mouth, constipation, ataxia, peripheral edema, orthostatic hypotension, and headache. The seizure threshold is lowered, and patients with a history of seizures are at risk. A unique side effect of amantadine is a temporary and benign skin reaction referred to as *livedo reticularis*, in which the skin becomes purple and locally edematous. As with other anticholinergic agents, blurred vision can develop.

Overdose and toxic effects are treated by stopping drug absorption. Induced vomiting, gastric lavage, and administration of activated charcoal all serve to decrease the entry of amantadine into systemic circulation. An anticholinergic syndrome is manifested by excitability, delirium, hallucinations, seizures, hypotension, urinary retention, and arrhythmias. Although acidifying the urine theoretically might hasten amantadine excretion, in practice, the problem of amantadine-induced urinary retention makes this approach risky. No specific antidote for amantadine toxicity exists, but physostigmine, a cholinesterase inhibitor traditionally used to treat atropine poisoning, may be beneficial.[38]

Adults are usually prescribed amantadine as an oral dose of 100 mg twice a day, up to 400 mg/day for EPSEs. Because the tablet is so large, many geropsychiatric patients are prescribed the syrup form (10 mg/ml) for easy swallowing.

Bromocriptine. Bromocriptine, a dopamine agonist, was originally prescribed to inhibit lactation. The mechanism for inhibition is worth noting because its understanding facilitates comprehension of several neuroleptic-related phenomena. Essentially, as dopamine levels increase, prolactin release by the pituitary is reduced (hence, lactation inhibition). On the other hand, as dopamine availability decreases (e.g., in antipsychotic therapy), prolactin levels increase, causing a number of bothersome symptoms (e.g., galactorrhea).

Bromocriptine directly stimulates dopaminergic postsynaptic receptors. It is prescribed for PD and has proven effective in the extrapyramidal-mediated NMS (Box 17-2). Bromocriptine is not well absorbed from the GI tract and undergoes extensive first-pass metabolism. Metabolism occurs in the liver, and excretion occurs via the bile into the feces.

Nausea is the most common side effect (approximately 50%) related to dopamine stimulation of the chemoreceptor trigger zone in the medulla. Hypotension is another major side effect of bromocriptine. Anxiety, hallucinations, depression, and confusion have been reported in approximately 30% of patients and are more common among those taking high dosages. Interaction with antipsychotic drugs may occur because by definition neuroleptics block dopamine receptors, the site of the agonistic effects of bromocriptine. If bromocriptine is needed for NMS, however, antipsychotics will have been discontinued. When combined with other antihypertensives, bromocriptine can potentiate hypotensive effects. Other bromocriptine interactions pertain more to longer-term use than those associated with the treatment of NMS. Overdose and toxic effects intensify the side effects mentioned previously. If overdose is suspected, the drug should be discontinued and supportive, symptomatic care should be instituted.

ANTICHOLINERGIC (ANTIPARKINSONISM) AGENTS

PD, according to the model proposed in Figure 17-7, can also be treated by decreasing the availability of ACh. Drugs that do this (anticholinergic drugs) have been used for more than 100 years to treat PD.[43] Anticholinergic agents cross the blood-brain barrier and block ACh. A more accurate term for these drugs is *antimuscarinic* because these drugs selectively block only one of the two overarching categories of ACh receptors—muscarinic and nicotinic receptors. All of these agents are similar in function to atropine, the prototypical antimuscarinic. However, they are not as potent in blocking muscarinic receptors as is atropine (Table 17-1).

Acetylcholine and Acetylcholine (Cholinergic) Receptors[31]

Acetylcholine is synthesized from choline and acetyl-coenzyme A and is degraded by acetylcholinesterase into acetate and choline. The choline reenters the presynaptic neuron to be exposed to more acetyl-coenzyme A, where they combine to form ACh again. ACh receptors are broadly divided into two major types: nicotinic and muscarinic. Nicotinic receptors are further divided into nicotinic-N receptors (at preganglionic autonomic synapses) and nicotinic-M receptors (at neuromuscular synapses).[28] Nicotinic-N receptor antagonists are rarely used because blockade of these receptors globally shuts down the autonomic system. Nicotinic-M receptor antagonists (e.g., succinylcholine [Anectine]) are used before electroconvulsive therapy to provide muscle relaxation.

Muscarinic receptors are also divided into subtypes. In fact, five subtypes have been identified: M-1, M-2, M-3, M-4, and M-5.[14,27,37] Although these muscarinic receptor distinctions have been observed, there is still much to learn about these subtypes, and only the muscarinic M-1 receptor is discussed here. M-1 receptors are located primarily in the cerebral cortex, hippocampus, and striatum; at the target organs of the parasympathetic system; and on blood vessels.[6] The M-1 receptor blockade accounts for the host of anticholinergic peripheral side effects associated with many psychotropic drugs. For example, blockade of the parasympathetic

Box 17-2 Neuroleptic Malignant Syndrome

Cause
A hypodopaminergic state

Offending agents
1. Primarily neuroleptics
2. Nonneuroleptics: lithium, antidepressants, antiemetics, other dopamine blockers, and withdrawal from dopaminergics (e.g., amantadine)
Incidence: Now known to be <1%
Mortality: 5%-20% of untreated cases

Demographics*
Gender: Male-to-female ratio 3:1
Age: 45% between ages 20 and 39

Cardinal symptoms
Mental changes
Rigidity
Hyperthermia
Diaphoresis
Tachypnea
Autonomic dysfunction

Other signs and symptoms
Agitation, hyperreflexia, impaired breathing, muteness, pallor

Laboratory findings
Elevated CPK,† hyperkalemia, hyponatremia, metabolic acidosis, elevated WBCs

Treatment‡
Bromocriptine
2.5-10 mg PO tid initially
If no improvement in 24 hr, increase up to 20 mg PO qid
Dantrolene
1-3 mg/kg/day IV in 4 divided doses; up to 10 mg/kg/day
Oral maintenance doses range from 50 to 200 mg/day

Rechallenging with neuroleptics§
Rechallenging a patient with a neuroleptic may be warranted in cases of unremitting psychosis. About 30% will develop NMS again. A 2-week washout period should be allowed, and the new neuroleptic should be a low-potency agent.

CPK, Creatinine phosphokinase; *WBCs,* white blood cells; *NMS,* neuroleptic malignant syndrome.
*From Reference 30.
†Most prominent laboratory finding.
‡Modified from Reference 41.
§From Reference 15.

Table 17-1 Anticholinergic Effect of Commonly Prescribed Psychotropic Drugs Compared with Trihexyphenidyl

Drug	Equivalent in milligrams	Typical use
Atropine	0.5	Given before surgery
Benztropine (Cogentin)	1.0	Antiparkinsonism
Trihexyphenidyl (Artane)	2.5	Antiparkinsonism
Biperiden (Akineton)	1.0	Antiparkinsonism
Amitriptyline (Elavil)	10	Antidepressant
Doxepin (Sinequan)	30	Antidepressant
Nortriptyline (Pamelor)	60	Antidepressant
Imipramine (Tofranil)	75	Antidepressant
Desipramine (Norpramin)	150	Antidepressant
Amoxapine (Asendin)	600	Antidepressant
Clozapine (Clozaril)	15	Antipsychotic
Thioridazine (Mellaril)	50	Antipsychotic
Chlorpromazine (Thorazine)	370	Antipsychotic
Diphenhydramine (Benadryl)	50	Antihistamine

Adapted from de Leon and others: A pilot effort to determine benztropine equivalents of anticholinergic medications, *Hosp Community Psychiatry* 45(6):606, 1994.
According to this table, 50 mg of thioridazine has the same anticholinergic effect as 1 mg of benztropine.

components of four cranial nerves (CNs) causes well-recognized symptoms. For example, blockade of CN III causes mydriasis, blockade of CN VII and CN IX causes dry mouth, and blockade of CN X causes tachycardia, constipation, and other smooth muscle effects (Table 17-2).

A central response to M-1 antagonism is caused by several commonly prescribed agents, including tricyclic antidepressants and some neuroleptics. A spectrum of cognitive disturbances can occur, ranging from mild "slippage" to a profound disorientation mimicking some of the symptoms of delirium and dementia. Interestingly, the major site of ACh synthesis, the basal nucleus of Meynert, is often found to be diminished in post mortem examinations of individuals with Alzheimer's disease. Furthermore, the hippocampus, critical in converting short-term memory to long-term memory, is a predominate site for M-1 receptors. The hippocampus is affected by Alzheimer's disease and contributes to the universal symptom of memory impairment found among these patients.

Anticholinergics and the Anticholinergic Prototype Trihexyphenidyl (Artane)

Anticholinergic agents are generally less effective than levodopa but are beneficial in the early stages of PD and in fact are the drugs most often prescribed. As the illness progresses, these agents become less beneficial and also lose appeal because of common noxious side effects related to toxicity: tachycardia, dry mouth, constipation, blurred vision, and urinary retention. Furthermore, CNS side effects such as memory problems and delirium (atropine poisoning) can be very troublesome and can compound dementia and depression, both of which can be associated with PD (Box 17-3). Although several of these drugs are used to treat PD, only three or four are routinely used to treat drug-induced parkinsonism and the related EPSEs. A management plan for EPSEs was developed by Bezchlibnyk-Butler and Remington.[7] An adaptation of their protocol is provided in Box 17-4.

Table 17-2 Anticholinergic Effect on Cranial Nerves with Parasympathetic Function

The parasympathetic system is driven by acetylcholine. Certain cranial nerves have a parasympathetic function, and those functions are blocked by anticholinergic agents such as those discussed in this chapter. Cranial nerves III, VII, IX, and X have parasympathetic functions, and many of the side effects associated with these drugs are caused by the effect on these four cranial nerves.

Cranial nerve	Parasympathetic function	Anticholinergic effect
III	Constricts pupils	Mydriasis (dilates pupils)—blurred vision
	Alters shape of lens	Impairs accommodation
VII	Salivation	Dry mouth
	Lacrimation	Decreased tearing
	Nasal mucus secretion	Dry nasal passage
IX	Salivation	Dry mouth
	Nasal mucus secretion	Dry nasal passage
X	Slows heart rate	Tachycardia
	Promotes peristalsis	Slows peristalsis—constipation
	Contracts bladder	Urinary hesitancy or urinary retention
	Constricts bronchi	Dilates bronchi

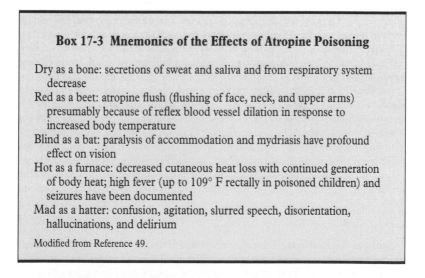

Box 17-3 Mnemonics of the Effects of Atropine Poisoning

Dry as a bone: secretions of sweat and saliva and from respiratory system decrease

Red as a beet: atropine flush (flushing of face, neck, and upper arms) presumably because of reflex blood vessel dilation in response to increased body temperature

Blind as a bat: paralysis of accommodation and mydriasis have profound effect on vision

Hot as a furnace: decreased cutaneous heat loss with continued generation of body heat; high fever (up to 109° F rectally in poisoned children) and seizures have been documented

Mad as a hatter: confusion, agitation, slurred speech, disorientation, hallucinations, and delirium

Modified from Reference 49.

The anticholinergic drugs used most often to treat drug-induced parkinsonism and other EPSEs are trihexyphenidyl (Artane) and benztropine (Cogentin). Less frequently used drugs include biperiden (Akineton), procyclidine (Kemadrin), and ethopropazine (Parsidol). In addition, the antihistamine diphenhydramine (Benadryl) has central anticholinergic effects and is often used substitutively for anticholinergic drugs. The antihistamines have fewer peripheral nervous system (PNS) side effects and may be better tolerated by elderly persons. Trihexyphenidyl is discussed as the prototypical anticholinergic drug. Table 17-3 summarizes the efficacy of these drugs for specific EPSEs.

**Box 17-4 Protocol for Treatment
of Extrapyramidal Side Effects (EPSEs)**

If EPSEs occur, the following steps can be used to reduce their intensity and
length:

1. Reduce the dosage of the neuroleptic if possible.
2. If the dosage cannot be decreased, change to a neuroleptic with less
   potential for causing EPSEs.
3. Add an anticholinergic based on efficacy for a particular EPSE.
4. If EPSEs continue, increase amount of anticholinergic or switch to a
   different agent.
5. If side effects of the anticholinergic become a concern, switch to another
   anticholinergic or use a nonanticholinergic agent.
6. Continue the anticholinergic for about 3 months, if the neuroleptic
   treatment is stable, and then start slowly decreasing the dosage amount
   until it is withdrawn.
7. If EPSEs recur, reinstitute the anticholinergic at the lowest possible
   effective dosage. Attempt to discontinue again in a few months.

Data from References 7, 11, and 36.

Table 17-3 Efficacy of Antiparkinsonism Drugs for Specific Extrapyramidal
Side Effects (EPSEs)

Drug	Tremor	Rigidity	Dystonia	Akinesia	Akathisia
Amantadine	xx	xx	xx	xxx	xx
Benztropine	xx	xxx	xxx	xx	xx
Biperiden	xx	xx	xx	xxx	xx
Diphenhydramine	xx	x	xx	—	xxx
Ethopropazine	xxx	xx	x	x	xx
Procyclidine	x	xxx	xx	xx	xx
Trihexyphenidyl	xx	xx	xx	xxx	xx

Modified from Reference 7.
—, No effect; *x*, some effect (20% response); *xx*, moderate effect (20% to 50% response); *xxx*,
50% response.

Pharmacologic effects. Trihexyphenidyl and the related anticholinergic drugs
inhibit the actions of ACh in the brain. Acetylcholine muscarinic M-1 receptors are
blocked by these drugs. These drugs also inhibit the reuptake of dopamine and more
weakly inhibit the reuptake of norepinephrine and serotonin.[6,38] Both effects
contribute to restoration of the acetylcholine-dopamine balance. When used to treat
PD, trihexyphenidyl is often given adjunctively with dopaminergic drugs; when used
to treat EPSEs, trihexyphenidyl is administered alone.

Pharmacokinetics. Trihexyphenidyl and the related drugs are usually given
orally. Little pharmacokinetic information is available on these drugs; however, it is
known that the half-lives range from 6 to 10 hours for trihexyphenidyl to up to 24

Table 17-4 Anticholinergic Treatment Dosages for EPSEs

Amantadine (Symmetrel)	PO: 100 to 400 mg/day
Benztropine (Cogentin)	1-4 mg, qd or bid PO or IM For acute dystonic reactions: 1-2 mg IM/IV, may repeat in 30 min, then 1-2 mg PO bid
Biperiden (Akineton)	2 mg 1-3 times per day
Diphenhydramine (Benadryl)	PO: 100-200 mg/day For acute dystonic reactions: 25-50 mg IM/IV
Ethopropazine (Parsidol)	Starting dose: 50 mg qd or bid Maximum dose: 600 mg/day
Procyclidine (Kemadrin)	Starting dose: 2.5 mg bid May increase to 30 mg/day
Trihexyphenidyl (Artane)	Starting dose: 2-5 mg/day Usual dose 5-15 mg/day May increase to 30 mg/day in younger patients

hours for biperiden. The peak concentration level is achieved in about 1 hour. These drugs are excreted by the kidneys. When trihexyphenidyl is used to treat EPSEs caused by antipsychotic drugs, 1 mg is given initially, with 1 mg added every few hours (2 to 5 mg/day) until the reaction is controlled (Table 17-4). The usual dosage is 5 to 15 mg/day, but dosages up to 30 mg/day have been prescribed for and tolerated by younger patients.[6] When an oculogyric crisis or other dystonic reaction occurs, a more aggressive approach must be pursued, using intramuscular or intravascular injections of agents such as benztropine.

Side effects. Anticholinergic drugs have the side effects associated with atropine. These drugs act both centrally and peripherally. About 20% to 30% of patients taking anticholinergics have CNS effects such as confusion, depression, delusions, and hallucinations. In addition, drowsiness and agitation are common central responses. Furthermore, the anticholinergic agents such as trihexyphenidyl can have euphoric side effects and are abused for that reason.

Because the cholinergic system is implicated in memory and learning, anticholinergic drugs have the potential to compromise both, particularly in elderly persons. PNS effects such as dry mouth, blurred vision, nausea, and nervousness occur in 30% to 50% of patients. Constipation, a problem for many patients taking antipsychotic drugs, can be worsened by anticholinergics. Urinary hesitancy and retention, decreased sweating, tachycardia, and mydriasis are other PNS effects. Decreased sweating (a sympathetic system function) contributes to hyperthermia, a side effect with a potentially serious outcome. Table 17-5 summarizes common anticholinergic side effects and appropriate intervention strategies.

An important consideration when prescribing anticholinergics for a patient is the presence of glaucoma. Mydriasis, or pupil dilation, blocks the flow of aqueous humor from the anterior chamber, causing increased intraocular pressure. In cases of undiagnosed acute-angle glaucoma, the anticholinergic effect could precipitate a very painful attack and cause blindness. Any eye pain associated with anticholinergics should be treated as an emergency. Elderly individuals are at greater risk for this complication. Amantadine, although having anticholinergic properties, is safe to use at low dosages for patients who have glaucoma.

Table 17-5 Side Effects, Interventions, and Suggestions for Cautious Use of Anticholinergics

Side effects	Appropriate interventions
Dry mouth	Encourage sugarless hard candy and chewing gum; frequent rinses.
Nasal congestion	Suggest over-the-counter nasal decongestant (but use with caution).
Urinary hesitancy	Suggest running water, privacy, warm water over perineum.
Urinary retention	Catheterize for residual urine; encourage fluid intake and frequent voiding.
Blurred vision, photophobia	Provide reassurance; normal vision typically returns in a few weeks; instruct patient to wear sunglasses and be cautious about driving.
Constipation	Order laxatives; encourage a diet with roughage.
Mydriasis	Instruct patient to report eye pain immediately.
Orthostatic hypotension	Request patient to get out of bed slowly, to sit on the edge of the bed a short while, then rise slowly.
Sedation	Help the patient get up early and get the day started.
Decreased sweating	Can lead to fever; take reading of temperature; if fever occurs, reduce body temperature (e.g., sponge baths); cases of fatal hyperthermia have been reported.

Precautions should be used in many situations. Be cautious in administering anti-cholinergics in these situations:

Situation	Rationale
Tachycardia or other arrhythmias	Anticholinergics take off the "brake" of the cholinergic system on the heart, leading to increased heart rates.
Prostatic hypertrophy	Anticholinergics inhibit the urinary system by relaxing the detrusor muscle of the bladder and contracting the trigone muscle and sphincter, thus creating significant mechanical barriers to urination.

Implications

Therapeutic versus toxic levels. The typical dosage range for trihexyphenidyl is 5 to 15 mg/day for drug-induced EPSEs. Overdose may result in CNS hyperstimulation, confusion, excitement, hyperpyrexia, agitation, disorientation, delirium, and hallucinations. Convulsions, sometimes fatal, can develop related to hyperthermia associated with atropine poisoning (see Box 17-3). Overdose can also result in CNS depression, drowsiness, sedation, or coma. The atropine-like effects summarized in Table 17-5 intensify. The mental symptoms of the patient receiving neuroleptics may also intensify. Circulatory collapse, cardiac arrest, and respiratory tract depression or arrest have been reported.

Treatment for anticholinergic drug overdose is similar to that for atropine overdose. The major emphasis is prevention of further absorption. Three mechanisms can be used: gastric lavage, induced vomiting, and ingestion of activated

Table 17-6 Drug Interactions with Anticholinergic Agents

Drug	Interaction
Antacids, antidiarrheals, and other absorbents	Decreased absorption of anticholinergics
Alcohol and other depressants	Increased drowsiness; avoid if possible
Anticholinergics	Additive effect; atropine-like effect, toxicity (leading to psychosis); cases of paralytic ileus reported
Caffeine	Can neutralize the antiparkinsonism effects of anticholinergics
Digoxin tablets	Anticholinergics can increase digoxin (tablets only) serum levels
Haloperidol	Decreased serum level of haloperidol; additive anticholinergic effect; may unmask tardive dyskinesia

charcoal. The literature supports gastric lavage as the preferred approach, particularly when the patient is conscious. Providing supportive care such as airway maintenance, assistance with breathing, and monitoring for hyperthermia (vitals and rectal temperatures) are important. The most effective antidote for antimuscarinic poisoning is physostigmine. More serious or life-threatening situations may require advanced supportive efforts such as treating hyperthermia with a cooling blanket, tepid baths, or ice packs; treating seizures with parenteral diazepam; using physostigmine to reverse cardiac and CNS effects; and using fluids and vasopressors for circulatory collapse.[38]

Use in pregnancy. Anticholinergics should be used cautiously during pregnancy. Theoretically, these drugs decrease milk flow during lactation. All of these agents except for diphenhydramine (category B) are placed in category C.

Interactions. Many over-the-counter drugs have anticholinergic properties and potentiate these drugs (Table 17-6). Antihistamines, commonly a component of cold medicines, are major interactants. Other major interactants with the potential for additive anticholinergic effects are amantadine, antiarrhythmics, antipsychotics, MAOIs, and tricyclic antidepressants. Elderly persons are most at risk for these additive effects.

RELATED ANTICHOLINERGIC DRUGS
Benztropine

Benztropine (Cogentin) is used to treat drug-induced EPSEs and is also prescribed prophylactically. It is the most commonly prescribed drug for EPSEs. An intramuscular form is available for noncompliant patients and for emergency intervention during an acute EPSE reaction such as oculogyric crisis. The oral form of the drug should be substituted for parenteral routes as soon as the patient's condition stabilizes. Because benztropine and trihexyphenidyl belong to different chemical classes, benztropine *may be* effective when trihexyphenidyl is not. Benztropine causes greater and longer-lasting muscle relaxation and sedation than does trihexyphenidyl. The more intense sedative effect may not be desirable for some patients but may make benztropine more desirable for others. Benztropine is less likely to cause a euphoric effect than is trihexyphenidyl, so it is less likely to be abused. These differences notwithstanding, benztropine should be considered the equivalent of trihexyphenidyl in peripheral anticholinergic effect.

Less Commonly Prescribed Anticholinergics

Biperiden. Biperiden (Akineton) is occasionally used to treat drug-induced EPSEs. It is chemically related to trihexyphenidyl. It is usually given orally but can be administered parenterally for acute drug-induced extrapyramidal reactions. There is some evidence that biperiden may actually ameliorate mild cases of tardive dyskinesia.[50] The half-life of biperiden is 18 to 24 hours.

Ethopropazine. Ethopropazine (Parsidol) is a phenothiazine derivative. Because phenothiazines block dopamine, it seems illogical to use this agent to treat neuroleptic-induced EPSEs. However, ethopropazine can be useful for drug-induced extrapyramidal disorders.

Procyclidine. Procyclidine (Kemadrin) is seldom used to treat drug-induced EPSEs but is particularly effective in alleviating rigidity. It is not effective in reducing tremor and may actually increase tremors early in treatment. Parenteral forms are not available. It is best given after meals. The half-life of procyclidine is approximately 12 hours.

Diphenhydramine. Diphenhydramine (Benadryl) is not a pure anticholinergic agent but is the prototypical antihistamine (H_1 antagonist). It has anticholinergic capabilities and appears to inhibit dopamine reuptake, providing two means of reestablishing the acetylcholine-dopamine balance. It is better tolerated in older patients who cannot tolerate the more potent anticholinergic agents. It is usually given orally but can be given parenterally. The half-life of diphenhydramine is 2 to 7 hours.

PATIENT EDUCATION ISSUES

Patient education is an important part of the care of patients taking anticholinergic agents to decrease drug-induced side effects. Patients should be taught the following:
- To report sudden, marked changes in bowel or bladder function
- Not to discontinue the drug suddenly because anxiety, depression, motor agitation, hallucinations, and cholinergic rebound (i.e., vomiting, malaise, sweating, excessive salivation, vivid dreams, and nightmares) can occur
- To avoid driving or other hazardous activities if drowsiness is a side effect
- To take with food if GI upset occurs
- To report eye pain immediately because it may be related to undiagnosed glaucoma
- To avoid strenuous activities in hot weather because of decreased sweating
- To avoid using over-the-counter and prescription drugs that contain anticholinergic properties (cold and hay fever medications) because of an additive effect

ISSUES IN ANTICHOLINERGIC DRUG ADMINISTRATION

A number of issues exist surrounding the use of anticholinergic agents to treat EPSEs. These issues are presented in the form of questions and answers.

Is Prophylactic Anticholinergic Treatment Necessary and Helpful?

Although it is known that these agents are therapeutic for acute EPSEs, it is not known whether they are beneficial as prophylaxis for drug-induced EPSEs. Both the prophylactic use and the duration of treatment concomitantly with neuroleptics are controversial.[19,33,52]

Arguments for prophylactic use

1. Rectifies poor assessment. Anticholinergic agents are particularly beneficial for akinesia, an extremely annoying EPSE that significantly contributes to noncompliance. Akinesia is often gradual in onset and can provoke listlessness, which in turn can be assessed as an exacerbation of psychosis. Prophylactic use might mitigate poor assessment practices.
2. Increases compliance. EPSEs are a major source of noncompliant behavior. If EPSEs can be minimized, the patient will be more likely to comply with the medication regimen.
3. Prevents frightening EPSEs. Anticholinergic agents can prevent the development of frightening dystonic reactions that both reinforce negative impressions of neuroleptic therapy and are health threatening. This is particularly true in young, male patients.
4. Mitigates the high rate of EPSEs. An estimated 60% to 90% of all patients taking antipsychotic drugs have some level of EPSEs.[2]
5. Decreases the high rate of EPSEs associated with depot and high-potency drugs. The use of depot and high-potency drugs increases the need for anticholinergics as prophylactic agents.
6. Prevents worsening of psychopathology. Anxiety, depression, motor agitation, and hallucinations have been reported after discontinuance of long-term anticholinergic drugs.[28]

Arguments against prophylactic use

1. It is not needed. Although most patients report EPSEs, only a few have severe symptoms.
2. New problems are created. Anticholinergic drugs cause additional side effects, including toxic anticholinergic psychosis, urinary retention, hyperthermia, and memory impairment.
3. These drugs have an unmasking effect. Anticholinergic drugs unmask latent TD or worsen the development of TD.
4. They are of questionable value. Even maintenance treatment is no guarantee EPSEs will not occur.[17]
5. The effects of neuroleptics are decreased. Anticholinergics interfere with the therapeutic effects of neuroleptics by impeding absorption.

Many clinicians believe the disadvantages of prophylactic use outweigh the advantages. Hence anticholinergic drugs are often not prescribed until EPSEs occur and then are discontinued as soon as possible (typically within 4 to 8 weeks). A common exception is use in young men receiving antipsychotic drugs.

What Is the Potential for Abuse or Misuse of Anticholinergic Drugs, and How Common Is Abuse or Misuse?

Anticholinergics have both hallucinogenic and euphorigenic properties. Hence, the major effects sought by abusers are (1) a toxic confusional state accompanied by hallucinations, paranoia, and impairment of recent memory or (2) a euphoriant, antidepressant, and socially stimulating state. Abusers use several routes: oral, intravenous, and mixed with tobacco for smoking.[13] Land, Pinsky, and Salzman reported that 1% to 17% of patients for whom these drugs are prescribed abuse or misuse them.[32] Abuse of anticholinergic drugs increases as the availability of other abused drugs decreases.

The first case of abuse of these drugs was reported by Bolin.[10] A woman being treated for torticollis with 2 mg four times a day of an anticholinergic started taking up to 30 mg/day to achieve a euphoric state; eventually, a full-blown toxic psychosis developed. Since that report, many other cases of anticholinergic abuse have been reported.

Misuse is different from abuse and is usually associated with a patient with negative symptoms who wants the sense of greater sociability.

Anticholinergic abuse can be deterred by the following[32]:

1. Avoid prophylactic use.
2. Do not use with low-potency antipsychotics that have high anticholinergic properties.
3. Treat EPSEs with nonanticholinergic medications when possible.
4. Prescribe the lowest effective dosage possible.

Does Abrupt Withdrawal from Anticholinergic Drugs Cause a Significant Reaction?

Anticholinergic drugs should never be discontinued abruptly, even when abuse is suspected. Abrupt withdrawal causes cholinergic rebound and withdrawal symptoms, including vomiting, malaise, sweating, excessive salivation, vivid dreams, and nightmares.

What Are the Characteristics of Toxic Anticholinergic Psychosis, and Who Is Most Susceptible?

Mild anticholinergic effects include those mentioned earlier in this chapter— drowsiness, dizziness, constipation, dry mouth, and nervousness. Anticholinergic psychosis or intoxication becomes evident with symptoms of agitation, visual and tactile hallucinations, nightmares, paranoid thinking, confusion, and impairment of recent memory. Toxic PNS symptoms include nausea and vomiting, diarrhea, tachycardia, arrhythmias, hypertension, and bronchospasm. Geriatric and pediatric patients are most sensitive to anticholinergic side effects.[26]

OTHER AGENTS USED TO TREAT EPSEs

Although anticholinergic antiparkinsonism drugs are most often used to treat neuroleptic-induced side effects, several other agents with antiparkinsonism capabilities have been successfully administered and continue to have their own advocates.

Benzodiazepines: Treatment of EPSEs

Benzodiazepines, especially lorazepam (Ativan) at 1.5 to 5 mg, diazepam (Valium) at 15 to 40 mg, and clonazepam (Klonopin) at 0.5 mg, have been used successfully to treat side effects.[24] These agents may be particularly useful for akinesia and akathisia.

Beta-Adrenergic Antagonists: Treatment of EPSEs

Propranolol (Inderal) at 20 to 100 mg and a few other beta-adrenergic antagonists have effectively reduced the side effects of neuroleptic drugs, particularly akathisia. These drugs are well tolerated and probably work through the antagonism of central beta-adrenergic receptors; however, in clinical trials, these agents are combined with antiparkinsonism drugs, so it is difficult to interpret their precise effects on EPSEs.

Clonidine: Treatment of EPSEs

Clonidine (Catapres) is a centrally acting alpha-2 agonist. Clonidine apparently works by decreasing CNS noradrenergic neurotransmission. Dosages from 0.15 to 0.8 mg have been used successfully to treat side effects of antipsychotic drugs, but Fleischhacker, Roth, and Kane found the alpha-2 agonists to be more difficult to use, with no advantage over other agents.[24] Tonda and Guthrie suggest clonidine as an alternative to anticholinergics in treatment-resistant akathisia.[52]

Nifedipine and Verapamil: Treatment of Tardive Dyskinesia

Nifedipine (Procardia) at 30 to 60 mg/day and verapamil (Calan) at 80 mg four times a day are calcium channel blockers that produce statistically significant improvement in patients with tardive dyskinesia.[4,20] The interaction between the dopamine system in the CNS and calcium antagonists probably explains the improvement noted in patients with TD.

Dantrolene: Treatment of Neuroleptic Malignant Syndrome

Dantrolene (Dantrium) has been prescribed successfully in patients with NMS and lethal catatonia.[40,48] Dantrolene interferes with the intracellular release of calcium necessary to initiate muscle contraction. Dantrolene also exerts a CNS effect.

REFERENCES

1. Agid Y: Parkinson's disease: pathophysiology, *Lancet* 337:1321, 1991.
2. American Psychiatric Association: *Practice guidelines for the treatment of patients with schizophrenia*, Washington DC, 1997, The Association.
3. Appleton M: Cytochrome P-450 isoenzymes. Nursing considerations, *J APNA* 5(1):15, 1999.
4. Barrow N, Childs A: An antitardive dyskinesia effect of verapamil, *Am J Psychiatry* 143: 1485, 1986.
5. Bassitt DP, Louza Neto MR: Clozapine efficacy in tardive dyskinesia in schizophrenic patients, *Eur Arch Psychiatry Clin Neurosci* 248(4):209, 1998.
6. Bezchilbnyk-Butler KZ, Jeffries JJ: *Clinical handbook of psychotropic drugs*, Seattle, 1997, Hogrefe and Huber.
7. Bezchlibnyk-Butler KZ, Remington GJ: Antiparkinsonian drugs in the treatment of neuroleptic-induced extrapyramidal symptoms, *Can J Psychiatry* 39(3):74, 1994.
8. Bitter I, Scheurer J, Volavka J: Are extrapyramidal symptoms necessary? *J Clin Psychopharmacol* 12(1):65, 1992 (letter).
9. Blair DT, Dauner A: Nonneuroleptic etiologies of extrapyramidal symptoms, *Clin Nurs Specialist* 7(4):225, 1993.
10. Bolin RR: Psychiatric manifestations of Artane toxicity, *J Nerv Ment Dis* 131:256, 1960.
11. Boodhoo JA, Sandler M: Anticholinergic antiparkinsonian drugs in psychiatry, *Br J Hosp Med* 46:167, 1991.
12. Borison RL, Diamond BL: Neuropharmacology of the extrapyramidal system, *J Clin Psychiatry* 48:9(suppl):7, 1987.
13. Brower KS: Smoking of prescription anticholinergic drugs, *Am J Psychiatry* 144:383, 1987.
14. Buckley NJ, Bonner TI, Buckley CM, Brann MR: Antagonists binding properties of five cloned muscarinic receptors expressed in CHO-K1 cells, *Mole Pharmacol* 35:469, 1989.
15. Buckley PF, Hutchinson M: Neuroleptic malignant syndrome, *Neurosurg Psychiatry* 58: 271, 1995.
16. Casey DE: Effects of clozapine therapy in schizophrenic individuals at risk for tardive dyskinesia, *J Clin Psychiatry* 59(suppl 3):31, 1998.
17. Comaty JE and others: Is maintenance antiparkinsonian treatment necessary? *Psychopharmacol Bull* 26(2):267, 1990.

18. Cummings JL: Depression and Parkinson's disease: a review, *Am J Psychiatry* 149(4): 443, 1992.

19. Double DB and others: Efficacy of maintenance use of anticholinergic agents, *Acta Psychiatr Scand* 88(5):381, 1993.

20. Duncan E and others: Nifedipine in the treatment of tardive dyskinesia, *J Clin Psychopharmacol* 10(6):414, 1990.

21. Dursun S, Oluboka OJ, Devarajan S, Kutcher SP: High-dose vitamin E plus vitamin B_6 treatment of risperidone-related neuroleptic malignant syndrome, *J Psychopharm* 12:220, 1998.

22. Factor SA, Friedman JH: The emerging role of clozapine in the treatment of movement disorders, *Movement Dis* 12(4):483, 1997.

23. Fleischhacker WW, Hummer M: Drug treatment of schizophrenia in the 1990s: achievements and future possibilities in optimizing outcomes, *Drugs* 53(6):915, 1997

24. Fleischhacker WW, Roth SD, Kane JM: The pharmacologic treatment of neuroleptic-induced akathisia, *J Clin Psychopharmacol* 10(1):12, 1990.

25. Foley JJ: Considerations in the use of benzodiazepines and antipsychotics in the emergency department, *J Emerg Nurs* 19(5):448, 1993.

26. Hamdan-Allen G, Nixon M: Anticholinergic psychosis in children: a case report, *Hosp Community Psychiatry* 42(2):191, 1991.

27. Hulme EC, Birdsall NJ, Buckley NJ: Muscarinic receptor subtypes, *Annu Rev Pharmacol Toxicol* 30:633, 1990.

28. Kandel ER, Schwartz JH, Jessell TM: *Principles of neural science,* ed 3, Norwalk, Conn, 1991, Appleton & Lange.

29. Keepers RSE, Casey DE: Clinical management of acute neuroleptic-induced extrapyramidal symptoms. In Masserman JH, editor: *Current psychiatric therapies,* New York, 1986, Grune & Stratton.

30. Kellam AM: The (frequently) neuroleptic (potentially) malignant syndrome, *Br J Psychiatry* 157:169, 1990.

31. Keltner NL: Neuroreceptor function and psychopharmacologic response, *Iss Mental Health Nurs* 21:31, 2000.

32. Land W, Pinsky D, Salzman C: Abuse and misuse of anticholinergic medications, *Hosp Community Psychiatry* 42(6):580, 1991.

33. Lavin MR, Rifkin A: Psychotic patients' interpretation of neuroleptic side effects, *Am J Psychiatry* 148(11):1615, 1991 (letter).

34. Lazarus A, Mann SC, Caroff SN: *The neuroleptic malignant syndrome and related conditions,* Washington, DC, 1989, American Psychiatric Press.

35. Liebman M: *Neuroanatomy made easy and understandable,* Gaithersburg, Md, 1991, Aspen.

36. Malhotra AK, Litman RE, Pickar D: Adverse effects of antipsychotic drugs, *Drug Saf* 9(6): 429, 1993.

37. Medina A and others: Effects of central muscarinic-1 receptor stimulation on blood pressure regulation, *Hypertension* 29:828, 1997.

38. Olin BR: *Drug facts and comparisons,* ed 49, St Louis, 1995, Wolters Kluwer.

39. Pelonero AL, Levenson JL, Pandurangi AK: Neuroleptic malignant syndrome: a review, *Psychiatric Serv* 49(9):1163, 1998.

40. Pennati A, Sacchetti E, Calzeroni A: Dantrolene in lethal catatonia, *Am J Psychiatry* 148(2):149, 1991 (letter).

41. Persing JS: Neuroleptic malignant syndrome: an overview, *SD J Med* 47(2):51, 1994.

42. Planansky K, Johnston R: The occurrence and characteristics of suidical preoccupation and acts in schizophrenia, *Acta Psychiatr Scand* 47:473, 1971.

43. Pletscher A, DaPrada M: Pharmacotherapy of Parkinson's disease: research from 1960 to 1991, *Acta Neurol Scand* 87(suppl 146):26, 1993.

44. Richards SS, Musser WS, Gershon S: *Maintenance pharmacotherapies for neuropsychiatric disorders,* Philadelphia, 1999, Brunner/Mazel.

45. Scherman D and others: Striatal dopamine deficiency in Parkinson's disease: role of aging, *Ann Neurol* 26:551, 1989.

46. Sedvall G: PET studies on the neuroreceptor effects of antipsychotic drugs, *Curr Approach Psychosis* 4:1, 1995.
47. Seeman P, Van Tol HH: Dopamine receptor pharmacology, *Trends Pharmacol Sci* 15(7): 264, 1994.
48. Shader RI, Greenblatt DJ: A possible new approach to the treatment of neuroleptic malignant syndrome, *J Clin Psychopharmacol* 12(3):155, 1992.
49. Shlafer M: *The nurse, pharmacology, and drug therapy,* ed 2, Redwood City, Calif, 1993, Addison-Wesley.
50. Silver H, Geraisy N, Schwartz M: No difference in the effect of biperiden and amantadine on parkinsonian- and tardive dyskinesia-type involuntary movements: a double-blind crossover, placebo-controlled study in medicated chronic schizophrenic patients, *J Clin Psychiatry* 56(4):167, 1995.
51. Spivak B and others: Clozapine treatment for neuroleptic-induced tardive dyskinesia, parkinsonism, and chronic akathisia in schizophrenic patients, *J Clin Psychiatry* 58(8): 403, 1997.
52. Tonda ME, Guthrie SK: Treatment of acute neuroleptic-induced movement disorders, *Pharmacotherapy* 14(5):543, 1994.
53. Van Putten T, Marder SR: Behavioral toxicity of antipsychotic drugs, *J Clin Psychopharmacol* 7:243, 1987.
54. Walters VL and others: New strategies for old problems; tardive dyskinesia (TD). Review and report on severe TD cases treated with 12, 8, and 5 years of video followup, *Schizophr Res* 28(23):231, 1997.

CHAPTER 18

Herbiceuticals in Psychiatry

DAVID G. FOLKS AND TERI GABEL

Herbs and related products are commonly used by patients who also seek conventional health care. A few herbs have been extensively studied, but little is known about the others. This chapter seeks to answer some of the questions regarding the clinical use of herbiceuticals in psychiatric conditions. The marketplace with respect to herbs is discussed, including websites that pertain to herbiceuticals.

THE HERBAL MARKET

The growing popularity and use of alternative medicine has created a need for clinicians to become informed about the use of herbal remedies. Herbiceuticals may be encountered by clinicians because herbs are used to treat psychiatric symptoms; produce changes in mood, thinking, or behavior as a side effect; or interact with other psychiatric medications. Most herbs that are used for psychiatric purposes are not well studied, and there are questions as to their efficacy and safety. On the other hand, the efficacy of St. John's Wort (for depression) or ginkgo (for memory impairment) is quite good.[21]

The reason there are so few controlled studies of herbal medicines is because they are not profitable. Thus little motivation is present for manufacturers to conduct randomized, placebo-controlled, double-blind clinical trials to prove efficacy because they are not required to do so and because they cannot patent the product to recoup the $350 million it would cost to prove the new drug effective and safe.[16] Despite these limitations, some scientific studies are being performed. Although additional research needs to be conducted to determine the appropriate use of herbs in psychiatric conditions, published information to date is useful in the process of diagnosing, counseling, and treating patients who may be taking these botanical remedies. Table 18-1 describes the major differences between herbs and approved drugs.

Herbs are divided into the following three groups:
1. Those that are commonly used to treat psychiatric symptoms
2. Those that have psychotropic effects
3. Those that may interact with either psychiatric illnesses or the drugs used to treat those illnesses[21]

Sources of Information about Herbs

As will be clear after reading this chapter, it is imperative for clinicians to incorporate knowledge of herbal drugs into their practices. However, it is also difficult to find good information about herbs. A clinician wanting nonbiased information on common herbs is advised to purchase a reference book that bases advice on published and critically reviewed literature. Of course, a comprehensive literature search will

Table 18-1 Difference between FDA-Approved Drugs and Herbs

Drug	Herbals
Dose established	Usually some guidelines
Proof of efficacy	Proof of efficacy not required
Monosubstance	Complex compound
FDA approval before marketing	No FDA preapproval; postmarketing notification for structure-function claims
Patentable	Not patentable
Potency standardized	Potency varies

ensure the most scientific, peer-reviewed information, but this process is impractical and time-consuming. Several avenues of information can now be accessed through traditional as well as Internet sources.

Traditional sources. Traditional sources for herbal information include the following:
1. *Physicians Desk Reference* version of Herbal Medicine (1998)
2. *Guide to Popular Natural Products:* Facts and Comparison (1999)
3. *The Review of Natural Products:* Facts and Comparison (2000)

Internet sources. Websites for herbal information are also available. The following are several sites providing information about herbs:
1. The U.S. Food and Drug Administration (FDA) access to "MedWatch," which provides herbal warnings under a specific nutritional adverse event monitoring system, is available at www.fda.gov.
2. The Aspet herbal and medicinal plant interest group features herb discussions among classic pharmacologists at www.faseb.org/aspet/.
3. The American Botanical Council, a respectable organization dedicated to the dissemination of factual herbal information, has established the Herb Research Foundation, which is located on the Internet at www.herbs.org.
4. Botanical.com, a somewhat biased website, has an emphasis on anecdotes and can be accessed at www.botanical.com.
5. The Herbal Information Center provides brief overviews on common herbs. It includes some warnings but seems mostly geared toward selling herbal drugs. It is located at www.kcweb.com/herb/herbmain/htm.
6. Herbnet links to other herb websites that appear to emphasize advertisements. Nonetheless, some good information can be found at www.herbnet.com.
7. The University of Washington Medicinal Herb Garden (with pictures of herbs) is cross-referenced to Medline abstracts and provides an excellent resource. It can be found at www.nnlm.nlm.nih.gov/pnr/uwmhg/.

Historical Perspective of Herbiceuticals

The earliest evidence of human use of plants for healing can be traced back to the Neanderthal period.[13] Chinese writings from 3000 BC contain more than 1000 herbal formulas.[10] In more recent times (i.e., during the 1500s), botanical gardens were created to grow "medicinal" plants for schools of medicine. Herbal medicine practice flourished until the seventeenth century when more "scientific" pharmacologic remedies were favored.[19]

In the United States, the history of herbal use began in early colonial days when health care was provided by women in the home. Initially, they used homemade botanical remedies and later purchased similar products as patent medicines. In the early nineteenth century, scientific methods became more advanced and preferred, and the practice of botanical healing was dismissed as quackery. In the 1960s, with concerns over the iatrogenic effects of conventional medicine and the desire for self-reliance, interest in "natural health" caused an increase in the use of herbal products.[19] Recognition of the rising use of herbal medicines and other nontraditional remedies led to the establishment of the Office of Alternative Medicine by the National Institutes of Health in 1992. Herbal use has also become a worldwide phenomenon; in 1974, the World Health Organization encouraged developing countries to use traditional plant medicines to "fulfill a need unmet by modern systems."[19] Thirty percent of all modern drugs are derived from plants, and some of the more familiar ones are listed in Box 18-1.

Use of Herbal Medicines

Internationally, the use of botanical medicines is generally higher than in the United States. Eighty percent of the world's population relies primarily on traditional medicines for their health care needs. Approximately 20% to 30% of the U.S. population uses herbiceuticals for one cause or another, most commonly in persons with chronic conditions.[7] An estimated $11 billion is spent annually on alternative medicine, and the growth rate of the industry, which includes herbal medicine, is estimated to be 20% annually.[12] It is certain that clinicians see patients who use herbs, and as is discussed, this use can affect the patient's health problems and the sought-after effects of conventional treatments as well.

Costs to the individual for herbal products can be substantial, albeit variable. Insurance plans and managed care organizations are beginning to offer reimbursement for some alternative treatments. Although reimbursements for herbal medicines is in its infancy, it is expected to grow tremendously along with the continued boom in sales of herbal products and alternative health care in general. Clinicians must become familiar with herbal medicine, because more insurance companies will expect their clinicians to make referrals or recommendations regarding herbal products.

Box 18-1 Conventional Medicines Derived from Plants

Atropine *(Atropa belladonna)*	Physostigmine *(Physostigma venenosum)*
Digoxin *(Digitalis purpurea)*	Senna *(Cassia acutifolia)*
Colchicine *(Colchicum autumnale)*	Ephedrine *(Ephedra sinica)*
Quinine *(Cinchona officinalis)*	Cocaine *(Erythroxylon coca)*
Codeine *(Papaver somniferum)*	Salicylin *(Salix purpurea)*
Vincristine *(Catharanthus roseus)*	Capsaicin *(Capsicum frutescens)*
Ipecac *(Cephaelis ipecacuanha)*	Scopolamine *(Datura fastuosa)*
Paclitaxel *(Taxus brevifolia)*	Reserpine *(Rauwolfia serpentina)*

Why People Use Herbs

There are multiple reasons why individuals turn to herbal therapies. Often cited is a sense of control, a mental comfort from taking action, which helps explain why many individuals taking herbs have diseases that are chronic or incurable (e.g., diabetes, cancer, arthritis, acquired immunodeficiency syndrome [AIDS]). In rural areas, additional cultural factors encourage the use of botanicals. Religious beliefs can be traced to the medieval doctrine of signatures, as "the good Lord has put these yerbs here for man to make hisself with. They is a yerb, could we but find it, to cure every illness" (sic).[18] Another argument is that natural plant products are perceived to be more healthful than manufactured medicines. In addition, reports of adverse effects of conventional medicines are found in the lay press at a much higher rate than reports of herbal toxicities, in part because mechanisms to track adverse effects exist for conventional medicines, whereas such data for self-treatment is harder to ascertain.

Clinicians often dismiss herbs as harmless placebos, whereas many consumers and clinicians mistakenly believe anything in a pill form has been approved by the FDA.[20] In 1993, the FDA began scrutinizing herbal and supplemental agents, which triggered a letter writing campaign organized by the health-food stores encouraging consumers to write to Congress. Under pressure, the FDA compromised its plans to regulate herbs and supplements, thus creating the "supplemental category" (e.g., vitamins, minerals, and herbs) and created the Dietary Supplement and Health Education Act of 1994. This legislation required that "no proof of efficacy, safety, or standards for quality control for products labeled as supplements was necessary." Although supplements may not promise a specific cure on the label, they may claim effect. If questions arise, the burden lies with the FDA to prove a product unsafe, rather than a company proving its products safe. Box 18-2 lists some herbs with hepatotoxic or carcinogenic properties.

In contrast, regulatory agencies in Germany, France, the United Kingdom, and Canada enforce standards of herb quality and safety assessment against manufacturers.[20] However, the amount of active ingredient per tablet may vary from one product to another, with striking differences found in some cases. This could have an impact

---

Box 18-2 Hepatotoxic, Carcinogenic, or Toxic Herbs

Avoid oral ingestion of the following:

Volatile oils: Toxicity is attributed to the phenyl allyl component. Important here is the concentration. Amount of some of these herbs (e.g., fennel, sweet basil, parsley) used in normal cooking is not dangerous.
  Calamus oil: *Toxic component*—beta-asarone (carcinogenic)
  Fennel, sweet basil, chervil oils: *Toxic component*—estragole (carcinogenic)
  Parsley oil: *Toxic component*—apiole (abortifacient and hepatotoxic)
  Pennyroyal oil: *Toxic component*—pulegone (abortifacient and hepatotoxic)
  Sassafras oil: *Toxic component*—safrole (abortifacient and hepatotoxic)

Pyrrolizidine alkaloids: Unsaturated nucleus of the pyrrolizidine ring metabolized to toxic metabolites. Examples of herbs: borage, colts foot, comfrey, liferoot.

Lignans: Use can result in irreversible hepatic and renal failure. Example herb: chapparal.

if a patient changed from one brand to another; for example, ginseng and other herbs have dose-dependent adverse effects, and variability of active ingredients can be problematic. Labels may also be incorrect, accidentally or intentionally. Further adding to this confusion, the same common name may be applied to different plants recommended for different illnesses. For example, some products labeled as ginseng may contain mandrake.

HERBS USED FOR PSYCHOTROPIC EFFECTS
St. John's Wort

The historical use of St. John's Wort *(Hypericum perforatum)* may be traced back to the texts of the ancient Greek physicians Hippocrates, Pliny, and Galen. Its contemporary use as an antidepressant reveals more rigorous evidence than for any other herbal agent. The active ingredients (hypericins) responsible for antidepressant action have been investigated, but there is no consensus regarding their mechanisms of action. Hypericins are absorbed within 2 hours in a dose-dependent manner. They are widely distributed, with a plasma half-life of 24 hours, allowing steady-state concentrations to be reached within 4 days. Hypericin extracts show affinity for a variety of neurotransmitter receptors, including adenosine, gamma-aminobutyric acid $(GABA)_A$, $GABA_B$, serotonin (5HT), central benzodiazepine, inositol, and triphosphate receptors, as well as for the MAO-A and MAO-B enzymes.[5] Serotonin reuptake inhibition, decreased serotonin receptor expression, altered receptor regulation, inhibition of benzodiazepine binding, and increased excretion of adrenergic metabolites as well as inhibition of MAO-A have been proposed to explain the observed antidepressant effects. Although the monoamine oxidase inhibitor (MAOI) activity is an attractive explanation for antidepressant action, studies are unable to confirm MAO inhibition is responsible for these effects.

Studies of St. John's Wort have yielded strong evidence of efficacy for mild to moderate depression.[15] St. John's Wort has been reported to be superior to placebo and comparable with conventional antidepressant drug treatment with both lower side effect and dropout rates. However, studies have included patients with variable degrees of depression, preparations that varied, and diagnostic classifications that varied among the various trials. In short, methodologic concerns still question as to whether St. John's Wort is comparable to commercially available antidepressant medications. Clearly, more research is needed to address the shortcomings in the literature.

Commercial St. John's Wort products are standardized extracts of 0.3% hypericin, of which 300 to 900 mg are given daily in three divided doses. This is approximately equivalent to 2 to 4 g of the dried herb. Fewer adverse effects are seen than with conventional antidepressants, but adverse effects may include photodermatitis, delayed hypersensitivity, gastrointestinal upset, dizziness, dry mouth, sedation, restlessness, and constipation. St. John's Wort is contraindicated in pregnancy (Box 18-3), during lactation, for individuals exposed to strong sunlight, and for those rare individuals with pheochromocytoma. In addition, the potential for MAOI-like drug interactions cannot be excluded given this presumed mechanism of action.

Valerian

Valerian *(Valeriana officinalis)* has a rich history of use throughout the world for various indications. Valerian ranks as one of the best characterized of the widely used herbs. Listed in the National Formulary until 1950, valerian has been described in human studies as possessing sedative and anxiolytic activity and is often combined

Box 18-3 Herbs That Should Not Be Used during Pregnancy

Alder buckthorn (*Rhamnus frangula*): laxative
Angelica (*Angelica archangelica*): stimulates menstruation
Barberry (*Berberis vulgaris*): uterine stimulant
Birthroot (*Trillium erectum*): uterine astringent
Blessed thistle (*Cnicus benedictus*): strong bitter
Butternut (*Juglans cinerea*): laxative
Cascara sagrada (*Rhamnus purshianua*): laxative
Colts foot (*Tussilago farfara*): possible fetal toxicity
Damiana (*Turnera diffusa*): nervous system and hormonal activity
Drug aloe (*Aloe vera*): cathartic
Ephedra/Ma-huang (*Ephedra sinica*): high alkaloid content, stimulant
Feverfew (*Tanacetum parthenium*): stimulates menstruation
Ginseng (*Panax ginseng*): estrogenic effects
Goldenseal (*Hydrastis canadensis*): uterine stimulant
Gotu Kola (*Centella asiatica*): affects nervous system
Juniper berries (*Juniperus communis*): possible fetotoxic, affects kidneys
Mugwort (*Artemisia vulargis*): stimulates menstruation
Osha (*Ligusticum porteri*): stimulates menstruation
Pennyroyal (*Mentha pulegium*): stimulates menstruation
Pleurisy root (*Asclepias tuberosa*): cardiac stimulant
Rhubarb (*Rheum palmatum*): laxative
Rue (*Ruta graveolens*): stimulates menstruation
Sarsaparilla (*Smilax* species): hormonal activity
Scotch broom (*Cytisus scoparius*): cardiac stimulant
Senna (*Cassia species*): laxative
Shepherd's purse (*Capsella bursa pastoris*): hemostatic
St. John's Wort (*Hypericum perforatum*): stimulant
Tansy (*Tanacetum vulgare*): stimulates menstruation
Wormwood (*Artemisia absinthium*): stimulates menstruation

with other sedative herbs such as hops. Extracts of valerian have affinity for $GABA_A$ receptors, release GABA, and inhibit its reuptake. Valerian may also have affinity for the $5HT_{1A}$ receptor, with possible anxiolytic or antidepressant effects.

Studies of valerian have involved a relatively small number of subjects that confirm a mild sedative effect. However, there is no evidence to suggest that valerian is superior to existing hypnotic medications. The dosage ranges recommended are from 2 to 3 g of dried root given three times daily or at bedtime. Adverse effects include hepatotoxic effects, although the offending preparations often contain other ingredients that may account for this reaction. Additives may be used but not listed on labels. Heavy metals are found in some preparations. Multiple reports in the literature include poisoning with lead, arsenic, cadmium, copper, and mercury found in herbal preparations from foreign countries.[20] There is currently insufficient information to recommend valerian in pregnancy and during lactation, although no reports of teratogenicity have been found. The sedative effects may potentiate the effects of other central nervous system (CNS) depressants, and the usual precautions taken with other sedating agents apply.

Kava (or Kava Kava)

Preparations made from the roots of kava *(Piper methysticum)* have been used extensively by the peoples of the South Pacific for medicinal and cultural purposes. This herb is reputed to have anxiolytic, anticonvulsant, sedative, and muscle relaxant properties. Conflicting evidence exists regarding the affinity of kava lactones (the primary bioactive constituents of kava root) for various GABA or benzodiazepine-binding sites. Kava has been reported to exhibit neuroprotective effects and anticonvulsant effects, and to produce changes in electroencephalograms similar to those seen with diazepam. Kava lactones, with a content of 70% or greater, may be beneficial in the management of anxiety or tension of nonpsychotic origin. Kava appears not to adversely effect cognitive function, mental acuity, or coordination in comparison with benzodiazepines such as oxazepam. Clinical trials have suggested 100 to 200 mg daily in divided dosage or a single dosage at bedtime is optional.[7] Long-term administration with larger doses such as 400 mg may result in scaling of the skin on the extremities. Kava may also produce a vitamin D deficiency that accounts for this scaling. Kava may interact with benzodiazepines, and consumptions of large amounts of alcohol may potentiate the herb.

Lemon Balm

Lemon balm *(Melissa officinalis)* has a history of use as an anxiolytic; however, no clinical studies demonstrate its hypnotic or anxiolytic effects, even though some individuals endorse the use of this product. A sleep-promoting effect is suggested with dosages ranging from 1 to 4 g daily. No side effects are reported; however, safety in pregnancy and during lactation has not been established. Lemon balm may potentiate the effects of other CNS depressants, including alcohol, and may interact with thyroid medications or thyroid disease.

Black Cohosh

Black cohosh *(Cimicifuga racemosa)* has a history of use among North American aboriginal peoples as a treatment for hot flashes, anxiety, and dysphoria associated with menopause; as an analgesic; and to promote lactation in menses. Its putative action affects the gonadotropin system through direct estrogen ligands that suppress luteinizing hormone release and through nonestrogen ligands that appear to decrease luteinizing hormone secretion with long-term use. Uncontrolled studies have demonstrated some clinical benefit in the treatment of ovarian insufficiency.

The dosage of black cohosh ranges from 40 to 200 mg daily. The onset of action is reported to take up to 2 weeks. Potential side effects include gastrointestinal upset, throbbing headaches, dysphoria, and cardiovascular depression. Caution is advised for those taking black cohosh with other hormonal therapies, and this herb should be avoided in pregnancy and during lactation.

German Chamomile

German chamomile *(Matricaria recutita)* has been used for the treatment of gastrointestinal tract discomfort, peptic ulcer disease, pediatric colic and teething, mild insomnia, and anxiety. The herb contains flavonoid apigenin, which may have an affinity for the benzodiazepine receptors and may interact with the histamine system.[1] A mild hypnotic effect has been reported, but no controlled studies are available to substantiate this claim. Dosages commonly range from 2 to 4 g of dried flower heads three times daily, normally prepared as a tea. A commercially available liquid extract exists and is dosed at 1 to 4 ml three times a day, or as a tincture, of which 3 to 10 ml is taken three times daily. Potentially adverse reactions are rare and mainly allergenic in nature.

Evening Primrose

The use of evening primrose *(Oenothera biennis)* in the treatment of schizophrenia, childhood hyperactivity, and dementia is based on reports of prostaglandin abnormalities in these disorders. Little scientific evidence or cultural tradition supports this use, but this herb appears to contain essential and nonessential fatty acids that presumably have therapeutic benefit. Most evening primrose oil supplements contain 8% *cis*-gaba-linolenic acid. The daily adult dosage ranges from 6 to 8 g, normally given in divided doses. Evening primrose oil is relatively safe but should be used with caution in mania and epilepsy, which may be exacerbated. Other adverse reactions include drug interactions that may occur with phenothiazines, nonsteroidal antiinflammatory drugs, cortical steroids, beta-blockers, and anticoagulants.

Hops

Hops *(Humulus lupulus)* are used in the brewing industry to produce beer, but the female flower of the plant has a long history for use as a mild sedative. Hops are therefore used as a mild hypnotic agent. No clinical studies of hops suggest its use as a single agent to treat insomnia or anxiety; hops are used adjunctively. Adverse effects of hops include allergy and disruption of the menstrual cycle. Hops are typically given three times daily and at bedtime in doses of 0.5 to 1 g of dried flowers, 0.5 to 1 ml of liquid extract, or 1 to 2 ml as a tincture. Hops should be avoided in depression, in pregnancy, and during lactation. Caution should also be advised in using hops along with sedative-hypnotic agents or with alcohol because potentiation of the agent may occur.

Passion Flower

Passion flower *(Passiflora incarnata)* is native to the Americas, where its perennial vine leaves have been used as a sedative by indigenous people such as the Aztecs. Passion flower's use as a sedative hypnotic is supported by the findings of some animal studies; however, the active ingredients and mechanisms of passion flower action are unknown. Passion flower is believed to be beneficial in the treatment of adjustment disorder with anxious mood.[2] Passion flower is given three times daily in doses of 0.25 to 1 g of dried herb commonly taken as a tea; 0.5 to 1 ml of liquid extract; or 0.5 to 2 ml of tincture. Hypersensitivity, vasculitis, and altered consciousness have been reported, and the flower may cause sedation, so the usual precautions regarding motor vehicle operation and other heavy machinery operation must be given. Excessive use during pregnancy and lactation is to be avoided, and interactions with other psychotropic medications have not been established.

Scullcap

Scullcap *(Scutellaria lateriflora)* has its roots in traditional Chinese medicine and more recently has been used in Western herbalism. Its primary use is as a sedative and anticonvulsant agent. The pharmacology and ingredients of scullcap are not well documented in the different species or with the different parts of the plant that are used.

Scullcap is available in dosage forms that are commonly taken three times daily as 1 to 2 g of dried herb or 2 to 4 ml of liquid extract. Adverse reactions include giddiness, confusion, sedation, seizures, and possibly hepatotoxic effects. Scullcap should be avoided in pregnancy and during lactation and may interact with other CNS drugs.

Ginkgo

The ginkgo *(Ginkgo biloba)* tree is one of the oldest deciduous tree species on earth. It has been used extensively for medicinal purposes in Europe and in traditional Chinese medicine. Indications are varied and include dementia, cerebral insufficiency, and cerebral trauma.[8]

The dosage of ginkgo for most indications is 40 mg of standardized extract three times daily, which must be given for 1 to 3 months before the full therapeutic effects are apparent. Ginkgo extracts may improve vascular protrusion by modulating vessel wall tone and can decrease thrombosis through antagonism of platelet-activating factor. Ischemic sites may benefit in particular from ginkgo treatment. The antioxidant properties that have been attributed to the flavonoid components found in ginkgo are believed to play an important role in its postulated neuroprotective and ischemia protective effects. A recent North American multicentered, randomized, controlled trial in patients with mild to severe Alzheimer's disease or vascular dementia followed 309 patients for 52 weeks and recorded improvements in memory and attention as well as clinical global impressions of improvement that were significant ($p < .005$). Improvements were observed as early as at 12 weeks in patients receiving ginkgo extract when compared with those receiving placebo.[14]

Ginkgo has been used as an antidote for patients with erectile dysfunction secondary to antidepressants as well as an augmentation drug in patients with treatment-resistant depression. Dried and fresh ginkgo leaves have MAO inhibitory activity; however, there is currently no evidence that ginkgo extracts ingested in normal dosage by humans will inhibit MAO activity in the brain. Side effects appear to be relatively uncommon and include headache, gastrointestinal upset, and skin allergy. Starting with a low dosage and gradually titrating to the required dosage will reduce the potential for headache and other adverse effects. Ginkgo erratically may potentiate other anticoagulants or increase bleeding time; however, these side effects rarely have clinically significant implications. Nonetheless, caution should be exercised when ginkgo is taken in conjunction with anticoagulant treatment, including aspirin, or when there is a risk of bleeding, for example, peptic ulcer disease or subdural hematoma. Subdural hematomas have occurred secondary to ginkgo ingestion.[17] This has been attributed to the inhibition of platelet-activating factor properties of ginkgo. Hence, concomitant use with aspirin or any of the nonsteroidal antiinflammatory drugs as well as anticoagulants such as dicumarol is ill advised. In addition, ginkgo toxin, in both the ginkgo leaf and seed, may be neurotoxic. Although the regular dosage is too low to exert a detrimental effect, it would be prudent to avoid the use of ginkgo in known epileptic patients.

Ginseng

Chinese ginseng. Chinese ginseng *(Panax ginseng)* is another widely used herb touted in Chinese traditional medicine as an "adaptogen" that allows the body to respond to physical and emotional stress. The mechanism of these effects is due to certain ginsenosides that appear to stimulate nitric oxide synthase and to increase nitric oxide production and release.

Chinese ginseng has a long list of indications, including the treatment of stress and fatigue and improvement of endurance. This variety of ginseng is white, peeled, dried, and cooled. It provides an energy boost and increases stamina. It probably affects the hypothalamic pituitary-adrenal axis, resulting in elevated plasma cortisol levels. One of the most common side effects is insomnia. Other side effects include hypertension, diarrhea, restlessness, anxiety, and euphoria. Chinese ginseng should be used with caution in patients with hypertension and diabetes and in conjunction with centrally acting medications. In addition, it may potentiate the effect of MAOIs, stimulants including caffeine, and pheno drugs such as haloperidol.

Siberian ginseng. Siberian ginseng *(Eleutherococcus senticosus)* is a native to the northern parts of China, Japan, and Eastern Russia and has been used for more than 400 years to treat fatigue and stress and to improve endurance. The Siberian ginseng is not a true ginseng species and has properties that are better tolerated than the other forms of ginseng. It should be used cautiously with sedative hypnotic agents; some studies have reported alterations of barbiturate induced sleeping time.[3]

Ginseng dosing. Ginseng is standardized at 4% to 5% ginsenosides (Chinese ginseng) and eleutherosides (Siberian ginseng) at dosages at 1 to 2g of root (or 100 to 300 mg extract) three times a day for 3 or 4 weeks (Table 18-2). The maximum recommended dose is 4 g/day. Dose-related nervousness and excitation may occur the first few days; thus it is necessary to start low and titrate accordingly as tolerated. Cyclic use, 2 months on and 2 to 4 weeks off, is commonly recommended. Overuse of ginseng will result in headache, insomnia, agitation, and palpitations. Patients are advised that ginseng may result in sustained hypertension, heart palpitations, anxiety, and diabetes. Ginseng is not recommended for use in pregnancy and may increase estrogen levels. If one species causes difficulty or does not work, another may be efficacious. Use within a year of purchase is also highly recommended.

Stimulant Herbs

A number of stimulant herbs are occasionally used for various purposes by psychiatric patients. Ephedra *(Ephedra sinica)* is sometimes used as a decongestant, for weight loss, to initiate menstruation, or simply for stimulant purposes. Its active constituent is ephedrine, which is dosed at $1/4$ to 1 teaspoon of tincture up to three times a day. Side effects include hypertension, tachycardia, palpitations, irritability, nervousness, insomnia, and dry mouth. Individuals are advised to beware of hypertension, cardiac conduct disorders, diabetes, hyperthyroidism, and glaucoma. It is not recommended for use in pregnancy or during lactation and may be additive to other stimulants. This agent is illegal in many states.

Yohimbe *(Pausinystalia yohimbe)*, as a botanical medicine, is an alkaloid agent with a derivative called *yohimbine*.[6] Yohimbine appears to have alpha-2-adrenoreceptor antagonist properties and is used in the treatment of erectile dysfunction. Its bark is reputed to have aphrodisiac properties, and it is widely sold for this purpose. It may cause anxiety, nervousness, palpitations, and restlessness, as well as elevated cortisol levels. It may provoke panic attacks and anxiety and is used as such in studies of pathophysiology of anxiety disorders. Its action is potentiated by tricyclic antidepressants, centrally acting sympathomimetics, alpha-2 antagonists, MAOIs, and antimuscarinic agents.

PRINCIPLES OF USE OF HERBS IN PSYCHIATRIC CONDITIONS

Most herbs fall into the category of agents that share pharmacologic mechanisms of action with already existing prescription or over-the-counter psychotropic drugs. Based on a logical consideration of the current state of herb standardization and pharmacokinetic evaluation, patients are best steered toward a regulated pharmaceutical preparation capable of predictable pharmacologic response.

Even the best-studied herbs carry certain risks. For example, St. John's Wort, an herb containing the potential MAOI hypericin, has been shown to have promising antidepressant action. However, it is unlikely patients can reliably make a diagnosis of endogenous depression, much less differentiate their condition from general medical conditions mimicking depression. In addition, there remains concern for hypertensive reactions resulting from concomitant ingestion of tyramine-containing foods and St. John's Wort. With St. John's Wort, the question is not whether the herb has therapeutic efficacy but whether it is safe and appropriate as a medicinal agent.

Herbal remedies for psychiatric conditions are commonly used by patients who also access conventional health care. As previously stated, few herbal remedies are shown to have beneficial effects beyond those of conventionally regulated products, and they may be costly. As shown in Box 18-2, adulterated with dangerous additives inherently toxic, some herbs may cause the patient to forego potentially curative care. For example, several herbal products may interact with anticoagulants; these include ginkgo, garlic, ginger, and ginseng.[9] Of course, all medications are potentially toxic under specific circumstances; there is always a risk that an adverse reaction will present a hazard to a particular patient. Licensed medications ensure the risk is small, and these drugs have been thoroughly evaluated for efficacy, safety, and quality (see Table 18-1). No such controls exist for herbal medicines. As stated by Brown and Marcy, the hazards of self-treatment with herbals are no less serious and may be greater than those for conventional medications.[4] If a patient does present with a significant problem that might be caused by an herb, clinicians should discontinue the product, watch for resolution, and consider referring to a reference book or website as previously outlined. The FDA provides readily available information at MEDWATCH, a toll-free number to which adverse effects of herbs may be reported (800-332-1088).[11]

Classically trained clinicians cannot ignore herbal medicines. We must realize that patients are using herbal medicines, and insurance companies are not only beginning to cover these costs but are asking clinicians to oversee the use of herbs. Thus asking patients about supplemental use during an initial history is imperative. Patient disclosure of herb use may provide an opportunity for the clinician to redirect the patient toward effective conventional health care, and by taking a complete drug and supplemental history, a dialog can be initiated to rationally compare the appropriateness of herbal remedies to regulated pharmaceuticals in relation to the severity of the patients' condition. Guidelines for purchasing herbal products include the following:

1. Avoid imported products.
2. Avoid products that contain multiple herbs.
3. Avoid herbs that claim to be "cure alls."
4. Use products from reputable, established companies.
5. Use organically grown products.
6. Use USP and/or ABC seal of approval herbal products.
7. Use 1-800 company phone numbers for obtaining additional information about a particular herb.
8. Consider noting lot numbers and expiration dates.
9. Read labels that should include standardization and dosage (see Table 18-2, column 5).

A number of other recommendations for the use of herbal medications are as follows:

1. If side effects occur, discontinue the herb and see health care professionals if side effects are serious.

Text continued on p. 466

Table 18-2 Overview of Herbiceuticals Used in Psychiatry

Herb	Indication/use	Reported active constituent/pharmacology	Side effects/caution/interactions	Usual dosing
Chamomile (*Matricaria recutita*; *Chamaemelum nobile*)	*Internal*: GI spasm and inflammatory diseases; menstrual cramps; sedative-hypnotic; colic *External*: eczema; wound healing	Volatile oil. *Activity*: antiinflammatory, spasmolytic, antimicrobial, CNS depression	Contact dermatitis; rare cross-reactivity with ragweed allergy *Caution*: may stimulate uterine contractions; *NOT* for use in large doses during pregnancy; may be abortifacient in very large doses; normal doses not considered a danger	*GI Problems and Anxiety*: Tea from 150 ml of hot water over 3 g (2-3 heaping tsp) dried flower heads steeped for 10-20 min, tid-qid. *Tincture*: 0.5-1 ml tid. *Encapsulated product*: 2-3 g tid. Take on an empty stomach/between meals. *Sleep*: Use a more potent tea (more flower heads/tea bags) at bedtime. *External*: Use a compress of the tea for wound healing; add essential oil or infusion to bath for relaxation. *Children <2 yr*: For colic, use weak infusion.
Ephedra/Ma-Huang (*Ephedra sinica*, *E. vulgaris*, *E. nevadensis*) Illegal in many states	Stimulant; decongestant; used for weight loss; used to initiate menstruation	Ephedrine; increases basal metabolic rate (BMR); stimulates uterine contractions	Increased blood pressure and heart rate, palpitations, irritability, nervousness, sleeplessness, dry mouth	1 tsp dried herb in 1 cup boiling water, simmer 10-15 min. Drink 1-2 cups a day. *Tincture*: 1/4 to 1 teaspoon up to 3 times a day.

Continued

GI, Gastrointestinal; *CNS*, central nervous system.

Table 18-2 Overview of Herbiceuticals Used in Psychiatry—cont'd

Herb	Indication/use	Reported active constituent/pharmacology	Side effects/caution/interactions	Usual dosing
Ephedra/ Ma-Huang—cont'd			*Caution:* not for use in patients with high blood pressure or conduction disorders, diabetes, hyperthyroidism, glaucoma; do *NOT* exceed recommended doses; not for use in children <2; patients >65 should use weaker doses *Pregnancy/Lactation:* not for use during pregnancy *Drug Herb Interaction:* additive stimulation with other stimulants	
Evening Primrose (*Oenothera biennis*)	Stress, atopic eczema	Converted to dihomo-GLA (*cis*-gamma linoleic acid) a prostaglandin precursor; metabolites: prostaglandin E_1 and 15-hydroxy-dihomo-GLA among others; contains essential fatty acids	Mild GI distress; headache	600-6000 mg a day for GLA supplementation in alcoholism and inflammation. Use 3-4 g twice a day for atopic eczema. Take with meals.
Ginkgo (*Ginkgo biloba*)	Cerebral vascular insufficiency, short-term memory impairment, tinnitus, depression	Free radical scavenger; promotes vasodilation and increased blood flow in capillaries and end arteries; increases brain tolerance to hypoxia; inhibits platelet activating	Minor GI disturbances; rarely causes headache, dizziness, and vertigo; not considered a problem in pregnancy and lactation	*Standardized Extract:* 24% flavonoid glycosides and 6% terpene lactones = GBE *Dosing:* 120-160 mg a day bid or tid (for intermittent

Herb	Uses	Action/Mechanism	Side Effects/Cautions	Dosage
		factor, decreases clotting time, relieves arteriolar spasm, stabilizes membranes; enhanced utilization of oxygen and glucose, activates Na$^+$-K$^+$- ATPase, stimulates release of endothelium-derived relaxing factor and prostacyclin, stimulates aerobic glycoysis, and promotoes lactate clearance		claudication; 240 mg a day for cerebral vascular insufficiency).
Ginseng (*Panax ginseng* [Chinese], *Panax quinquefolius* [American], *Eleutherococcus senticosus* [Siberian])	Adaptogen, stress, fatigue	Stimulates protein and cholesterol production in the liver; slow carbohydrate-sparing and stamina-increasing activity in muscle tissue; increases enzymatic activity and fatty acid production; may decrease blood sugar and cholesterol levels; prevents depletion of stress fighting hormones; may increase brain levels of neurotransmitters	Dose-related nervousness, sleeplessness, nausea, and headache; extreme doses (>15 g) may exacerbate hypertension *Caution:* stage II and higher hypertension, anxiety, diabetes *Drug-Herb Interaction:* Warfarin—decreased INR; digoxin—increased digoxin levels (1 patient report)	*Standardized:* 4%-5% ginsenosides, all ginsengs. *Panax Ginseng:* 1-2 g a day. *Tea:* 3 tsp of dried sliced root per cup of water, simmer 45 min. *Tincture:* 0.5 tsp per cup of water. *Eleutherococcus:* 2-3 g a day tid. A 2- to 3-wk interval off the herb after use for a 2-month period, then restarting use is recommended.
Gotu Kola (*Centella asiatica*)	*Internal:* a relaxing restorative for the nervous system	Does not contain caffeine	Rash, headache *Caution:* discontinuation is recommended if the rash develops; not for use in children <2; use is not recommended during pregnancy and lactation; do not exceed recommended doses	*Tincture:* ½ tsp in a cup of water (insomnia). The tea has a bitter taste, and honey and lemon are added to make it palatable. It is recommended that it be taken for 4-6 wk with a 2-wk break before reinitiating therapy. *For Wounds and Psoriasis:* Use a compress made from the infusion.

GBE, Ginkgo biloba extract.

Continued

Table 18-2 Overview of Herbiceuticals Used in Psychiatry—cont'd

Herb	Indication/use	Reported active constituent/pharmacology	Side effects/caution/interactions	Usual dosing
Hops (*Humulus lupulus*)	*Internal:* sedative	CNS depression	Sedation; dermatitis on direct contact with plant. *Caution:* not for use in children <2 yr, in pregnancy, or in women with estrogen-dependent breast cancer (may have estrogenic effects)	An infusion of 2 tsp of herb in a cup of boiling water steeped for 5 min is useful for sleep, 2 ml of the tincture or a weaker infusion tid is used for anxiety and digestive disorders; 1.5 ml on a sugar cube is recommended for a nervous stomach. Adjust dosage as necessary. *Standardization:* Equivalent to 60-120 mg kava pyrones. Give 100 mg PO bid or less as an initial dose.
Kava (or Kava Kava) (*Piper methysticum*)	Anxiety, stress, restlessness	Arylethylene pyrones similar to myristicin found in nutmeg (called *kava lactones*)	None reported with usual doses except a temporary yellow coloring of the skin, hair and nails; if this develops, discontinuation of the herb is recommended; rarely, allergic skin reactions have occurred; intoxication at higher dosages; chronic use may result in dermatitis; not recommended for continued use past 3 mo without medical advice. *Drug-Drug Interactions:* kava may interact with other CNS depressant agents	

Kudzu (*Pueraria lobata*)	Chronic alcoholism through inhibition of alcohol and aldehyde dehydrogenases; hypertension	Puerarin, antioxidant (100× more powerful than vitamin E); Isoflavones inhibit alcohol dehydrogenases	Disulfiram-like reaction with ingestion of alcohol (ethanol)	*Dosing:* approx 1.2 g of kudzu root bid.
St. John's Wort (*Hypericum perforatum*)	Treatment of mild to moderate depression; sedative; antiviral	Anthraquinones: hypericin and pseudohypericin; antiinflammatory; serotonin reuptake inhibition; MAOI activity	Fatigue, pruritus, weight gain, photodermatitis *Caution:* not to be used during pregnancy or lactation; no data on need for tyramine-free diet; minimize use of restricted foods, drink, and medication combinations; do not combine with traditional antidepressants	*Standardization:* 0.3% hypericin. *Dosing:* 300 mg tid is the initial dose for depression. *Average Therapeutic Dosing Range:* 2–4 g a day in divided doses.
Valerian (*Valeriana officinalis*)	Sedative-hypnotic, antispasmodic	Valepotriatesa; augmentation of the actions of GABA: weak antagonist of $GABA_A$ receptors; improves sleep quality and decreases sleep latency	Safe, mild with no morning hangover; no dependency has been noted; excessive initial doses (person dependent) may cause excitation; no potentiation of alcohol *Caution:* data in pregnancy are scarce; *NOT* recommended at this time	*Standardized Form:* 0.5% essentil oil. *Dosing:* 300–400 mg hs in capsule or tablet form, 2.5–5 ml of the tincture or a tea of 2–3 g of the herb in 1 cup of boiling water. Additional doses (200–300 mg) can be added during the day for anxiety.

MAOI, Monoamine oxidase inhibitor.

Continued

Table 18-2 Overview of Herbiceuticals Used in Psychiatry—cont'd

Herb	Indication/use	Reported active constituent/pharmacology	Side effects/caution/interactions	Usual dosing
Yohimba (*Pausinystalia yohimbe*) Prescription: Yohimbine hydrochloride (Yocon, Yohimex)	Impotence—erectile dysfunction	Actions attributed to yohimbine, an alpha-2-adrenergic blocker; stimulates salivation and erection	Anxiety, increased pulse and blood pressure, flushing, hallucinations, headache (especially with the use of the natural bark product). Yohimbine prescription formulation has far fewer side effects *Caution:* use of raw herb does *NOT* exacerbate psychiatric conditions	*Dosing:* Yohimbine Rx 5.4-10.8 mg/day in divided doses.
Niacin (Vitamin B$_3$)	Hyperlipidemias (triglycerides and cholesterol): decrease total cholesterol up to 25%; decrease triglycerides up to 50%	Unknown mechanism	Itching, flushing, warmth (attenuated with low-dose aspirin); hyperglycemia; hepatotoxicity (associated with slow-release formulations)	Give 500-3000 mg/day in divided doses.

| Melatonin (Melatonin) | Jet lag; insomnia (see Chapter 10) | Melatonin is a hormone secreted by the pineal gland in response to daily light/dark cycles (circadian rhythm); taking melatonin purportedly "resets" this cycle to allow normalization of sleep patterns | Mostly absent of adverse effects at doses <80 mg; minor side effects with these doses include "heavy head," headache, and transient depression; avoid use in small children and in pregnancy; at high dosages has contraceptive effects *Drug Interactions:* because melatonin is structurally related to serotonin, patients taking antidepressant medications should avoid concurrent use | *Jet Lag:* 5-10 mg (at sleep time) upon arrival at destination and 3-4 days thereafter. *Insomnia:* 0.3-5 mg administered 1 hr before sleep. Best for patients having difficulty getting to sleep. For patients having trouble staying asleep, melatonin will probably not be effective. |

2. Use in mild to moderate disease states only after correct diagnosis is made.
3. Use with appropriate monitoring by a health care professional.
4. If no improvement occurs in an appropriate amount of time, discontinue and see a health care professional.
5. Recognize that herbal medication is not the same as homeopathic medication or agents.
6. Use in recommended dosages only; more is not necessarily better.
7. Ask questions.
8. Double-check health claims with multiple reference sources that are not attempting to sell you something.
9. During pregnancy and lactation, women should avoid the use of most herbs.
10. Children younger than 2 years of age and individuals older than 65 should use herbs with caution and in smaller doses if at all.

REFERENCES

1. Berry M: The chamomiles, *Pharm J* 254:191, 1995.
2. Bourin M and others: A combination of plant extracts in the treatment outpatients with adjustment disorder with anxious mood: controlled study versus placebo, *Fundam Clin Pharmacol* 11:127, 1997.
3. Bradley P: *British herbal compendium,* Bournemouth, England, 1992, British Herbal Medicine Association.
4. Brown JS, Marcy SA: The use of botanicals for health purposes by members of a prepaid health plan, *Res Nurs Health* 14:339, 1991.
5. Cott JM: In vitro receptor binding and enzyme inhibition by *Hypericum perforatum* extract, *Pharmacopsychiatry* 30:108, 1997.
6. De Smet PAGM and others: *Adverse effects of herbal drugs,* Berlin, Germany, 1997, Springer Verlag.
7. Eisenberg DM and others: Unconventional medicine in the United States: prevalence, costs and patterns of use, *N Engl J Med* 328:246, 1993.
8. Gaby AR: Ginkgo biloba extract: a review, *Altern Med Rev* 1:236, 1996.
9. Gianni L, Dreitlein WB: Some popular OTC herbals can interact with anticoagulant therapy, *USP* 23:5:80, 1998.
10. Guiness AE: *Family guide to natural medicines,* Pleasantville, NY, 1993, Reader's Digest Association.
11. Kessler DA: Introducing MEDWATCH: a new approach to reporting medication and device adverse effects and product problems, *JAMA* 269:2765, 1993.
12. Khaliq Y: Alternative medicine: what pharmacists need to know, *Pharm Pract* 13:44, 83, 1997.
13. Kleiner SM: The true nature of herbs, *Phys Sports Med* 23:13, 1995.
14. LeBars PL and others: A placebo-controlled, double blind randomized trial of an extract Ginkgo biloba for dementia, *JAMA* 278:1327, 1997.
15. Linde K and others: St. John's Wort for depression: an overview and meta-analysis of randomised clinical trials (see comments), *BMJ* 313:253, 1996.
16. Marwick C: Growing use of medicinal botanicals forces assessment by drug regulators, *JAMA* 273:607, 1995.
17. Miller LG: Herbal medicinals. Selected clinical considerations focusing on known or potential drug-herb interactions, *Arch Intern Med* 158:2200, 1998.
18. Price E: Root digging in the Appalachians: the geography of botanical drugs, *Geogr Rev* 50: 1, 1960.
19. Trevelyan J: Herbal medicine, *Nurs Times* 89:36, 1993.
20. Winslow LC, Kroll DJ: Herbs as medicine, *Arch Intern Med,* 158:2192, 1998.
21. Wong Albert HC and others: Herbal remedies in psychiatric practice, *Arch Gen Psychiatry* 55:1033, 1998.

UNIT IV

Developmental Issues Related
to Psychotropic Drugs

CHAPTER 19

Psychopharmacology for Children

LAWRENCE SCAHILL

SCOPE OF THE PROBLEM

The mental illnesses of childhood are often classified according to broad categories, including disruptive behavior disorders, mood disorders, anxiety disorders, developmental disorders, tic disorders, and psychotic disorders. Collectively, these disorders affect as many as 20% of children younger than 18 years of age. Of these, roughly half are considered to have serious emotional or behavioral disturbances.[22] This estimate translates into approximately 8 million children and adolescents with serious disturbance, exacting an enormous cost to society. Increasingly, children with psychiatric disorders are being treated with medication to reduce their emotional and behavioral problems.[17,94] This trend has raised concern among policy makers and in the popular press.[14,135] The empirical foundation for using psychotropic drugs in children is not as solid as it is for adults. Nonetheless, an accumulating body of evidence provides some guidance for the practitioner faced with the clinical management of children and adolescents taking psychotropic medications.

Although there may not be important differences in absorption in children compared to adults, there are differences in distribution, metabolism, and excretion of drugs (pharmacokinetics) in children. Because of these differences, simple weight-based extrapolations of child dosages from adult dosages are generally inaccurate.[123] There is also evidence that the developing brain may respond differently to psychotropic drugs, which could account for differences in therapeutic effects and side effects in children. As children grow, the reactions and responses to drugs begin to approximate those of adults. Consequently, this text provides separate chapters on child and adolescent psychopharmacology.

The history of pediatric psychopharmacology is brief. Box 19-1 displays important benchmarks in this chronology. The establishment of the Research Units in Pediatric Psychopharmacology by the National Institute of Mental Health is a recent milestone in this chronology and reflects the recognition that the research base in child psychopharmacology in not adequate to guide a rapidly changing clinical practice.

GENERAL PRINCIPLES

The *first principle* of pediatric psychopharmacology is to identify clear target symptoms for drug therapy. Of course, accurate diagnosis is a prerequisite for initiating pharmacotherapy, but diagnosis alone is not sufficient for selecting an appropriate medication. It is the identification of target symptoms that is fundamental to the choice of medication and the assessment of response. Diagnosis, target symptoms, and their severity are determined by clinical observation and interviews with the child, parents, and other important informants (e.g., teachers). Measurement of symptom severity can also be aided by using standardized rating

---

Box 19-1 History of Pediatric Psychopharmacology

1937	Bradley uses benzedrine to treat behavioral disorders in children.
1950	Methylphenidate is used to treat hyperactive children.
1953	First reported use of chlorpromazine in children.
1965	Tricyclic antidepressants are used to treat children with major depressive disorder.
1969	Haloperidol is used in childhood psychosis.
1970	Lithium is used in children and adolescents with mania.
1978	Haloperidol is approved to treat tic disorders in children.
1979	First reported use of clonidine to treat tic disorders and disruptive behavior problems.
1989	Double-blind study of clomipramine to treat obsessive-compulsive disorder.
1990	First reported use of fluoxetine in children with obsessive-compulsive disorder.
1994	National Institute of Mental Health sponsored multicenter trial of methylphenidate for children with attention-deficit hyperactivity disorder.
1995	Risperidone used for the first time in children with various disorders.
1996	Efficacy of fluoxetine in children and adolescents with depression is demonstrated.
1996-1997	National Institute of Mental Health establishes Research Units in Pediatric Psychopharmacology for anxiety disorders and for autism.
1997	Food and Drug Administration policy supports increased clinical pharmacologic research in pediatric populations.
1999	Published results from the "Multimodal Treatment of ADHS ($N = 579$)" (see 1994 above).

---

scales.[106] Another issue that can affect the identification of target symptoms and therapeutic effects is that young children may not be able to describe their internal states. Furthermore, children may not understand words and concepts in the same way that adults do. Bearing this in mind, clinicians should explain relevant concepts in a developmentally appropriate way and establish a common vocabulary for discussing symptoms with children.

The *second principle* in child psychopharmacology is that children are physiologically different from adults. Developmental immaturity not only affects dosage calculations but may also influence efficacy. Surprisingly, on a milligram-per-kilogram basis, children often require larger doses of psychotropic drugs than adults to achieve similar drug serum levels and therapeutic effects.[35] The reasons for this are not completely clear but are assumed to be because liver metabolism and the glomerular filtration rate are more efficient in children. Drug effects (pharmacodynamics) may be altered in children as well because of immature neural pathways. For example, the catecholamine systems (norepinephrine and dopamine) are not fully developed until early adulthood.[4,127]

Parent education is the *third* important *principle* of pediatric psychopharmacology. Because parents are ultimately responsible for compliance with dosage schedules, they are essential collaborators in medication management. Simply stated, if the drug regimen is not followed, the clinician cannot determine whether the drug is effective or make rational decisions about dosage adjustments. Assuming good compliance is achieved, parents are also essential in determining therapeutic response and adverse effects. Parents may harbor unrealistic expectations about the potential benefits of the medication. Failure to address such expectations may contribute to noncompliance, attrition, and biased reporting about response. Finally, some parents may underestimate the potency of psychotropic drugs and fail to inform clinicians about concomitant medications. This unwitting omission could lead to risky drug-drug interactions.[27] For all these reasons, parents should be thoroughly educated about the child's medication, including any delay in positive effects, side effects, the potential for overdose, and relevant drug interactions. General guidelines for parent education are provided in Box 19-2.

Several factors can influence compliance:
- Parental ambivalence concerning the need for medication
- Inadequate parental supervision of drug administration
- Parental misunderstanding of drug serum levels and the importance of consistency in drug doses
- Parental misconceptions about how drugs work, for example, not understanding that antidepressant drugs may take several weeks to show benefit

PSYCHOTROPIC MEDICATIONS USED WITH CHILDREN
STIMULANTS
Indications: Attention-Deficit Hyperactivity Disorder

Stimulants are indicated for managing attention-deficit hyperactivity disorder (ADHD) and are considered the standard treatment for this disorder. ADHD is a relatively common psychiatric disorder of childhood, affecting 2% to 10% of school-aged children.* Boys are affected more often than girls. Studies of clinical populations indicate that the symptoms of ADHD are among the most common reasons children are referred to mental health agencies. ADHD is characterized by inattention, impulsiveness, and hyperactivity. The DSM-IV allows clinicians to distinguish between a primarily inattentive type, a primarily impulsive/hyperactive type, or a combined type.[3] Children with ADHD are described as overactive, restless, easily distracted, and easily frustrated. They are often socially unsuccessful because they are unable to take turns in games, tend to intrude into the affairs of others, and may misinterpret the intentions of others. Children with ADHD are also at greater risk for conduct disorder, depression, anxiety disorders, and learning disabilities.

The most commonly used stimulants for the treatment of ADHD include methylphenidate (Ritalin), dextroamphetamine (Dexedrine), and an amphetamine mixture including dextroamphetamine, levamphetamine, and other amphetamine salts with the trade name of Adderall.[87] Methylphenidate and dextroamphetamine are also available in sustained-release formulations. Each of these stimulants has shown short-term efficacy in placebo-controlled trials. Methylphenidate and dextroamphetamine have been extensively studied for more than two decades. The recently marketed formulation of mixed amphetamines (Adderall) is slightly longer acting than methylphenidate but is still considered an immediate-release preparation.[116] Pemoline (Cylert) is another long-acting stimulant. Because of concern

---

*References 9, 23, 50, 101, 119, and 133.

Box 19-2 Parent Education for Specific Psychotropic Drugs

Stimulants

Stimulants can decrease appetite and may affect growth. Hence parents should monitor appetite, height, and weight.

Short-acting stimulants may cause rebound hyperactivity.

Stimulants can result in an increase in motor and phonic tics or stereotypic behavior.

Stimulants can improve inattention, hyperactivity, and impulsiveness but may not improve interpersonal relationships.

In children with suspected growth retardation, drug holidays may be needed to evaluate impact on appetite and growth.

Antidepressants

Tricyclics can be fatal in overdose. Drug administration should be supervised and the drug should be securely stored.

Other medications, including antibiotics and over-the-counter agents, may interact with antidepressants. Hence all medications should be reviewed with the primary clinician.

The selective serotonin reuptake inhibitors (SSRIs) can cause motor restlessness, insomnia, and irritability.

The SSRIs alone may not be sufficient in obsessive-compulsive disorder (OCD). Addition of cognitive-behavioral therapy is often indicated.

In OCD and depression, there may be a lag between initiation of treatment and clinical response.

Antipsychotic agents

Antipsychotic drugs are part of a comprehensive program to treat psychosis.

Traditional antipsychotic medications can cause dystonic reactions, especially early in treatment.

Watch for muscle rigidity, inability to remain still, and new abnormal movements.

Review the risk of tardive dyskinesia and withdrawal dyskinesia before treatment.

In treating tic disorders, the goal is to reduce tics as eradication is rarely achievable.

about hepatotoxicity, the use of pemoline appears to be declining.[77] Of the stimulant medications, methylphenidate is used most often. This clear preference for methylphenidate over the other stimulants cannot be attributed to greater effectiveness but may be the result of familiarity and a presumed better side effect profile.[30]

Empirical Support

Placebo-controlled trials have shown that stimulants improve sustained attention, impulse control, and overactivity.[85,89,90] These effects can also result in decreased disruption in the classroom and better academic performance.[24] Some studies also suggest that stimulants can improve parent-child interactions and peer relationships.[29,45]

Mechanism of Action

Although stimulants have become the standard treatment for ADHD, the mechanism of action is not clearly understood. It is clear that stimulants enhance dopaminergic function in the brain. This enhancement is caused by blocking the reuptake of dopamine and norepinephrine by presynaptic neurons. Stimulants may also promote release of dopamine into the synaptic cleft. These effects are proposed to enhance inhibitory subcortical-cortical pathways, resulting in better concentration and impulse control, as well as decreased motor activity.[29]

Pharmacokinetics

Standard preparations of methylphenidate, dextroamphetamine, and the combined preparation Adderall are readily absorbed and begin exerting behavioral effects 30 to 60 minutes after ingestion. The peak level of methylphenidate occurs approximately 90 to 150 minutes after ingestion, and the clinical effects last 3 to 5 hours. Methylphenidate is broken down in the liver, and the parent compound and metabolites are excreted in the urine within 24 hours. Dextroamphetamine and Adderall show similar patterns of absorption, each achieving peak levels between 1 and 3 hours, with duration of action of 5 to 7 hours. Recent data suggest that Adderall has a slightly longer duration of action than standard dextroamphetamine.[116] The amphetamines are also broken down in the liver and excreted in the urine. The available forms of sustained-release methylphenidate and dextroamphetamine are absorbed more slowly, and beneficial effects are not observed until 60 to 90 minutes after the oral dose, but last up to 8 hours.[85]

Clinical Management

Table 19-1 provides information about dosages for dextroamphetamine, methylphenidate, Adderall, and pemoline. Before initiating a trial of a stimulant, it is useful to obtain behavior ratings such as Conners Parent and Teacher Questionnaires or the ADHD rating scales at baseline, during the dosage adjustment phase, and after the medication has been stabilized.[29,106] Also, if there are unanswered questions

Table 19-1 Dosing Guidelines for Commonly Used Stimulants

Drug name	Typical starting dose (mg)	Typical daily dose range (mg)	Doses per day
MPH	5	15-60	2-3
DEX	2.5-5	10-40	2
Adderall	2.5-5	10-40	2
Pemoline	18.75	37.5-112.5	1
MPH-SR	20	20-40	1
DEX-S	10	5-30	1

MPH, Methylphenidate; *DEX*, dextroamphetamine; *Adderall*, amphetamine mixture; *MPH-SR*, methylphenidate sustained-release; *DEX-S*, DEX-Spansule.

about the child's capacity to learn, a psychoeducational evaluation should be considered.

Methylphenidate. Methylphenidate (Ritalin) is not approved for use in children younger than 6 years of age, although recent data suggest that it might be useful in preschool-aged children.[72] Depending on weight, children older than age 5 can be started on 2.5 to 10 mg twice daily (just before breakfast and lunch). As a crude guide, clinicians typically use 0.3 mg/kg/dose as the starting dosage. The dosage may be increased to 5 to 10 mg twice daily after 4 to 6 days and then adjusted upward in increments of 5 to 10 mg every 4 to 6 days. Doses are given 3.5 to 4 hours apart on two- or three-times-daily schedule. The third dose, if given, is typically half that of the first and second dose to minimize the *rebound* effects.[45]

The optimal daily dose of methylphenidate has been disputed by some researchers, who argue that high dosages impair cognitive performance.[45,87] These disparate views may be due to differences in outcome measures used and heterogeneity within ADHD.[24,29] Current dosage recommendations for methylphenidate range between 0.6 and 1.5 mg/kg of body weight per day in two or three divided doses, that is, approximately 0.3 to 0.8 mg/kg/dose.[45] The milligram-per-kilogram calculation is only a crude guide. Dosages higher than 35 mg/day in younger children and 60 mg/day in older children are not recommended. A single daily dose of the sustained-release form (Ritalin-SR) can be used instead of divided doses of the regular product.

Dextroamphetamine and the amphetamine mixture (Adderall). Dextroamphetamine (Dexedrine) is not commonly used in children younger than 5 years of age. The initial dosage may be a single 2.5-mg dose in younger children or a 5-mg dose in older children. After 4 to 6 days, the medication may be raised 2.5 mg/day (5 mg in older children) and given in two doses. Thereafter, the dosage may be raised every 4 to 6 days to a total of 15 to 20 mg/day in younger children and 40 mg/day in older children. The medication is typically given with or immediately before or after meals to prevent loss of appetite. The total daily dose is usually between 0.3 and 1.0 mg/kg of body weight.[87] If the slow-release preparation is used, the same total dose would be given once daily in the morning. The amphetamine mixture (Adderall) is dosed similarly to dextroamphetamine.

Pemoline. Pemoline (Cylert) differs chemically from the amphetamines and from methylphenidate. It is used exclusively for ADHD, whereas amphetamines and methylphenidate are occasionally prescribed for narcolepsy. Pemoline is well absorbed and has a 12-hour half-life. A total of 50% of the agent is excreted unchanged in the urine.

Pemoline causes less cerebral stimulation than do the other two central nervous system (CNS) stimulants. Its side effects are similar to those of the amphetamines and methylphenidate. However, several cases of choreoathetoid movements have been reported with pemoline. Although rare, liver toxicity ranging from mild to severe has been reported with pemoline, and its use is declining. Liver function should be checked at baseline every 4 to 6 months in children maintained on pemoline. In addition, families should be educated about the signs and symptoms of liver toxicity such as abdominal pain, vomiting, jaundice, dark urine, clay-colored stool. Because of the 12-hour half-life, pemoline can be given once per day. The daily dose may be increased by 18.75 mg every 4 to 5 days, up to a maximum of 112.5 mg/day in smaller children and 150 mg/day in larger children.[87] A recent study suggests that beneficial effects can be observed at relatively low dosages such as 37.25 to 75 mg/day.[85]

Side Effects of Central Nervous System Stimulants

Growth retardation secondary to decreased appetite is a common concern among clinicians and families of children treated with stimulants. Research evidence indicates that slowed growth may be temporary and that children with ADHD may be shorter than their agemates before puberty but catch up after puberty.[115] Appetite suppression can be managed by giving the stimulant with or immediately before or after meals. Height and weight should be monitored regularly in children treated with stimulants.

Another commonly reported side effect is insomnia. This can be difficult to solve because many children with ADHD have trouble falling asleep before receiving stimulant medication. In addition, although it is plausible that sleep problems could be related to the rebound effects associated with stimulant withdrawal, a recent study found that the third dose of methylphenidate did not cause more sleep problems when compared with a placebo dose.[54] At baseline, it is important to obtain a careful sleep history and then to monitor sleep during treatment. As noted, it is common practice for the third dose of methylphenidate to be lower than the first two doses to minimize the rebound effect. It is increasingly common to add clonidine at night as an aid for sleep, but it has not been studied carefully and has become controversial.[117,132]

Several case reports and controlled studies have shown that some children will show a worsening or emergence of tics upon exposure to a stimulant.[108] As many as 10% of children with no history of tics will manifest tics when treated with stimulants.[7,67] In addition, some children with preexisting tics will show an increase in tics after exposure to stimulant medication.[98] However, several recent studies in children with ADHD and tic disorders have shown that tics do not invariably worsen when children affected with a tic disorder are treated with stimulants.[19,37,38] Nonetheless, children with tic disorders should be monitored carefully when treated with stimulants. In some cases, dosage reduction may be sufficient, but discontinuation may be called for in other cases.[61]

Toxic Effects

Dextroamphetamine overdose can be fatal. In overdose the child appears hyperalert; is talkative; and may have tremors, exaggerated startle reflex, paranoia, hallucinations, confusion, and tachyarrhythmias. A child with this clinical presentation requires hospitalization.

Abuse of Stimulants

The abuse potential of methylphenidate, dextroamphetamine, and the amphetamine mixture is probably overestimated. Indeed, evidence from a recent follow-up study suggests that by facilitating better functional outcomes, stimulant treatment may actually decrease the risk of substance abuse in late adolescence.[13] Nonetheless, the U.S. Food and Drug Administration (FDA) classifies these stimulants as Schedule II drugs. In many states, these drugs require a new prescription each month.

ANTIDEPRESSANTS
Indications: Depression, Anxiety, Obsessive-Compulsive Disorder

Antidepressant medications are approved for use in individuals with depression who are older than 12 years of age. Three chemically unrelated antidepressants—clomipramine (Anafranil), fluvoxamine (Luvox), and sertraline (Zoloft)—are approved for treating obsessive-compulsive disorder (OCD) in pediatric patients.

The tricyclic medication imipramine (Tofranil) is approved for treating children with enuresis.

Antidepressant drugs include a long list of chemically diverse compounds that have all been effective in treating adults with depression. Common sense categories include the tricyclic antidepressants (TCAs), so named because of their characteristic three-ring structure; monoamine oxidase inhibitors (MAOIs), which are rarely used in children or adolescents; selective serotonin reuptake inhibitors (SSRIs), a group of chemically unrelated compounds that are grouped together because of their common mechanism; and novel antidepressants such as bupropion (Wellbutrin), venlafaxine (Effexor), nefazodone (Serzone), and mirtazapine (Remeron).

Depression. Depression is characterized by profound sadness, loss of interest in usual activities, loss of appetite with weight loss, sleep disturbance, loss of energy, feelings of worthlessness or guilt, irritability, tearfulness, and recurrent thoughts of death or suicide. To meet DSM-IV criteria, at least some of these symptoms must be present daily and must persist for at least 2 weeks. Depression in childhood is similar in presentation to depression in adulthood.[5] One important difference is that children may be less able to describe their feelings.

The prevalence of depression in children and adolescents is estimated to range from 1% to 5%, with adolescents being at the higher end of this range and school-age children at the lower end. Boys appear to be at higher risk for depression until adolescence, when it becomes more common in girls.

Separation anxiety. Separation anxiety disorder is a disorder of childhood characterized by extraordinary distress when faced with routine separations from the mother (or primary caretaker) such as going to school. In most cases, children with separation anxiety disorder express worry about harm or permanent loss of their mothers. The DSM-IV specifies childhood onset of excessive anxiety upon separation from the home or major attachment figure as evidenced by acute distress, frequent nightmares about separation, and reluctance or refusal to separate. These symptoms must be present for at least a month and cause clinically significant impairment in social or academic functioning.

The prevalence of separation anxiety disorder is estimated at 4% of school-aged children and is equally common among boys and girls. The most common manifestation of separation anxiety disorder is school refusal. However, school refusal may be part of general anxiety, social phobia, OCD, depression, or conduct disorder. Cases of school phobia have also been reported as a side effect of haloperidol. Thus school refusal warrants careful assessment.

Obsessive-compulsive disorder. OCD is characterized by recurring thoughts or worries (obsessions) that the child is unable to dislodge and/or repetitive habits (compulsions) that are performed in a ritualistic fashion. DSM-IV requires that either the obsessions or the compulsions waste time, cause distress, and interfere with functioning. Additional criteria include recognition that the obsessions and compulsions are excessive (not a required criterion for children).

OCD is relatively common in older adolescents and adults, with estimates of occurrence in the range of 2% to 3%.[52,124] By contrast, it appears to be less common in prepubertal children, with estimates of occurrence less than 1%.[23] Common obsessions include worries about contamination (e.g., with dirt, germs, chemicals), worries about harm coming to the self or family members, concerns about illness, and concerns about acting on unwanted impulses.[96,118] Common compulsions include handwashing or other cleaning rituals, ordering and arranging objects over and over again, checking, repeating routine activities such as picking up an object and setting it back down again, and going in and out of doorways. The relationship between obsessive worry and compulsive habit may be complex. For example, some OCD patients clearly state that a concern about germs prompts the excessive handwashing. Other patients deny specific worries. Instead, they may describe a need to repeat an action to achieve a vague sense of completion or mollify a fundamental feeling of discomfort.[62]

TRICYCLIC ANTIDEPRESSANTS
Empirical Support

TCAs have been used in child and adolescent psychiatry for more than 30 years. TCAs are used to treat several psychiatric disorders of childhood, including depression, ADHD, OCD, separation anxiety, and enuresis.[11,28,56,57,92,114]

Although TCAs are commonly used in clinical practice, evidence for their efficacy in treating children with depression is unconvincing.[1] Geller and colleagues have conducted several studies with nortriptyline (Pamelor) and have shown that some children and adolescents do have a positive response to it; however, clear superiority of active drug over placebo has yet to be demonstrated.[39,40] Nonetheless, it appears that at least some children with depression benefit from nortriptyline. For example, in the study by Geller and others, approximately 60% of the patients (ages 6 to 12) responded favorably.[39] Responders had a daily dosage range of 0.64 to 1.57 mg/kg. In contrast, double-blind, placebo-controlled studies have demonstrated the effectiveness of desipramine for treating ADHD and clomipramine for treating children and adolescents with OCD.[11,28,64,113] The evidence supporting the use of TCAs in separation anxiety is modest, and treatment appears to be bolstered by behavioral therapy.[56]

Mechanism of Action

The primary mechanism of action of the TCAs is to block the reuptake of norepinephrine and serotonin. Precisely how this known pharmacologic property brings about positive effects in depression or ADHD is unclear. In addition to blocking the reuptake of norepinephrine, clomipramine also potently blocks serotonin reuptake and is referred to as an *SRI* (serotonin reuptake inhibitor). The positive effect of imipramine on enuresis may be related to its anticholinergic properties, although other mechanisms have been proposed.

Pharmacokinetics

Children can show tremendous variation in serum level at the same dose of these drugs. Thus, even though therapeutic ranges for TCAs in children are not well established, serum levels can be useful in regulating the dose of the agents and in identifying slow metabolizers. Suggested levels for these compounds are imipramine at 125 to 250 ng/ml (includes imipramine and metabolite, desipramine), desipramine at 115 ng/ml, nortriptyline at 60 to 100 ng/ml, and for the combined level of clomipramine and desmethylclomipramine, 150 to 450 ng/ml.[126]

Clinical Management

Table 19-2 provides dosing guidelines for the most commonly used TCAs in children. As shown in the table, dosing instructions are somewhat different across

Table 19-2 Dosing Guidelines for Tricyclic Antidepressants Commonly Used in Children

Drug name	Typical starting dose (mg)	Typical daily dose range (mg)	Doses per day
Imipramine	25	25-150	1-2
Desipramine	10-25	25-125	1-2
Nortriptyline	10-25	20-100	1-2
Clomipramine	25	50-100	1-2

these TCAs. Imipramine is typically begun with a dosage of 25 mg and increased every fourth day to a range of 2 to 5 mg/kg/day, but usual doses are less than this maximum.[56,92] In younger children, nortriptyline may be introduced with a 10-mg dose, with increases every 4 to 6 days to a range of 50 to 75 mg/day in divided doses. Clomipramine is usually given initially at a dosage of 25 mg, with gradual increases every 4 or 5 days to a maximum of 100 mg/day in younger children. The use of desipramine in children is declining in the wake of reports of sudden death in a few children (see the following discussion).

Side Effects

Side effects of the TCAs include fatigue, dizziness, dry mouth, sweating, weight gain, urinary retention, tremor, and agitation. These common side effects can sometimes be addressed by lowering the dosage or changing the dosing schedule.

Of greater concern is the potential for these medications, especially desipramine, to alter electrical conduction through the heart.[93] Although evidence from one controlled study shows that the cardiac effects of desipramine are minimal, many clinicians avoid using desipramine in children because of a report of the sudden deaths of four children who had been taking the drug.[12] Currently, most attention is focused on the potential of TCAs, especially desipramine, to prolong the QT interval, which is believed to increase the risk of fatal ventricular tachycardia in susceptible individuals.[93] Accepted guidelines for monitoring cardiac effects of TCAs include a PR interval less than 210 ms, a QRS interval within 30% of baseline, a QT interval less than 450 ms, a heart rate less than 130 beats/min, and blood pressure less than 130 mm Hg for systolic or less than 85 mm Hg for diastolic.[44,126]

Before treatment with a TCA is initiated, a child should have an electrocardiogram (ECG) performed. The ECG should be repeated during the dosage adjustment phase, when the maintenance dose is achieved, and semiannually during therapy.[44] The baseline assessment should also include resting blood pressure and pulse, a review of medical and family history (e.g., syncope, sudden death), and evidence of a recent normal physical examination. Discussion with the family should also include a review of the potential cardiac effects.

Interactions

As with most other psychotropic drugs, TCAs are metabolized in the liver by enzymes of the cytochrome P-450 system.[35] Several psychotropic (fluoxetine, fluvoxamine, paroxetine) and nonpsychotropic drugs (cisapride, cimetidine, erythromycin) inhibit the action of one or more of these liver enzymes. Because TCAs can be toxic at high dosages, inhibition of enzyme activity that results in dramatic increases in the level of the TCA may have fatal results. See Chapter 6 and the Part II (Drug Profiles) for a discussion of individual TCAs.[35]

Toxic Effects

Children are thought to be more sensitive to overdoses of TCAs than adults. Although deaths of children for whom TCAs were prescribed have been reported, TCA poisoning in children may be caused by taking another family member's (usually a parent's) medication. The long-acting preparation imipramine pamoate (Tofranil-PM) is not recommended for children because the smallest available unit dose is 75 mg. Because TCAs have a narrow therapeutic index, compliance with the dosage regimen warrants close monitoring, and these drugs must be made inaccessible to children. Treatment guidelines for TCA overdose are presented in Chapter 6.

SELECTIVE SEROTONIN REUPTAKE INHIBITORS

The current SSRIs marketed in the United States include fluoxetine (Prozac), sertraline (Zoloft), paroxetine (Paxil), fluvoxamine (Luvox), and citalopram (Celexa). As noted earlier, clomipramine is a TCA that acts similarly to the SSRIs. The SSRIs (fluoxetine, sertraline, paroxetine, fluvoxamine, and citalopram) are not chemically related to one another nor are they chemically related to the older TCAs. As a group, they are also more specific in their action, and consequently, they are called *SSRIs*.

Indications: Primarily OCD

All of the SSRIs in current use have shown efficacy for treating depression in adults. In controlled trials, fluoxetine, sertraline, fluvoxamine, paroxetine, and citalopram have also been effective for OCD.

Empirical Support

Several recent controlled studies have shown that these newer SSRIs are effective in reducing the intensity of OCD symptoms in adults.[46] Pharmacotherapy of OCD in the pediatric population has also made considerable gains in recent years. Following the early clinical trials with clomipramine in children and adolescents, several controlled clinical trials with fluoxetine, fluvoxamine, and sertraline have been conducted.[43] Large, multisite trials have been completed with sertraline and fluvoxamine.[74,99] Several smaller studies have been done with fluoxetine, and a large-scale, double-blind, placebo-controlled study is currently under way with paroxetine. To date, only one open-label study has been done in children with the recently released SSRI citalopram.[121]

Mechanism of Action

The SSRIs inhibit the return of serotonin into the presynaptic neuron. Although the precise mechanism is not completely understood, it is known to be complex. Blocking the reuptake of serotonin produces a cascade of events that ultimately enhances serotonergic function. Moreover, available evidence suggests that this action accounts for the effectiveness of these agents in treating OCD.[15]

Table 19-3 Dosing Guidelines for Selective Serotonin Reuptake Inhibitors in Children

Drug name	Typical starting dose (mg)	Typical daily dose range (mg)	Half-life* (days)
Fluoxetine	5-10	5-40	2-4
Sertraline	12.5-25	25-150	1
Fluvoxamine	12.5-25	50-200	1
Paroxetine	5-10	10-40	1
Citalopram	5	5-40	1.5

*Long half-life allows single dose per day. Does not include active metabolite.

Pharmacokinetics

All five of the SSRIs have relatively long half-lives, permitting single daily dosing. The half-lives of sertraline, fluvoxamine, and paroxetine are each about 24 hours in adults. Recent data indicate that children may metabolize these medications faster than adults.[33] Citalopram and fluoxetine have longer half-lives. For example, citalopram has a half-life of 35 hours, and fluoxetine has a half-life of 2 to 4 days and has an active metabolite with an even longer half-life (up to 10 days or more). In addition, fluoxetine and paroxetine inhibit their own breakdown, resulting in nonlinear kinetics at higher dosages. Table 19-3 presents dosing guidelines for SSRIs for children.

Clinical Management

Fluoxetine. Fluoxetine (Prozac) comes in a 10-mg tablet or a 20-mg capsule and in a liquid preparation. The typical starting dosage is 5 to 10 mg/day. Because of its long half-life, fluoxetine should be increased slowly to avoid overshooting the optimal dose. The dosage range for children and adolescents is 5 to 60 mg/day, but most children will fall between 10 and 40 mg/day.

The most common side effect of fluoxetine is behavioral activation, which is characterized by motor restlessness, insomnia, and disinhibition. This side effect is especially prevalent early in treatment but may also be seen with dosage increases.[97] Other side effects include abdominal pain, heartburn, diarrhea, and decreased appetite. There have also been reports of suicidal ideation and self-injurious behavior.[55] Currently, it is unclear whether fluoxetine confers greater risk for suicidal ideation than the other SSRIs. Thus, as with all antidepressants, clinicians should be vigilant for suicidal thoughts or self-injurious behavior in children and adolescents treated with fluoxetine.

Sertraline. Sertraline (Zoloft) is available in 25-, 50-, and 100-mg tablets that easily break in half. A therapeutic trial might begin with a 12.5- to 25-mg dose, with weekly increases to a range of 25 to 150 mg in children and slightly higher dosages in older adolescents. Evidence from adult studies suggests that some patients may respond to low dosages of sertraline; hence clinicians should review symptomatic response before proceeding with additional dose increases. Sertraline can be given in a single daily dose.

The side effects of sertraline are similar to those of fluoxetine and include activation, insomnia, diarrhea, and sedation. In a review of 33 children and adolescents being treated for depression, Tierney and others reported two cases of sertraline-induced mania.[122]

Fluvoxamine. Fluvoxamine (Luvox) is available in a 25-, 50-, and 100-mg scored tablets. Treatment usually begins at 12.5 to 25 mg/day and is increased by 25 mg every 5 to 7 days as tolerated, for example, in the absence of diarrhea, sedation, or activation. The medication can be given once daily; the typical dose range is 50 to 200 mg/day. The side effects are similar to those of fluoxetine and sertraline.

Paroxetine. Paroxetine (Paxil) comes in 10-, 20-, and 30-mg tablets that can be divided in half. Pediatric dosing guidelines have been aided by a recent pharmacokinetic study that showed that although pediatric patients metabolize the medication more efficiently than adults, it can still be given as a once daily drug.[33] A reasonable starting dosage is 5 to 10 mg/day, with gradual increases as needed and as tolerated to a total daily dose of 10 and 40 mg. Limited clinical experience in pediatric populations indicates that paroxetine is generally well tolerated, with side effect profiles similar to those of the other SSRIs.[16]

Withdrawal of SSRIs and Duration of Therapy

Although relatively few side effects are associated with the SSRIs, several case studies have reported dizziness, nausea, vomiting, and diarrhea upon withdrawal of sertraline and paroxetine.[8,69] A recent controlled study in 220 adults showed that paroxetine and sertraline, but not fluoxetine, were associated with discontinuation-emergent symptoms such as irritability, agitation, fatigue, insomnia, confusion, dizziness, and nervousness.[100] These differences are probably the result of the longer half-life of fluoxetine and its active metabolite norfluoxetine, which results in a gradual taper even when the oral dose is stopped abruptly. Thus a slow withdrawal of the shorter-acting SSRIs such as paroxetine, sertraline, and fluvoxamine is warranted. No data are available for citalopram.

A related question that parents often ask concerns the duration of treatment with an SSRI. Unfortunately, very little evidence exists on which to base a clear answer. Many clinicians suggest discontinuation after a symptom-free period of 8 to 12 months. Evidence from one of the few follow-up studies in 54 children and adolescents indicated that about 70% (39/54) were maintained on medication for more than 2 years, suggesting that OCD can be chronic.[65] Thus children and parents should be informed that symptoms may return after discontinuation of an SSRI.

Augmentation Strategies

Although the SSRIs offer great promise for children and adolescents with OCD, not all children will have a positive response. Studies in adults show that 30% to 40% of patients with OCD will demonstrate only partial or no response to monotherapy with an SSRI. A similar rate of nonresponse was observed in a recent multicenter trial of sertraline in children and adolescents.[74] Thus clinicians often resort to adding another medication to produce positive effects on OCD symptoms. Studies by McDougle and others have shown that drugs such as lithium and buspirone, which enhance serotonergic function, are not effective as adjunctive agents.[81] However, the addition of low-dose neuroleptics can be effective in refractory OCD.[81,82]

Based on these findings in adults, many clinicians are beginning to explore augmentation strategies in children who do not have an optimal response to an SSRI. To date, however, this strategy has not been well studied in pediatric populations. Before placing a child on a neuroleptic agent to augment ongoing treatment with an SSRI, the clinician should weigh several issues.

First, although the transition can be difficult, an alternative SSRI should at least be considered.

Second, the SSRI may influence hepatic metabolism of the neuroleptic, which may affect the level of the neuroleptic. In most instances, this interaction results in an increase in the neuroleptic level and elevates the risk of adverse effects. For example, oculogyric events have been reported in two youngsters when a neuroleptic was added to ongoing treatment with paroxetine.[47,68] These adverse events are almost certainly the result of paroxetine's inhibition of CYP 2D6, which is the enzyme that metabolizes risperidone. This inhibition of the liver enzyme causes a rise in the neuroleptic level. To varying degrees, the SSRIs all have the capacity to reduce the activity of (inhibit) one or more of these enzymes. Thus care is required when combining drugs with the SSRIs, including psychotropics and drugs used in primary care.[35,91]

Third, neuroleptic medications have both short-term side effects such as cognitive dulling, fatigue, weight gain, and akathisia and long-term side effects such as tardive dyskinesia. In view of these concerns, other interventions should be considered. For example, cognitive-behavioral therapy has shown promise for treating children and adolescents with OCD.[73,106]

SSRIs and Depression

Fluoxetine and sertraline have been studied for the treatment of depression in children and adolescents.[2,31,110,122] The fluoxetine study by Emslie and colleagues is the only published controlled study to date in which an antidepressant was superior to placebo for the treatment of depression in children and adolescents.[31] A placebo-controlled, multicenter trial with paroxetine has recently been completed, but results are not yet available. The open-label sertraline studies by Tierney and others and Ambrosini and others included more than 80 subjects collectively and showed promising preliminary results.[2,122] An industry-sponsored, placebo-controlled study is now under way. Thus, although more evidence is needed, these findings suggest that the SSRIs are the first-line agents for depression in children. Dosing guidelines are similar to those described earlier for OCD.

OTHER ANTIDEPRESSANT MEDICATIONS

Bupropion (Wellbutrin) is not related to the TCAs or any other currently available antidepressant. It is approved for use in adults with depression. A recent placebo-controlled study showed that it is effective in the treatment of children and adolescents with ADHD at dosages ranging from 50 to 200 mg/day in divided doses. Side effects include agitation, insomnia, skin rashes, nausea, vomiting, constipation, and tremor. Bupropion has been associated with a low risk of seizures. Venlafaxine (Effexor) inhibits the reuptake of both norepinephrine and serotonin. To date, there is one placebo-controlled trial in children with depression. The study, which included 32 youngsters, found that the drug was no better than placebo in relieving depression.[71] A large multisite study is now under way, but the results are not yet available. Several other new antidepressants, including nefazodone (Serzone), mirtazapine (Remeron), and reboxetine, have entered the marketplace. These newer antidepressants have not been well studied in children or adolescents.[76]

ANTIPSYCHOTIC DRUGS

Antipsychotic drugs are discussed in detail in Chapter 5. In this chapter, only those antipsychotic agents that are commonly used in pediatric psychopharmacology are reviewed.

Indications: Psychosis, Pervasive Developmental Disorders, and Tourette's Syndrome

Antipsychotic agents are used for the treatment of psychosis, severe aggression, and complex behavioral problems associated with autism and other developmental disorders in children and adolescents. Haloperidol, pimozide, and fluphenazine are commonly used for tics.

Psychotic disorders. Although rare, schizophrenia can occur in children younger than 12 years of age.[78] As defined in the DSM-IV, the prevalence of childhood schizophrenia is estimated at 2 cases per 100,000 and is more common in boys than in girls. Symptoms may include hallucinations, delusions, disordered thinking, and inappropriate affect. Speech idiosyncrasies such as neologisms, echolalia, and an inability to use verbal communication in an age-appropriate fashion are usually present. These symptoms cause substantial dysfunction in all domains, and affected children may also exhibit other developmental delays.

The cause is unknown, but genetic vulnerability is assumed to play an important role. The diagnosis of childhood schizophrenia follows a careful assessment in which other disorders such as autism and neurodegenerative disorders have been ruled out.[78]

Pervasive developmental disorders. The pervasive developmental disorders (PDDs) are a group of syndromes that are characterized by severe developmental delays in several areas of functioning, including socialization, communication, and interpersonal relationships. The DSM-IV describes several subtypes of PDD, including autism, Asperger's disorder, and PDD-not otherwise specified.[128]

Autism. The child with autism appears uninterested in social contact, has great difficulty with change, and exhibits both delayed and deviant language development. Autism is differentiated from schizophrenia by the earlier age of onset and the absence of hallucinations and delusions. Stereotypic behaviors such as rocking, hand flapping, and head banging are common; self-injurious behavior such as hitting and biting are commonly observed. These children tend to have a narrow range of interests and seemingly prefer inanimate objects to social contact. Approximately half of children with autism are mentally retarded, and about 25% have seizures.

Asperger's disorder. Children with Asperger's disorder may have normal intelligence and typically exhibit higher verbal, rather than nonverbal, intelligence. Although their linguistic skills may not be as impaired when compared with children who have autism, children with Asperger's disorder have profound social delays. They show deficits in initiating social interactions and reading social cues and have a predilection to be concrete in their interpretation of language. Stereotypic behaviors such as rocking and hand flapping may be present. These children typically exhibit intense preoccupation with peculiar topics such as fans, geography, train schedules, or dates of historical events.

PDD—not otherwise specified. Children with PPD—not otherwise specified are probably a heterogeneous group who are inflexible, intolerant of change, and prone to behavioral outbursts in response to modest environmental demands or changes in routine. They are socially delayed, deficient in performing daily living tasks, often preoccupied with narrow fields of interest, and may have significant difficulty with regulating anxiety. Stereotypic behaviors may also be observed.[21,58]

Tourette's syndrome. Tourette's syndrome (TS) is a movement disorder characterized by a changing repertoire of motor tics and vocalizations. The symptoms begin in childhood, exhibit a fluctuating course, and often decline in adulthood. Typical motor tics include eye blinking, head jerking, grimacing, and shrugging. Vocal tics include throat clearing, grunting, snorting, barking, hooting, and repetitive words or parts of words. Uncontrollable swearing (coprolalia) and obscene gestures (copropraxia) are present in a minority of patients. In addition to tics, many children also have significant problems with ADHD and obsessive-compulsive symptoms.[109]

TS is not a common disorder, but recent evidence suggests that it is not as rare as once believed. Current estimates are that TS occurs in approximately 1 to 3 cases per 1000 in school-age children, with a two to four times higher frequency in boys.[23] Although the cause of TS is unknown, recent evidence converges on dysregulation of brain circuits connecting the cortex, basal ganglia, and thalamus.[62] Family genetic studies and twin studies provide compelling evidence that TS is an inherited disorder with variable expression in other family members, including chronic tic disorder, TS, and some forms of OCD. Despite the evidence of genetic transmission in families, the mode of inheritance has yet to be determined. Recent studies suggest that TS may not be caused by a single gene as previously believed.[83,84,130]

Mechanism of Action

The neuroleptics can be classified according to chemical family, for example, the phenothiazines, or by potency, that is, low versus high (see Chapter 5). The primary action of the traditional antipsychotic medications is postsynaptic dopamine blockade at D_2 receptors.[32,107] The newer so-called atypical antipsychotics are exceptions to this rule. These medications include clozapine, olanzapine, risperidone, quetiapine, and ziprasidone, which are described later in this chapter and in Chapters 5 and 20. Differences in action and side effects of the standard neuroleptics appear to be related to regional specificity of binding in the brain. For example, striatal binding is correlated with extrapyramidal side effects (EPSEs).

Antipsychotic medications also have anticholinergic and antihistaminergic effects. They block adrenergic pathways as well. The relative strength of these pharmacologic properties influences their side effect profile. Hence low-potency neuroleptics such as chlorpromazine and thioridazine cause more sedation, dry mouth, and constipation (anticholinergic effects). In contrast, the high-potency agents such as haloperidol and fluphenazine have greater EPSE liability. In this chapter, representative agents from different chemical families and of different potencies are presented.

Pharmacokinetics

Most of the antipsychotic drugs have relatively long half-lives; for example, pimozide has a half-life of 55 hours, and risperidone has a half-life of 20 to 24 hours. Nonetheless, plasma blood levels at a given milligram-per-kilogram dosage can vary substantially. This observation, coupled with the goal of averting unwanted side effects, favors a twice-daily dosing schedule.

Clinical Management and Empirical Support

Chlorpromazine. Chlorpromazine (Thorazine) is an aliphatic phenothiazine that was the first neuroleptic used in children. An early controlled study showed that at dosage ranges between 120 and 430 mg/day, chlorpromazine was superior to a placebo on crude measures of behavioral disturbance. Despite modest improvement in children taking this drug, the children remained severely impaired.[57] With the introduction of newer agents, chlorpromazine has not been used as often as in the past.

Chlorpromazine is usually prescribed at 10 to 25 mg on the first day and gradually increased over 2 weeks to a total of 150 to 300 mg/day in divided doses. For acutely disturbed children who require immediate treatment, an intramuscular dose of 0.5 mg/kg of body weight every 6 to 8 hours is appropriate. A 2- to 5-year-old child should not receive more than 40 mg/day, and a 5- to 12-year-old child should not receive more than 75 mg/day intramuscularly.

Thioridazine. Thioridazine (Mellaril) is a piperidine phenothiazine that is also a low-potency neuroleptic. Compared with chlorpromazine, thioridazine is currently more commonly used for severe behavioral problems and psychotic symptoms. The dosage for treating psychosis in 3- to 12-year-old children is 0.5 to 3.0 mg/kg/day, which translates into 10 to 50 mg two or three times per day.[78,107]

Haloperidol. Haloperidol (Haldol), a high-potency antipsychotic, is a butyrophenone and is structurally unrelated to the phenothiazines. It is used to treat children between ages 3 and 12 with psychosis, aggressive behavior, and tics, as well as behavioral dyscontrol associated with PDD.

Haloperidol is the most thoroughly studied of the neuroleptics in children, with both open-label and double-blind studies conducted in children with autism, schizophrenia, severe aggressive behavior, and tics. These studies show that haloperidol is effective, although not free of side effects.[18,80,109] As a high-potency neuroleptic, haloperidol is more likely to cause EPSEs compared with chlorpromazine or thioridazine. On the other hand, haloperidol is less sedating. Table 19-4 shows typical dosages for haloperidol by symptom cluster.

Fluphenazine. Fluphenazine (Prolixin), a commonly used piperazine in adults, is not approved for children younger than 12. In one of the few studies of fluphenazine in prepubertal children, Joshi, Capozzoli, and Coyle found that low dosages (i.e., 0.04 mg/kg/day) were effective in decreasing aggressive behavior,

Table 19-4 Recommended Doses of Haloperidol in Children

Clinical problem	Starting dose (mg)	Dose range (mg/day)
Psychosis	0.5	1-6
Tics (Tourette's syndrome)	0.25	0.5-2.0
Behavioral dyscontrol (pervasive developmental disorder)	0.25-0.5	0.5-3.0
Aggression	0.5	1-6

hyperactivity, and stereotypic behavior in a sample of 12 children with PDD.[51] The initial dosage might be 0.5 mg/day, with increases every 3 to 5 days as tolerated and according to clinical response. The total daily dose of 1 to 3.0 mg can be given in two divided doses.

Fluphenazine has also been used in the treatment of tic symptoms in TS. At dosages ranging from 2 to 15 mg/day in divided doses (mean dosage, 7 mg/day), Goetz and colleagues reported that fluphenazine was effective and generally well tolerated.[41] The study of 21 TS patients included both children and adults.[41] Unfortunately, the dosing schedule and response was not separately reported for the pediatric patients.

Thiothixene. Thiothixene (Navane) is a thioxanthene and is structurally related to phenothiazines. It is approved for treating psychosis in children older than 12. The meager evidence that is available for children younger than 12 indicates that thiothixene is less sedating than low-potency neuroleptics and may cause fewer EPSEs than the high-potency neuroleptics. The medication can be initiated with a 1- to 2-mg dose given two to three times per day. Thereafter, the dosage can be increased to 5 to 40 mg/day in two or three divided doses.[78,107]

Pimozide. Pimozide (Orap) is a diphenylbutylpiperidine that is not related to the phenothiazines or to haloperidol. It is a potent blocker of dopamine at the D_2 postsynaptic receptors, and it is used to treat TS.

In an open study of 66 children with TS, Sallee, Sethuraman, and Rock found pimozide and haloperidol were equally effective in reducing tics at mean dosages of 3.7 and 1.5 mg/day, respectively.[102] In that study, children were randomly assigned to receive either haloperidol, pimozide, or no medication. The children treated with pimozide performed significantly better on computerized tests of attention. Haloperidol appeared to show decreased performance on these tests. Differences in the type and frequency of side effects between the two drugs were not reported.

Pimozide is available in a 2-mg tablet. The typical starting dosage is 0.5 (half a tablet every other day) to 1 mg/day (half a tablet every day), with increases every 5 to 7 days in 0.5- to 1-mg increments over a 3-week period. The total dose typically ranges from 2 to 4 mg/day. Common side effects include fatigue, cognitive dulling, dysphoria, akathisia, and dystonic reactions. An additional concern with pimozide is that it can cause cardiac conduction abnormalities such as prolonged QT interval and inverted T waves. These abnormalities are probably rare in the typical dosage range for tics. Nonetheless, an ECG should be obtained at baseline, following dosage adjustment, and annually during maintenance therapy.[109]

Risperidone. Risperidone (Risperdal) is a neuroleptic medication that not only blocks dopamine postsynaptically but also acts as a serotonin antagonist at the $5HT_2$ site. The dual action is similar to that of clozapine and appears to protect against EPSEs.[66] Although risperidone has some pharmacologic features in common with clozapine, it has not been associated with agranulocytosis. Risperidone has been extensively studied in adults with schizophrenia and appears to be safe and effective for treating psychosis, with fewer side effects than haloperidol.[75] However, the data supporting its use in children and adolescents are limited.

In the last 5 years, several open-label studies in various pediatric populations have been published with risperidone.[80,104] These data suggest that risperidone may be useful for the treatment of children and adolescents with thought disorder, behavioral dyscontrol in PDD, and tic disorders.[6,34,68,79,82] In most of these studies, the drug was initiated at 0.5 mg/day and increased by 0.5 mg every 5 to 7 days to a range of 1 to 3.5 mg/day in two divided doses. At these dosage levels, risperidone was well tolerated, with increased appetite and weight gain being the most commonly observed side effect. By contrast, reports from other open trials indicate that when more aggressive dosing schedules are used, children and adolescents are at greater risk for EPSEs.[70,112] Limited data are available for quetiapine, olanzapine, or ziprasidone in children and adolescents.[104]

Side Effects

Side effects of antipsychotic drugs that are relevant to pediatric patients are discussed here. Side effects of neuroleptics are also discussed in Chapters 5 and 20.

Drowsiness is a common side effect that may be especially prominent with chlorpromazine and thioridazine, that is, the low-potency antipsychotic agents. Anticholinergic side effects such as dry mouth, constipation, and blurred vision are also common. Dystonic reactions, rigidity, and akathisia (i.e., EPSEs) are more common with the high-potency neuroleptics such as haloperidol, fluphenazine, and pimozide.

Toxic Effects

Deaths resulting from antipsychotic drug overdoses are rare in any age group. Overdose causes CNS depression, hypotension, and EPSEs. Treatment guidelines for overdose are outlined in Chapter 5.

Tardive Dyskinesia

Long-term use of neuroleptics carries a small risk for tardive dyskinesia (TD). A few cases of TD in pediatric patients have been reported.[18,95] Thus children and adolescents treated with neuroleptics should be monitored for abnormal movements. In some cases, it may be difficult to discriminate between dyskinesia, stereotypies, and tics. Referral to a consultant with expertise in movement disorders may be helpful in making this determination.

Because of the concern about withdrawal dyskinesia, the question of when and how to discontinue neuroleptic medication is a critical one. Dosage reductions should be done gradually to minimize withdrawal dyskinesia and to evaluate changes in symptom severity. Attempts at discontinuation should be considered annually. If symptoms persist, the maintenance dose of the neuroleptic should be reduced to the lowest possible dosage to minimize overall exposure.[78]

The atypical neuroleptics do indeed seem to have a lower risk of EPSEs during short-term treatment. Based on the collective experience with clozapine, the atypicals probably also have lower risks of TD. A recurring side effect that has been reported for olanzapine, quetiapine, and risperidone is weight gain. Virtually all open-label studies with risperidone, olanzapine, and quetiapine have reported weight gain.[53] In some cases, the gain is substantial. The mechanism for the increased weight appears to be through an increase in appetite. Because the health consequences can be significant, families need to be educated about the possibility of weight gain and weight should be monitored. Rare cases of hepatotoxicity have been reported with risperidone, prompting some investigators to recommend periodic measurement of liver enzyme levels.[59,60]

LITHIUM
Indications: Bipolar Disorder and Aggressiveness

Lithium is not approved for use for children younger than 12. Nonetheless, several published studies document its use in prepubertal children with bipolar illness or severe aggressive behavior. A brief description of lithium is provided here; more detailed descriptions are presented in Chapters 6 and 20.

Bipolar disorder. Whether mania exists in children is a matter of considerable controversy.[126] For example, questions remain about the presentation of bipolar illness in children. Available data suggest that bipolar disorder resembling the adult form of the illness is rare in prepubertal children.[36,131] If an expanded phenotype is accepted, however, the disorder may be more common.[25,134] Until these questions are resolved, the identification of bipolar illness in children will continue to be controversial.

Severe aggressive behavior. Aggressive behavior is a feature of several child and adolescent psychiatric disorders such as ADHD, conduct disorder, and perhaps bipolar disorder as well. Significant, unprovoked aggressive behavior often leads to consultation and to hospitalization in some cases. Both behavioral therapy and medication have been used to treat aggressive behavior in children.

Empirical Support

There are very few controlled studies of lithium in prepubertal children with bipolar illness. The best empirical support comes from a large open study that showed that 39 of 59 (66%) children benefited from lithium treatment.[26] A recent placebo-controlled study of 50 children (mean age, 9.4 years) showed that lithium was effective in reducing severe aggressive behavior.[18]

Clinical Management

For children younger than 12, a dosage of 30 mg/kg/day is typical. Thus, for a 30-kg child, the dosage would be 900 mg/day in divided doses. The optimal serum level range is 0.6 to 1.2 mEq/L.

Before a trial of lithium is initiated, a child should have a physical examination; screening laboratory tests such as a complete blood count, electrolytes, blood urea nitrogen, creatinine, liver function tests, and thyroid indices; and an ECG. Lithium decreases free thyroxine and triiodothyronine, but increased thyroid-releasing hormone generally compensates in euthyroid patients. Nonetheless, thyroid function and renal function should be checked every 6 months. Lithium levels should be monitored several times during the dosage adjustment phase and then periodically after the dosage is stabilized. Levels above 1.4 mEq/L are associated with signs of toxicity.

Side Effects

Common side effects of lithium include weight gain, nausea, vomiting, polydipsia, polyuria, tremor, fatigue, and diarrhea.

ALPHA-2 ADRENERGIC AGONISTS
Indications: Unapproved Treatment of TS, Tics, ADHD, and Aggressiveness

The alpha-2 adrenergic agents (clonidine and guanfacine) are approved only for use in adults with hypertension. Beginning with the early studies of clonidine for TS, these drugs have become increasingly common in child psychiatry for treating tics, ADHD, and aggressive behavior.[105,108]

Empirical Support

Clonidine. A recent double-blind study showed that clonidine (Catapres) can be effective in reducing the severity of tics in some patients.[63] Other studies provide modest evidence for efficacy in ADHD, but these findings were not replicated in a recent controlled study.[49,113]

Guanfacine. Guanfacine (Tenex) is another alpha-2 adrenergic agonist that was introduced more recently. Interest in guanfacine was prompted by its longer duration of action compared with clonidine, and it appears to be less sedating. To date, only three open studies have evaluated guanfacine in children.[20,47,48] These studies included a total of 38 children with ADHD. All three groups of investigators reported that guanfacine reduced the target symptoms of ADHD. The study by Chappell and others also included children with TS, and guanfacine appeared to have a modestly beneficial effect on tics.[20] A recent controlled study has confirmed these preliminary results. In that study of 34 youngsters, guanfacine was superior to placebo for ADHD symptoms and tics.[108] The typical starting dosage of guanfacine is 0.5 mg at bedtime; then it is increased by 0.5 mg every 3 to 4 days to a total of 1.5 to 3.0 mg/day in three divided doses.

Mechanism of Action

These drugs stimulate presynaptic noradrenergic receptors, resulting in decreased sympathetic output over time. Guanfacine appears to have postsynaptic effects in the frontal cortex.[105]

Clinical Management

Clonidine is usually introduced with a single 0.05-mg dose (half of a 0.1-mg tablet) and then increased by half-tablet increments every 3 to 4 days to a total of 0.15 to 0.2 mg/day. To ensure even blood levels across the entire day, clonidine is typically given three to four times per day. Sedation, which is most evident early in therapy, is the most common side effect. Other side effects include dry mouth, headache, irritability, and occasionally, sleep disturbance. Blood pressure should be monitored, but it is rarely a problem. Clonidine should be tapered slowly, however, because abrupt discontinuation can cause a rebound increase in blood pressure, tics, and anxiety.

Clonidine is being used increasingly as an adjunct to other medications, especially the stimulants.[88] Clinicians may resort to combined pharmacotherapy either to augment the positive effects of the first medication, offset the side effects caused by the primary medication, or treat another set of target symptoms.[129] Unfortunately, there is very little research support for combination pharmacotherapies in the pediatric age group, and clinicians must rely on experience, case reports, and extrapolation from adult studies.[81] The limitations of case reports are illustrated by the recent report of three deaths of children treated with the combination of clonidine and methylphenidate. A careful review of these cases showed that neither medication nor the combination played a role in the deaths of these children.[88] Nonetheless, combination pharmacotherapy calls for careful reconsideration of the target symptoms, the dose and timing of the primary medication, and a thorough discussion with the family regarding treatment alternatives.

Treatment with guanfacine may be initiated with a 0.5-mg dose in the evening and increased every 3 to 5 days to 0.5 mg three times per day. The common dosage range is 1.0 to 3.0 mg/day in two or three divided doses. Side effects include sedation, irritability, and midsleep awakening. These side effects can sometimes be managed by lowering the dosage or adjusting the times of doses.

OTHER AGENTS USED IN THE TREATMENT OF CHILDREN WITH PSYCHIATRIC DISORDERS

Desmopressin. Desmopressin (Stimate) is a synthetic, antidiuretic hormone that inhibits the production of urine. It is administered intranasally. A recent review suggests that desmopressin helps approximately 25% of children who use it, with minimal risk of adverse effects.[120] Although desmopressin is usually well tolerated, the beneficial effects often do not endure over time. The most effective treatment for enuresis is the use of a pad and buzzer. In this method, the bed is equipped with a pad that sets off a buzzer when the child wets. The buzzer wakes up the child.

Carbamazepine. Carbamazepine (Tegretol) is an anticonvulsant that has been used in many psychiatric disorders. In adults, it has been effective in treating lithium-resistant mania and impulsive behavior. The drug has been used in prepubertal children, but very few studies have been placebo controlled. The meager evidence to date suggests that carbamazepine may be useful in severe aggressive behavior.[25,126] Dosages may begin with 100 mg given twice a day and then gradually increased to a total of 200 to 600 mg/day in three divided doses (10 to 20 mg/kg/day). Side effects include fatigue, dizziness, blurred vision, mild ataxia, slurred speech, skin rash, and rarely, blood dyscrasias such as leukopenia, aplastic anemia, or thrombocytopenia. Another concern regarding the use of carbamazepine in pediatric populations is the potential for drug-drug interactions.

Buspirone. Buspirone (BuSpar) is an anxiolytic agent that is not related to the benzodiazepines. Its mechanism of action differs from the benzodiazepines and the SSRIs and appears to be a result of its ability to reduce the release of serotonin by presynaptic neurons.[125] Buspirone does not cause physical dependence and does not cover benzodiazepine withdrawal. A study in 15 children with anxiety disorders showed that dosages of 10 to 20 mg/day given in two divided doses resulted in significant improvement as measured by a global scale. This improvement was evident within 3 to 4 weeks of starting the medication. Side effects included tiredness, sleep disturbance, abdominal discomfort, and headache.[111] In a group of 25 hospitalized children with anxiety and aggressive behavior, Pfeffer, Jiang, and Domeshek noted improvement in anxiety and aggression in about 75% of the patients.[86] Approximately 16% ($n = 8$) worsened and four developed hypomania. In prepubertal children, buspirone may be initiated at 2.5 to 5 mg/day and increased thereafter every 3 to 4 days to a total of 20 to 30 mg/day in three divided doses.[125] If there is no evidence of improvement after 6 weeks, buspirone should be discontinued.

Clonazepam. Clonazepam (Klonopin) is a long-acting benzodiazepine that is approved as an anticonvulsant. In adults, it is also used to treat anxiety disorders and tics. A recent study of 15 prepubertal children showed that clonazepam can be useful in anxiety disorders in some children, but side effects were common and problematic. The most common side effects were disinhibited behavior, irritability, and drowsiness.[42] Thus clonazepam does not appear to be a first-line agent for the treatment of anxiety disorders in pediatric populations. Treatment might begin with 0.25 mg in the morning and increasing to 0.25 mg twice daily after 3 to 4 days. Thereafter, the dosage may be increased slowly to a maximum of 2 mg/day in divided doses. Upon discontinuation, clonazepam should be tapered gradually.

Secretin. Secretin is a peptide that regulates pH in the small intestine. It is also used as a diagnostic probe to assess pancreatic function. Spectacular and much publicized results in a child with autism produced tremendous interest and hope in secretin.[10] Results from a recent placebo-controlled study casts serious doubts on the usefulness of secretin in autism.[103] In that study, 60 children were randomly assigned to receive an intravenous infusion of saline or secretin (0.4 µg/kg) under double-blind conditions. Subjects were systematically evaluated over a 4-week posttreatment period. There was no evidence of a treatment effect for secretin compared with placebo on any of the outcome measures. These results suggest that a single dose of secretin is unlikely to be effective in the treatment of autism.

REFERENCES

1. Ambrosini PJ and others: Antidepressant treatments in children and adolescents. Part I: affective disorders, *J Am Acad Child Adolesc Psychiatry* 32:1, 1993.
2. Ambrosini PJ and others: Multicenter open-label sertraline study in adolescent outpatients with major depression, *J Am Acad Child Adolesc Psychiatry* 38:566, 1999.
3. American Psychiatric Association: *Diagnostic and statistical manual of mental disorders-TR*, ed 4, Washington, DC, 2000, The Association.
4. Anderson GM, Cook EH: Pharmacogenetics: promise and potential in child and adolescent psychiatry, *Child Adolesc Psychiatr Clin North Am* 9:23, 2000.
5. Angold A and others: Puberty and depression: the roles of age, pubertal status and pubertal timing, *Psychol Med* 28:51, 1998.
6. Armenteros JL and others: Risperidone in adolescents with schizophrenia: an open pilot study, *J Am Acad Child Adolesc Psychiatry* 36:694, 1997
7. Barkley RA and others: Side effects of methylphenidate in children with attention deficit hyperactivity disorder: a systematic, placebo-controlled evaluation, *Pediatrics* 86:184, 1992.
8. Barr LC, Goodman WK, Price LH: Physical symptoms associated with paroxetine discontinuation, *Am J Psychiatry* 151:289, 1994.
9. Baumgaertel A, Wolraich ML, Dietrich M: Comparison for diagnostic criteria for attention deficit disorders in a German elementary school sample, *J Am Acad Child Adolesc Psychiatry* 34:629, 1995.
10. Beck G, Beck V: *Unlocking the potential of secretin: information and questions for parents and physicians who want to learn more about secretin as its use is explored in autism and other disorders,* San Diego, 1998, Autism Research Institute.
11. Biederman J and others: A double-blind placebo-controlled study of desipramine in the treatment of ADD. Part I: efficacy, *J Am Acad Child Adolesc Psychiatry* 28:777, 1989.
12. Biederman J and others: A naturalistic study of 24-hour electro-cardiographic recordings and echocardiographic findings in children and adolescents treated with desipramine, *J Am Acad Child Adolesc Psychiatry* 32:805, 1993.
13. Biederman J and others: Systematic chart review of the pharmacologic treatment of comorbid attention deficit hyperactivity disorder in youth with bipolar disorder, *J Child Adolesc Psychopharmacol* 9:247, 1999.

14. Blackman A and others: The age of Ritalin, *Time,* 152 (November), 1998.
15. Blier P, de Montigny C: Possible serotonergic mechanisms underlying the antidepressant and anti-obsessive-compulsive disorder responses, *Biol Psychiatry* 44:313,1998.
16. Boyer WF, Blumhardt CL: The safety profile of paroxetine, *J Clin Psychiatry* 53(suppl): 61, 1992.
17. Campbell M, Cueva JE: Psychopharmacology in child and adolescent psychiatry: a review of the past seven years, Part I, *J Am Acad Child Adolesc Psychiatry* 34:1124, 1995.
18. Campbell M and others: Lithium in hospitalized aggressive children with conduct disorder: a double-blind and placebo-controlled study, *J Am Acad Child Adolesc Psychiatry* 34:445, 1995.
19. Castellanos FX and others: Controlled stimulant treatment of ADHD and comorbid Tourette's syndrome: effects of stimulant and dose, *J Am Acad Child Adolesc Psychiatry* 36: 589, 1997.
20. Chappell PB and others: Guanfacine treatment of comorbid attention deficit hyperactivity disorder and Tourette's syndrome: preliminary clinical experience, *J Am Acad Child Adolesc Psychiatry* 34:1140, 1995.
21. Cohen DJ, Volkmar FR: *Handbook of autism and pervasive developmental disorders,* ed 2, New York, 1997, John Wiley.
22. Costello EJ, Angold A, Burns BJ: The Great Smoky Mountains study of youth: functional impairment and serious emotional disturbance, *Arch Gen Psychiatry* 53:1137, 1996.
23. Costello EJ, Angold A, Burns BJ: The Great Smoky Mountains study of youth: goals, design, methods, and the prevalence of DSM-III-R disorders, *Arch Gen Psychiatry* 53:1129, 1996.
24. Cunningham CE, Siegel LS, Offord DR: A dose-response analysis of the effects of methylphenidate on the peer interaction and simulated classroom performance of ADD children with and without conduct problems, *J Child Psychol Psychiatry* 32(3):439, 1991.
25. Davanzo PA, McCracken JT: Mood stabilizers in the treatment of juvenile bipolar, *Child Adolesc Psychiatr Clin North Am* 9(1):159, 2000
26. DeLong GR, Aldershof AL: Long-term experience with lithium treatment in childhood: correlation with clinical diagnosis, *J Am Acad Child Adolesc Psychiatry* 26:389, 1987.
27. Desta Z, Kerbusch T, Flockhart DA: Effect of clarithromycin on the pharmacokinetics and pharmacodynamics of pimozide in healthy and extensive metabolizers of cytochrome P450 2D6 (CYP2D6), *Clin Pharmacol Ther* 65:10, 1999.
28. DeVeaugh-Geiss J and others: Clomipramine in child and adolescent obsessive-compulsive disorder: a multicenter trial, *J Am Acad Child Adolesc Psychiatry* 31:45, 1992.
29. DuPaul GJ, Connor, D Barkley RA: Medication therapy. In Barkley RA, editor: *Attention deficit hyperactivity disorder: a handbook for diagnosis and treatment,* ed 2, New York, 1998, Guilford.
30. Efron D, Jarman F, Barker M: Side effects of methylphenidate and dextroamphetamine in children with attention-deficit hyperactivity disorder: a double-blind cross-over trial, *Pediatrics* 100:662, 1997.
31. Emslie GJ and others: A double-bind, randomized, placebo-controlled trial of fluoxetine in children and adolescents with depression, *Arch Gen Psychiatry* 54: 1031, 1997.
32. Findling RL and others: Venlafaxine in adults with attention-deficit/hyperactivity disorder: an open clinical trial, *J Clin Psychiatry* 57:184, 1996.
33. Findling RL and others: Paroxetine pharmacokinetics in depressed children and adolescents, *J Am Child Adolesc Psychiatry* 38:952, 1999.
34. Fisman S and others: Use of risperidone in pervasive developmental disorders: a case series, *J Child Adolesc Psychopharmacol* 6:177, 1996.
35. Flockhart DA, Oesterheld JR: Cytochrome P450-mediated drug interactions, *Child Adolesc Psychiatr Clin North Am* 9(1):43, 2000.
36. Fristad MA, Weller EB, Weller RA: The Mania Rating Scale: can it be used in children? A preliminary report, *J Am Acad Child Adolesc Psychiatry* 31:252, 1992.
37. Gadow KD and others: Efficacy of methylphenidate for attention-deficit hyperactivity disorder in children with tic disorder, *Arch Gen Psychiatry* 152:444, 1995.

Gadow KD and others: Long-term methylphenidate therapy in children with comorbid attention-deficit hyperactivity disorder and chronic multiple tic disorder, *Arch Gen Psychiatry* 56:330, 1999.

39. Geller B and others: Preliminary data on the relationship between nortriptyline plasma level and response in depressed children, *Am J Psychiatry* 143:1283, 1986.

40. Geller B and others: Pharmacokinetically designed double-blind placebo-controlled study of nortriptyline in 6- to 12-year-olds with major depressive disorder, *J Am Acad Child Adolesc Psychiatry* 31:34, 1992.

41. Goetz C, Tanner CM, Klawans HL: Fluphenazine and multifocal tic disorders, *Arch Neurol* 41:271, 1984.

42. Graae F and others: Clonazepam in childhood anxiety disorders, *J Am Acad Child Adolesc Psychiatry* 33:372, 1994.

43. Grados M, Scahill L, Riddle MA: Pharmacotherapy in children and adolescents with obsessive-compulsive disorder, *Child Adolesc Psychiatr Clin North Am* 8:617, 1999.

44. Green WH: *Child and adolescent clinical psychopharmacology,* Baltimore, 1995, Williams & Wilkins.

45. Greenhill LL and others: Medication treatment strategies in the MTA study: relevance to clinicians and researchers. *J Am Acad Child Adolesc Psychiatry* 35(10):1304, 1996

46. Greist JH and others: Efficacy and tolerability of serotonin transport inhibitors in obsessive-compulsive disorder, *Arch Gen Psychiatry* 52:53, 1995.

47. Horrigan JP, Barnhill LJ: Guanfacine for treatment of attention-deficit hyperactivity disorder in boys, *J Child Adolesc Psychopharmacol* 5:215, 1995.

48. Hunt RD, Arnsten AFT, Asbell MD: An open trial of guanfacine in the treatment of attention deficit hyperactivity disorder, *J Am Acad Child Adolesc Psychiatry* 34:50, 1995.

49. Hunt RD, Minderaa RB, Cohen DJ: Clonidine benefits children with attention deficit disorder and hyperactivity: report of a double-blind placebo-crossover therapeutic trial, *J Am Acad Child Adolesc Psychiatry* 24:617, 1985.

50. Jensen PS and others: A 14-month randomized clinical trial of treatment strategies for attention-deficit/hyperactivity disorder, *Arch Gen Psychiatry* 56:1073, 1999.

51. Joshi PT, Capozzoli JA, Coyle JT: Low-dose neuroleptic therapy for children with childhood onset pervasive developmental disorder, *Am J Psychiatry* 145:335, 1988.

52. Karno M, Golding JM, Sorenson SB, Burnam A: The epidemiology of obsessive-compulsive disorder in five US communities, *Arch Gen Psychiatry* 45:1094, 1988.

53. Kelly DL and others: Weight gain in adolescents treated with risperidone and conventional antipsychotics over six months, *J Child Adolesc Psychopharmacol* 8:151, 1998.

54. Kent JD and others: Effects of late-afternoon methylphenidate administration on behavior and sleep in attention-deficit hyperactivity disorder, *Pediatrics* 96:320, 1995.

55. King RA and others: Emergence of self-destructive phenomena in children and adolescents during fluoxetine treatment, *J Am Acad Child Adolesc Psychiatry* 30:179, 1991.

56. Klein RG, Koplewicz HS, Kanner A: Imipramine treatment of children with separation anxiety disorder, *J Am Acad Child Adolesc Psychiatry* 31(1):21, 1992.

57. Klein DF and others: *Diagnosis and drug treatment of psychiatric disorders: adults and children,* ed 2, Baltimore, 1980, Williams & Wilkins.

58. Koenig K, Scahill L: Pharmacotherapy in children and adolescents with pervasive developmental disorders, *J Child Adolesc Psychiatr Nurs* 12:41, 1999.

59. Kumra S and others: Case study: risperidone-induced hepatotoxicity in pediatric patients, *J Am Acad Child Adolesc Psychiatry* 35:701, 1997.

60. Landau J, Martin A: Is liver function monitoring warranted during risperidone treatment? *J Am Acad Child Adolesc Psychiatry* 37;1007, 1998.

61. Law SF, Schachar RT: Do typical clinical doses of methylphenidate cause tics in children treated for attention-deficit hyperactivity disorder? *J Am Child Adolesc Psychiatry* 38: 944, 1999.

62. Leckman JF, Cohen DJ: *Tourette's syndrome, tic disorders, obsessions and compulsions,* New York, 1999, Wiley.

63. Leckman JF and others: Clonidine treatment of Gilles de la Tourette syndrome, *Arch Gen Psychiatry* 48:324, 1991.

64. Leonard HL and others: Treatment of obsessive-compulsive disorder with clomipramine and desipramine in children and adolescents, *Arch Gen Psychiatry* 46:1088, 1989.

65. Leonard HL and others: Tics and Tourette's disorder: a 2- to 7-year follow-up of 54 obsessive-compulsive children, *Am J Psychiatry* 149:1244, 1993.

66. Leysen JE and others: Risperidone: a novel antipsychotic with balanced serotonin-dopamine antagonism, receptor occupancy profile, and pharmacologic activity, *J Clin Psychiatry* 55: 5, 1994.

67. Lipkin PH, Goldstein IJ, Adesman AR: Tics and dyskinesias associated with stimulant treatment in attention-deficit hyperactivity disorder, *Arch Pediatr Adolesc Med* 148:859, 1994.

68. Lombroso PJ and others: Risperidone treatment of children and adolescents with chronic tic disorders: a preliminary report, *J Am Acad Child Adolesc Psychiatry* 34:1147, 1995.

69. Louie AK, Lannon RA, Ajari LJ: Withdrawal reaction after sertraline discontinuation, *Am J Psychiatry* 151(3):450, 1994.

70. Mandoki MW: Risperidone treatment of children and adolescents: increased risk of extrapyramidal side effects, *J Child Adolesc Psychopharmacol* 5:49, 1995.

71. Mandoki MK and others: Venlafaxine in the treatment of children and adolescents with major depression, *Psychopharmacol Bull* 33:149, 1997.

72. Manos MJ, Short EJ, Findling RL: Differential effectiveness of methylphenidate and Adderall in school-age youths with attention-deficit/hyperactivity disorder, *J Am Acad Child Adolesc Psychiatry* 38:7, 1999.

73. March JS, Mulle K, Herbel B: Behavioral psychotherapy for children and adolescents with obsessive-compulsive disorder: an open trial with a new protocol driven treatment package, *J Am Acad Child Adolesc Psychiatry* 33:333, 1994.

74. March JS and others: Sertraline in children and adolescents with obsessive-compulsive disorder: a multicenter randomized trial, *JAMA* 280:1752, 1998.

75. Marder SR, Meibach RC: Risperidone in the treatment of schizophrenia, *Am J Psychiatry* 151:825, 1994.

76. Martin A, Kaufman J, Charney D: Pharmacotherapy of early-onset depression: update and new directions, *Child Adolesc Psychiatr Clin North Am* 9: 135, 2000.

77. Marotta PJ, Roberts EA: Pemoline hepatotoxicity in children, *Pediatrics* 132:894, 1998.

78. McClellan J, Werry J: Practice parameters for the assessment and treatment of children and adolescents with schizophrenia, *J Am Acad Child Adolesc Psychiatry* 33:616, 1994.

79. McDougal and others: Risperidone treatment of children and adolescents with pervasive developmental disorders: a prospective open-label study, *J Am Acad Child Adolesc Psychiatry* 36:685, 1997.

80. McDougal and others: Research units on pediatric psychopharmacology (RUPP): background and rationale for an initial controlled study of risperidone, *Child Adolesc Psychiatr Clin North Am* 9:201, 2000.

81. McDougle CJ and others: Haloperidol addition in fluvoxamine-refractory obsessive-compulsive disorder: a double-blind, placebo-controlled study in patients with and without tics, *Arch Gen Psychiatry* 51:302, 1994.

82. McDougle CJ and others: A double-blind, placebo-controlled study of risperidone addition in serotonin reuptake inhibitor-refractory obsessive-compulsive disorder, *Arch Gen Psychiatry* 57:794, 2000.

83. Pauls DL: A complete genome scan in sib pairs affected by Gilles de la Tourette Syndrome, *Am J Hum Genet* 63:1428, 1999.

84. Pauls DL and others: A family study of Gilles de la Tourette syndrome, *Am J Hum Genet* 48:154, 1991.

85. Pelham WE and others: Relative efficacy of long-acting stimulants on children with attention deficit-hyperactivity disorder: a comparison of standard methylphenidate, sustained-release methylphenidate, sustained-release dextroamphetamine, and pemoline, *Pediatrics* 86: 226, 1990.

Pfeffer CR, Jiang H, Domeshek LJ: Buspirone treatment of psychiatrically hospitalized prepubertal children with symptoms of anxiety and moderately severe aggression. *J Child Adolesc Psychopharmacol* 7:145, 1997.

87. Pliszka SR: The use of psychostimulants in the pediatric patient, *Pediatr Clin North Am* 45:1085, 1998.

88. Popper CW: Combining methylphenidate and clonidine: pharmacologic questions and news reports about sudden death, *J Child Adolesc Psychopharmacol* 5:157, 1995.

89. Porrino LJ and others: A naturalistic assessment of the motor activity of hyperactive boys. Part I, *Arch Gen Psychiatry* 40:681, 1983.

90. Porrino LJ and others: A naturalistic assessment of the motor activity of hyperactive boys. Part II. *Arch Gen Psychiatry* 40:688, 1983.

91. Preskorn SH: Pharmacokinetics of antidepressants: why and how they are relevant to treatment, *J Clin Psychiatry* 54(suppl):14, 1993.

92. Puig-Antich J and others: Imipramine in prepubertal major depressive disorders, *Arch Gen Psychiatry* 44:81, 1987.

93. Riddle MA, Geller B, Ryan N: Another sudden death in a child treated with desipramine, *J Am Acad Child Adolesc Psychiatry* 32:792, 1993.

94. Riddle MA, Lebellarte MJ, Walkup JT: Pediatric psychopharmacology: problems and prospects, *J Child Adolesc Psychopharmacol* 8:87, 1998.

95. Riddle MA and others: Tardive dyskinesia following haloperidol treatment in Tourette's syndrome, *Arch Gen Psychiatry* 44:98, 1987.

96. Riddle MA and others: Obsessive compulsive disorder in children and adolescents: phenomenology and family history, *J Am Acad Child Adolesc Psychiatry* 29:766, 1990.

97. Riddle MA and others: Behavioral side effects of fluoxetine, *J Child Adolesc Psychopharmacol* 3:193, 1991.

98. Riddle MA and others: Effects of methylphenidate discontinuation and re-initiation in children with Tourette's syndrome and ADHD, *J Child Adolesc Psychopharmacol* 5:205, 1995.

99. Riddle MA and others: *A controlled trial of fluvoxamine for OCD in children and adolescents,* Boca Raton, FL, 1996, NCDEU.

100. Rosenbaum JF and others: Selective serotonin reuptake inhibitor discontinuation syndrome: a randomized clinical trial, *Biol Psychiatry* 44:77, 1998.

101. Safer DJ, Krager JM: A survey of medication treatment for hyperactive/inattentive students, *JAMA* 260:2256, 1988.

102. Sallee FR, Sethuraman G, Rock CM: Effects of pimozide on cognition in children with Tourette syndrome: interaction with comorbid attention-deficit hyperactivity disorder, *Acta Psychiatr Scand* 90:4, 1994.

103. Sandler AD and others: Lack of benefit of a single dose of synthetic human secretin in the treatment of autism and pervasive developmental disorder, *N Engl J Med* 341:1801, 1999.

104. Scahill L, Lynch KA: Atypical neuroleptics in children and adolescents, *J Child Adolesc Psychiatr Nurs* 11:38, 1998.

105. Scahill L, Barloon L, Farkas L: Alpha-2 agonists in the treatment of attention deficit hyperactivity disorder, *J Child Adolesc Psychiatr Nurs* 12:168, 1999.

106. Scahill L, Ort SI: Clinical ratings in child psychiatric nursing, *J Child Adolesc Psychiatr Nurs* 8:33, 1995.

107. Scahill L, Skrypeck A: The use of traditional neuroleptics in children and adolescents, *J Child Adolesc Psychiatr Nurs* 10:41, 1997.

108. Scahill L and others: A placebo-controlled study of guanfacine in the treatment of attention deficit hyperactivity disorder and tic disorders. Presented at the Annual Meeting of the American Academy of Child and Adolescent Psychiatry, Chicago, October 1999.

109. Scahill L and others: Pharmacological treatment of tic disorders, *Child Adolesc Psychiatr Clin North Am* 9:99, 2000.

110. Simeon JG and others: Adolescent depression: a placebo controlled treatment study and follow-up, *Prog Neuropsychopharmacol Biol Psychiatry* 14:791, 1990.

111. Simeon JG and others: Buspirone therapy of mixed anxiety disorders in childhood and adolescence: a pilot study, *J Child Adolesc Psychopharmacol* 4:29, 1994.

112. Simeon JG and others: Risperidone effects in treatment-resistant adolescents: preliminary case reports, *J Child Adolesc Psychopharmacol* 5:69, 1995.

113. Singer HS and others: The treatment of attention-deficit hyperactivity disorder in Tourette's syndrome: a double-blind placebo-controlled study with clonidine and desipramine, *Pediatrics* 95:74, 1995.

114. Spencer T and others: Nortriptyline treatment of children with attention-deficit disorder and tic disorder or Tourette's syndrome, *J Am Acad Child Adolesc Psychiatry* 32:205, 1993.

115. Spencer TJ and others: Growth deficits in ADHD children revisited: evidence for disorder-associated growth delays? *J Am Acad Adolesc Psychiatry* 35:1460, 1996.

116. Swanson JM and others: Analog classroom assessment of Adderall in children with ADHD, *J Am Acad Child Adolesc Psychiatry* 37:519, 1998.

117. Swanson JM and others: Combining methylphenidate and clonidine: ill-advised, *J Am Acad Child Adolesc Psychiatry* 38:617, 1999.

118. Swedo SE and others: Obsessive-compulsive disorder in children and adolescents, *Arch Gen Psychiatry* 46:335, 1989.

119. Szatmari P, Offord DR, Boyle MH: Ontario Child Health Study: prevalence of attention deficit disorder with hyperactivity, *J Child Psychol Psychiatr* 30:219, 1989.

120. Thompson S, Rey JM: Functional enuresis: is desmopressin the answer? *J Am Acad Child Adolesc Psychiatry* 34:266, 1995.

121. Thomsen PH: Child and adolescent obsessive-compulsive disorder treated with citalopram: findings from an open trial of 23 cases, *J Child Adolesc Psychopharmacology* 7:157, 1997.

122. Tierney E and others: Sertraline for major depression in children and adolescents: preliminary clinical experience, *J Child Adolesc Psychopharmacol* 5:13, 1995.

123. Tosyali MC, Greenhill LL: Child and adolescent psychopharmacology: Important developmental issues, *Pediatr Clin North Am* 45:1021, 1998.

124. Valeni-Basile LA and others: Frequency of obsessive-compulsive disorder in a community sample of young adolescents, *J Am Acad Child Adolesc Psychiatry* 33:782, 1994.

125. Velosa JF, Riddle MA: Pharmacologic treatment of anxiety disorders in children and adolescents, *Child Adolesc Psychiatr Clin North Am* 9:119, 2000.

126. Viesselman JO: Antidepressant and antimanic drugs. In JS Werry, MG Aman, editors: *Practitioner's guide to psychoactive drugs for children and adolescents*, ed 2, New York, 1999, Plenum.

127. Vitiello B, Jensen P: Psychopharmacology in children and adolescents: current problems, future prospects—summary notes in the 1995 NIMH-FDA Conference, *J Child Adolesc Psychopharmacology* 5:5, 1995.

128. Volkmar FR and others: Field trial for autistic disorder in DSM-IV, *Am J Psychiatry* 151: 1361, 1994.

129. Walkup JT: Clinical decision making in child and adolescent psychopharmacology, *Child Adolesc Psychiatr Clin North Am* 4:23, 1995.

130. Walkup JT and others: Evidence for a mixed model of inheritance in Tourette's syndrome, *Am J Human Genetics*, 59:684, 1996.

131. Weller EB, Weller RA, Fristad MA: Bipolar disorder in children: misdiagnosis, underdiagnosis, and future directions, *J Am Acad Child Adolesc Psychiatry* 34:709, 1995.

132. Wilens TE, Spencer TJ: Combining methylphenidate and clonidine: a clinically sound medication option, *J Am Acad Child Adolesc Psychiatry* 38:614, 1999.

133. Wolraich ML, Hannah JN, Baumgaertel A, Feurer ID: Examination of DSM-IV criteria for attention deficit/hyperactivity disorder in a county-wide sample, *J Dev Behav Pediatr* 19: 162, 1998.

134. Wozniak J and others: Mania-like symptoms suggestive of childhood onset bipolar disorder in clinically referred children, *J Am Acad Child Adolesc Psychiatry* 34:867, 1995.

135. Zito JM and others: Trends in the prescribing of psychotropic medications to preschoolers, *JAMA* 283:1025, 2000.

CHAPTER 20

Psychopharmacology for Adolescents

Lawrence Scahill

SCOPE OF THE PROBLEM

Serious mental illness afflicts an estimated 8 million children younger than 18 in the United States.[14,29] A recent national survey indicates that nearly 500,000 of the 3 to 4 million adolescents (ages 13 to 18) with mental disorders use inpatient or outpatient mental health services.[48] This obvious discrepancy between the estimated number of adolescents with mental illness and those using services indicates that many adolescents with mental disorders are not using mental health services.[29] Several factors may explain this, including limited access to services for some segments of the population and the use of primary health care systems for psychosocial and pharmacologic (e.g., methylphenidate) interventions.[28,48,80] Nonetheless, psychopharmacologic interventions are being used with increasing frequency in child and adolescent psychiatry, often without sufficient research data to inform practitioners.[51] Finally, the proliferation of new medications poses an extraordinary research challenge to the clinician in child and adolescent psychiatry to guide clinical care. This chapter provides specific information about treating adolescents with psychotropic drugs. For example, medications such as lithium and valproic acid are used more commonly in adolescents compared with prepubertal children, but treatment guidelines for adolescents may not be the same as those for adults.[12] Although some repetition of content from previous chapters is unavoidable, readers are referred to those chapters when appropriate.

GENERAL PRINCIPLES OF ADOLESCENT PSYCHOPHARMACOLOGY

As with other age groups, psychotropic drug intervention for adolescents should be viewed as one aspect of a multidimensional treatment approach. Drug therapy alone is unlikely to ensure optimal development in youths who have serious emotional or behavioral problems. Moreover, in addition to concerns such as the complex pharmacokinetics of the developing child, other issues such as treatment compliance, risk of drug abuse, and the emotional vicissitudes of adolescence are crucial variables for successful pharmacotherapy in this age group.

Strategies for Effective Pharmacotherapy

Evaluation. A careful review of presenting problems, their onset, course, and current severity, as well as any prior treatments and the adolescent's response to those interventions, is the foundation of a comprehensive evaluation. Other essential elements include the patient's medical history; developmental history; family history; and school, social, and family functioning. The collection of these data can be aided with the use of clinical ratings, parent and teacher checklists, and self-reports.[4,58]

The clinician should also ensure that the adolescent has had a recent physical examination, and depending on the medication being considered, screening blood tests and an electrocardiogram (ECG) are often indicated as well.

Collaboration. The goal of the assessment is to identify the source of greatest impairment and define the target symptoms for intervention. Obviously, there should be a good fit between the target symptoms and the intervention. Identifying target symptoms involves careful collaboration among the clinician, the family, and the adolescent. Failure to include the adolescent and the family in this negotiation can be a threat to the treatment alliance and perhaps the treatment plan as well.

Education. The adolescent patient and his or her parents should be thoroughly educated about the medication chosen and the reasons for its selection. This session may include a mutual identification of treatment goals, a review of common side effects, clarification of any delay in therapeutic response (e.g., with antidepressants), and a review of alternative treatments. The clinician should also explore the expectations of the adolescent and the family regarding the medication trial to make certain that these expectations are appropriate.

Assessment and ongoing monitoring. Some aspects of assessment and monitoring are drug specific. For example, adolescent boys appear to be at greater risk for acute dystonic reactions to neuroleptics compared with adults.[20,25] To avoid alarm and to promote early detection of a dystonic reaction, both the parents and the youth should be informed about this possible side effect.

In the early phase of treatment with any psychotropic agent, the adolescent should have frequent follow-ups to review body systems and to evaluate activity, appetite, sleep, elimination, and energy level. Following this initial phase of treatment, attention should be paid to both therapeutic and adverse effects.

Other Issues of Adolescent Pharmacotherapy

Compliance. The efficacy and safety of any psychotropic medication cannot be evaluated if the patient does not take the drug consistently. Although parental monitoring is essential to treatment compliance, parents may not monitor their adolescent children as closely as they might a younger child. Thus it may be necessary to negotiate a system of reminders and medication monitoring with the adolescent patient and the parents to ensure optimal compliance with the medication schedule. This negotiation often includes the clinician's pledge to adjust the dose of medication to promote therapeutic effects and to minimize side effects.

Suicide and overdose. Drug-related emergencies among 6- to 17-year-old adolescents accounted for more than 21,000 emergency room visits in 1988.[32] A recent national survey in Sweden found that prescribed psychotropic drugs were implicated in nearly half of the suicides in individuals younger than 30 years of age.[31] Suicide remains among the leading causes of death among adolescents, with as many as 8.6% of adolescents acknowledging suicidal behavior.[33] This national survey reported that tricyclic antidepressants (TCAs) and lithium were among the agents commonly used in intentional or accidental overdose. Although the TCAs have declined in use over the past few years, lithium use in adolescents may be increasing. Both the TCAs and lithium can be fatal. The emergence of suicidal ideation has been reported in adolescents being treated with the now commonly used antidepressants such as fluoxetine.[35] For these reasons, clinicians should be vigilant about suicidal thought and action in adolescents being treated with psychotropic drugs.

Toxic effects. Toxic effects occur when drug level surpasses therapeutic level. This is especially relevant for medications such as TCAs, lithium, and to a lesser extent, the selective serotonin reuptake inhibitors (SSRIs) and the neuroleptics. Toxicity may occur intentionally (deliberate overdose), inadvertently (accidental overdose), by drug-drug interaction, or by unduly rapid dose escalation. Safe clinical management of these agents requires monitoring for signs of toxicity and informing parents (and adolescents to the extent that is developmentally appropriate) about these signs. In recent years, there has been increased attention to drug-drug interaction, particularly those affecting the cytochrome P-450 system of enzymes that metabolize drugs in the liver. It is now well established that combining certain drugs increases the risk of adverse events as a result of inhibitory or inducing effects on this metabolic system.[22]

Abuse. Abuse of drugs is another important issue when working with adolescent patients. The patient, a friend, or a sibling may experiment with prescribed agents. In addition, the adolescent may be experimenting with or using illicit drugs while in treatment. These concerns require that a therapeutic alliance be developed with the adolescent and the family so that ongoing monitoring is perceived as helpful rather than imperious.

PSYCHOTROPIC MEDICATIONS USED WITH ADOLESCENTS
STIMULANTS
Indications: Attention-Deficit Hyperactivity Disorder

The stimulants methylphenidate, dextroamphetamine, and the combined amphetamine Adderall are the primary agents used to treat attention-deficit hyperactivity disorder (ADHD) (Box 20-1).

ADHD is a heterogeneous, relatively common disorder of childhood onset that is characterized by inattention, impulsiveness, and hyperactivity. The DSM-IV permits further subclassification of ADHD into the primarily inattentive type, primarily impulsive/hyperactive type, or combined type.[3] Depending on the definition and methods of case identification, ADHD affects an estimated 2% to 10% of the school-age population.[6,15,70,78]

Until recently, many clinicians and researchers believed that children outgrow ADHD. Although fidgeting and restlessness may be more prominent in adolescents than is hyperactivity, evidence from several prospective studies refutes the notion that children outgrow ADHD.[4] These studies show that 40% to 70% of children with ADHD continue to meet criteria for diagnosis in adolescence. Moreover, adolescents with ADHD often demonstrate continued impairment across several domains, including academic, family, and interpersonal, and are at greater risk for legal trouble. Finally, those with comorbid conduct disorder have the poorest outcomes.[27]

Empirical Support

The efficacy and safety of methylphenidate, dextroamphetamine, the amphetamine mixture, and pemoline have been replicated in numerous controlled studies (see Chapter 19). These studies show that stimulants decrease hyperactivity and motor

---

Box 20-1 Commonly Used Stimulants to Treat Adolescents with ADHD

Methylphenidate (Ritalin)
  Dosage: The total daily dose ranges from 0.6 to 2 mg/kg/day given in 2 or 3 divided doses. Methylphenidate is typically started at 5 mg qd or bid and increased by 5 to 10 mg every 3-6 days. Dosages >70 mg are not recommended.
  Available dose forms: 5- and 10-mg tablets; 20-mg sustained-release tablets.

Dextroamphetamine (Dexedrine)
  Dosage: The total daily dose ranges from 0.3 to 1.5 mg/kg/day in 2, or occasionally, 3 divided doses. Dextroamphetamine is usually started at 5 mg/day and increased by 5 mg every 3-6 days. Dosages >50 mg/day are not recommended.
  Available dose forms: 5- and 10-mg tablets; 5-, 10-, and 15-mg sustained-release tablets.

Amphetamine mixture (Adderall)
  Dosage: The total daily dose ranges from 0.3 to 1.5 mg/kg/day in 2 divided doses. Treatment is initiated at 5 mg/day and is increased by 5 mg every 3-6 days. Dosages >50 mg/day are not recommended.
  Available dose forms: 5- and 10-mg tablets

Side effects related to these stimulants
  Insomnia, loss of appetite, weight loss, behavioral rebound (as medication wears off), increased heart rate and blood pressure, involuntary movements, mood lability, and cognitive rigidity. Psychotic reactions can occur but are rare.

---

restlessness and increase sustained attention. Stimulants may also improve antisocial behavior and interpersonal conflict. However, most studies have considered only the short-term benefits of stimulants; longer-term benefits are more difficult to show.[26,62]

Mechanism of Action

Although the precise mechanism by which stimulants exert their positive effect is not completely clear, it is presumed that the capacity of stimulants to increase the levels of dopamine and norepinephrine in the brain is central to this mechanism.[67]

Clinical Management

Contemporary clinical management of an adolescent being treated with a stimulant includes a thorough evaluation to rule out other causes of behavioral disturbances. In addition, psychologic testing may be indicated if there are questions about intellectual functioning or learning disability. Assessment of general health status, sleep and appetite, and vital signs are also necessary. Finally, assessing the severity of the patient's symptoms and response to the medication can be aided by the use of parent and teacher checklists.[4,58]

ANTIDEPRESSANTS
Indications: Depression, Obsessive-Compulsive Disorder, and ADHD

Antidepressant medications are approved for treating depression in youths older than 12. A small group of chemically unrelated antidepressants, including clomipramine (Anafranil), fluoxetine (Prozac), fluvoxamine (Luvox), and sertraline (Zoloft), are approved for treating obsessive-compulsive disorder (OCD). Imipramine (Tofranil) is also approved for treating enuresis. Although not officially approved for use in ADHD, desipramine and bupropion have shown benefit for treating both children and adolescents with the disorder. Fluoxetine and paroxetine have demonstrated efficacy for the treatment of depression in pediatric populations (Table 20-1).

Table 20-1 Antidepressants Commonly Used with Adolescents

| Name of drug | Class | Dosage range (mg/day)* | Disorder and level of empirical support | |
			Modest†	Strong†
Imipramine (Tofranil)	TCA	50-200	Separation anxiety	Enuresis
Desipramine (Norpramin)	TCA	50-150	—	ADHD
Nortriptyline (Pamelor)	TCA	50-125	Depression	—
Clomipramine (Anafranil)	TCA/SRI	50-150	—	OCD
Fluoxetine (Prozac)	SSRI	10-60	—	OCD, depression
Sertraline (Zoloft)	SSRI	50-200	Depression	OCD
Fluvoxamine (Luvox)	SSRI	50-200	—	OCD
Paroxetine (Paxil)	SSRI	10-40	—	OCD,‡ depression‡
Citalopram (Celexa)	SSRI	5-40	OCD	—
Bupropion (Wellbutrin)	Aminoketone	100-250	—	ADHD

TCA, Tricyclic antidepressant; *ADHD*, attention-deficit hyperactivity disorder; *SRI*, serotonin reuptake inhibitor; *OCD*, obsessive-compulsive disorder; *SSRI*, selective serotonin reuptake inhibitor.
*Administered in a single or divided dose, depending on agent.
†Modest = large open-label study, small controlled study, mixed results across studies; strong = large controlled study or two smaller controlled studies with similar results.
‡Results from large clinical trials in children and adolescents are pending.

Empirical Support

Depression. All currently available antidepressants have demonstrated efficacy and safety in treating adults with depression. The effectiveness of these agents has been less convincing in children and adolescents with depression. To date, there have been only about 15 controlled trials of antidepressants in depressed children and adolescents. In a recent review of these studies, Martin, Kaufman, and Charney noted that only two studies have shown that an antidepressant medication was superior to placebo in treating youngsters with depression.[43] In the first study of 96 children between the ages of 8 and 18 years, 20 mg/day of fluoxetine was significantly better than placebo in an 8-week randomized clinical trial.[19] The second study was an industry-sponsored study of paroxetine compared with placebo in adolescents.[34] That study included 275 subjects between 12 and 19 years of age. The subjects were randomly assigned to paroxetine (20 to 40 mg/day), imipramine (200 to 300 mg/day), or placebo. Paroxetine was superior to placebo, but imipramine was not.

Encouraging (although preliminary) results are now available for sertraline and venlafaxine for depression. Sertraline was evaluated in a multicenter, open-label study involving 53 adolescents.[2] Of these, data were available on 47 subjects. At an average dose of 127 ± 45 mg, just over half of the subjects were classified as responders. A large-scale, multicenter study of sertraline for the treatment of children and adolescents with depression is now under way. Mandoki conducted a placebo-controlled study of venlafaxine in 32 adolescents. In that study, venlafaxine was no better than placebo in reducing symptoms of depression.[40]

There are probably several reasons why medication studies of depression in pediatric populations have so often showed negative results. First, some of these studies have included too few subjects. A second contributing factor, which is clearly related to the issue of sample size, is the high placebo response rates in pediatric depression studies (as high as 50% in some studies). Third, there may be important differences in neurotransmitter systems in children, adolescents, and adults.[37,43]

Obsessive-compulsive disorder. Results from large clinical trials have shown that sertraline, fluvoxamine, and clomipramine are effective for the treatment of OCD.[17,41,49] Two smaller studies support the use of fluoxetine for treating children and adolescents with OCD.[53,59,60] Data from a large-scale, placebo-controlled study with paroxetine will soon become available. To date, only one open-label study has been reported with citalopram for the treatment of OCD in children and adolescents.[71] In that study, 23 subjects were treated for 10 weeks with dosages ranging from 10 to 40 mg/day. Citalopram was associated with improvement in OCD symptoms in 11 of the 23 youngsters. Table 20-1 displays common uses and level of empirical support for selected antidepressants.[24]

Attention-deficit hyperactivity disorder. Several TCAs and bupropion have been studied for their effectiveness in treating ADHD. Available evidence suggests that desipramine and bupropion are effective against ADHD.[5,7,13,65] Nortriptyline is commonly used in adolescents with ADHD, but empirical support is limited; only retrospective evidence from one study is available.[66] In general, these agents have not produced the same level of improvement as that shown by stimulants but may be considered if stimulants are not effective or are not tolerated.[55]

Mechanism of Action

To varying degrees, the TCAs block the reuptake of norepinephrine and serotonin by the presynaptic neuron. This action is presumed to enhance noradrenergic function.

The SSRIs and clomipramine inhibit the reuptake of serotonin, which ultimately enhances serotonergic functioning. For both the standard TCAs and the SSRIs, however, other neurotransmitters are also involved. The precise mechanism of bupropion remains unclear, although it appears to have both noradrenergic and dopamine-enhancing properties.

Several other antidepressants have entered the marketplace in recent years, including nefazodone, mirtazapine, and reboxetine. These new agents have not been studied in children or adolescents.

Clinical Management

Specific guidelines for dosing the various types of antidepressants are provided in Chapter 19. General principles include starting at low dosages followed by gradual increases. The upper dosage limit for TCAs ranges from a low of 1.5 mg/kg/day for nortriptyline to 3 mg/kg/day for others. Daily dosages of the SSRIs vary so widely that it is difficult to provide a milligram-per-kilogram formula. The average daily dose of bupropion may be as high as 5 mg/kg and is typically given in divided doses.

Side Effects

The frequency and seriousness of adverse effects vary greatly among the different classes of antidepressants (see Chapters 6 and 19). TCAs are associated with several side effects such as dry mouth, blurred vision, sweating, tremor, and urinary retention. Central nervous system (CNS) side effects include dizziness, drowsiness, agitation, and rarely, seizures. The cardiovascular side effects are of particular concern with TCAs.[25,50,56,73] Although controversy continues concerning the degree of risk for cardiac arrhythmias attributable to TCAs, available evidence suggests that pulse, blood pressure, and the ECG should be monitored in adolescents receiving TCAs. Vital signs and an ECG should be obtained before initiating treatment and repeated during upward dosage adjustment, after reaching a stable dose, and periodically during treatment. (See Chapter 19 for specific guidelines.)

SSRIs appear to be better tolerated than TCAs, and there is no evidence of serious cardiac effects with these newer agents. Common side effects include decreased appetite, diarrhea, abdominal pain, and fatigue. Perhaps the most common side effect in pediatric populations is behavioral activation. This adverse effect may be accompanied by hyperactivity, impulsiveness, insomnia, and expansive mood. It has been documented for fluoxetine but may occur with the other SSRIs as well.[24,52] Behavioral activation is most likely to occur early in treatment or with dosage increases. There have also been reports of suicidal ideation and self-injurious behavior, but this has also been observed with other types of antidepressants.[35]

The side effects of bupropion include skin rash, dry mouth, insomnia, agitation, headache, constipation, tremor, and tics. Although apparently rare, more serious adverse effects such as serum sickness and seizures have been reported.[13,25,63]

In summary, the best available evidence suggests that fluoxetine or paroxetine is the first choice for treating depression in adolescents. Nortriptyline is a second-line agent. Fluvoxamine, sertraline, paroxetine, fluoxetine, and clomipramine appear to be equally effective for the treatment of OCD in children and adolescents. Concern about cardiac conduction abnormalities with the TCAs (clomipramine, desipramine, nortriptyline, imipramine) and about the low, but increased, risk of skin rash and seizures associated with bupropion cause many clinicians to select the SSRIs as the first-line treatment for depression and OCD. Preliminary evidence indicates SSRIs may have also be useful in anxiety disorders.[72]

ANTIPSYCHOTICS

Antipsychotic drugs are also discussed in Chapters 5 and 19. This chapter focuses on the treatment of adolescents with psychotic disorders.

Indications: Primarily Psychosis

Psychotic disorders such as schizophrenia are the primary indication for antipsychotic drugs. They are also used to treat aggressive behavior, tic disorders, and severe behavioral problems associated with autism and mental retardation (see Chapter 19).

Psychotic disorder is a broad term that embraces a group of heterogeneous conditions that have multiple etiologies. The best-described psychotic disorder is schizophrenia, although it too is probably heterogeneous with respect to etiology. Schizophrenia may emerge in childhood, but more often it begins in late adolescence.[36] Symptoms include hallucinations, delusions, disordered thinking, blunted affect, idiosyncratic speech, concrete thinking, and profound social deficits. In children, diagnostic uncertainty can be present between schizophrenia and autism, but this ambiguity is less problematic during adolescence, when schizophrenia resembles the adult form of the disorder. However, the hallucinations, delusions, and thought disorder seen in schizophrenia can be present in psychotic depression, bipolar disorder, metabolic disorders such as Wilson's disease, or drug-induced psychosis. Thus careful assessment is essential when evaluating an adolescent with psychotic symptoms.

Schizophrenia in childhood is considered rare (approximately 2 cases per 100,000). In contrast, the prevalence of schizophrenia among older adolescents is several-fold more common, affecting between 0.5% and 1% of the general population. Schizophrenia is more common in males, tends to be chronic, and is associated with significant disability.

Empirical Support

The phenothiazines were the first drugs used to treat psychoses in adolescents. Since then, several other classes of antipsychotic drugs have been introduced. Numerous randomized clinical trials with neuroleptics have been conducted in adults with schizophrenia. These studies provide a convincing body of evidence concerning the effectiveness of neuroleptics to treat adults with schizophrenia. Unfortunately, the number of controlled studies in adolescents is far fewer.[25,44,57,59] Currently, there is little or no evidence to support the use of one antipsychotic agent over another; however, the newer atypical neuroleptics appear to be better tolerated.[20,57] Compared with the traditional neuroleptics, these newer neuroleptic drugs have lower risk of neurologic side effects such as dystonia, akathisia, and dyskinesia. Thus the newer atypical neuroleptics are becoming first-line treatments for psychosis in both pediatric and adult populations.

Mechanism of Action

The traditional neuroleptics such as thioridazine, thiothixene, and haloperidol block dopamine at the postsynaptic D_2 receptor. However, to varying degrees, antipsychotic agents also block histamine, norepinephrine, and acetylcholine receptors. In addition, antipsychotic drugs differ in their affinity for specific dopamine receptor subtypes. The blocking of these additional neurotransmitters and differences in affinity for dopamine receptor subtypes among the various antipsychotic agents influence their potency and side effect profiles. For example, the low-potency neuroleptics such as thioridazine are less D_2 selective and more anticholinergic than haloperidol. Not surprisingly, thioridazine is used at higher dosages, and more anticholinergic side effects are associated with its use than with haloperidol.

The atypical antipsychotic agents, including clozapine (Clozaril), risperidone (Risperdal), olanzapine (Zyprexa), quetiapine (Seroquel), and ziprasidone (Zeldox), differ in their relative affinity for D_2 receptors, but all are potent serotonin antagonists. For example, risperidone and ziprasidone are relatively potent dopamine blockers, whereas clozapine and quetiapine have relatively weak dopamine-blocking properties. The serotonin antagonism is believed to reduce the risk of extrapyramidal side effects (EPSEs) and may protect against tardive dyskinesia as well (see Chapters 5 and 19).

Clinical Management

An overview of drugs used to treat psychotic disorders is presented in Table 20-2 and in Box 20-2. For additional discussion of antipsychotic drugs, see Chapter 5; for information related to pediatric use, see Chapter 19.

As shown in Table 20-2, the dosages of these neuroleptics vary tremendously. In general, the low-potency neuroleptics such as chlorpromazine and thioridazine require higher dosages and are more likely to be accompanied by sedation and anticholinergic effects. The high-potency compounds such as thiothixene, trifluoperazine, and haloperidol are effective at much lower dosages. However, these agents are also associated with an increased risk of dystonic reactions, akathisia, and parkinsonism.

Clozapine, which is not recommended for use with children younger than 16, has proved effective in treating patients with schizophrenia who have failed to respond to standard antipsychotic medications. However, clozapine can cause life-threatening agranulocytosis and hence is generally not used unless standard antipsychotic medications have failed.

Risperidone, an atypical antipsychotic medication that has not been associated with agranulocytosis, has shown promise for treating adolescents with psychosis.[40,64] These open-label studies show that although effective, risperidone is not free of EPSEs. For example, 6 of 10 youngsters (age range 7 to 17 years) treated by

Table 20-2 Commonly Used Antipsychotic Agents for the Treatment of Psychosis and Severe Behavior Disturbance in Adolescents

Name of drug	Class	Typical dose range (mg/day)	Studied in adolescents
Chlorpromazine (Thorazine)	Phenothiazine	50-400	Yes
Thioridazine (Mellaril)	Phenothiazine	50-400	Yes
Fluphenazine (Prolixin)	Phenothiazine	2-8	Minimal
Haloperidol (Haldol)	Butyrophenone	2-10	Yes
Thiothixene (Navane)	Thioxanthene	8-40	Yes
Loxapine (Loxitane)	Dibenzoxazepine	60-100	Yes
Clozapine (Clozaril)	Dibenzodiazepine	100-700	Yes
Risperidone (Risperdal)	Benzisoxazole	2-8	Yes
Olanzapine (Zyprexa)	Thienobenzodiazepine	2.5	No
Quetiapine (Seroquel)	Dibenzothiazepine	100-400	Minimal

Box 20-2 Guidelines for Selected Antipsychotic Drugs Used to Treat Adolescents with Psychotic Disorders

Thioridazine (Mellaril)
Start with 25 to 50 mg bid or tid depending on severity of presenting symptoms. Dosage can be gradually increased over 1-3 wk as tolerated to bring about symptomatic relief. A typical dose is 200 mg/day in 2 or 3 divided doses. Common side effects include sedation, weight gain, dry mouth, and blurred vision. Extrapyramidal effects are not common.

Trifluoperazine (Stelazine)
Start with 1 to 5 mg bid, with gradual increases over 2-3 weeks up to 15 mg/day in 2 divided doses. Common side effects include dystonic reactions, akathisia, and drowsiness.

Thiothixene (Navane)
Start with 2 mg tid and gradually increase to 5 mg tid or higher if necessary. Typical dosage is 15-20 mg/day in 3 divided doses. Common side effects include drowsiness, dystonic reactions, weight gain, and akathisia.

Haloperidol (Haldol)
Start with 0.5 to 2 mg bid or tid. Higher starting dosage may be required in acutely disturbed adolescents. The dosage can then be adjusted upward to achieve symptomatic control or decrease to manage side effects. Average dosage is about 10 mg/day in 2 or 3 divided doses. The maintenance dose can usually be given twice daily. Common side effects include muscle rigidity, dystonic reactions, akathisia, weight gain, and cognitive blunting.

Loxapine (Loxitane)
Start with 10 mg bid and adjust according to therapeutic and adverse effects. Typical dosage is 80 mg/day. Higher dosages may be required in some cases, but dosage does not usually exceed 100 mg/day. Common side effects include muscle rigidity and sedation.

Clozapine (Clozaril)
Start with 25 mg qd or bid and increase daily over a 2-wk period to a target dose range of 300 to 450 mg/day. The dosage is then increased more slowly as needed to achieve benefit. A dosage of 700 mg/day is usually considered the maximum daily dose for adolescents. Side effects include weight gain (which can be substantial), tachycardia, orthostatic hypotension, seizures (risk appears to be dose related), and agranulocytosis, which occurs in as many as 2% of patients (adults).

Risperidone (Risperdal)
Start with 0.5 mg bid and increase in 0.5-mg every 3-4 days to a total dose of 3 mg/day in 2 divided doses. Thereafter, the dosage should be increased more slowly, (e.g., weekly). The average dose range is 2-4 mg/day. Side effects include weight gain, drowsiness, dystonic reactions (especially if the dosage increased too rapidly), dizziness, tachycardia, and anxiety.

Mandoki experienced EPSEs such as dystonia, muscle rigidity, dyskinesia, and oculogyric crises.[40] Comparing these observations with other open-label studies of risperidone in children and adolescents for other problems, it appears that the risk of EPSEs with risperidone is related to the rate of dosage increase. With slower upward dosage schedules, EPSEs can usually be avoided.[21,39,45]

The other newer atypical neuroleptics, olanzapine, quetiapine, and ziprasidone, have been described in several recent reviews.[20,36,57]

LITHIUM
Indications: Bipolar Disorder

Lithium is a naturally occurring element that is indicated for treating bipolar disorder. A full discussion of lithium can be found in Chapter 6.

The DSM-IV identifies two broad types: bipolar I and bipolar II. Bipolar I is characterized by the occurrence of a manic episode but may occur in the absence of depression. In contrast, bipolar II disorder is marked by a history of major depression and hypomanic episodes.[3] A manic episode is defined by the presence of elevated or irritable mood and three or more additional clinical features (Box 20-3).

The occurrence of bipolar illness in young children is presumed to be rare. By late adolescence, the prevalence appears to be similar to that observed in adults. The prevalence of bipolar illness in adolescents has recently been estimated at approximately 1%.[38] In a large community survey, the authors identified 18 cases of bipolar illness, 11 of which were bipolar II cases; that is, the subjects had histories of depression. Girls were affected more often than boys. The mean age of onset for the whole group was about 12 years, with depression being the most common feature present at onset. This finding is consistent with a prospective study of 79 children with major depression in which nearly a third went on to develop bipolar illness.[23]

Two other findings from the community survey by Lewinsohn, Klein, and Seeley are worth noting.[38] First, the authors identified 97 youth with "core symptoms" of bipolar illness but who did not meet the full criteria for bipolar illness. Although these youngsters (55 girls and 42 boys) did not meet the criteria for bipolar illness, a high percentage of these youngsters showed evidence of functional impairment. Second, of the 18 bipolar cases identified, only one had been treated with lithium. These findings underscore the importance of careful assessment before initiating therapy so that subclinical cases are not treated inappropriately and true cases are not overlooked.

Box 20-3 Definition of a Manic Episode

A manic episode includes three or more of the following:
- Grandiosity
- Pressured speech or excessive talking
- Decreased need for sleep
- Flight of ideas or racing thoughts
- Distractibility
- Hyperactivity
- Excessive pleasure-seeking behavior

The findings of this study are relevant to the current controversy about bipolar illness in children and adolescents. Several authors have described case series of children and adolescents with bipolar illness.[11,23,69,79] Although all these studies ascertained the subjects from clinical settings, the case definition was not uniform across these studies. This lack of uniformity suggests some authors may have included cases from the *subclinical* cases identified by Lewinsohn, Klein, and Seeley, whereas others applied more strict diagnostic criteria.[38] It is unclear what portion of this subclinical group will go on to manifest a full bipolar picture. Similarly, it is unclear whether this potential *subclinical* variant of bipolar illness is responsive to mood-stabilizing drugs. An answer to the first question awaits results of community-based and clinic-based prospective studies. An answer to the second question regarding response of bipolar core symptoms to mood-stabilizing drugs also awaits further study. On one hand, it may be argued that identification of adolescents with core symptoms of bipolar illness represents early detection of a serious psychiatric disorder. If so, treatment could slow the progress of bipolar illness. On the other hand, not all *subclinical cases* will go on to develop the full syndrome. These adolescents could be exposed to potent drug treatment unnecessarily. Given this uncertainty, it is essential that treatment studies of adolescents with core symptoms of bipolar illness be prospective in design, with clear descriptions of the target symptoms.

Empirical Support

The evidence supporting the use of lithium in adolescents with bipolar disorder derives from case reports, open trials, and a small number of controlled trials. These studies suggest that lithium is effective and safe in adolescents with bipolar illness. Nonetheless, for reasons that are not clear, lithium is not always successful in treating adolescents with bipolar illness.[1] A naturalistic study by Strober and others showed that youngsters with bipolar illness who discontinued lithium were three times more likely to relapse compared with those who remained on maintenance therapy.[68] This finding suggests, as is seen in adults with bipolar illness, that lithium may have prophylactic value for preventing future manic episodes.

Mechanism of Action

Lithium is an alkali metal and is in the same chemical family as sodium and potassium. Although it has been used to treat psychiatric disorders for more than four decades, only recently have its complex neurophysiologic effects begun to be understood. Lithium is known to enhance several neurotransmitter systems, including serotonin, norepinephrine, and dopamine. In addition, lithium has other neurobiologic effects on ion channels and other cellular activity.[1,16]

Clinical Management

Before starting a trial of lithium, the adolescent with bipolar illness should have a thorough medical evaluation, including a physical examination and a careful medical history. Laboratory screening measures to assess thyroid and renal function, as well as an ECG and complete blood count, should also be obtained. Lithium is excreted by the kidneys; thus renal impairment could affect dosing and drug levels. Lithium can decrease free thyroxine and triiodothyronine, but increased thyroid-releasing hormone typically compensates in euthyroid patients. Cardiac complications of lithium are not common, but it has been reported to alter cardiac conduction in some cases. Occasionally, lithium also causes elevated white blood cell and platelet counts. Thus renal function, thyroid function, ECG, and blood count should be monitored every 6 months or so during maintenance therapy. Girls of childbearing age should be counseled about the importance of preventing pregnancy while taking lithium because of the elevated risk for birth defects following fetal exposure.

Healthy adolescents usually tolerate lithium well, and the dosage can be increased rapidly to therapeutic levels (between 0.6 and 1.2 mEq/L). The initial dose of 300 to 600 mg may be given after a meal to decrease gastrointestinal (GI) side effects. Thereafter, the dosage can be increased by 300 to 600 mg every 4 to 5 days to the typical dosage range of 1500 to 1800 mg/day in two divided doses. Levels should be checked 3 to 4 days after dose increases and every 2 months after the typical dose range has been reached. The maintenance dose of lithium is usually lower, for example, 900 to 1200 mg/day, than the initial dose required to achieve therapeutic blood levels.[25,73] How long an adolescent patient should remain on lithium following the resolution of a manic episode is unclear, but most researchers recommend 18 months to 2 years of stability before beginning a gradual withdrawal of the drug.[16,73]

Side Effects

Lithium can have serious side effects, but children and adolescents appear to tolerate it well. Common side effects include weight gain, tremor, headache, and GI upset (nausea, vomiting, and diarrhea). The stomach upset can often be reduced by administering the medication after meals. Other side effects include polydipsia, polyuria, ataxia, weakness, dysarthria, and mental confusion. Lithium may also exacerbate acne.

Interactions

Drugs with the ability to interact with lithium are discussed in Chapter 6.

Toxic Effects

Lithium has a low therapeutic index, necessitating frequent serum level analysis. Adolescents should be advised that they might be required to measure lithium blood levels frequently. Lithium levels can be determined from saliva specimens, although saliva-to-serum ratios show tremendous individual variation. Because dehydration can lead to toxic levels of lithium, parents and adolescents should also be advised to maintain adequate hydration. Parents should be instructed to hold the medication if the child has a GI illness accompanied by frequent vomiting or diarrhea. Other toxic effects of lithium are discussed in Chapter 6.

OTHER DRUGS USED IN THE TREATMENT OF BIPOLAR DISORDER
Valproate

Lithium is the drug of choice for bipolar disorder in adolescents, but a substantial minority of patients do not respond to lithium.[1] Valproate (Depakote) is an anticonvulsant medication that has been effective in treating adults with acute mania. To date, there have been only a few case reports in adolescents.[75,76] In these two studies, West and others treated a total of 16 adolescents with bipolar illness, all of whom had failed on standard treatment. Of these 16 patients, 13 responded positively to valproate, with a minimum of adverse effects. In the second of these open trials, the investigators used a relatively large initial dose (20 mg/kg) in the hope of achieving more rapid stabilization.[75] This strategy achieved clinically meaningful response in four of the five patients within several days as opposed to several weeks with more conservative dosage increases. However, these findings should be regarded with caution because of the small sample size and the nonblinded design of the study.

Donovan and colleagues evaluated the effectiveness of valproate on 10 adolescents with disruptive and frequent bouts of out of control behavior.[18] This open-label study reflects a growing sentiment in the field that valproate may be useful for the core symptoms of bipolar disorder. The support for using valproate for these target symptoms is extremely limited.

Following a careful workup as described for lithium, the medication may be initiated at 100 mg twice daily and gradually increased to reach serum levels of 50 to 100 µg/ml. Side effects include GI upset, tremor, and skin eruptions. In children being treated for seizure disorders, there have been reports of cognitive dulling and a few cases of fatal liver toxicity. These cases had acute onsets and occurred in children younger than 10. Safety monitoring during maintenance therapy should include complete blood counts, liver function tests, and drug levels. There have also been reports of polycystic ovary disease in women being treated with valproate for seizure disorders.[31] In their sample of 78 women, 23 had polycystic ovaries. Patients who began treatment in their teen years were more likely to develop this complication. The potential for developing polycystic ovaries in adolescent girls raises serious questions about the risk-to-benefit ratio of valproate for the treatment of core symptoms of bipolar illness versus the full syndrome.

Carbamazepine

Carbamazepine (Tegretol) is an anticonvulsant that has been used in children and adolescents with seizure disorders for many years. It has also been shown to be an effective alternative for mood stabilization in adults. Unfortunately, there are very few studies demonstrating its efficacy in adolescents with bipolar illness.[16,25] The mechanism of action is not clear, but it is believed to reduce firing from the amygdala and turn down the limbic system.[73]

The medical assessments just described for lithium are also appropriate before initiating a trial of carbamazepine. The starting dose for adolescents is usually 100 to 200 mg daily and is gradually increased weekly by 200 mg to reach a blood level of 4 to 12 µg/ml. This blood level has not been established as the therapeutic range for adolescents with bipolar illness; however, experience with adult patients who have bipolar illness and children with seizure disorders suggests that levels above this range can result in toxicity. The usual maintenance dose range is 10 to 20 mg/kg/day given in two or three divided doses.[16]

Side effects include dizziness, sedation, irritability, nausea and vomiting, and diplopia. These side effects are most likely to occur early in treatment, especially if the dosage is increased too rapidly. Skin rashes occur in 10% to 15% of patients. Carbamazepine has also been reported to cause reversible agranulocytosis in 2% to 3% of patients. Aplastic anemia is a rare adverse effect.

DRUGS USED IN THE TREATMENT OF AGGRESSIVE BEHAVIOR

A substantial percentage of children and adolescents referred for emotional or behavioral problems exhibit aggressive behavior. Indeed, aggressive behavior is associated with several different psychiatric diagnoses, including ADHD, schizophrenia, bipolar disorder, conduct disorder, paranoid thinking, and seizure disorders.[42] Control of aggressive behavior is also a critically important clinical management issue for adolescent inpatient psychiatric units.

Several different classes of psychopharmacologic agents have been used to treat aggressive states. Information presented in Chapter 11 is appropriate for older adolescents. A brief review is provided here as additional guidance to managing younger adolescents.

Neuroleptics

Neuroleptics are used for managing acute aggressive behavior and as an ongoing treatment approach. Youths who require immediate treatment can be given an intramuscular dose of chlorpromazine at 0.5 mg/kg every 6 to 8 hours as needed. For severely agitated adolescents, an intramuscular dose of 25 mg may be given and repeated in 1 hour. Thereafter, injections should be spaced at least 4 to 6 hours apart. A 12-year-old child should not receive more than 75 mg intramuscularly per day.

For the longer-term treatment of aggressive behavior, several studies have shown that chlorpromazine, thioridazine, haloperidol, and risperidone are useful. To date, no controlled studies of risperidone have been published, but open-label data in various pediatric populations suggest that it is likely to be an effective treatment. For each of these neuroleptics, dosages tend to be lower than those used for psychosis. Side effects are similar to those described earlier in the section on psychotic disorders.

Lithium

A series of double-blind studies showed that lithium was as effective as chlorpromazine and haloperidol, although better tolerated, for treating aggressive behavior.[8,9] More recently, lithium was examined in a double-blind study of 50 children and adolescents and was found to be superior to placebo.[10] The clinical management of lithium for aggression is essentially the same as that described earlier in the section on bipolar disorders.

Alpha-2 Adrenergic Agonists

The alpha-2 adrenergic drugs clonidine (Catapres) and guanfacine (Tenex) were developed as antihypertensive agents. Beginning with the early studies of clonidine for Tourette's syndrome, these drugs have become increasingly common in child psychiatry for tics, ADHD, and aggressive behavior (see Chapter 19).[46,54,55] Despite evidence of increased use, the alpha-2 agonists have not been well studied in children or adolescents for the treatment of aggression.

The typical starting dose of clonidine is 0.05 mg at bedtime; then it is increased by 0.05 mg every 3 to 4 days to a total of 0.15 to 0.2 mg/day in three or four divided doses.

Guanfacine is a newer alpha-2 agonist medication that has a slightly longer duration of action than clonidine. To date, it has shown promise in three open studies in children with ADHD, many of whom also had tics.[54,55,61] A recent controlled study has confirmed these preliminary results. In that study of 34 youngsters, guanfacine was superior to placebo for ADHD symptoms and tics.[55] Guanfacine has not been studied for effectiveness in treating aggressive behavior. The typical starting dose of guanfacine is 0.5 mg at bedtime; then it is increased by 0.5 mg every 3 to 4 days to a total of 1.5 to 3.0 mg/day in three divided doses.

TIC DISORDERS

The treatment of tic disorders is reviewed in detail in Chapter 19.

USE OF COMBINED DRUG THERAPIES

Another trend in pediatric psychopharmacology that warrants mention concerns the increasing use of combined drug therapies.[47,74] Concern about this trend has provoked controversy with the recent report of the deaths of three children who had been treated with methylphenidate and clonidine. A careful review ruled out a causal role for either the combination or the individual medications in these deaths. Nonetheless, because the combination of methylphenidate and clonidine appears to be fairly common, many clinicians and parents were troubled by these reports.[47]

There are various reasons for adding a second medication to treat children and adolescents with psychiatric disorders. First, a second agent may diminish the severity of unwanted side effects produced by the primary therapeutic agent. The addition of benztropine for side effects from neuroleptic medications is an example of this type of combined treatment.

Second, an additional medication is sometimes administered because clinically important symptoms remain that are not addressed by the first medication. For example, some clinicians recommend clonidine at bedtime to reduce the sleep problems in children or adolescents with ADHD. (It should be noted that this practice, although often effective, has become a matter of controversy.[77])

Third, the second medication may be selected in the hope of boosting the treatment benefit of a partially effective medication for the target symptoms. The addition of a neuroleptic to ongoing treatment with an SSRI in refractory OCD and the addition of lithium to an antidepressant for a partial response in depression are examples of this line of reasoning.

Unfortunately, there are very few studies on which to base such difficult clinical decisions. The meager information that is available on combined pharmacotherapies comes primarily from adult studies. As emphasized by Walkup, in lieu of clear evidence on how to proceed with additional strategies, it is essential to be thorough in gathering history and systematic in approaching rational polypharmacy.[74] Careful thought is warranted concerning the potential for drug-drug interaction. On these complex clinical decisions, consulting with colleagues also can be helpful.

REFERENCES

1. Alessi N and others: Update on lithium carbonate therapy in children and adolescents, *J Am Acad Child Adolesc Psychiatry* 33:291, 1994.
2. Ambrosini PJ and others: Multicenter open-label sertraline study in adolescent outpatients with major depression, *J Am Acad Child Adolesc Psychiatry* 38:566, 1999.
3. American Psychiatric Association: *Diagnostic and statistical manual of mental disorders-TR*, ed 4, Washington, DC, 2000, The Association.
4. Barkley RA: *Attention deficit hyperactivity disorder: a handbook for diagnosis and treatment*, ed 2, New York, 1998, Guilford.
5. Barrickman LL and others: Bupropion versus methylphenidate in the treatment of attention-deficit hyperactivity disorder, *J Am Acad Child Adolesc Psychiatry* 34:649, 1995.
6. Baumgaertel A, Wolraich ML, Dietrich M: Comparison for diagnostic criteria for attention deficit disorders in a German elementary school sample, *J Am Acad Child Adolesc Psychiatry* 34:629, 1995.
7. Biederman J and others: A double-blind placebo controlled study of desipramine in the treatment of ADD, Part I: efficacy, *J Am Acad Child Adolesc Psychiatry* 28:777, 1989.

8. Campbell M, Cohen I, Small AM: Drugs in aggressive behavior, *J Am Acad Child Adolesc Psychiatry* 21:107, 1982.

9. Campbell M and others: Behavioral efficacy of haloperidol and lithium carbonate, *Arch Gen Psychiatry* 41:650, 1984.

10. Campbell M and others: Lithium in hospitalized aggressive children with conduct disorder: a double-blind and placebo-controlled study, *J Am Acad Child Adolesc Psychiatry* 34:445, 1995.

11. Carlson GA: Identifying prepubertal mania, *J Am Acad Child Adolesc Psychiatry* 34:750, 1995.

12. Carlson GA, Lavelle J, Bromet EJ: Medication treatment in adolescents vs. adults with psychotic mania, *J Child Adolesc Psychopharmacol* 9:221, 1999.

13. Conners C and others: Bupropion hydrochloride in attention deficit disorder with hyperactivity, *J Am Acad Child Adolesc Psychiatry* 35:1314, 1996.

14. Costello EJ: Prevalence and impact of parent-reported disabling mental health conditions among US children, *J Am Child Adolesc Psychiatry* 38;5, 1999.

15. Costello EJ, Angold A, Burns BJ: The Great Smoky Mountains study of youth: Goals, design, methods, and the prevalence of DSM-III-R disorders, *Arch Gen Psychiatry* 53:1129, 1996.

16. Davanzo PA, McCracken JT: Mood stabilizers in the treatment of juvenile bipolar disorders: Advances and controversies, *Child Adolesc Psychiatr Clin North Am* 9:159, 2000.

17. DeVeaugh-Geiss J and others: Clomipramine in child and adolescent obsessive-compulsive disorder: a multicenter trial, *J Am Acad Child Adolesc Psychiatry* 31:45, 1992.

18. Donovan SJ and others: Divalproex treatment of disruptive adolescents: a report of 10 cases, *J Clin Psychiatry* 58:12, 1997.

19. Emslie GJ and others: A double-bind, randomized, placebo-controlled trial of fluoxetine in children and adolescents with depression, *Arch Gen Psychiatry* 54:1031, 1997.

20. Findling RL and others: The antipsychotics: a pediatric perspective, *Pediatr Clin North Am* 45:1205, 1998.

21. Fisman S, Steele M: Use of risperidone in pervasive developmental disorders: a case series, *J Child Adolesc Psychopharmacol* 6:177, 1996.

22. Flockhart DA, Oesterheld JR: Cytochrome P450-mediated drug interactions, *Child Adolesc Psychiatr Clin North Am* 9:43, 2000.

23. Geller B, Fox LW, Clark KA: Rate and predictors of prepubertal bipolarity during follow-up of 6- to 12-year-old depressed children, *J Am Acad Child Adolesc Psychiatry* 33:461, 1994.

24. Grados, Scahill, Riddle: Pharmacotherapy in children and adolescents with obsessive-compulsive disorder, *Child Adolesc Psychiatr Clin North Am* 8:617, 1999.

25. Green WH: *Child and adolescent clinical psychopharmacology,* Baltimore, 1995, Williams & Wilkins.

26. Greenhill LL and others: Medication treatment strategies in the MTA study: relevance to clinicians and researchers, *J Am Acad Child Adolesc Psychiatry* 35(10):1304, 1996

27. Hechtman L: Long-term outcome in attention-deficit hyperactivity disorder, *Child Adolesc Psychiatr Clin North Am* 1:553, 1992.

28. Horwitz SM and others: Identification and management of psychosocial and developmental problems in community-based primary care pediatric practices, *Pediatrics* 89:480, 1992.

29. Institute of Medicine: *Research on children and adolescents with mental, behavioral, and developmental disorder,* Washington, DC, 1989, National Academy Press.

30. Isacsson G and others: Psychotropics and suicide prevention: implications from toxicological screening of 5281 suicides in Sweden 1992-1994, *Br J Psychiatry* 174:259, 1999.

31. Isojarvi JI and others: Polycystic ovaries and hyperandrogenism in women taking valproate for epilepsy, *N Engl J Med* 329:1383, 1993.

32. Kalogerakis MG: Emergency evaluation of adolescents, *Hosp Community Psychiatry* 43(6): 617, 1992.

33. Kann L and others: Youth risk behavior surveillance: United States, 1993, *J Sch Health* 65: 163, 1995.

34. Keller MB and others: Paroxetine and imipramine in the treatment of adolescent depression. In Program and Abstracts on New Research from the 151st Annual Meeting of the American Psychiatric Association. Toronto, Ontario, American Psychiatric Association, 1998.

35. King RA and others: Emergence of self-destructive phenomena in children and adolescents during fluoxetine treatment, *J Am Acad Child Adolesc Psychiatry* 30:179, 1991.

36. Kumra S: The diagnosis and treatment of children and adolescents with schizophrenia, *Child Adolesc Psychiatr Clin North Am* 9:183, 2000.

37. Laraia MT: Current approaches to the psychopharmacologic treatment of depression in children and adolescents, *J Child Adolesc Psychiatr Nurs* 9:15, 1996.

38. Lewinsohn PM, Klein DN, Seeley JR: Bipolar disorders in a community sample of older adolescents: prevalence, phenomenology, comorbidity, and course, *J Am Acad Child Adolesc Psychiatry* 34:454, 1995.

39. Lombroso PJ and others: Risperidone treatment of children and adolescents with chronic tic disorders: a preliminary report, *J Am Acad Child Adolesc Psychiatry* 34:1147, 1995

40. Mandoki MW: Risperidone treatment of children and adolescents: increased risk of extrapyramidal side effects, *J Child Adolesc Psychopharmacol* 5:49, 1995.

41. March JS and others: Sertraline in children and adolescents with obsessive-compulsive disorder: a multicenter randomized controlled trial, *JAMA* 280:1752, 1998.

42. Marohn RC: Management of the assaultive adolescent, *Hosp Community Psychiatry* 43(6): 622, 1992.

43. Martin A, Kaufman J, Charney D: Pharmacotherapy of early-onset depression: update and new directions, *Child Adolesc Psychiatr Clin North Am* 9:135, 2000.

44. McClellan J, Werry J: Practice parameters for the assessment and treatment of children and adolescents with schizophrenia, *J Am Acad Child Adolesc Psychiatry* 33:616, 1994.

45. McDougal and others: Risperidone treatment of children and adolescents with pervasive developmental disorders: a prospective open-label study, *J Am Acad Child Adolesc Psychiatry* 36:685, 1997.

46. McDougal and others: Research Units on Pediatric Psychopharmacology (RUPP): background and rationale for an initial controlled study of risperidone, *Child Adolesc Psychiatr Clin North Am* 9:201, 2000.

47. Popper CW: Combining methylphenidate and clonidine: pharmacologic questions and news reports about sudden death, *J Child Adolesc Psychopharmacol* 5:157, 1995.

48. Pottick K and others: Factors associated with inpatient and outpatient treatment for children and adolescents with serious mental illness, *J Am Acad Child Adolesc Psychiatry* 34:425, 1995.

49. Riddle MA and others: *A controlled trial of fluvoxamine for OCD in children and adolescents,* Boca Raton, FL, 1996, NCDEU.

50. Riddle MA, Geller B, Ryan N: Another sudden death in a child treated with desipramine, *J Am Acad Child Adolesc Psychiatry* 32:792, 1993.

51. Riddle MA, Lebellarte MJ, Walkup JT: Pediatric psychopharmacology: problems and prospects, *J Child Adolesc Psychopharmacol* 8:87, 1998.

52. Riddle MA and others: Behavioral side effects of fluoxetine, *J Child Adolesc Psychopharmacol* 3:193, 1991.

53. Riddle MA and others: Double-blind, crossover trial of fluoxetine and placebo in children and adolescents with obsessive compulsive disorder, *J Am Acad Child Adolesc Psychiatry* 31: 1062, 1992.

54. Scahill L, Barloon L, Farkas L: Alpha-2 agonists in the treatment of attention deficit hyperactivity disorder, *J Child Adolesc Psychiatric Nurs* 12:168, 1999.

55. Scahill L, Koenig K: Pharmacotherapy in children and adolescents with pervasive developmental disorders, *J Child Adolesc Psychiatr Nurs* 12:41, 1999.

56. Scahill L, Lynch KA: Tricyclic antidepressants: cardiac effects and clinical implications, *J Child Adolesc Psychiatr Nurs* 7:37, 1994.

57. Scahill L, Lynch KA: Atypical neuroleptics in children and adolescents, *J Child Adolesc Psychiatr Nurs* 11:38, 1998.

58. Scahill L, Ort SJ: Clinical ratings in child psychiatric nursing, *J Child Adolesc Psychiatr Nurs* 8:33, 1995.

59. Scahill L, Skrypeck A: The use of traditional neuroleptics in children and adolescents, *J Child Adolesc Psychiatr Nurs* 10:41, 1997.

60. Scahill L and others: Fluoxetine has no marked affect on tic symptoms in patients with Tourette's syndrome: a double-blind placebo-controlled study, *J Child Adolesc Psychopharmacol* 7:75, 1997.
61. Scahill L and others: A placebo-controlled study of guanfacine in the treatment of attention deficit hyperactivity disorder and tic disorders. Presented at the Annual Meeting of the American Academy of Child and Adolescent Psychiatry, Chicago, IL, October 1999.
62. Schachar R, Tannock R: Childhood hyperactivity and psychostimulants: a review of extended treatment studies, *J Child Adolesc Psychopharmacol* 3:81, 1993.
63. Sikich LM and others: Allergic reactions to bupropion in child psychiatric inpatients: a case series. Poster presentation at the annual meeting of the American Academy of Child and Adolescent Psychiatry, New Orleans, October 1995.
64. Simeon JG and others: Risperidone effects in treatment-resistant adolescents: preliminary case reports, *J Child Adolesc Psychopharmacol* 5:69, 1995.
65. Singer HS and others: The treatment of attention-deficit hyperactivity disorder in Tourette's syndrome: a double-blind placebo-controlled study with clonidine and desipramine, *Pediatrics* 95:74, 1995.
66. Spencer T and others: Nortriptyline treatment of children with attention-deficit hyperactivity disorder and tic disorder or Tourette's syndrome, *J Am Acad Child Adolesc Psychiatry* 32: 205, 1993.
67. Spencer T and others: Pharmacotherapy of attention deficit hyperactivity disorder, *Child Adolesc Psychiatr Clin North Am* 9:77, 2000.
68. Strober M and others: Relapse following discontinuation of lithium maintenance therapy in adolescents with bipolar-I illness: a naturalistic study, *Am J Psychiatry* 147:457, 1990.
69. Strober and others: Recover and relapse in adolescents with bipolar affective illness: a five year naturalistic, prospective follow-up, *J Am Acad Child Adolesc Psychiatry* 34:724, 1995.
70. Szatmari P, Offord DR, Boyle MH. Ontario Child Health Study: prevalence of attention deficit disorder with hyperactivity, *J Child Psychol Psychiatr* 30:219, 1989.
71. Thomsen PH: Child and adolescent obsessive-compulsive disorder treated with citalopram: findings from an open trial of 23 cases, *J Child Adolesc Psychopharmacology* 7:157, 1997.
72. Velosa JF, Riddle MA: Pharmacologic treatment of anxiety disorders in children and adolescents, *Child Adolesc Psychiatr Clin North Am* 9:119, 2000.
73. Viesselman JO: Antidepressant and antimanic drugs. In Werry JS, Aman MG, editors: *Practitioner's guide to psychoactive drugs for children and adolescents,* ed 2, New York, 1999, Plenum.
74. Walkup JT: Clinical decision making in child and adolescent psychopharmacology, *Child Adolesc Psychiatr Clin North Am* 4:23, 1995.
75. West SA, Keck PE, McElroy SL: Oral loading doses in the valproate treatment of adolescents with mixed bipolar disorder, *J Child Adolesc Psychopharmacol* 5:225, 1995.
76. West SA and others: Open trial of valproate in the treatment of adolescent mania, *J Child Adolesc Psychopharmacol* 4:263, 1994.
77. Wilens TE, Spencer TJ: Combining methylphenidate and clonidine: a clinically sound mediation option, *J Am Acad Child Adolesc Psychiatry* 38:5, 1999.
78. Wolraich ML, Hannah JN, Baumgaertel A, Feurer ID: Examination of DSM-IV criteria for attention deficit/hyperactivity disorder in a county-wide sample, *J Dev Behav Pediatr* 19: 162, 1998.
79. Wozniak J and others: Mania-like symptoms suggestive of childhood onset bipolar disorder in clinically referred children, *J Am Acad Child Adolesc Psychiatry* 34:867, 1995.
80. Zito JM and others: Trends in the prescribing of psychotropic medications to preschoolers, *JAMA* 283:1025, 2000.

CHAPTER 21

———— ● ————

Psychopharmacology for Elderly Persons

Pharmacotherapy in older patients may be complicated by multiple factors, including the following:

1. Physiologic effects of aging
2. Pharmacokinetic and pharmacodynamic changes
3. Polypharmacy and resultant drug interactions
4. Variability of treatment settings
5. Coexisting medical conditions
6. Cognitive impairment
7. Reduced functional capacity
8. Decreased life expectancy
9. Compliance issues

All the factors listed above are important considerations in the effective pharmacologic approach to treating a geriatric patient. When pharmacologic treatment is indicated for an older patient, specific knowledge of drug actions and effects are essential. The following are the ultimate goals of psychotropic drug therapy for an older patient:

1. To improve symptoms
2. To improve functioning and quality of life
3. To decrease morbidity
4. To decrease rates of health care utilization and decrease mortality

The enhancement of communication and understanding between an older patient and the clinician can significantly improve the overall quality of care provided to elderly patients.

The psychopharmacologic treatment of geriatric patients requires knowledge of psychiatric and nonpsychiatric conditions that are prevalent in these patients. An appreciation of coexistent medical conditions may be critical to safe and effective drug treatment. Knowledge of bioepidemiologic differences among older adults will enable the clinician to individualize treatment plans and evaluate responses to drug intervention. Most data on older populations report the following:

1. Elderly individuals are taking unnecessary drugs.
2. Drug dosage can be decreased.
3. A safer alternative drug can be substituted.[2,14]

SCOPE OF THE PROBLEM

The geriatric population is growing at a remarkable rate. Several factors are chiefly responsible for the disproportionate rate of growth that is occurring in this segment of the population:

1. Decreased infant mortality
2. Declining birth rates
3. Increased life expectancy
4. Declining death rates for those older than 65

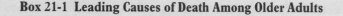

Box 21-1 Leading Causes of Death Among Older Adults

Heart disease
Cancer, malignant neoplasms
Stroke, cerebrovascular disease
Alzheimer's disease and related disorders

Infection: influenza, pneumonia
Accidents: falls and motor-pedestrian
  fatalities
Suicide

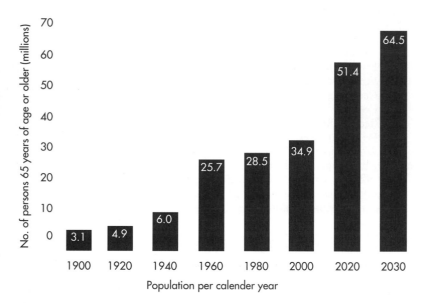

Figure 21-1 Geriatric population demographics through the year 2030. The disproportionate growth rate for the geriatric population in the United States is evident. (From Folks DG: Clinical approaches to anxiety in the medically ill elderly, *Drug Ther Suppl* Aug:72, 1990.)

As depicted in Figure 21-1, the significant rate of growth among the elderly population has occurred steadily since 1900, when about 3.1 million people, or 4% of the population in the United States, were older than 65. Currently, approximately 15% of the population, or 35 million individuals, have reached their 65th birthday. This age group accounts for 25% to 50% of a primary care practitioner's caseload. By 2030, when the last of the "baby boomers" reach their 65th birthdays, it is estimated 65 million people (approximately 20% to 25% of the U.S. population) will be older than 65. The declining death rate for those older than 65 and increased longevity is primarily responsible for the rapid growth of the "true elderly segment," that is, those older than 85. This subsegment of the elderly population will continue to be the most rapidly growing of all age groups. It is staggering to realize that this elderly subsegment of the population will more than double in the next decade, with a growth rate many times greater than that of the adolescent segment of our population.

Psychiatric disorders are not generally encountered in isolation in geriatric patients. Acute, life-threatening illness and prevalent chronic general medical

---

Box 21-2   Chronic General Medical Conditions in Older Adults

Arthritis and rheumatologic disease
Neurosensory loss: hearing disturbance, visual disturbance
Cardiovascular disease: congestive heart failure, ischemic heart disease,
    hypertension, peripheral vascular disease
Gastrointestinal disorders
Chronic sinusitis and upper respiratory disturbances
Genitourinary tract problems
Chronic obstructive pulmonary disease
Adult-onset diabetes mellitus
Thyroid disease, endocrinopathy
Dermatologic disturbances

Box 21-3   Psychobiologic Changes with Aging

Autonomic nervous system	Hearing and vision
Behavioral and personality function	Immune function
Bone density	Pulmonary function
Body composition	Renal function
Cognitive function	Skin
Glucose tolerance	Systolic blood pressure

---

conditions require careful consideration with respect to intervention with psychiatric agents. Multiple disease processes, common environmental influences, and genetic variation often combine with the physiologic or psychobiologic effects of aging to significantly influence pharmacologic treatment outcomes (Boxes 21-1, 21-2, and 21-3). Of course, physiologic aging does not necessarily parallel chronologic aging. Apart from the prominent effects of overt disease states, physiologic aging more often underlies the age-related differences observed in the action of psychotropic drugs.

GENERAL FACTORS PERTINENT TO PSYCHOTROPIC DRUG THERAPY

This section outlines the pharmacokinetic, pharmacodynamic, and nontherapeutic effects of drugs as they relate to psychotropics used to treat geriatric patients. In addition, issues relating to compliance are outlined. These factors determine many of the general principles that are useful in the clinical approach to common psychiatric syndromes encountered in late life.

Pharmacokinetics

Pharmacokinetics refers to what the body does to a drug with respect to absorption, distribution, metabolism, and elimination. Altered pharmacokinetics in elderly individuals results in part from physiologic changes that accompany aging. The predictable age-related changes in body composition and organ function in older adults also result in altered pharmacokinetics. These changes include diminished renal function, diminished hepatic blood flow, decreased serum albumin level and lean muscle mass, decreased total body water, and increased alpha-1 acid glycoprotein (AGP) concentrations. Thus age-related differences and drug disposition are multifactorial and are significantly influenced by environmental, genetic, physiologic, and pathologic factors.

Most studies of older populations and pharmacokinetics are cross sectional and merely provide information about the average age-related differences. Because of the difficulties in design, administration, and cost of longitudinal studies, few studies have provided a precise picture of the changes in pharmacokinetics that occur within an aging cohort. Whereas some age-related physiologic changes profoundly affect drug kinetics, for example, renal function, others, such as gastrointestinal (GI) absorption, do not appear to alter pharmacokinetic values consistently.

Absorption. Changes in absorption of drugs related to aging include the following:

1. Increased gastric pH
2. Decreased absorptive surface area
3. Decreased splanchnic blood flow
4. Decreased GI motility
5. Delayed gastric emptying

Despite several age-related alterations that occur in the GI tract, such as increased gastric pH, delayed gastric emptying, diminished blood flow, and impaired intestinal motility, few psychotropic drugs actually show any delayed rates of GI tract absorption after oral administration. Thus the anatomic and physiologic changes that occur with aging in the GI tract have little effect on drug metabolism.

The term *bioavailability* refers to the relative amount of drug reaching the systemic circulation after absorption. The bioavailability of a drug is determined not only by the extent of absorption through the GI tract but also by the presystemic drug elimination in the liver as the drug passes from the portal circulation. The bioavailability of drugs is generally unchanged in older adults, except in the case of those drugs that are abstracted at a high rate by the liver. Decreased presystemic hepatic extraction leads to modest increases in the bioavailability of certain drugs, for example, beta-blockers. However, these findings have no real clinical significance. In contrast, pathologic and surgical alterations in the GI tract and interactions between psychotropics and drugs such as laxatives, antacids, and agents that decrease gastric emptying may alter absorption.

Distribution. Changes in distribution of drugs related to aging include the following:

1. Increased body fat
2. Decreased lean body mass
3. Decreased total body water
4. Decreased serum albumin
5. Decreased cardiac output

Changes in body composition (Figure 21-2) and blood flow may profoundly affect drug distribution in an older adult.[16] A decrease in total body water and lean body mass, combined with a proportional increase in body fat, undoubtedly affects the volume of distribution of many drugs. Water-soluble drugs (e.g., ethanol, lithium) have a reduced volume of distribution in elderly individuals, with increased initial concentrations in the central compartment and resultant higher plasma concentrations. Lipid-soluble drugs (e.g., the benzodiazepines) tend to have a much greater

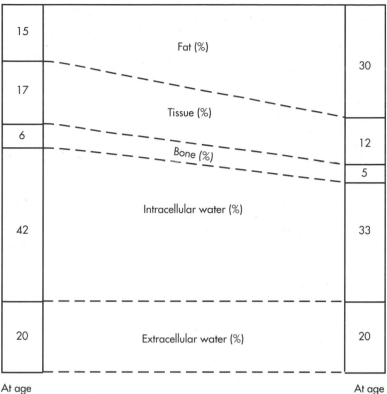

At age 25 years		At age 75 years
15	Fat (%)	30
17	Tissue (%)	
6	Bone (%)	12
		5
42	Intracellular water (%)	33
20	Extracellular water (%)	20

Figure 21-2 Representation of changes in body composition in the "average" individual, comparing body composition at 25 and 75 years of age. (From Folks DG: Clinical approaches to anxiety in the medically ill elderly, *Drug Ther Suppl* Aug:92, 1990.)

distribution in older persons because of the average increase in body fat. Interestingly, some lipophilic drugs, most notably lorazepam (Ativan) and amobarbital (Amytal), do not have significantly different volumes of distribution with increased age. When the volume of distribution is increased for an anxiolytic or another psychotropic, as is the case with diazepam (Valium), the result may be a prolonged action because of an even longer elimination half-life, as discussed in Chapter 7.

Free and unbound drug concentrations are important determinants of both drug distribution and elimination. Thus alterations in the binding of drugs to plasma proteins, red blood cells, and metabolic organs can and do alter pharmacokinetic properties in elderly persons. Theoretically, the age-driven tendency is toward lower protein binding of drugs related to decline in serum albumin concentrations and alterations in albumin receptor configuration. However, the clinical impact resulting from alteration of plasma proteins is not thought to be marked in most cases. In fact, the equilibrium between bound and unbound drug does not change significantly in most elderly patients. Thus the amount of free unbound psychotropic drug available (and necessary) to produce desired clinical effects often remains unchanged, although the total amount of protein binding is diminished.

In contrast, chronic diseases may be associated with substantial reductions in serum albumin levels. In this case, it is important to note that weakly acidic drugs (e.g., barbiturates, phenytoin [Dilantin]) bind primarily to plasma albumin. Weak bases such as propranolol (Inderal) are bound primarily to AGP, so some degree of variability would exist in the concentration of this specific agent (i.e., propranolol) because AGP concentrations tend to increase with age. Thus, in elderly persons, the decrease in albumin and the increase in AGP concentrations may be associated with both reduced and increased protein bindings of drugs.

Metabolism. Changes in the metabolism of drugs related to aging include the following:
1. Decreased hepatic blood flow
2. Decreased hepatic mass
3. Decreased activity of hepatic enzymes

Metabolism of drugs by the liver depends on the activity of enzymes that carry out biotransformation. This process is influenced by the extent of hepatic blood flow. Hepatic blood flow determines the rate of delivery of drugs to the liver. Drugs that are metabolized slowly and have a low intrinsic clearance are processed proportionately to the rate of hepatic metabolism. Because hepatic mass decreases with age in absolute terms and in proportion to body weight, the metabolism of drugs with low intrinsic clearance is reduced. Generally, this includes drugs that to a great extent depend on oxidation, that is, those that use oxidative pathways of drug metabolism.

Drugs with a rapid rate of metabolism and high intrinsic clearance are extracted rapidly by the liver. The rate-limiting step in this case is hepatic blood flow. This relationship is particularly pertinent to drugs that are administered intravenously, for example, diazepam. Advancing age is associated with reduction in the presystemic metabolism of drugs having a relatively higher rate of extraction. Thus the bioavailability of certain drugs such as beta-blockers is increased, and accordingly, other drugs with high rates of hepatic extraction, for example, antipsychotics or tricyclic antidepressants (TCAs), will have higher serum levels and should be administered with great caution and with careful monitoring for side effects.

Liver metabolism may be classified based on biotransformation reactions as phase 1, with oxidation, reduction, and hydrolysis; and phase 2, with conjugation reactions that include glucuronidation, acetylation, and sulfation. Microsomal and nonmicrosomal enzymes are involved in both processes. Phase 1 pathways of metabolism may be reduced in elderly persons, whereas phase 2 pathways are not altered and are more predictable. Benzodiazepines undergo both types of metabolism.[3] For example, chlordiazepoxide (Librium), diazepam, clorazepate (Tranxene), and prazepam (Centrax) all undergo oxidative metabolism, and therefore their elimination tends to be prolonged in elderly persons. Furthermore, each of these drugs is converted to an active metabolite, for example, desmethyldiazepam, which in turn has other active metabolites for which the half-life is substantially longer (up to 220 hours) than that of the parent compound (e.g., 20 to 80 hours for diazepam). Other benzodiazepines, oxazepam (Serax), lorazepam, and temazepam (Restoril), undergo conjugation reactions; the metabolism of these agents remains unaltered by age. Thus these compounds do not give rise to active metabolites and represent safer compounds within the benzodiazepine class for use with elderly persons.[9]

Age is only one of many factors that potentially affect drug metabolism. For example, cigarette smoking, alcohol intake, dietary considerations, drugs, illness, and caffeine consumption may all affect the rate of drug metabolism. Enzyme induction through smoking and alcohol consumption and hepatic enzyme inhibition through decreased drug clearance by other drugs (e.g., cimetidine) may also affect drug metabolism in older individuals. In short, hepatic metabolism is a complex process and psychotropic agents that are more easily metabolized are preferred in the elderly.

Elimination. Changes in the elimination of drugs related to aging include the following:

1. Decreased renal blood flow
2. Decreased glomerular filtration rate
3. Decreased tubular secretion
4. Decreased number of nephrons

Perhaps the best documented and the most predictable alteration in pharmacokinetics with advancing age is the reduction in the rate of renal elimination or excretion. This reduction is caused by a decline in both the glomerular filtration rate (GFR) and the tubular secretion rate, which accounts for the decreased creatinine clearance that results from aging. Beginning with the fourth decade of life, a 6% to 10% reduction in GFR and renal blood flow occurs every 10 years. Thus, by age 70, an individual may have as much as a 50% decrease in renal function in the absence of renal disease.

Drug elimination in patients who have normal *serum creatinine* concentrations is affected because creatinine production decreases with age. Thus measuring *creatinine clearance* is useful in determining a dosage. Direct measurement can be difficult to achieve, but an estimate for men may be derived from the following formula:

$$\text{Creatinine clearance} = \frac{140 - \text{Age} \times \text{Body weight (kg)}}{72} \times \text{Serum creatinine}$$

For example, a 70-year-old man weighing 70 kg (150 pounds) with a serum creatinine of 1.4 would be estimated to have a creatinine clearance of 95 ml/min

$$[((140 - 70) \times 70 \div 72) \times 1.4 = 95]$$

For women, this result should be multiplied by 0.85. As a caveat, this formula has been shown to be less than accurate in estimating creatinine clearance among nursing home patients.[8] Thus this method of assessment may provide only a crude estimate of dosage requirements.

Drugs that are eliminated predominantly through renal excretion and that have untoward pharmacologic effects are even more potentially serious with respect to toxic effects in older persons. Amantadine (Symmetrel), lithium, beta-blockers, clonidine (Catapres), and several nonpsychotropic drugs such as aminoglycosides, digoxin, antiarrhythmics, diuretics, nonsteroidal antiinflammatory drugs (NSAIDs), and angiotensin-converting enzyme inhibitors are noteworthy examples.[26] The discussion of lithium excretion in kidney function, as noted in Chapter 6, is of particular concern in elderly persons.[20]

Drug Interactions

The pharmacokinetic effects outlined in this section prominently affect interactions with other drugs. Absorption may be affected significantly by antacids. Distribution of drugs may be affected by the competition for binding proteins among various drugs. Metabolism of drugs that use the oxidative cytochrome P-450 enzyme system, for example, barbiturates, anticonvulsants, and oral hypoglycemics, may induce drug metabolism of other drugs utilizing this system. Other compounds may inhibit metabolism, for example, cimetidine, beta-blockers, certain antidepressants, and

Table 21-1 Cytochrome P-450 Induction, Inhibition, and Substrates

Isoenzyme	Substrate	Inducer	Inhibitor
CYP 1A1	Chlorinated benzenes	Polycyclic hydrocarbons	Propofol, nitric oxide
CYP 1A2	Caffeine, phenacetin TCA, R-warfarin Erythromycin Haloperidol, antipyrine Theophylline, paracetamol Ropivacaine	Phenytoin Phenobarbital Omeprazole Polycyclic hydrocarbons	Quinolone Antibiotics Cimetidine
CYP 2C8	TCA, diazepam Hexabarbitone	Rifampicin Phenobarbital	Cimetidine
CYP 2C9-9/10	Phenytoin, S-warfarin Diclofenac, tolbutamide		Sulfaphenazole
CYP 2C19	Mephenytoin, diazepam, TCA	Phenobarbitol	Sulfaphenazole
CYP 2D6	Debrisoquine, sparteine Codeine, dextromethorphan Beta-blockers, SSRIs, TCA	Pregnancy	Cimetidine Quinidine Methadone
CYP 2E1	Paracetamol, isoflurane Sevoflurane, methoxyflurane Enflurane, trichlorethylene	Ethanol, isoniazid, benzene	Disulfiram
CYP 3A4	Nifedipine, TCA Dextromethorphan Alfentanil, sufentanil Fentanyl, erythromycin Lignocaine, ropivacaine Midazolam, codeine Granisetron, diltiazem Hydrocortisone	Rifampicin Glucocorticoid Carbamazepine Phenobarbitol	Cimetidine Troleandomycin Propofol Grapefruit juice Ketoconazole
CYP 3A5	Caffeine, diltiazem	Dexamethasone	Troleandomycin
CYP 3A7	Midazolam		
CYP 7	Cholesterol		
CYP 11A1	Cholesterol		
CYP 17	Pregnolone		
CYP 19	Testosterone		
CYP 21A2	17-Hydroxyprogesterone		

TCA, Tricyclic antidepressants; *SSRI,* selective serotonin reuptake inhibitors.

methylphenidate (Ritalin) (Table 21-1).[6,16] Excretion of psychotropic agents, especially lithium, may be significantly affected by proximal loop and potassium-sparing diuretics. NSAIDs may also be responsible for disrupting excretions of lithium and other psychotropic agents.

Overall, the pharmacokinetic changes of aging may have a profound influence on psychotropic drug therapy. GI tract diseases may affect absorption; diseases affecting volume of distribution may result from altered concentrations of binding proteins; hepatic disease may affect metabolism; and renal disease may affect excretion. A comprehensive review of pharmacokinetic factors including the effects of aging is found in Chapter 3.

Pharmacodynamics

Pharmacodynamics refers to what a drug does to the body and to the study of effects of drugs on the target site. More broadly, pharmacodynamics reflects the physiologic or psychologic response to a drug or combination of drugs. Pharmacodynamics have been examined less extensively in elderly persons than have pharmacokinetics, largely because of the difficulty of such investigations. Older patients are generally more responsive to the effects of psychotropic agents, perhaps because of changes in neurotransmitter systems or receptor site sensitivity.[25]

Geriatric patients can be extremely sensitive to the effects of psychotropic drugs but less so to nonpsychotropic agents such as cardiovascular preparations. In support of pharmacodynamic changes related to aging, the beta-adrenergic receptor is most promising.[1,22] It has been observed that beta-blockers are less effective in older individuals. It is theorized that either beta-receptors are decreased in number or have become less sensitive with age. Other drugs, known to produce more intense effects, are thought to do so because of receptor upregulation. Thus receptor changes result in a differential (sometimes exaggerated or diminished) response in older individuals.

Other significant age-related neurophysiologic changes include cholinergic degeneration that is known to occur in older adults and that can affect memory function and presumably predispose patients to the effects of drugs that potentially exacerbate disorders of cognitive impairment (i.e., anticholinergic agents). The degeneration of the nigrostriatal pathways and resultant declines in dopamine concentrations may also result in an older individual's predisposition to extrapyramidal side effects (EPSEs) or to the development of tardive dyskinesia with use of a neuroleptic.[15,24] Moreover, the sedation threshold and unfavorable effects on memory in response to benzodiazepines or other sedative-hypnotic class agents may be exaggerated in older patients. The effects of TCAs on cardiac conduction in patients with cardiac disease and neuroleptics in patients with Parkinson's disease or Lewy body dementia may also be accentuated. These pharmacodynamic changes may intensify drug-drug interactions as well. For example, it is thought there is a greater potential for TCAs to interact with an older person's antihypertensive agents, antiarrhythmics, and other agents that possess anticholinergic properties. Similarly, low-potency neuroleptics such as thioridazine may affect response to antihypertensives; specifically, alpha-receptor blockade may be accentuated as a result of pharmacodynamic changes.

Drug Reactions

Nontherapeutic drug reactions are commonly encountered in older adults. Many side effects are simply related to sedation (excessive daytime drowsiness, cognitive impairment, motor impairment, or fatigue). Sedating psychotropic drugs can compound the sedation resulting from alcohol or other classes of agents, both prescribed and over the counter. The high prevalence of dizziness reported in the elderly in association with certain psychotropics may predispose these individuals to falls resulting in hip fracture or head injury. Psychotropic agents mentioned most often in this regard are benzodiazepines, TCAs, newer antidepressants, and antipsychotic agents.

Psychotropic agents used safely in younger patients require closer attention when prescribed for older individuals because of greater risk of clinically important adverse drug reactions. Older individuals generally have higher plasma concentrations (pharmacokinetic changes) of many prescribed medications and are more sensitive (pharmacodynamic changes) to a given plasma concentration relative to dose. Risk factors for adverse drug reactions include the following:

1. Multiple medications
2. Increased number of illnesses
3. Severe illness or frailty
4. History of increased sensitivity to drug effects

The incidence of adverse drug reactions or nontherapeutic effects ranges between 10% and 20% among older adult patients.[7] Patients taking NSAIDs have an increased risk of hyperkalemia, renal failure, or death resulting from GI hemorrhage. Patients receiving diuretic therapy are more susceptible to fluid and electrolyte disorders, including volume depletion, hypokalemia, hyponatremia, and hypomagnesemia. As mentioned previously, disease states may also alter the disposition or effect of a drug, and because geriatric patients often suffer from more than one disease, careful attention to concomitant illnesses and medications must be given when prescribing any medication.

Compliance

Noncompliance with drug therapy is reported to occur in one third to half of geriatric patients.[18] Factors that account for lower rates of compliance include the following:

1. Poor communication with the health care professional
2. Decline in cognitive function coupled with complicated dosing regimens
3. Lack of support and reinforcement from the clinician or family.

Using the fewest possible drugs at the minimum effective dosages in convenient combinations usually enhances compliance. Once a therapeutic goal has been achieved, a dosage of a particular drug may be able to be reduced or discontinued. Of course, full dose continuation therapy is perhaps more common and is often followed by maintenance throughout the period in which the patient is considered to be most susceptible to recurrence or relapse. Maintenance therapy may continue in perpetuity; thus long-term side effects must be considered carefully and compliance strategies must be reinforced. Compliance is enhanced when dosage schedules are kept simple, drug regimens are uncomplicated, family members and caregivers are involved, uncomplicated written instructions are provided, containers are easy to open, and liquid formulations are available for individuals who have difficulty swallowing. Various aids and devices can also be improvised or obtained to assist older patients and their families with accurate self-administration.

PSYCHIATRIC DISTURBANCES PREVALENT IN LATE LIFE

Psychotropics are the second most commonly prescribed class of drugs in geriatric patients. *Symptoms* that become a focus of treatment include anxiety, insomnia, agitation, aggression, and other disruptive behaviors. *Syndromes* or *disorders* commonly treated include anxiety, depression, mood cycling, psychoses, and cognitive disorders. Irrespective of the condition, pharmacologic treatment is best combined with other appropriate interventions. Prescribing a psychotropic drug to an older patient is generally preceded by an adequate assessment that seeks to optimize the patient's medical and physiologic condition while providing some documentation of the patient's baseline mental and psychosocial status. Generally, this assessment should seek to answer the following questions:

1. What is the patient's medical status?
2. What is the patient's mental status?
3. What is the patient's functional status and capacity to carry out daily activities?

4. What is the patient's psychosocial status and ability to function socially, occupationally, and interpersonally?
5. What is the patient's or caregiver's potential to comply with the medical regimen?

MOOD DISORDERS
Depressive Disorders

Depressive disorders are commonly encountered among geriatric patients. Epidemiologic data suggest that about half of all major depression is encountered initially by an individual older than 65. Of community-dwelling elderly persons, 13% are found to have clinically significant symptoms within the depressive spectrum. For example, medical illnesses are often associated with depression (20% to 35% of patients within medical-surgical settings are found to have coexisting symptoms of depression). Furthermore, mortality rates are increased for geriatric patients with depression, and the suicide rate among elderly individuals is disproportionate. The current geriatric population accounts for at least 25% of all completed suicides, but elderly persons attempt suicide at least three times less often than do nongeriatric patients. Simply put, suicide attempts made by older adults are more often successfully completed.[11] Thus effective drug treatment of depression, careful monitoring of response, and an appreciation of suicide risk are imperative for depressed geriatric patients.

Selection and use of antidepressant medications in late life requires consideration of dosing and titration, pharmacokinetic factors, and cost benefit. Among the antidepressants, selective serotonin reuptake inhibitors (SSRIs) are the most commonly prescribed antidepressants for older patients. Citalopram (Celexa) and sertraline (Zoloft) have pharmacokinetic advantages over other SSRIs, that is, linear pharmacokinetics and less potential for drug interactions.

Other new generation antidepressants, bupropion (Wellbutrin) and venlafaxine (Effexor), are well tolerated by geriatric patients, possess excellent pharmacologic profiles, and have fewer side effects than do older agents. Bupropion and venlafaxine may be beneficial for patients who are not responsive to SSRIs. Bupropion has been touted as being useful in patients with a history of bipolar disorder or in those who require maintenance antidepressant therapy after electroconvulsive therapy. Bupropion has virtually no anticholinergic or cardiotoxic effects and lacks sedative properties that may contribute to daytime drowsiness. Venlafaxine extended-release (Effexor XR) also has good tolerability and has been effective in treatment-resistant depression. The anxiolytic effects, linear kinetics, and lack of interference with P-450 isoenzymes are also a tremendous advantage in older, medically ill patients. Nefazodone (Serzone) and mirtazapine (Remeron) are also drugs that are well tolerated in geriatric patients. As discussed in Chapter 6, nefazodone enhances sleep, rapidly reduces anxiety, and lacks significant potential for orthostatic or anticholinergic symptoms. Drug-drug interactions may occur with nefazodone with agents metabolized by the P-450 3A4 enzyme system. Mirtazapine is sedating, stimulates appetite, an advantage in some cases, and is presumed not to interfere with the metabolism of other drugs.

When TCAs are selected, the secondary amine tricyclics, desipramine (Norpramin) and nortriptyline (Pamelor), are generally preferred because of their more favorable side effect profiles. When acute antidepressant drug treatment results in remission of symptoms, it is typically recommended that therapy continue for at least 6 to 12 months. This recommendation stems from research indicating more than 50% of successfully treated patients either relapse or develop recurrence in the first year.[21] Many older patients with depression need maintenance antidepressant therapy. This is especially true when the patient presents with a history, severe episodes, or persistent symptoms of depression.

Monoamine oxidase inhibitors (MAOIs) may be effective for depressed or severely anxious elderly patients who are refractory to SSRIs or other antidepressant intervention. Because MAO enzyme activity increases with advancing age, a special niche for these agents in the geriatric population is implied, particularly in dementia complicated by depression. However, orthostatic hypotension or other adverse reactions, as outlined in Chapter 6, may emerge. Some geriatric patients may also be at risk for noncompliance with the relatively rigid dietary precautions.

Although activating antidepressants such as desipramine, fluoxetine, or bupropion are useful in geriatric patients who are abulic, motor retarded, or cognitively impaired, psychostimulants have gained popularity as an initial or adjunctive treatment of depression among geriatric patients. Psychostimulants such as dextroamphetamine or methylphenidate may be used safely for initial or sustained treatment of major depression; for treatment of depression complicated by general medical illness, apathy or amotivational symptoms; or for depressive symptoms in patients with dementia. Surprisingly, psychostimulants have few serious adverse or nontherapeutic effects. The use of methylphenidate in doses of 5 to 40 mg is generally preferred. It can be administered both as a short-term agent (with or without concomitant administration of a conventional antidepressant) and as an adjunct in the long-term treatment of treatment-refractory cases. The stimulant challenge test, in which a test dose of a stimulant is given before initiating conventional antidepressant therapy, has been reported as a useful way of predicting potential responses to antidepressant drug therapy.[12] However, when in doubt regarding the presence of depression, treat.

Bipolar Disorder

Using lithium to treat bipolar disorder in geriatric patients is a well-documented and accepted treatment strategy.[6] It can also be useful for augmenting antidepressant agents. The dose-response relationship for using lithium in bipolar illness in geriatric cases is different. A therapeutic response or maintenance prophylaxis occurs at lower therapeutic plasma levels (i.e., at 0.4 to 0.8 mEq/L versus 0.6 to 1.2 mEq/L in younger adults). This lower-dose treatment is preferred because side effects and adverse reactions are more commonly encountered among older adult patients, including the potential for neurotoxic effects and dyskinesias. Interestingly, many older patients who seek medical attention with an apparent agitated depression may actually have mixed bipolar disorder that is ultimately responsive to lithium or other mood-stabilizing agents in concert with antidepressant therapy. For 30% to 50% of older patients who are either nonresponders to lithium or intolerant of its side effects, valproic acid (Depakote), carbamazepine (Tegretol), or other mood stabilizers may be used as alternatives. Valproic acid is well tolerated, especially in the form of divalproex (Depakote), and is gaining popularity as a first-line agent in geriatric patients with bipolar disorder. These alternative mood-stabilizing compounds do not lower the seizure threshold or significantly interfere with cognitive function; thus they may also be useful in cognitively impaired patients who have prominent symptoms of mood instability or aggression.

PSYCHOTIC DISORDERS

Psychotic disorders in older patients may include schizophrenia or other disorders that are potentially manageable with antipsychotic agents (as they are in younger patients). The choice of drug often entails selection of an atypical antipsychotic agent because of better tolerability and the lowered risk of tardive dyskinesia, as discussed in Chapter 5. The relative efficacy versus the side effect profile of an antipsychotic agent generally includes consideration of whether the patient has any preexisting general medical conditions that might result in a greater risk for side effects. For some patients, sedation associated with an agent such as quetiapine (Seroquel) at dosages of 50 to 400 mg may represent a "therapeutic fringe benefit," whereas clozapine (Clozaril) may be beneficial for geriatric conditions that are treatment refractory.[23] Clozapine may be particularly beneficial in elderly persons with Parkinson's disease.

Older patients with schizophrenia or other psychoses constitute one of several groups for whom depot neuroleptics have a special role. Both fluphenazine decanoate (Prolixin decanoate) and haloperidol decanoate (Haldol decanoate) have proved to be useful, especially in cases involving noncompliance. Moreover, for patients in institutional settings, lower dosages of depot rather than oral neuroleptic agents may ultimately be required to maintain the antipsychotic effect.[13] Antipsychotic agents may also be generally useful for patients with sundowning, confusional episodes, agitation, delirium, transient psychosis, agitation, or behavioral disturbances secondary to dementia.[10] Furthermore, these agents may be beneficial for patients at risk for harm to themselves or others or for those individuals unable to carry out essential daily activities without some degree of tranquilization.

Anxiety Disorders and Acute Insomnia

Anxiety disorders represent one of the more common problems encountered in later life.[4] Pharmacologic treatment usually involves a benzodiazepine, an antidepressant, or buspirone (see Chapter 7). Benzodiazepines and nonbenzodiazepine sedatives (e.g., zolpidem [Ambien] or zaleplon [Sonata]), trazodone, or the short-term use of chloral hydrate may be useful for treating acute insomnia.

The pharmacology and pharmacologic properties of anxiolytics and sedatives have been discussed in preceding chapters. Differential drug effects related to drug metabolism and pharmacokinetics in elderly persons may be exaggerated because of changes in plasma protein binding, increased volume of distribution, diminished hepatic biotransformation, and impaired renal clearance.

Hepatic biotransformation and renal clearance are significant pharmacokinetic considerations that often account for differences in drug response to benzodiazepines or sedative-hypnotics. For example, reduced hepatic biotransformation and reduced renal clearance in elderly persons both lead to metabolic accumulation, diminished clearing of the drug, and a resultant higher blood level of drug or active metabolite or both. This is indeed why short-acting benzodiazepines that undergo metabolism through conjugation pathways in the liver (oxazepam, lorazepam, and temazepam) are preferred.

A number of treatment issues and guidelines must be considered with the use of anxiolytics or sedative-hypnotics in geriatric patients. These primarily relate to the potential for nontherapeutic effects of the drugs in relation to the effects of aging (see Chapter 10). Diazepam and other benzodiazepines, that is, alprazolam (Xanax), oxazepam, and lorazepam, are known to have increased risk of causing disinhibition; this phenomenon is characterized by an episode of violence or increasing agitation that is clearly drug induced. Thus the loss of behavioral control and explosive or violent behavior may also occur during the course of benzodiazepine treatment. Triazolam (Halcion) occasionally has shown this effect but more often produces other significant adverse effects in an older patient, for example, amnestic episodes. Benzodiazepines have well-known amnestic properties, which are more prominent in elderly persons. The potential for lorazepam, alprazolam, and triazolam to produce amnestic effects is discussed in Chapter 10.

Drug accumulation with long-acting benzodiazepines is thought to explain the higher incidence of falls in elderly persons. Moreover, the benzodiazepines with longer half-lives pose the greatest risk for resultant falls that may be complicated by hip fracture, head injury, or both. The potential adverse effects of sedation and the negative influence on cognition are also compounded in elderly patients with dementia or cognitive impairment, creating additional risk for accidents.

The clinical approach to acute insomnia requires prudent selection of a drug with the most suitable pharmacologic profile. The dose should preserve normal sleep architecture to the extent possible. The pharmacokinetic profile should meet the clinical requirement to shorten sleep onset, to reduce nocturnal wakefulness, and to provide the anxiolytic effect required during the following day. This approach should result in the patient being as free as possible from untoward effects on daytime functioning. The utility and clinical appropriateness of any hypnotic agent must depend to some extent on whether the therapeutic profile solves the clinical problems.

Benzodiazepines used as hypnotics are likely to have some side effects. However, unnecessarily high dosages for long periods are the more significant clinical issue. Impaired daytime performance, anterograde amnesia, and other adverse effects occur with the benzodiazepines. Anterograde amnesia can be associated with rage or psychosis. A 20% incidence of amnesia is associated with triazolam, but approximately 45% of patients with insomnia who do not receive treatment also complain of memory problems, making it difficult to establish the clinical significance of triazolam's effect on memory.[10] Also, on cessation of sedative treatment, insomnia may arise as a rebound phenomenon, particularly when short-acting agents are withdrawn suddenly. Rebound insomnia occurs more often when a relatively high dosage of a rapidly eliminated drug is prescribed and used nightly. Generally, this phenomenon is not observed when these drugs are used in recommended dosages for limited periods.

The possibility of dependence can be minimized by intermittent use of low dosages together with limited duration of prescription and gradual withdrawal in the event that continuous treatment has been given for more than 1 month. Indeed, withdrawal of hypnotics after long-term use may lead to a recrudescence of the original symptoms, as well as to rebound insomnia.[19] Zolpidem or zaleplon are ideal hypnotics for elderly individuals, especially in doses of 5 to 10 mg. Long-term use seems to result in little accumulation. Minimal daytime drowsiness and lack of drug interaction makes these drugs preferable among elderly persons.

Mixed Anxiety-Depression

Mixed anxiety-depression is often diagnosed in older adults who receive treatment in primary care settings. Clinical presentations may not meet the full syndromal criteria for either a mood or anxiety disorder, and anxiety or depression may not be distinguishable as the overriding disorder. Elderly individuals come to medical attention with clinical symptoms for which diagnostic criteria are not clearly identifiable or for which the clinical setting or brief nature of the assessment may not lend itself to a definitive diagnosis, for example, the nursing home or emergency department. Nonetheless, these patients exhibit clinically significant symptoms that are potentially responsive to anxiolytics.

The pharmacotherapy of mixed anxiety-depression is best accomplished with a broad-spectrum, first-line agent such as an SSRI, venlafaxine, nefazodone, buspirone, or alprazolam. Mixed anxiety-depression is best treated with a benzodiazepine or venlafaxine when anxiety is associated with an acute stressor or with overwhelming situational factors. Buspirone, venlafaxine, nefazodone, or an

SSRI represents an ideal drug in patients requiring long-term therapy and may ultimately alleviate several target symptoms of anxiety-depression while diminishing agitation, improving concentration, and enhancing functional ability. A full discussion of these agents is provided in Chapters 6 and 7.

Agitation and Aggression

Older patients, particularly those who may be cognitively impaired or institutionalized, often receive treatment for agitation or aggression. In many cases, when agitation is the result of psychosis or delirium, the best pharmacologic choice is an antipsychotic or neuroleptic. However, the benzodiazepines (e.g., oxazepam, lorazepam) offer advantages when sedation is needed. Lorazepam is the best choice and offers significant pharmacokinetic advantages, especially when given intramuscularly.

In long-term care settings, the Omnibus Budget Reconciliation Act of 1987 (OBRA) guidelines restrict the prescription of antipsychotic medications and "tranquilizing" anxiolytics.[17] These guidelines require that nursing home patients be appropriately diagnosed. Patients can then receive treatment in adherence to federal guidelines that mandate that specific psychiatric conditions be appropriately treated with a selected psychotropic agent. OBRA guidelines require both a rationale and a justification for using a psychotropic drug, including documentation and monitoring. In addition, drug selection, dosage, duration of therapy, and discontinuation of prescription when potential dependency and addiction are present are addressed by OBRA guidelines. Thus anxiolytic drug therapy with benzodiazepines and antipsychotics in long-term care settings is subject to OBRA guidelines. Also, as a result of the OBRA legislation, the incidental use of anxiolytics or antipsychotics in long-term care settings is discouraged and may even be prohibited. Antidepressants and other classes of drugs such as valproic acid and buspirone are not subject to the drug holidays, tapering, and monitoring required with tranquilizing agents.

Antipsychotic or neuroleptic drugs have been both vigorously recommended and condemned for treating chronically agitated or anxious elderly patients in any clinical setting. Although high-potency neuroleptics such as haloperidol are often used for this purpose, drugs with strongly sedating properties may be preferred. For example, thioridazine may be prescribed at low dosages, in the range of 10 to 50 mg one to four times per day. Although using a neuroleptic agent avoids the risk of drug dependency, the risk of tardive dyskinesia and the emergence of other equally problematic side effects are concerns. Thus neuroleptics are not recommended for simple anxiety or agitation. Newer, atypical antipsychotics (e.g., olanzapine, risperidone, quetiapine) confer less risk of EPSEs, tardive dyskinesia, or other more significant adverse effects; these agents are more acceptable in the treatment of severe agitation and psychosis.

The availability of anxiolytics, for example, short-acting benzodiazepines or buspirone, should be considered as therapeutic in the context of risks versus benefits for treating agitation and aggression. Buspirone in doses of 15 to 60 mg; low dosages of short-acting benzodiazepines such as alprazolam, lorazepam, and oxazepam; and other agents may be useful alone or as adjuncts for treating agitation. Trazodone, lithium, valproic acid, carbamazepine, gabapentin, and the beta-blockers have also been reported most often to be potentially useful. SSRIs have been reported to be useful in agitated patients with cognitive impairments and psychosis.[5] One or more of these alternative agents may be necessary for long-term treatment when persistent agitation, aggression, or suicidality poses a significant risk. Agitated, aggressive, or disruptive behavior in the context of dementia, delirium, or other disorders of cognitive impairment are further addressed in Chapter 8.

REFERENCES

1. Abrass IB, Scarpace PJ: Human lymphocyte beta-adrenergic receptors are unaltered with age, *J Gerontol* 36:298, 1981.
2. Avorn J and others: A randomized trial of a program to reduce the use of psychoactive drugs in nursing homes, *N Engl J Med* 327:168, 1992.
3. Bellatuono C and others: Benzodiazepines: clinical pharmacology and therapeutic use, *Drugs* 19:195, 1980.
4. Burke WJ, Folks DG, McNeilly DP: Effective use of anxiolytics in the elderly, *Clin Geriatr Med* 14(1):47, 1998.
5. Burke WJ and others: The use of selective reuptake inhibitors for depression and psychosis complicating dementia, *Int J Geriatr Psychiatry* 12:519, 1997.
6. Catterson ML, Preskorn SH, Martin RL: Pharmacodynamic and pharmacokinetic considerations in geriatric psychopharmacology, *Psychiatr Clin North Am Geriatr Psychiatry* 20(1): 205, 1997.
7. Cusack BJ: Polypharmacy and clinical pharmacology. In Beck J, editor: *Geriatrics review syllabus: a core in geriatric medicine*, New York, 1989, American Geriatrics Society.
8. Drusano GL and others: Commonly used methods of estimating creatinine clearance are inadequate for elderly debilitated nursing home patients, *J Am Geriatr Soc* 36:437, 1988.
9. Folks DG: Clinical approaches to anxiety in the medically ill elderly, *Drug Ther Suppl* Aug: 72, 1990.
10. Folks DG, Burke WJ: Sedative hypnotics and sleep in geriatric patients, *Clin Geriatr Med* 14(1):67, 1998.
11. Folks DG, Ford CV: Clinical features of depression and dysthymia in older adults. In Blazer D, editor: *Principles and practice of geriatric psychiatry*, West Sussex, England, 1994, John Wiley & Sons.
12. Goff DC: The stimulant challenge test in depression, *J Clin Psychiatry* 47:538, 1986.
13. Gottlieb G, McAllister T, Gur R: Depot neuroleptics in the treatment of behavioral disorders in patients with Alzheimer's disease, *J Am Geriatr Soc* 36:619, 1988.
14. Gurwitz JH: Suboptimal medication use in the elderly: the tip of the iceberg, *JAMA* 272:316, 1994 (editorial).
15. Jeste DV and others: Incidence of tardive dyskinesia in early stages of low-dose treatment with typical neuroleptics in older patients, *Am J Psychiatry* 156(2):309, 1999.
16. Keltner NL, Folks DG: Pharmacokinetics and psychopharmacology: application to the geropsychiatric patient, *Perspect Psychiatr Care* 29:34, 1993.
17. Keltner NL, Folks DG: The Omnibus Budget Reconciliation Act: impact on psychotropic drug use in long-term care facilities, *Perspect Psychiatr Care* 31:30, 1995.
18. Morrow D, Leirer V, Sheikh J: Adherence and medication instructions: review and recommendations, *J Am Geriatr Soc* 36:1147, 1988.
19. Nicholson AN: Hypnotics: rebound insomnia and residual sequelae, *Br J Clin Pharmacol* 9: 223, 1980.
20. Ragheb M, Ban TA, Buchanan D, Frohlich JC: Interaction of indomethacin and ibuprofen with lithium in manic patients under a steady-state lithium level, *J Clin Psychiatry* 41:397, 1980.
21. Rubin EH, Kinscherf BA, Wehrman SA: Response to treatment of depression in the old and very old, *J Geriatr Psychiatry Neurol* 4:65, 1991.
22. Scarpace PJ: Decreased beta-adrenergic responsiveness during senescence, *Fed Proc* 45: 51, 1986.
23. Small JG and others: Treatment outcome with clozapine in tardive dyskinesia, neuroleptic sensitivity, and treatment-resistant psychosis, *J Clin Psychiatry* 48:263, 1987.
24. Sweet RA and others: Duration of neuroleptic treatment and prevalence of tardive dyskinesia in late life, *Arch Gen Psychiatry* 52:478, 1995.
25. Swift CG: Pharmacodynamics: changes in homeostatis mechanisms, receptor and target organ sensitivity in the elderly, *Br Med Bull* 46:36, 1990.
26. Williams L, Lowenthal DT: Drug therapy in the elderly, *South Med* 85(2):127, 1992.

PART TWO

PSYCHOTROPIC
DRUG PROFILES

Acetazolamide

AK-ZOL, DAZAMIDE, DIAMOX
(a-set-a-zole´-a-mide)

Functional classifications: Diuretic, anticonvulsant
Chemical classification: Carbonic anhydrase inhibitor
FDA pregnancy category: C

Indications: *Diuretic:* not discussed here (e.g., edema related to CHF, glaucoma); *anticonvulsant:* especially petit mal and tonic-clonic seizures, particularly in children

Contraindications: Known hypersensitivity to acetazolamide; depressed sodium or potassium levels; kidney and liver disease or dysfunction; suprarenal gland failure

Pharmacologic Effects: Inhibition of carbonic anhydrase, which apparently slows abnormal firing of CNS neurons; anticonvulsant effect not truly understood

Pharmacokinetics: Absorbed from GI tract; distributed to body tissues and CNS; eliminated unchanged in urine

Side Effects: *CNS:* convulsions, weakness, malaise, fatigue, nervousness, sedation, depression; *peripheral:* nausea, vomiting, constipation, hematuria, urinary frequency, hepatic insufficiency, blood dyscrasias, skin problems, weight loss, fever, acidosis

Interactions
- *Amphetamines:* because it alkalinizes urine, might increase effect of amphetamines (and ephedrine, pseudoephedrine, flecainide, and quinidine)
- *Digitalis:* might sensitize patient to digitalis toxicity r/t hypokalemia
- *Primidone:* might delay primidone absorption
- *Salicylates:* together, might cause metabolic acidosis

Implications
Assess
- Weight, I&O for fluid loss, respirations, BP
- Potassium, sodium, and other electrolyte levels

Teaching
- To increase fluid, if indicated
- To rise slowly when orthostatic hypotension is a problem

Evaluate
- For seizure activity, CNS side effects, confusion in elderly, signs of metabolic acidosis, signs of hypokalemia

Treatment of Overdose: Lavage for oral doses, monitor electrolytes and fluid profile, assess renal function, give dextrose in saline, give bicarbonate for acidosis.

Administration
- *Epilepsy:* 8-30 mg/kg/day in divided doses; optimal range 375-1000 mg/day
- *Concomitant antiepileptic dosage:* start with 250 mg/day and increase to levels for epilepsy
- *Available forms:* tabs 125, 250 mg; caps sus-rel 500 mg; inj 500 mg/vial

Acetophenazine*

TINDAL
(a-set-oh-fen´-a-zeen)

Functional classification: Antipsychotic
Chemical classification: Piperazine phenothiazine
FDA pregnancy category: C

Indications: Management of psychotic disorders

Contraindications: See Trifluoperazine

Pharmacologic Effects: See Trifluoperazine

Pharmacokinetics: See Trifluoperazine

Side Effects: *CNS:* see Trifluoperazine; *peripheral:* see Trifluoperazine

Interactions: See Trifluoperazine

Implications: See Chlorpromazine

Treatment of Overdose: See Trifluoperazine

Administration
- 20 mg tid; if insomnia present, give last tablet 1 hr before bedtime; usual daily dosage 40-80 mg
- *Hospitalized patients:* optimally 80-120 mg/day in divided doses
- *Severe schizophrenia:* up to 400-600 mg/day
- *Available forms:* tabs 20 mg

Alprazolam

XANAX
(al-pray´-zoe-lam)

Functional classification: Antianxiety agent
Chemical classification: Benzodiazepine
Controlled substance schedule IV
FDA pregnancy category: D

Indications: Anxiety, panic disorders

Contraindications: Hypersensitivity to benzodiazepines; narrow-angle glaucoma; psychosis; nursing women; child <18 yr, and use with ketoconazole and itraconazole, because these drugs impair the oxidative metabolism of CYP-450 3A
Cautious use: Elderly or debilitated patients; hepatic or renal disease

---

*Infrequently used.　†Available in Canada only.

Pharmacologic Effects: Increases the affinity of GABA molecules for their specific receptor increasing the frequency with which chloride channels open in response to GABA; might also decrease norepinephrine and serotonin turnover rates

Pharmacokinetics

- *Speed of onset:* intermediate
- *PO:* onset 30 min, peak 1-2 hr, duration 4-6 hr, therapeutic response 2-3 days; metabolized by liver; excreted by kidneys; crosses placenta, breast milk; half-life 12-15 hr

Side Effects: *CNS:* drowsiness, dizziness, confusion, headache, anxiety, tremor, stimulation, fatigue, depression, insomnia; paradoxic agitation can occur; *peripheral:* photophobia caused by mydriasis; blurred vision caused by cycloplegia; sleeplike slowing of respirations with therapeutic doses; cough; orthostatic hypotension; tachycardia; hypotension; constipation, dry mouth

Interactions

- *Alcohol and other CNS depressants:* increased risk of excessive CNS depression
- *Cimetidine:* potentiation of CNS depression
- *Digoxin:* increased risk of cardiac side effects
- *Levodopa:* decreased antiparkinson effect
- *Phenytoin:* increased phenytoin serum levels

Implications: For Benzodiazepines
  Assess
- Patient's level of anxiety and method of coping
- BP, VS
- Establish baseline physical assessment data before medications are started
- Periodically perform CBC, UA
- Reassess need for treatment q4mo

Planning/Implementation

- Monitor patient's response to medication.
- Observe elderly, very young, and debilitated patients for paradoxic excitement.
- Reduce dosage of other depressant drugs.
- Observe for signs of withdrawal when discontinuing antianxiety medication; discontinue by gradual tapering.

Teaching

- To avoid operating dangerous machinery and other tasks requiring good reflexes
- To report ocular pain and any other visual disturbances at once
- To take drug with food

Evaluate

- Whether patient achieves lower levels of anxiety without undue sedation
- Whether patient can follow prescribed regimen
- For signs of physical dependence: withdrawal symptoms include headache, nausea, vomiting, muscle pain, and weakness after long-term use

Treatment of Overdose: Lavage, VS, supportive care, administer flumazenil, a specific benzodiazepine receptor antagonist; few deaths, if any, reported from benzodiazepine overdose alone; deaths occur when benzodiazepines are mixed with other drugs (i.e., alcohol).

Administration

- *Adult:* PO 0.25-0.5 mg tid, not to exceed 4 mg/day in divided doses; *geriatric:* PO 0.25 mg bid-tid
- *Available forms:* tabs 0.25, 0.5, 1 mg

Amantadine HCl

SYMMETREL
(a-man´-ta-deen)

Functional classification: Antiparkinson agent, antiviral

Chemical classification: Tricyclic amine

FDA pregnancy category: C

Indications: Extrapyramidal reactions, parkinsonism, antiviral (A)

Contraindications: Hypersensitivity, lactation, child <1 yr
  Cautious use: Epilepsy, CHF, orthostatic hypotension, psychiatric disorders, hepatic or renal disease

Pharmacologic Effects: Causes release of dopamine from neurons

Pharmacokinetics: *PO:* onset 48 hr, peak 4 hr, half-life 15 hr in normal renal function, not metabolized, excreted in urine (90%) unchanged, crosses placenta, excreted in breast milk

Side Effects: *CNS:* confusion, headache, dizziness, drowsiness, fatigue, anxiety, psychosis, depression, hallucinations, tremors, convulsions, insomnia; *peripheral:* orthostatic hypotension, CHF, photosensitivity, dermatitis, livedo reticularis, blurred vision, leukopenia, nausea, vomiting, constipation, dry mouth, urinary frequency, retention

Interactions

- *Atropine, other anticholinergics:* increased anticholinergic responses
- *CNS stimulants:* increased CNS stimulation

Implications
  Assess
- EPSEs

Planning/Implementation

- Give at least 4 hr before bedtime to prevent insomnia.
- Give after meals for better absorption to decrease GI symptoms.
- Give in divided doses to prevent CNS disturbances: headache, dizziness, fatigue, drowsiness.

Teaching

- To change body position slowly to prevent orthostatic hypotension
- To report dyspnea, weight gain, dizziness, poor concentration, behavioral changes
- To avoid hazardous activities when dizziness occurs
- To take drug exactly as prescribed; if drug is discontinued abruptly, parkinsonian crisis might occur

Evaluate

- Therapeutic response: decrease in EPSEs

Treatment of Overdose: Withdraw drug; empty stomach; maintain airway; administer O_2, IV corticosteroids; use appropriate antiarrhythmic and vasopressor therapy as needed.

Administration

- *Extrapyramidal reaction and parkinsonism: adult:* PO 100 mg bid, up to 300 mg/day for EPSEs in divided doses; *geriatric:* 100 mg/day
- *Influenza type A:* not addressed here
- *Available forms:* caps 100 mg; syr 50 mg/5 ml
- A *suggested dosing guideline* for patients with impaired renal function is available

Amitriptyline HCl

ELAVIL, ENDEP, ENOVIL, LEVATE,† MERAVIL,† NOVOTRIPTYN,† ROLAVIL† (a-mee-trip´-ti-leen)

Functional classification: Antidepressant
Chemical classification: Tricyclic, tertiary amine
FDA pregnancy category: C

Indications: Depression

Contraindications: Hypersensitivity to TCAs, recovery phase of myocardial infarction, use with MAOIs
Cautious use: Suicidal patients, ECT, child <12 yr, MAOI therapy

Pharmacologic Effects: Blocks reuptake of norepinephrine (+) and serotonin (+++) into presynaptic neurons; also thought to be r/t downregulation of beta-adrenergic receptors; receptor antagonist of ACh (+++), histamine (++++), alpha-1 (+++); therapeutic plasma levels 110-250 ng/ml

Pharmacokinetics: PO/IM onset 45 min, peak 2-12 hr, therapeutic response 2-3 wk; metabolized by liver; excreted in urine and feces; crosses placenta; excreted in breast milk; half-life 31-46 hr; protein binding >95%

Side Effects for Most TCAs: *CNS:* sedation, ataxia, confusion, delirium, insomnia, excitement, headache; *peripheral:* anticholinergic (blurred vision, dry mouth, decreased tearing, constipation,

difficulty urinating, decreased sweating); CV (orthostatic hypotension, dizziness, tachycardia, palpitations, arrhythmias); EPSEs; weight gain; sexual dysfunction; eyes (photophobia, increased intraocular pressure); diarrhea
Specifically for amitriptyline: Dry mouth (~30%), blurred vision (~10%), constipation (~10%), sedation (~30%), orthostasis (~10%), tachycardia (~10%), sexual disturbance (~2%)

Interactions

- *Alcohol:* acute use decreases first-pass metabolism, increasing TCA level; chronic use causes enzyme induction, speeding TCA metabolism
- *Antiarrhythmic* (e.g., quinidine): additive effect, heart block possible
- *Anticholinergic agents:* additive anticholinergic effects
- Atropine
- Antihistamines (H_1 blocker)
- Antiparkinson drugs
- Antipsychotics
- OTC cold and allergy drugs
- *Cigarettes:* decreased TCA serum as a result of enzyme (P-450 1A) induction
- *Cimetidine:* reduced metabolism leading to delayed elimination and increased steady-state concentration of TCA
- *CNS depressants:* additive depressant effect
- **Drugs metabolized by CYP-450 2D6* (e.g., SSRIs, TCAs, beta-blockers, codeine): increased plasma levels of TCAs
- *Guanethidine, clonidine:* decreased antihypertensive effect
- *Lithium:* additive antidepressant effect
- *MAOIs:* hypertensive crisis; atropine-like poisoning
- *Oral contraceptives:* inhibit metabolism of TCAs
- *Phenothiazines:* might increase TCA serum level
- *Sympathomimetics:* potentiates sympathomimetic effects
- *Thyroid preparations:* tachycardia, arrhythmias; might increase TCA effect

Implications: For TCAs
Assess

- Establish baseline data to aid recognition of adverse responses to medication: liver enzyme levels, VS, renal function, mental status, speech patterns, affect, weight
- Assess for signs of noncompliance: poor therapeutic response
- Observe for major symptoms of depression: apathy, sadness, sleep disturbances, hopelessness, guilt, decreased libido, spontaneous crying
- Review history for contraindicated conditions: glaucoma, CV disease, GI conditions, urologic conditions, seizures, pregnancy

---

Planning/Implementation

- Monitor for "cheeking" or hoarding; chcck drug dosage carefully—a small overdose might cause toxicity.
- Monitor for suicidal ideations; suicidal thought content might increase as antidepressants begin to "energize" patient.
- Monitor vital signs; withhold TCAs when hypotension, tachycardia, or arrhythmias occur
- Give most TCAs in a single dose hs.
- Observe for early signs of toxicity: drowsiness, tachycardia, mydriasis, hypotension, agitation, vomiting, confusion, fever, restlessness, sweating.
- Discontinue drug when CNS overstimulation occurs: hypomania, delirium.

Teaching

- That these drugs have a lag time of up to 1 mo
- To adhere to drug regimen
- To avoid OTC drugs, particularly those containing sympathomimetics or anticholinergics
- To avoid drugs listed in Interactions section
- About ways to deal with minor side effects, as follows: *dry mouth:* hard candies, sips of water, mouth rinses; *visual disturbances:* artificial tears, sunglasses, assistance with ambulation; *constipation:* bulk-forming foods, increased fluids; *urinary hesitancy:* adequate fluids, privacy; *decreased perspiration:* appropriate clothing, avoidance of unnecessary exercise; *orthostatic hypotension:* slow positional changes, avoidance of hot baths and showers; *drowsiness:* take single dose hs with physician approval, avoid driving
- That abrupt discontinuance might result in cholinergic rebound: nausea, vomiting, insomnia, headache

Evaluate

- Desired therapeutic serum level
- Verbalized decrease in subjective symptoms
- Observed decrease in objective symptoms
- Minimal to no adverse drug effects
- Stable VS

Treatment of Overdose: ECG monitoring; induce emesis; lavage, activated charcoal; treat anticholinergic effects; administer anticonvulsants if needed.

Administration

- *Adult:* PO 40-100 mg hs, may increase to 200 mg qd, not to exceed 300 mg/day; IM 20-30 mg qid; maintenance dose typically 50-100 mg/day; *for outpatients:* 75 mg/day in divided doses, may be increased to 150 mg/day; *alternative therapy:* 50-100 mg hs, can be increased by 25-50 mg to a total of 150 mg/day; *hospitalized patients:* might require 100 mg/day, which can be increased gradu-

ally to 200 mg/day; some patients might require 300 mg/day
- *Adolescent/geriatric:* PO 30 mg/day in divided doses, may add 20 mg hs
- *Available forms:* tabs 10, 25, 50, 75, 100, 150 mg; IM 10 mg/ml

Amobarbital/ amobarbital sodium
AMYTAL, AMYTAL SODIUM, ISOBEC
(am-oh-bar´-bi-tal)

Functional classifications: Sedative, hypnotic
Chemical classification: Amylobarbitone
Controlled substance schedule II
FDA pregnancy category: B

Indications: Sedation, preanesthetic sedation, anticonvulsant

Contraindications: Hypersensitivity to barbiturates, respiratory depression, addiction to barbiturates, severe liver dysfunction, porphyria

Pharmacologic Effects: Depresses activity in reticular activating system; when used as anticonvulsant, inhibits CNS neural firing

Pharmacokinetics: Onset within 45-60 min after PO dose, with duration of action of 6-8 hr; metabolized by liver, excreted by kidneys; highly protein bound; half-life 16-40 hr; excreted in breast milk; onset in 5 min when given IV (e.g., for seizures)

Side Effects: *CNS:* lethargy, drowsiness, barbiturate hangover, dizziness, paradoxic stimulation of children and elderly patients on occasion, CNS depression, slurred speech, physical dependence; *peripheral:* nausea, vomiting, diarrhea, constipation, skin eruptions (e.g., rashes), hypotension, bradycardia, respiratory depression, apnea, blood dyscrasias

Interactions

- *CNS depressants:* increased CNS depression
- *MAOIs:* CNS depression
- *Oral anticoagulants, corticosteroids, quinidine, oral contraceptives:* decreased effect of these drugs
- *Phenytoin:* unpredictable effect
- *Valproic acid:* decreased half-life of valproic acid

Implications
Assess

- If given parenterally, check VS q30min for 2 hr

Planning/Implementation

- Have staff assist patient in walking after dose is given to prevent falls.
- Maintain safety.

Teaching

- To avoid long-term use (i.e., potential for physical dependence)
- To avoid alcohol and other CNS depressants
- To notify other prescribers about amobarbital

Evaluate

- Therapeutic responses
- Mental status
- Tendencies toward dependence
- Toxic effects
- Respiratory depression
- Blood dyscrasias

Treatment of Overdose: In general, 1 g causes serious poisoning in adults; lavage if taken orally, alkalinize urine; warm with blankets if needed; supportive measures, including monitoring VS; hemodialysis might be required.

Administration

- *Sedation: adult:* PO 30-50 mg bid or tid; range from 15-120 mg bid-qid; *child:* PO 2 mg/kg/day in 4 divided doses
- *Anticonvulsant: adult:* give IV 65-500 mg over several minutes, not to exceed 100 mg/min, do not exceed 1 g; *child <6 yr:* IV/IM 3-5 mg/kg over several minutes
- *Available forms:* tabs 30, 50, 100 mg; caps 65, 200 mg; powder for inj IM, IV 250, 500 mg/vial

Amoxapine

ASENDIN
(a-mox´-a-peen)

Functional classification: Novel antidepressant
Chemical classification: Dibenzoxazepine derivative (i.e., a metabolite of loxapine), heterocyclic, secondary amine
FDA pregnancy category: C

Indications: Depression

Contraindications: Hypersensitivity to TCAs, recovery phase of myocardial infarction
    Cautious use: Seizure disorders, elderly patients, patients receiving MAOI therapy, NMS, child <16 yr

Pharmacologic Effects: Blocks reuptake of norepinephrine (+++) and serotonin (+) into presynaptic neuron; also blocks dopamine receptors and can produce EPSEs (it is a metabolite of the antipsychotic loxapine); also receptor antagonist of ACh (++), histamine (+++), and alpha-1 (+++); therapeutic plasma levels 200-500 ng/ml

Pharmacokinetics: *PO:* steady state 2-7 days, metabolized by liver, excreted by kidneys, crosses placenta, half-life 8-30 hr; protein binding >90%

Side Effects: *CNS:* sedation (~10%), ataxia; confusion, delirium, tardive dyskinesia, NMS; *peripheral:* blurred vision (~2%), photophobia, increased intraocular pressure, decreased tearing, orthostatic hypotension (~10%), arrhythmias, tachycardia (~10%), palpitations, dry mouth (~30%), constipation (~30%), diarrhea, decreased sweating, urinary retention and hesitancy, nausea

Interactions

- *Anticholinergic agents:* additive anticholinergic effects with atropine, antihistamines (H$_1$ blockers), antiparkinson drugs, antipsychotics, OTC cold and allergy drugs
- *CNS depressants:* additive depressant effect
- *Guanethidine, clonidine:* decreased antihypertensive effect
- *MAOIs:* hypertensive crisis, atropine-like poisoning
- *Oral contraceptives:* inhibit effects of TCAs
- *Phenothiazines:* might increase TCA serum level, EPSEs
- *Quinidine:* additive effect, heart block possible
- *Sympathomimetics:* potentiates sympathomimetic effects
- *Thyroid preparations:* tachycardia, arrhythmias; might increase TCA effect

Implications: See Amitriptyline

Teaching

- That amoxapine has a shorter lag time (4-7 days) than other TCAs

Treatment of Overdose: ECG monitoring; induce emesis; lavage; consider prophylactic antiepileptics; support respirations.

Administration

- *Adult:* 16 yr: PO 100-150 mg/day in divided doses, may increase to 300 mg/day or may give daily dose hs
- *Geriatric:* PO 50-75 mg/day, may increase to 150 mg/day
- *Available forms:* tabs 25, 50, 100, 150 mg

---

*Infrequently used.   **†Available in Canada only.**

Amphetamine combination (dextroamphetamine and other amphetamines)

ADDERALL
(am-fet´-a-meen)

Functional classification: Cerebral stimulant
Chemical classification: Amphetamine
Controlled substance schedule II
FDA pregnancy category: C

Indications: Narcolepsy, exogenous obesity, ADHD

Contraindications: Hypersensitivity to sympathomimetic amines, hyperthyroidism, hypertension, glaucoma, severe arteriosclerosis, nephritis, angina pectoris, parkinsonism, drug abuse, CV disease, anxiety, MAOI use
Cautious use: Tourette's syndrome, lactation, child <3 yr, diabetes mellitus, elderly patients

Pharmacologic Effects: Mechanism of action not clearly understood; stimulates dopamine function in the brain, probably as a result of blocking of both dopamine and norepinephrine reuptake; might also promote release of dopamine into synaptic cleft; theoretically, these effects enhance inhibitory subcortical-cortical pathways, resulting in better concentration and impulse control, with a subsequent decrease in motor activity; therapeutic plasma levels 5-10 mg/dl

Pharmacokinetics: *PO:* onset 30 min, peak 1-3 hr, duration 4-20 hr, metabolized by liver, excreted by kidneys, crosses placenta, excreted in breast milk, half-life 10-30 hr

Side Effects: *CNS:* hyperactivity, insomnia, restlessness, talkativeness, dizziness, headache, chills, stimulation, dysphoria, irritability, aggressiveness; *peripheral:* nausea, vomiting, anorexia, dry mouth, diarrhea, constipation, weight loss, metallic taste, cramps, erectile dysfunction, change in libido, palpitations, tachycardia, hypertension, hypotension

Interactions

- *Acetazolamide, antacids, sodium bicarbonate, ammonium chloride, phenothiazines, haloperidol:* increased half-life of amphetamine
- *Guanethidine, other antihypertensives:* decreased effects of these drugs
- *MAOIs or within 14 days of MAOIs:* hypertensive crisis
- *Urinary acidifiers:* decreased half-life of amphetamines

Implications

Assess

- VS, BP because this drug might reverse antihypertensives; check patients with cardiac disease more often
- CBC, urinalysis; in diabetes: blood and urine glucose levels; insulin changes might need to be made because eating decreases
- Height, growth rate in children (growth rate might be decreased)

Planning/Implementation

- Give at least 6 hr before bedtime to prevent sleeplessness.
- Give with meals or immediately after to prevent loss of appetite.
- For obesity only when patient is on weight-reduction program that includes dietary changes, exercise; tolerance develops, and weight loss will not occur without additional methods.
- Instruct patient to chew sugarless gum, suck on hard candies, or take frequent sips of water for dry mouth.
- If drug is for obesity, give 30-60 min before meals.
- Dispense least amount feasible to minimize risk of overdose.

Teaching

- To decrease caffeine consumption (coffee, tea, cola, chocolate), which might increase irritability, stimulation
- To avoid OTC preparations unless approved by physician
- To taper off drug over several weeks, or depression, increased sleeping, lethargy might occur
- To avoid alcohol ingestion
- To avoid hazardous activities until patient's condition is stabilized on medication regimen
- To get needed rest; patients feel more tired than usual at end of day
- To check to see that PO medication has been swallowed

Evaluate

- Mental status: mood, sensorium, affect, stimulation, insomnia; aggressiveness might occur
- Physical dependency: should not be used for extended time; drug should be discontinued gradually
- Withdrawal symptoms: headache, nausea, vomiting, muscle pain, weakness
- Drug tolerance: develops after long-term use; if develops, dosage not to be increased

Treatment of Overdose: Gastric evacuation if overdose <4 hr old; otherwise, acidify urine, administer fluids until urine flow is 3-6 ml/kg/hr; hemodialysis or peritoneal dialysis might be helpful; antihypertensives for increased BP; ammonium chloride for increased excretion; chlorpromazine for CNS stimulation.

Administration

- *ADHD: child <5 yr:* PO initially 2.5 mg hs, after 4-6 days may be raised to 2.5 mg/day and given in 2 doses; *child >5 yr:* initially 5 mg and after 4-6 days may increase by 5 mg/day; total dose 15-20 mg/day; total daily dose usually between 0.3 and 1.0 mg/kg of body weight

Benztropine

COGENTIN
(benz´-troe-peen)

Functional classification: Anticholinergic
FDA pregnancy category: C

Indications: Parkinsonism, EPSEs

Contraindications: Hypersensitivity, narrow-angle glaucoma, duodenal obstruction, peptic ulcer, prostatic hypertrophy, myasthenia gravis, megacolon

Pharmacologic Effects: Block cholinergic receptors, might inhibit the reuptake and storage of dopamine

Pharmacokinetics: Little pharmacokinetic information is known

Side Effects: *CNS:* depression develops in 19% to 30% of patients; disorientation, confusion, memory loss, hallucinations, psychoses, agitation, delusions, nervousness; *peripheral:* tachycardia, palpitations, hypotension, orthostatic hypotension, dry mouth, nausea, vomiting, constipation, paralytic ileus, blurred vision, mydriasis, diplopia, urinary retention and hesitancy, elevated temperature

Interactions

- *Amantadine:* increased anticholinergic effect
- *Digoxin:* increased digoxin serum levels
- *Haloperidol:* worsening of schizophrenia, decreased haloperidol serum levels
- *Levodopa:* Possible reduction of levodopa efficacy
- *Phenothiazines:* increased anticholinergic effect, decreased antipsychotic effect

Implications

Assess
- VS, BP
- For glaucoma
- Mental status

Planning/Implementation

- Provide instructions for anticholinergic responses: dry mouth, constipation, urinary hesitancy, decreased sweating.

Teaching

- To take with meals
- To emphasize safety because might cause drowsiness, blurred vision, dizziness
- To avoid alcohol and other CNS depressants
- To notify physician of rapid or pounding heartbeat
- To use caution in hot weather

Evaluate

- EPSE improvement
- For adverse effects
- Mental status: confusion, delirium, memory

Treatment of Overdose: Induce emesis; lavage, activated charcoal; treat respiratory depression, hyperpyrexia.

Administration

- *EPSEs: adult:* PO/IM 1-4 mg qd-bid
- *Acute EPSEs: adult:* IM/IV 1-2 mg, followed by 1-2 mg PO, taken twice to prevent recurrences
- *Prophylactic: adult:* PO 1-2 mg bid-tid
- *Available forms:* tabs 1, 2 mg; sol 1mg/ml

Biperiden

AKINETON
(bye-per´-i-den)

Functional classification: Anticholinergic
FDA pregnancy category: C

Indications: Parkinsonism, EPSEs

Contraindications: Hypersensitivity, narrow-angle glaucoma, duodenal obstruction, peptic ulcer, prostatic hypertrophy, myasthenia gravis, megacolon

Pharmacologic Effects: Block cholinergic receptors, might inhibit reuptake and storage of dopamine

Pharmacokinetics: Peak 1-1½ hr, half-life 18.4-24.3 hr; little pharmacokinetic information is known

Side Effects: *CNS:* depression (19%-30%); disorientation, confusion, memory loss, hallucinations, psychoses, agitation, delusions, nervousness; *peripheral:* tachycardia, palpitations, hypotension, orthostatic hypotension, dry mouth, nausea, vomiting, constipation, paralytic ileus, blurred vision, mydriasis, diplopia, urinary retention and hesitancy, elevated temperature

Interactions

- *Amantadine:* increased anticholinergic effect
- *Digoxin:* increased digoxin serum levels
- *Haloperidol:* worsening of schizophrenia, decreased haloperidol serum levels

---

- *Levodopa:* possible reduction of levodopa efficacy
- *Phenothiazines:* increased anticholinergic effect, decreased antipsychotic effect

Implications: See Benztropine

Treatment of Overdose: Induce emesis; lavage, activated charcoal; treat respiratory depression, hyperpyrexia.

Administration
- *EPSEs: adult:* PO 2 mg qd-tid
- *Acute EPSEs: adult:* IM/IV 2 mg q30min prn, up to 4 doses in 24 hr
- *Available forms:* tabs 2 mg; IM/IV 5 mg/ml

Bromocriptine mesylate
PARLODEL
(broe-moe-krip´-teen)

Functional classification: Dopamine receptor agonist
Chemical classification: Ergot alkaloid derivative
FDA pregnancy category: C

Indications: Female infertility, Parkinson's disease, prevention of postpartum lactation, amenorrhea, galactorrhea caused by hyperprolactinemia, acromegaly, treatment of NMS, cocaine withdrawal and craving

Contraindications: Hypersensitivity to ergot, severe ischemic disease, pregnancy

Pharmacologic Effects: Inhibits prolactin release by activating postsynaptic dopamine receptors; activation of dopamine receptors is the reason for improvement in Parkinson's disease and NMS (symptom of primary interest in this text)

Pharmacokinetics: PO: peak 1-3 hr, duration 4-8 hr, 90%-96% protein bound, half-life 3-8 hr, metabolized by liver (inactive metabolites), excreted in feces (85%-98%) and urine (2.5%-5.5%)

Side Effects: *CNS:* headache, abnormal involuntary movements, depression, restlessness, anxiety, nervousness, confusion, convulsions, hallucinations; *peripheral:* frequency, retention, incontinence, diuresis, blurred vision, diplopia, burning eyes, nausea, vomiting, anorexia, cramps, constipation, diarrhea, dry mouth, rash on face or arms, alopecia, orthostatic hypotension, decreased BP, palpitation, shock, arrhythmias, shortness of breath

Interactions
- *Antihypertensives, levodopa:* Increase effect of these drugs
- *Phenothiazines, haloperidol, droperidol, oral contraceptives:* decrease action of bromocrip-

tine, thus increasing likelihood of conception in women taking estrogen-containing oral contraceptives

Implications: For NMS treatment only
Assess
- BP; this drug decreases BP

Planning/Implementation
- Instruct patient to take dose with meals to prevent GI symptoms.
- Administer hs so that dizziness, orthostatic hypotension are not problems.

Teaching
- To prevent orthostatic hypotension, change position slowly
- To use barrier contraceptives during treatment with this drug; pregnancy might occur
- To avoid hazardous activity when dizziness occurs

Evaluate
- Therapeutic response (NMS): decreased fever, sweating, rigidity, decreased slow movements, drooling

Administration
- *Parkinson's disease: adult:* PO 1.25 mg bid with meals, may increase q2-4wk, not to exceed 100 mg qd
- *NMS:* although standardized dose not established for this unlabeled use, dosages of 2.5-10 mg tid have been reported to be effective; if no improvement in 24 hr, increase to 20 mg PO qid (for other uses see PDR)
- *Cocaine withdrawal:* 1.25 mg tid for 7 days, then discontinue
- *Available forms:* caps 5 mg; tabs 2.5 mg (must be cut in half for 1.25-mg dose)

Buprenorphine
BUPRENEX
(byoo-pre-nor´-feen)

Functional classification: Opioid agonist/antagonist
Controlled Substance Schedule V
Pregnancy category: C

Indications: Management of moderate to severe pain; opioid detoxification

Contraindications: Hypersensitivity
Cautious use: Increased intracranial pressure; severe renal, hepatic, or pulmonary disease; hypothyroidism; undiagnosed abdominal pain; elderly; prostatic hypertrophy; pregnancy; children <13 yr

Pharmacologic Effects: A partial agonist at mu receptors and an antagonist at kappa receptors; by binding to opioid receptors, alters perception of pain and precipitates a withdrawal reaction in individuals dependent upon opioids

Pharmacokinetics: Well absorbed (IM), metabolized primarily by liver, half-life 2-3 hr, patients develop tolerance to analgesia

Side Effects: *CNS:* sedation, confusion, headache, euphoria, unusual dreams, hallucinations, dysphoria, dizziness; *peripheral:* miosis at high dosages, blurred vision, can cause respiratory depression but not severe as with morphine, hypotension, hypertension, nausea, vomiting, constipation, dry mouth, sweating

Interactions
- *Antihypertensives:* additive hypotensive effect
- *Anticholinergic:* additive to dry mouth, constipation, and others
- *CNS depressants:* additive CNS depression
- *MAOIs:* use with caution because of potential for respiratory depression and hypotension
- *Opioid analgesics:* decreased effectiveness of these drugs

Implications
Assess
- Establish baseline BP, pulse, and respirations

Planning/Implementation
- Inject IM preparation deep into muscle and rotate injection sites.
- Know it can precipitate withdrawal symptoms.

Teaching
- This drug might cause drowsiness
- To avoid concurrent use with alcohol and other CNS depressants
- To know the symptoms of orthostatic hypotension and to sit or lie down if they occur

Treatment of Overdose: In overdose, respiratory depression may be partially reversed with naloxone (Narcan); however, buprenorphine is tightly bound to receptors, and naloxone does not easily replace it.

Administration: *Adult:* Opioid detoxification: 2-8 mg sublingually qd

---

Bupropion HCl

WELLBUTRIN, ZYBAN (FOR SMOKING CESSATION)
(byoo-proe´-pee-on)

Functional classification: Novel antidepressant, selective dopamine reuptake inhibitor (SDRI)
Chemical classification: Aminoketone
FDA pregnancy category: B

Indications: Depression; smoking cessation; for sexual side effects of other drugs (e.g., SSRIs)

Contraindications: Hypersensitivity, concomitant use of MAOIs, seizure history, children <18 yr, patients with prior diagnosis of bulimia or anorexia (high incidence of seizures in these patients)

Cautious use: Psychoses, suicidal patients, CV disorders, hepatic or renal disorders, elderly patients

Pharmacologic Effects: Not clear but thought to result from inhibition of dopamine and norepinephrine reuptake; considered an "activating" antidepressant

Pharmacokinetics: Peak levels 2 hr; metabolized in liver, excreted in urine (87%) and feces (10%), half-life 15 hr, metabolized by CYP-450 2D6

Side Effects: *CNS:* seizures that are dose related (dosages <450 mg/day reduce risk of seizures); agitation, confusion, insomnia, headache, sedation, tremor; *peripheral:* blurred vision, dizziness, tachycardia, arrhythmias, dry mouth, constipation, weight loss or gain, nausea and vomiting, anorexia, excessive sweating, menstrual complaints, rash, erectile dysfunction, upper respiratory tract complaints

Interactions
- *Carbamazepine, phenytoin, cimetidine, phenobarbital:* slow metabolism of bupropion
- *Drugs that lower seizure threshold* (phenothiazines, TCAs): increased risk of seizures
- *Levodopa:* increased incidence of adverse effects of bupropion
- *MAOIs and alcohol:* increased toxicity of bupropion and seizures (alcohol)

Implications
Assess
- Blood studies: CBC, leukocyte count, cardiac enzyme levels
- Liver function tests before and during therapy: bilirubin level, AST, ALT
- ECG: flattening of T wave; bundle branch block; AV block; arrhythmias in cardiac patients

Planning/Implementation
- Treat constipation and dry mouth.
- Instruct patient to take dose with food or milk to prevent GI upset.
- Instruct patient to take last dose no later than 4 PM to minimize effects on sleep.

Teaching
- Therapeutic effects take 2-4 wk
- To use caution in driving or other hazardous activities
- To avoid alcohol; when alcohol is consumed, to wait until next morning to take bupropion
- Not to discontinue use abruptly

Evaluate
- Therapeutic response: level of depression; ability to perform activities of daily living; ability to sleep
- Mental status: mood, suicidal ideation

Treatment of Overdose: Hospitalize; give emetic if patient is conscious; activated charcoal; provide adequate fluids; treat seizures with IV benzodiazepines.

Administration

- *Adult:* 100 mg bid to start (AM and PM); based on clinical response, may be increased to 300 mg/day in divided doses no sooner than 3 days after beginning therapy; usual dose 300 mg/day, maximum dose 450 mg/day, with never more than 150 mg given in single dose; Wellbutrin SR: target dose 300 mg/day (150 mg bid)
- *Available forms:* tabs 75, 100 mg

Buspirone HCl

BUSPAR
(byoo-spear´-own)

Functional classification: Antianxiety agent
Chemical classification: Azaperone
FDA pregnancy category: B

Indications: Anxiety disorders

Contraindications: Hypersensitivity, psychosis
Cautious use: Lactation, child <18 yr, elderly patients, impaired hepatic or renal function

Pharmacologic Effects: Uncertain but thought to be related to partial agonist effects at postsynaptic $5HT_{1A}$ and full agonist effect presynaptically at these receptors; at high dosages, might increase dopamine activity; does not affect GABA systems; active metabolite, 1-2 pyrimidinyl piperazine (1PP), probably accounts for its therapeutic effect

Pharmacokinetics: Rapidly absorbed and undergoes extensive first-pass metabolism with 1%-4% becoming bioavailable, peak serum levels within 90 min, almost completely bound to serum proteins (~95%) excreted in urine and feces, half-life 2-11 hr, metabolized by CYP 3A4

Side Effects: *CNS:* dizziness, headache, depression, stimulation, insomnia, nervousness, lightheadedness, numbness, paresthesia, incoordination, tremors, excitement, involuntary movements, confusion, akathisia; *peripheral:* nausea, dry mouth, diarrhea, constipation; tachycardia, palpitations, hypotension; sore throat, tinnitus, blurred vision, nasal congestion; urinary frequency and hesitancy; muscle cramps; hyperventilation, chest congestion, shortness of breath; rash, edema, pruritus, alopecia, dry skin

Interactions

- *Alcohol:* do not mix, even though serious interactions have not been documented
- *Haloperidol:* increased haloperidol serum levels
- *MAOIs:* increased BP
- *Trazodone:* increased ALT

Implications

Assess

- BP, pulse; if systolic BP drops 20 mm Hg, withhold drug
- Hepatic studies: AST, ALT, bilirubin, creatinine, LDH, alkaline phosphatase levels
- Mental status

Planning/Implementation

- Assist with ambulation during beginning of therapy; drowsiness, dizziness occur.
- Have safety measures available, including side rails, when drowsiness occurs.

Teaching

- To allows 3-6 wk for optimal results (some improvement within 7-10 days)
- To take with food or milk for GI symptoms; food might decrease absorption but increase bioavailability
- To avoid driving and engaging in activities requiring alertness because drowsiness might occur
- To avoid alcohol or other CNS depressant medications unless prescribed by physician
- Not to discontinue medication abruptly after long-term use
- To rise slowly to prevent fainting
- To notify physician if chronic abnormal movements occur (restlessness, involuntary movements)

Evaluate

- Therapeutic response: decreased anxiety

Treatment of Overdose: Basically a very safe drug; gastric lavage, VS, supportive care; no deaths from overdose have been reported.

Administration

- *Adult:* PO 5 mg tid, may increase 5 mg/day every 2-3 days, not to exceed 60 mg/day; *initial dose:* 15 mg/day (7.5 mg bid, therapeutic response achieved by increasing dose 5 mg/day every 2-3 days)
- *Available forms:* tabs 5, 10, 15 mg (may be bisected or trisected)

Butabarbital/ butabarbital sodium*

**BUTATRAN, BUTICAPS, BUTISOL,
BUTISOL SODIUM, MEDARSED**
(byoo-ta-bar´-bi-tal)

Functional classifications: Sedative, hypnotic
Chemical classification: Barbitone
Controlled substance schedule II
FDA pregnancy category: D

Indications: Sedation, insomnia

Contraindications: See Amobarbital

Pharmacologic Effects: See Amobarbital

Pharmacokinetics: Onset 45-60 min, duration 6-8 hr; metabolized by liver, excreted in urine; half-life 66-140 hr

Side Effects: *CNS:* see Amobarbital; *peripheral:* see Amobarbital

Interactions: See Amobarbital

Implications: See Amobarbital

Treatment of Overdose: See Amobarbital

Administration
- *Insomnia:* PO 50-100 mg hs
- *Available forms:* tabs 15, 30, 50, 100 mg; caps 15, 30 mg; elix 30, 33.3 mg/5 ml

Caffeine

NO DOZ, TIREND, VIVARIN
(kaf´-een)

Functional classification: Cerebral stimulant
Chemical classification: Xanthine
FDA pregnancy category: C

Indications: Mild CNS stimulation to stay awake or increase mental alertness, used with analgesics

Contraindications: Gastric or duodenal hypersensitivity
Cautious use: Arrhythmias, lactation

Pharmacologic Effects: Promotes accumulation of cAMP by increasing calcium permeability and causes CNS stimulation; constricts cerebral blood vessels and relaxes smooth muscles in blood vessels to bronchi

Pharmacokinetics: *PO:* Readily absorbed, onset 15 min, peak ½-1 hr, metabolized by liver, excreted by kidneys, crosses placenta, excreted in breast milk, half-life 3-4 hr

Side Effects: *CNS:* hyperactivity, insomnia, restlessness, talkativeness, dizziness, headache, stimulation, irritability, aggressiveness, tremors, twitching; *peripheral:* nausea, vomiting, anorexia, diuresis, tachycardia

Interactions
- *Oral contraceptives, cimetidine:* increased effects of caffeine
- *Smoking:* enhanced caffeine elimination

Implications
Assess
- VS, BP

Planning/Implementation
- Do not give to patient who has peptic ulcer disease.

Teaching
- To decrease other caffeine consumption

(coffee, tea, cola, chocolate), which might increase irritability, stimulation
- To taper off drug over several weeks after long-term use
- Not to use as a substitute for regular sleep

Evaluate
- Therapeutic response: increased CNS stimulation, decreased drowsiness
- Mental status: stimulation, insomnia, irritability
- Tolerance or dependency: an increased amount may be used to get same effect
- Overdose: pain, fever, dehydration, insomnia, hyperactivity

Treatment of Overdose: Lavage, activated charcoal; monitor electrolyte levels, VS; administer anticonvulsants if needed.

Administration
- *Adult:* PO 100-200 mg q4h prn; *infant or child:* 8 mg/kg, not to exceed 500 mg
- *Available forms:* tabs 100, 200 mg; time-rel caps 200, 250 mg

Carbamazepine

CARBATROL (EXTENDED RELEASE), MAZEPINE,† TEGRETOL
(kar-ba-maz´-e-peen)

Functional classification: Antiepileptic
Chemical classification: Iminostilbene derivative
FDA pregnancy category: D

Indications: Tonic-clonic, psychomotor, mixed seizures; pain-associated trigeminal neuralgia
Unlabeled uses: Bipolar illness, schizoaffective illness, resistant schizophrenia, PTSD

Contraindications: History of bone marrow depression; hypersensitivity to carbamazepine and TCAs; concomitant use of MAOIs
Cautious use: History of hematologic reaction to any drug, glaucoma, psychosis history, child <6 yr, lactation

Pharmacologic Effects: Unrelated to other antiepileptics but structurally related to TCAs; mechanism of action unknown but it reduces high-frequency actions potentials, thus preventing the spread of seizures; appears to do this by normalizing sodium channel activity and sodium influx; also affects other neurotransmitters systems, including norepinephrine, dopamine, ACh, and GABA; therapeutic serum levels 4-12 mg/ml

Pharmacokinetics: PO peak serum in 4-5 hr, metabolized in liver, excreted in urine (72%) and feces (28%), half-life 12-17 hr with repeated doses, protein binding 75%; metabolized by P-450 2D6 and 3A4

Side Effects: *CNS:* drowsiness, dizziness, unsteadiness, confusion, fatigue, paralysis, headache, hallucinations; *peripheral:* nausea, vomiting, diarrhea, blood dyscrasias that lead to fatalities (i.e., aplastic anemia, leukopenia, agranulocytosis, thrombocytopenia, bone marrow depression), hepatitis, urinary frequency and retention, pulmonary hypersensitivity, fever, dyspnea, CHF, hypertension, hypotension, transient diplopia, fever and chills, rash

Interactions
- *Barbiturates; primidone:* lower serum level of carbamazepine
- *Carbamazepine:* increases the metabolism of acetaminophen and oral anticoagulants
- *Cimetidine, danazol, diltiazem, erythromycin, isoniazid, nicotinamide, propoxyphene, verapamil:* elevate carbamazepine serum levels
- *Doxycycline:* reduces half-life of doxycycline
- *Haloperidol:* decreases effect of haloperidol
- *Hydantoins:* decreases carbamazepine levels; both increases and decreases hydantoin serum levels
- *Lithium:* increases CNS intoxication or enhanced antimanic effects
- *Nondepolarizing muscle relaxants:* resist or reverse muscle relaxants
- *Succinimides:* reduces succinimide levels
- *Theophylline:* for both drugs, decreased effects
- *Valproic acid:* decreases serum levels of valproic acid

Implications
Assess
- Renal studies, blood studies, hepatic studies for baseline data and to determine whether carbamazepine therapy is appropriate

Planning/Implementation
- Instruct patient to take dose with food or milk to decrease GI upset (might enhance absorption).

Teaching
- To avoid driving or operating hazardous machinery when dizzy, drowsy, or experiencing blurred vision
- To notify physician of unusual bleeding or bruising, jaundice, abdominal pain, pale stools, darkened urine, erectile dysfunction, CNS disturbances, edema, fever, chills, sore throat, or ulcer in mouth
- To wear MedicAlert identification bracelet
- Not to discontinue drug abruptly because doing so can cause seizures

Evaluate
- Therapeutic responses: decreased seizure activity, decreased flashbacks, and the like
- Mental status
- Blood dyscrasias: fever, sore throat, rash, bruising

- Toxic effects: bone marrow depression, nausea and vomiting

Treatment of Overdose: *Symptoms:* neuromuscular disturbances, irregular breathing, hypotension or hypertension, respiratory depression; treat symptoms with lavage, charcoal; maintain airway; elevate legs and administer plasma volume expander for hypotension; monitor breathing, heart rate (ECG), BP, kidney function.

Administration
- *Seizures: adult and child >12 yr:* initially 200 mg bid; increase at weekly intervals by up to 200 mg/day in 3-4 doses; not to exceed 1000 mg/day in children 12-15 yr; not to exceed 1200 mg/day in children >15 yr; maintenance usually 800-1200 mg/day; *child 6-12 yr:* initially 100 mg bid; increase at weekly intervals by adding 100 mg/day in 3-4 doses; do not exceed 1000 mg/day; maintenance dose usually 400-800 mg/day
- *Available forms:* tabs, chewable 100 mg; tabs 200 mg; suspension 100 mg/5 ml, XR; tabs 100, 200, 400 mg

Carbidopa-levodopa

SINEMET

(kar-bi-doe´-pa lee-voe-doe´-pa)

Functional classification: Antiparkinson drug
Chemical classification: Catecholamine
FDA pregnancy category: C

Indications: Parkinsonism

Contraindications: Narrow-angle glaucoma, hypersensitivity, undiagnosed skin lesions, MAOI therapy

Pharmacologic Effects: Carbidopa prevents metabolism of levodopa to dopamine in periphery; dopamine cannot cross blood-brain barrier in significant amounts, so more levodopa enters CNS

Pharmacokinetics: Peak blood level 1-3 hr; excreted in urine

Side Effects: *CNS:* tremors of hand, fatigue, involuntary movements, headache, anxiety, twitching, confusion, agitation, insomnia, nightmares, hallucinations; *peripheral:* nausea, vomiting, GI symptoms, gas, dysphagia, skin eruptions, orthostatic hypotension, tachycardia, palpitations, blurred vision, dilated pupils, dark urine, urinary retention

Interactions
- *Antacids, metoclopramide:* Increased effects of levodopa
- *Anticholinergics, hydantoins, papaverine, pyridoxine, haloperidol:* Decreased effect of levodopa

- *Antihypertensives:* orthostatic hypotension
- *MAOIs:* hypertensive crisis
- *TCAs:* hypertension
Consult PDR for the many other interactions.

Implications
Assess
- BP, respirations, mental status

Planning/Implementation
- Assist patient with ambulation until condition is stabilized on drug regimen.

Teaching
- To change positions slowly
- Not to discontinue use abruptly, because parkinsonian crisis can occur
- Not to be alarmed by dark urine or sweat
- To allow 3-4 mo for therapeutic effect

Evaluate
- Mental status, therapeutic response

Treatment of Overdose: No reports of overdosage with carbidopa; for levodopa, provide supportive care with immediate gastric lavage; monitor for airway, development of arrhythmias.

Administration
- *Adult:* PO 3-6 tabs of 25 mg carbidopa/250 mg levodopa per day in divided doses; maximum dose not to exceed 8 tabs/day
- *Available forms:* tabs 10 mg (carbidopa)/100 mg (levodopa), 25/100, 25/250 mg

Chloral hydrate

AQUACHLORAL SUPPRETTES, NOCTEC, NOVOCHLORHYDRATE†
(klor-al hy´-drate)

Functional classifications: Sedative, hypnotic
Controlled substance schedule IV
FDA pregnancy category: C

Indications: Sedation, insomnia

Contraindications: Hypersensitivity to chloral hydrate, severe renal and hepatic disease, GI problems

Pharmacologic Effects: Mechanism of action not clear; hypnotic dose causes mild CNS depression

Pharmacokinetics: Metabolized to trichloroethanol, an active metabolite that has a half-life of 7-10 hr; protein binding 35%-41%; trichloroethanol metabolized to trichloroacetic acid, an inactive metabolite; trichloroacetic acid excreted in urine and bile and has protein binding capacity of 71%-88%; can displace other acidic drugs from protein binding sites

Side Effects: *CNS:* somnambulism, disorientation, incoherence, paradoxic excitement, delirium, drowsiness, ataxia; *peripheral:* nausea and vomiting; other GI disturbances; blood dyscrasias; skin eruptions (e.g., rashes, hives)

Interactions
- *Alcohol:* synergistic effect with disulfiram-like reactions (i.e., tachycardia, flushing)
- *CNS depressants:* additive effect
- *Furosemide:* sweating, hot flashes, tachycardia
- *Hydantoins:* reduced effect of hydantoin
- *Oral anticoagulants:* slight increased effect

Implications
Assess
- Blood studies

Planning/Implementation
- Maintain safety (e.g., prevent falls, keep side rails up).
- Instruct patient to take dose ½-1 hr before bedtime for insomnia.
- Instruct patient to take dose after meals to decrease GI effect.

Teaching
- To avoid driving and use of alcohol and other CNS depressants
- That there is a potential for dependence
- Not to discontinue use abruptly
- Not to chew capsules

Evaluate
- Therapeutic response, mental status, respiratory difficulties, monitor for blood dyscrasias

Treatment of Overdose: Symptoms similar to those for barbiturate overdose; doses >2 g might produce intoxication; deaths have occurred with dosages as low as 1.25-3 g; dosages as high as 36 g have been tolerated; treatment is gastric lavage or induced emesis; activated charcoal might retard absorption; hemodialysis might be helpful; other supportive care as needed.

Administration
- *Insomnia: adult:* PO/REC 500 mg-1 g ½-1 hr before bedtime; *child:* PO/REC 25-50 mg/kg in 1 dose, up to 1 g (hypnotic) or 500 mg (sedative)
- *Available forms:* caps 250, 500 mg; syr 250, 500 mg/5 ml; supp 324, 500, 648 mg

Chlordiazepoxide HCl

**A-POXIDE, CHLORDIAZEPOXIDE HCL,
LIBRITABS, LIBRIUM, MEDILIUM,†
NOVOPOXIDE,† SOLIUM†**
(klor-dye-az-e-pox´-ide)

Functional classification: Antianxiety agent
Chemical classification: Benzodiazepine
Controlled substance schedule IV
FDA pregnancy category: D

Indications: Short-term management of anxiety, acute alcohol withdrawal; preoperatively for relaxation

Contraindications: Hypersensitivity to benzodiazepines, narrow-angle glaucoma, psychosis, child <6 yr (oral), child <12 yr (inj)
Cautious use: Elderly or debilitated patients, hepatic or renal disease

Pharmacologic Effects: Increases affinity of GABA molecules for their specific receptor, increasing the frequency with which chloride channels open in response to GABA; might also decrease norepinephrine and serotonin turnover rates

Pharmacokinetics
- *Speed of onset:* intermediate
- *PO:* onset 30 min, peak 0.5-4 hr, duration 4-6 hr, metabolized by liver, excreted by kidneys, crosses placenta, excreted in breast milk, half-life 5-30 hr (average 18 hr)

Side Effects: *CNS:* drowsiness, dizziness, confusion, headache, anxiety, tremor, stimulation, fatigue, depression, insomnia; *peripheral:* photophobia caused by mydriasis, blurred vision caused by cycloplegia, sleeplike slowing of respirations with therapeutic doses, cough, orthostatic hypotension, tachycardia, hypotension, constipation, dry mouth

Interactions
- *Alcohol and other CNS depressants:* increased risk of excessive CNS depression
- *Cimetidine:* potentiation of CNS depression
- *Digoxin:* increased risk of cardiac side effects from digoxin
- *Levodopa:* decreased antiparkinson effect
- *Oral anticoagulants:* increases or decreases anticoagulant effect
- *Phenytoin:* increased phenytoin serum levels

Implications: See Alprazolam

Treatment of Overdose: Lavage, VS, supportive care; few deaths, if any, reported as resulting from benzodiazepine overdose alone; deaths occur when benzodiazepines are mixed with other drugs, especially alcohol.

Administration
- *Mild anxiety: adult:* PO 5-10 mg tid or qid;

child >6 yr: 5 mg bid-qid, not to exceed 10 mg bid-tid; *geriatric:* 5 mg bid-qid
- *Severe anxiety: adult:* PO 20-25 mg tid-qid
- *Alcohol withdrawal: adult:* PO/IM/IV 50-100 mg, not to exceed 300 mg/day; is poorly absorbed
- *Available forms:* caps 5, 10, 25 mg; tabs 5, 10, 25 mg; powder for IM inj 100-mg ampule

Chlorpromazine HCl

**CHLORPROMANYL, ORMAZINE,
THORAZINE**
(klor-proe´-ma-zeen)

Functional classifications: Traditional antipsychotic (low potency), neuroleptic
Chemical classification: Phenothiazine, aliphatic
FDA pregnancy category: D

Indications: *Psychiatric:* psychotic disorders, mania, schizophrenia; *other:* intractable hiccups, nausea, vomiting, preoperatively for relaxation, acute intermittent porphyria

Contraindications: Hypersensitivity, liver damage, cerebral arteriosclerosis, coronary disease, severe hypertension or hypotension, blood dyscrasias, coma, child <6 mo, brain damage, bone marrow depression, presence of alcohol and barbiturate
Cautious use: Lactation, seizure disorders, hypertension, hepatic disease, cardiac disease, respiratory impairment, especially in children

Pharmacologic Effects: Traditional antipsychotic drugs produce a neuroleptic effect characterized by sedation, emotional quieting, psychomotor slowing, and affective indifference; exact mode of action is not fully understood; blocks D_2 receptors (+++) in the basal ganglia, hypothalamus, limbic system, brainstem, and medulla; blockade of these receptors accounts for both therapeutic and adverse responses; because of their nonselective actions, many other neurotransmitters systems are affected as well; acetylcholine (+++), histamine (+++), and alpha-1 (++++); therapeutic plasma levels are 30-500 ng/ml

Pharmacokinetics
- *PO:* onset erratic, peak 2-4 hr; *IM:* onset 15-30 min, peak 15-20 min, provides 4-10 times more active drug than do oral doses; *IV:* onset 5 min, peak 10 min; PO, IM, and IV forms might be detected for up to 6 mo after last dose; *REC:* onset erratic, peak 3 hr; metabolized by liver, excreted in urine, crosses placenta, excreted in breast milk; 95% bound to plasma proteins; elimination half-life 16-30 hr

Side Effects for Traditional Antipsychotics:
CNS: parkinsonism, akathisias, dystonias, tardive

dyskinesia, oculogyric crisis, weight gain; *peripheral:* blurred vision (cycloplegia or paralysis of accommodation), ocular pain, photophobia, mydriasis, impaired vision; intolerance of extreme heat or cold, possible heat stroke or fatal hyperthermia; nasal congestion, wheezing, dyspnea; hypotension, especially orthostatic, leading to dizziness, syncope, tachycardia, irregular pulse, arrhythmias; dry mouth, constipation, jaundice, abdominal pain, urinary retention and hesitancy, galactorrhea, gynecomastia, impaired ejaculation, amenorrhea

Specific for chlorpromazine: Sedation (~30%), EPSEs (~10%), orthostasis (~30%), anticholinergic (~30%), weight gain (~30%), sexual dysfunction (min)

Interactions

- *Alcohol and other CNS depressants* (barbiturates, antihistamines, antianxiety or antidepressant drugs): increased CNS depression, increased risk of EPSEs
- *Amphetamines:* possible decreased antipsychotic effect
- *Antacids* (magnesium and aluminum products): possible decreased antipsychotic effect
- *Anticholinergics* (e.g., atropine, benztropine, H_1-type antihistamines, antidepressants): increased risk of excessive atropine-like side effects or toxic effects
- *Anticonvulsants:* phenytoin causes decreased serum level of phenothiazines, haloperidol, and clozapine
- *Antidepressants:* cyclics (amitriptyline, trimipramine, trazodone) cause additive sedation, hypotension, and anticholinergic effects; SSRIs (fluoxetine, paroxetine, fluvoxamine) cause increased neuroleptic plasma levels
- *Antihistamines* (terfenadine, astemizole): can cause prolongation of QT interval for thioridazine and pimozide
- *Buspirone:* might increase EPSEs
- *Cigarettes:* decreased plasma level of neuroleptic because of CYP induction
- *Diazoxide:* possible severe hyperglycemia, prediabetic coma
- *Guanethidine:* poor control of hypertension by guanethidine
- *Hypoglycemia drugs* (insulin, oral hypoglycemia agents): poor diabetic control
- *Lithium:* poor control of psychosis with combined therapy; can mask lithium intoxication; neurotoxic effects with confusion, delirium, seizures, encephalopathy
- *Meperidine, morphine:* increased risk of severe CNS depression, respiratory depression, hypotension
- *Propranolol:* increased pharmacologic effects of either drug

Implications: For traditional antipsychotics
Assess
- Establish baseline VS, laboratory values to aid in assessing side effects, allergic or hypersensitivity reactions
- Physiologic and psychologic status before therapy to determine needs and evaluate progress
- For early stages of tardive dyskinesia by use of Abnormal Involuntary Movement Scale
- Identify concurrent symptoms that might be aggravated by antipsychotics (e.g., glaucoma, diabetes)

Planning/Implementation

- Ensure that drug has been taken; check mouth for "cheeking."
- When giving liquid antipsychotics, use at least 60 ml of compatible beverage to mask taste; dilute and give immediately; take drug with food to minimize GI upset; give IM injections in lateral thigh.
- Keep patient quiet after injection to prevent falls associated with postural hypotension.
- For dry mouth, give chewing gum, hard candies, lip balm; monitor urinary output; check for bladder distension in inactive patients, older men, and patients receiving high dosages.
- Assist patient with ambulation when blurred vision occurs; dim room lights for photosensitivity.
- Ensure safety with hypotension; have patient sit on side of bed before rising, head-low position for dizziness, avoid hot showers, wear elastic stockings.
- Check BP (supine, sitting, standing) and pulse before and after each dose when possible; observe for side effects.
- Monitor body temperature for indications of muscle rigidity, fever, depressed neurologic status; ensure adequate hydration, nutrition, and ventilation.
- Protect patient from exposure to extreme heat or cold.
- Recognize impending hypersensitivity: pruritus or jaundice with hepatitis, flulike or coldlike symptoms, evidence of bleeding with blood dyscrasia.
- Observe for involuntary movements.

Teaching

- About benefits and potential harm of antipsychotic drugs; weigh need to know against causing apprehension
- To comply with drug treatment
- To avoid activities requiring clear vision for a few weeks after treatment starts; to report eye pain immediately
- To understand importance of exercise, fluids, and fiber in the diet
- To watch for symptoms of heart failure: weight gain, dyspnea, distended neck veins, tachycardia
- Possible male sexual performance failure; suggest relaxed, stress-free environment

---

*Infrequently used.   †Available in Canada only.

- To avoid conception; women should practice effective contraception; phenothiazines might cause false-positive results in pregnancy tests
- To avoid exposure to sunlight; keep skin covered but with temperature-appropriate clothing
- That patient cannot become addicted to antipsychotic drugs
- To avoid overheating and dehydration; should be advised regarding appropriate care in avoiding both

Evaluate
- Whether patient follows prescribed regimen, takes medications as ordered
- Avoids injury; reports dizziness or need for assistance
- Verbalizes reduced anxiety
- Experiences minimal or no adverse responses
- Uses appropriate interventions to minimize side effects
- Achieves improved mental status; most problems occur during first 2 wk of therapy
- For agranulocytosis, especially within 4-10 wk after initiation of chlorpromazine therapy

Treatment of Overdose: Lavage, if orally ingested; provide an airway; do not induce vomiting; control EPSEs and hypotension.

Administration: Psychiatric indications
- *Psychiatry: adult:* PO 10-50 mg q1-4h initially, then increase up to ≈800 mg/day (up to 2000 mg/day); IM 10-50 mg q1-4h; *child:* PO 0.25 mg/lb q4-6h or 0.5 mg/kg; IM 0.25 mg/lb q6-8h or 0.5 mg/kg; REC 0.5 mg/lb q6-8h or 1 mg/kg; *other uses:* see PDR
- *Available forms:* tabs 10, 25, 50, 100, 200 mg; time-rel caps 30, 75, 150, 200, 300 mg; syr 10 mg/5 ml; conc 30, 100 mg/ml; supp 25, 100 mg; inj IM, IV 25 mg/ml

Chlorprothixene
TARACTAN
(klor-proe-thix´-een)

Functional classifications: Traditional antipsychotic (low potency), neuroleptic
Chemical classification: Thioxanthene
FDA pregnancy category: C

Indications: Psychotic disorders, schizophrenia

Contraindications: Hypersensitivity, liver damage, cerebral arteriosclerosis, coronary disease, severe hypertension or hypotension, blood dyscrasias, coma, child <6 yr (PO), child <12 yr (IM), brain damage, bone marrow depression, alcohol and barbiturate withdrawal states

Cautious use: Lactation, seizure disorders, hypertension, hepatic disease, cardiac disease

Pharmacologic Effects: Traditional antipsychotic drugs produce a neuroleptic effect characterized by sedation, emotional quieting, psychomotor slowing, and affective indifference; exact mode of action not fully understood; blocks D_2 receptors (++++) in the basal ganglia, hypothalamus, limbic system, brainstem, and medulla; blockade of these receptors accounts for both therapeutic and adverse responses; because of their nonselective actions, many other neurotransmitters systems are affected as well: acetylcholine (+++), histamine (+++++), and alpha-1 (++++)

Pharmacokinetics: PO: onset erratic, peak 2-4 hr; duration might be detected for up to 6 mo after last dose; metabolized by liver, excreted in urine (metabolites), crosses placenta, excreted in breast milk

Side Effects: See Chlorpromazine; *specific for chlorprothixene:* sedation (~10%), EPSEs (~10%), CV (~30%), anticholinergic (~30%), weight gain (~10%), sexual dysfunction (min)

Interactions: See Chlorpromazine
Implications: See Chlorpromazine

Treatment of Overdose: Lavage, if orally ingested; provide an airway; do not induce vomiting.

Administration
- *Adult:* PO 25-50 mg tid or qid, increased to desired response, maximum dosage 600 mg/qd
- *Geriatric:* start at 10-25 mg tid or qid; IM 25-50 mg tid or qid
- *Child >6 yr:* PO 10-25 mg tid or qid; IM not recommended for children <12 yr
- *Available forms:* tabs 10, 25, 50, 100 mg; conc 100 mg/5 ml; inj IM 12.5 mg/ml

Citalopram
CELEXA
(sy-tal´-oh-pram)

Functional classification: SSRI antidepressant
Chemical classification: Bicyclic phthalane derivative

Indications: Depression

Contraindications: MAOIs, sensitivity to citalopram
Cautious use: Patients with reduced hepatic function, reduced renal function, elderly, mania or hypomania, seizure disorder, suicide risk, diseases with altered metabolism or hemodynamic response, myocardial infarction

Pharmacologic Effects: Inhibits the neuronal reuptake of serotonin with minimal effects on norepinephrine and dopamine reuptake mechanisms; clinical response in ~2 wk

Pharmacokinetics: Peak 4 hr, steady state achieved in 1 wk, absorption not affected by food, primarily metabolized by liver, excreted by kidneys, protein binding 80%; weak inhibitor of P-450 1A2, 2D6, and 2C19; primarily metabolized by P-450 3A4 and 2C19

Side Effects: CNS: dizziness, insomnia (++), sleepiness (++), fatigue (+); *peripheral:* nausea (+++), dry mouth (++), increased sweating (++), diarrhea (+), delay in ejaculation (+), tremor (+), vomiting (+), anorexia (+), anxiety (+), agitation (+), dysmenorrhea (+), erectile dysfunction (+), abdominal pain (+), decreased libido (+)

Interactions: Because of its weaker inhibition of CYP isoenzymes, citalopram is thought to have fewer problematic interactions

- *Alcohol:* increased drowsiness
- *Carbamazepine:* ? increased clearance of citalopram
- *Cimetidine:* increased levels when combined with citalopram
- *CNS drugs:* increased drowsiness
- *MAOIs:* potential for hypertensive crisis
- *Lithium:* increased serotoninergic effect
- *TCAs:* toxic effects of TCAs increased
- *Warfarin:* pharmacokinetics not affected but prothrombin time increased by 5%

Implications
Assess:
See Sertraline

Planning/Implementation: See Sertraline for general planning concepts

Teaching
- To avoid driving a car or operating hazardous machinery
- To avoid alcohol or other CNS depressants
- To check with prescriber before starting OTC medications

Evaluate
- Monitor therapy (i.e., side effects, mood)
- Be aware of the potential for suicide as patient is energized

Treatment of Overdose: Deaths have occurred when SSRIs have been combined with other serotonergic drugs; for overdose, establish and maintain an airway; administer oxygen prn, charcoal might inhibit absorption and might be more effective than induced vomiting.

Administration: Usual initial dose of citalopram 20 mg qd with an increase to 40 mg daily
- *Adult:* up to 60 mg/day
- *Elderly and those with liver damage:* typically 20 mg/day
- *Available forms:* tabs 20 mg, 40 mg

Clomipramine*
ANAFRANIL
(klom-ip´-ra-meen)

Functional classification: Antidepressant (serotonin reuptake inhibitor [SRI])
Chemical classification: Tricyclic, tertiary amine
FDA pregnancy category: C

Indications: Obsessive-compulsive disorder

Contraindications: Hypersensitivity to TCAs; acute recovery phase following MI; concomitant use with MAOIs; children <10 yr

Pharmacologic Effects: Blocks serotonin reuptake (++++) while the active metabolite desmethylclomipramine blocks norepinephrine reuptake (+); also receptor antagonist of ACh (+++), histamine (+++), and alpha-1 (+++); therapeutic plasma level 150-300 ng/ml

Pharmacokinetics: Metabolized by liver, excreted in urine; half-life 19-37 hr

Side Effects: CNS: sedation, headache (52%), insomnia (25%), libido change (21%), nervousness (18%), myoclonus (13%), increased appetite (11%), ataxia, confusion, delirium; *peripheral:* blurred vision, photophobia, increased intraocular pressure; decreased tearing; orthostatic hypotension; arrhythmias, tachycardia, palpitations; dry mouth (84%), constipation (47%), diarrhea; increased sweating; urinary retention and hesitancy; ejaculation failure (42%), erectile dysfunction (20%); fatigue (39%); weight gain (18%)

Interactions
- *Alcohol and other CNS depressants:* increased CNS depression
- *Anticholinergics:* increased anticholinergic effect
- *Estrogens:* decreased or increased effects of clomipramine
- *Ethchlorvynol:* delirium
- *Haloperidol, cimetidine:* toxic effects r/t increased plasma levels of clomipramine
- *MAOIs:* hypertensive crisis, convulsions
- *Phenytoin, phenobarbital:* decreased seizure threshold
- *Sympathomimetics:* increased risk of sympathomimetic effect

Implications: See Amitriptyline

Administration
- *Adult:* 25 mg/day to start, gradually increase to 100-200 mg/day during first 2 wk; give in divided doses and with food to reduce GI upset; maximum dose 250 mg/day; eventually total doses can be given hs
- *Child and adolescent:* 25 mg/day to start,

gradually increase in first 2 wk to 3 mg/kg or 200 mg, whichever is smaller; can be given once a day hs
- *Available forms:* caps 25, 50, 75 mg

This drug is also available under the name Clomicalm for use in animals exhibiting obsessive behavior.

Clonazepam

KLONOPIN
(kloe-na´-zi-pam)

Functional classification: Anticonvulsant
Chemical classification: Benzodiazepine
Controlled substance schedule IV
FDA pregnancy category: D

Indications: Absence, Lennox-Gastaut syndrome, atypical absence, akinetic, myoclonic seizures
Unlabeled use: Panic attacks, benzodiazepine withdrawal

Contraindications: Hypersensitivity to benzodiazepines, acute narrow-angle glaucoma
Cautious use: Open-angle glaucoma, chronic respiratory disease, impaired hepatic and renal function

Pharmacologic Effects: Inhibits spike and wave formation in absence seizures (petit mal), decreases amplitude, frequency, duration, and spread of discharge in minor motor seizures; effects probably related to enhancing the effects of GABA-mediated neuronal inhibition

Pharmacokinetics: PO: peak 1-2 hr, metabolized by liver, excreted in urine, half-life 18-60 hr; therapeutic plasma level 20-80 mg/ml; 85% bound; CYP 3A might play an important role in reduction and oxidation; absolute bioavailability 90%

Side Effects: *CNS:* drowsiness (50%), ataxia (30%), dizziness, confusion, behavioral changes, tremors, insomnia, headache, suicidal tendencies; *peripheral:* nausea, constipation, diarrhea; polyphagia, anorexia; rash, alopecia, hirsutism; increased salivation; nystagmus, diplopia, abnormal eye movements; sore gums; respiratory depression, dyspnea, congestion (from increased salivation); palpitations, bradycardia; thrombocytopenia, leukocytosis, eosinophilia

Interactions
- *Alcohol, CNS depressants, and other anticonvulsants:* increased CNS depression
- *Carbamazepine:* increased carbamazepine serum level
- *Valproic acid:* increased potential for seizures

Implications
Assess
- Renal studies: urinalysis, BUN and urine creatinine levels
- Blood studies: RBC, hematocrit, hemoglobin level, reticulocyte counts qwk for 4 wk, then qmo
- Hepatic studies: ALT, AST, bilirubin, and creatinine levels
- Drug serum levels during initial treatment

Planning/Implementation
- Instruct patient to take dose with milk or food to decrease GI symptoms.
- Have patient suck on hard candy and rinse mouth and gums frequently for dry mouth.
- Assist with ambulation during early part of treatment; dizziness occurs.

Teaching
- To carry MedicAlert identification bracelet
- To avoid driving or other activities that require alertness
- To avoid ingestion of alcohol or CNS depressants; increased sedation might occur
- Not to discontinue medication quickly after long-term use; taper off over several weeks (can precipitate status epilepticus)

Evaluate
- Therapeutic response: decreased seizure activity, document on patient's chart
- Mental status
- Eye problems: need for ophthalmic examinations before, during, and after treatment
- Allergic reaction: red raised rash; if rash occurs, drug should be discontinued
- Blood dyscrasias: fever, sore throat, bruising, rash, jaundice
- Toxic effects: ataxia, hypotension, hypotonia

Treatment of Overdose: Lavage; activated charcoal; monitor electrolyte levels, VS; administer vasopressors.

Administration
- *Lennox-Gastaut, akinetic, myoclonic seizures: adult:* PO: first start with 1.5 mg/day in 3 divided doses; may be increased 0.5-1 mg every 3 days until desired response, not to exceed 20 mg/day; *infant or child <10 yr or 30 kg:* PO 0.01-0.03 mg/kg/day in divided doses q8h, not to exceed 0.05 mg/kg/day; may be increased by no more than 7.5 mg/wk; maximum dose is 60 mg/day; not recommended for children <9 yr.
- *Available forms:* tabs 0.5, 1, 2 mg

Clorazepate dipotassium

TRANXENE
(klor-az´-e-pate)

Functional classification: Antianxiety agent
Chemical classification: Benzodiazepine
Controlled substance schedule IV
FDA pregnancy category: D

Indications: Anxiety, acute alcohol withdrawal, adjunct in partial seizure treatment

Contraindications: Hypersensitivity to benzodiazepines, narrow-angle glaucoma, psychosis, child <9 yr
   Cautious use: Elderly or debilitated patients, hepatic or renal disease, lactation

Pharmacologic Effects: Increases affinity of GABA molecules for their specific receptor, increasing the frequency with which chloride channels open in response to GABA

Pharmacokinetics
- *Speed of onset:* fast
- *PO:* onset 15 min, peak 1-2 hr, duration 4-6 hr, metabolized by liver, excreted by kidneys, crosses placenta, excreted in breast milk, half-life 30-100 hr

Side Effects: *CNS:* drowsiness, dizziness, confusion, headache, anxiety, tremor, stimulation, fatigue, depression, insomnia; *peripheral:* photophobia caused by mydriasis, blurred vision caused by cycloplegia; sleeplike slowing of respirations with therapeutic doses, cough; orthostatic hypotension, tachycardia, hypotension; constipation; dry mouth; decreased hematocrit; transient skin rash

Interactions: See Alprazolam

Implications: See Alprazolam

Treatment of Overdose: Lavage, VS, supportive care; few deaths, if any, reported as resulting from benzodiazepine overdose alone; deaths occur when benzodiazepines are mixed with other drugs, especially alcohol.

Administration
- Not recommended for use in patients <9 yr of age
- *Anxiety: adult:* PO 15-60 mg/day, usual daily dose 30 mg; *geriatric:* 7.5-15 mg/day
- *Alcohol withdrawal: adult:* PO 30 mg, then 30-60 mg in divided doses; day 2, 45-90 mg in divided doses; day 3, 22.5-45 mg in divided doses; day 4, 15-30 mg in divided doses; then reduce daily dose to 7.5-15 mg
- *Seizure disorders: adult and child >12 yr:* PO 7.5 mg tid, may increase by ≤7.5 mg/wk, not to exceed 90 mg/day; *child 9-12 yr:* PO 7.5

mg bid; increase by 7.5 mg/wk, not to exceed 60 mg/day
- Tranxene SD (half dose) 11.25 and 22.5 may be administered as a single dose q24h; Tranxene SD should not be used to initiate therapy
- *Available forms:* caps 3.75, 7.5, 15 mg; tabs 3.75, 7.5, 11.25, 15, 22.5 mg

Clozapine

CLOZARIL
(kloz´-a-peen)

Functional classifications: Atypical antipsychotic, neuroleptic, serotonin/dopamine antagonist
Chemical classification: Dibenzodiazepine
FDA pregnancy category: B

Indications: Management of schizophrenia refractory to other antipsychotics

Contraindications: History of clozapine-induced agranulocytosis; myeloproliferative disorders; concomitant use with other agents that can depress bone marrow function; severe CNS depression; coma; child <16 yr; lactation
   Cautious use: Patients with hepatic, renal, or cardiac disease

Pharmacologic Effects: Interferes with binding of dopamine at D_1 and D_4 receptors and serotonin at $5HT_2$ receptors; preferentially more active at limbic than at striatal dopamine receptors, probably accounting for the relative lack of EPSEs; weakly blocks D_2 receptors

Pharmacokinetics: Metabolized in liver, excreted in urine and feces, half-life 4-12 hr, 97% protein bound

Side Effects: Clozapine has relatively few EPSEs; *CNS:* drowsiness (39%), dizziness or vertigo (19%), headache (7%), tremor (6%), syncope (6%), disturbed sleep or nightmares (4%), restlessness (4%), akinesia (4%), agitation (4%), dose-related seizures (3%), rigidity (3%), akathisia (3%), confusion (3%); *peripheral:* salivation (31%), sweating (6%), dry mouth (6%), visual disturbances (5%), tachycardia (25%), hypotension (9%), hypertension (4%), constipation (14%), nausea (5%), fever (5%), agranulocytosis (1%); fatalities have occurred often enough to necessitate a special monitoring system

Interactions
- *Agents that suppress bone marrow function:* agranulocytosis
- *Anticholinergics:* increased anticholinergic effect
- *Antiepileptics:* might diminish efficacy of clozapine

- *Antihypertensives:* increased hypotensive effect
- *CNS depressants:* additive effect
- *Epinephrine:* severe hypotension
- *Protein-binding drugs:* potentiation of clozapine or the other drug

Implications
Assess
- Blood studies
- Concomitant illness
- Fever; flulike symptoms might indicate agranulocytosis

Planning/Implementation
- Monitor WBC and granulocyte count weekly
- Monitor ECG
- Monitor BP (standing and sitting) for hypotension

Teaching
- To be aware of risk of agranulocytosis and need for weekly blood tests
- To be aware of significant risk of seizures
- To avoid driving or operating hazardous machinery
- To be aware of risk of orthostatic hypotension
- Not to become pregnant
- Not to breast-feed

Evaluate
- Blood values
- Mental status
- Seizure activity

Treatment of Overdose: Symptoms of altered states of consciousness (i.e., drowsiness, delirium, coma, tachycardia, respiratory depression); establish and maintain airway, ensure adequate ventilation and oxygenation; give activated charcoal; provide supportive care; do not use epinephrine or its derivatives for hypotension.

Administration
- *Adult:* PO: begin with 12.5 mg qd or bid, then increase by 25-50 mg/day; target dose is 300-450 mg/day by the end of 2 wk, if tolerated; some patients might require 600-900 mg/day
- *Available forms:* tabs 25, 100 mg

Dantrolene sodium

DANTRIUM, DANTRIUM IV
(dan´-troe-leen)

Functional classification: Skeletal muscle relaxant, direct acting
Chemical classification: Hydantoin
FDA pregnancy category: C

Indications: Spasticity caused by upper motor neuron disorders, malignant hyperthermia and NMS

Contraindications: Hypersensitivity, active hepatic disease, impaired myocardial function, lactation, children <5 yr
Cautious use: Peptic ulcer disease, renal or hepatic disease, stroke, seizure disorder, diabetes mellitus, impaired pulmonary function

Pharmacologic Effects: Produces skeletal muscle relaxation by affecting the muscle directly; this effect probably associated with interference with the release of calcium

Pharmacokinetics: PO: peak 5 hr, half-life 8 hr, metabolized in liver, excreted in urine (metabolites)

Side Effects: *CNS:* dizziness, weakness, fatigue, drowsiness, headache, disorientation, insomnia, paresthesias, tremors, decreased seizure threshold; *peripheral:* nasal congestion, blurred vision, mydriasis, eosinophilia, hypotension, chest pain, palpitations, nausea, constipation, vomiting, abdominal pain, dry mouth, anorexia, urinary frequency, rash, pruritus

Interactions
- *Alcohol and CNS depressants:* CNS depression
- *Warfarin and clofibrate:* reduced plasma protein binding of dantrolene

Implications: For treatment of NMS
Assess
- For increased seizure activity in patient with epilepsy
- Hepatic function by frequent determination of AST, ALT

Planning/Implementation
- Have patient take with meals to prevent GI symptoms.
- Have patient chew sugarless gum and take frequent sips of water for dry mouth.
- Assist with ambulation when dizziness or drowsiness occurs.

Teaching
- To avoid discontinuing medication quickly because hallucinations, spasticity, tachycardia might occur; drug should be tapered off over 1-2 wk
- To avoid alcohol or other CNS depressants
- To avoid prolonged exposure to sunlight; photosensitivity may occur
- To be aware that muscle weakness may occur
- To avoid hazardous activities when drowsiness or dizziness occurs
- To avoid using OTC medication such as cough preparations and antihistamines unless directed by physician
- To exercise caution at mealtimes because choking and difficulty swallowing have been reported

Evaluate
- Therapeutic response: for NMS, decreased fever, sweating, rigidity
- Allergic reactions: rash, fever, respiratory distress
- Severe weakness, numbness in extremities
- CNS depression: dizziness, drowsiness, psychiatric symptoms

Treatment of Overdose: Induce emesis in conscious patient, lavage, dialysis.

Administration
- *Spasticity: adult:* PO 25 mg/day for 7 days then 25 mg tid for 7 days, 50 mg tid for 7 days, to 100 tid; not to exceed 400 mg/day; *child:* PO 0.5 mg/kg/day bid; may increase gradually, not to exceed 100 mg qid
- *Malignant hyperthermia: adult and child:* IV 1 mg/kg, may repeat to total dose of 10 mg/kg; PO 4-8 mg/kg/day in 4 divided doses for 1-3 days to prevent further hyperthermia
- *NMS:* 1-3 mg/kg/day in 4 divided doses, up to 10 mg/kg/day
- *Available forms:* caps 25, 50, 100 mg; powder for inj IV 20 mg/vial

Desipramine HCl
NORPRAMIN, PERTOFRANE
(dess-ip′-ra-meen)

Functional classification: Antidepressant
Chemical classifications: Tricyclic, secondary amine
FDA pregnancy category: C

Indications: Depression
Unlabeled use: Cocaine withdrawal

Contraindications: Hypersensitivity to TCAs, recovery phase of myocardial infarction, narrow-angle glaucoma
Cautious use: Convulsive disorders, prostatic hypertrophy, child <12 yr; suicidal patients, elderly patients, thyroid disease, MAOI therapy, ECT

Pharmacologic Effects: Blocks reuptake of norepinephrine (+++++) and serotonin (+) in presynaptic neurons; also thought related to downregulation of beta-adrenergic receptors; also receptor antagonist of acetylcholine (++), histamine (++), and alpha-1 (++); therapeutic plasma level 125-300 ng/ml

Pharmacokinetics: PO: steady state 2-11 days; metabolized by liver, 70% excreted by kidneys, crosses placenta, half-life 12-24 hr, protein binding 90%-95%

Side Effects: *CNS:* sedation, ataxia; confusion, delirium; *peripheral:* blurred vision, photophobia, increased intraocular pressure, decreased tearing; orthostatic hypotension, arrhythmias, tachycardia, palpitations; dry mouth; constipation, diarrhea; decreased sweating; urinary retention and hesitancy
Specific for desipramine: Dry mouth (~10%), blurred vision (~2%), constipation (~2%), sedation (~2%), orthostasis (~2%), tachycardia (~10%), sexual disturbance (~2%)

Interactions: See Amitriptyline

Implications: See Amitriptyline

Treatment of Overdose: Hospitalization, ECG monitoring; monitor cardiac function for at least 5 days, induce emesis, lavage, support airway.

Administration
- *Adult:* PO 100-200 mg/day in divided doses, may increase to 300 mg/day or may give daily dose; *adolescent/geriatric:* PO 25-100 mg/day, may increase to 150 mg/day
- *Available forms:* tabs 10, 25, 50, 75, 100, 150 mg; caps 25, 50 mg

Dextroamphetamine sulfate
DEXEDRINE, FERNDEX, OXYDESS II, SPANCAP NO. 1
(dex-troe-am-fet′-a-meen)

Functional classification: Cerebral stimulant
Chemical classification: Amphetamine
Controlled substance schedule II
FDA pregnancy category: C

Indications: Narcolepsy, exogenous obesity, ADHD

Contraindications: Hypersensitivity to sympathomimetic amines, glaucoma, severe arteriosclerosis, drug abuse, CV disease, anxiety, hyperthyroidism, MAOI use
Cautious use: Tourette's syndrome, lactation, child <3 yr

Pharmacologic Effects: Mechanism of action not clearly understood; stimulates dopamine function in the brain probably because of blocking of both dopamine and norepinephrine reuptake; might also promote release of dopamine into synaptic cleft; theoretically, these effects enhance inhibitory subcortical-cortical pathways, resulting in better concentration and impulse control, with a subsequent decrease in motor activity; therapeutic plasma levels 5-10 mg/dl

Pharmacokinetics: PO: onset 30 min, peak 1-3 hr, duration 4-20 hr, metabolized by liver, excreted by kidneys, crosses placenta, excreted in breast milk, half-life 10-30 hr

Side Effects: See Amphetamine combination

Interactions: See Amphetamine combination

Implications: See Amphetamine combination

Treatment of Overdose: Administer fluids, hemodialysis or peritoneal dialysis; antihypertensive for increased BP, ammonium chloride for increased excretion, chlorpromazine for CNS stimulation.

Administration

- *Narcolepsy:* PO 5-60 mg qd in divided doses; *adult and adolescent >12 yr:* PO 10 mg qd, increasing by 10 mg/day at weekly intervals; *child 6-12 yr:* PO 5 mg qd, increasing by 5 mg/day at weekly intervals, up to 60 mg/day
- *ADHD: child ≤5 yr:* PO initially 2.5 mg hs, after 4-6 days may be raised to 2.5 mg/day and given in 2 doses; *child >5 yr:* initially 5 mg and after 4-6 days may increase by 5 mg/day; total dose should be 15-20 mg/day; total daily dose usually between 0.3 and 1.0 mg/kg of body weight
- *Obesity: adult:* PO 5-30 mg qd in divided doses 30-60 min before meals
- *Available forms:* tabs 5, 10 mg; caps time-rel 5, 10, 15 mg; elix 5 mg/5 ml

Diazepam

D-TRAN,† E-PAM,† MEVAL,† NOVODIPAM,† STRESS-PAM,† VALIUM, VALRELEASE, VIVOL† DIASTAT (RECTAL) (dye-az´-e-pam)

Functional classification: Antianxiety agent
Chemical classification: Benzodiazepine
Controlled substance schedule IV
FDA pregnancy category: D

Indications: Anxiety, acute alcohol withdrawal, status epilepticus

Contraindications: Hypersensitivity to benzodiazepines, narrow-angle glaucoma, psychosis, child <6 mo (oral)
Cautious use: Elderly or debilitated patients, hepatic or renal disease

Pharmacologic Effects: Increases affinity of GABA molecules for their specific receptor, increasing the frequency with which chloride channels open in response to GABA; might also decrease norepinephrine and serotonin turnover rates

Pharmacokinetics

- *Speed of onset:* very fast
- *PO:* onset ½ hr, duration 2-3 hr; *IM:* onset 15-30 min, duration 1-1½ hr; *IV:* onset 1-5 min, duration 15 min; metabolized by liver, excreted by kidneys, crosses placenta, excreted in breast milk, half-life 20-80 hr

Side Effects: *CNS:* drowsiness, dizziness, confusion, headache, anxiety, tremor, stimulation, fatigue, depression, insomnia; *peripheral:* photophobia caused by mydriasis, blurred vision caused by

cycloplegia; sleeplike slowing of respirations with therapeutic doses, cough; orthostatic hypotension, tachycardia, hypotension; constipation; dry mouth

Interactions: See Alprazolam

Implications: See Alprazolam

Treatment of Overdose: Lavage, VS, supportive care; few deaths, if any, reported as resulting from benzodiazepine overdose alone; deaths occur when benzodiazepines are mixed with other drugs, especially alcohol.

Administration

- *Anxiety: adult:* PO 2-10 mg tid-qid or time-rel 15-30 mg qd; *child >6 mo:* PO 1-2.5 mg tid-qid
- *Acute alcohol withdrawal:* 10 mg tid-qid during first 24 hr; then reduce to 5 mg tid-qid prn
- *Status epilepticus: adult:* IV 5-10 mg at 2-5 mg/min up to a maximum dose of 30 mg; may repeat in 2-4 hr; *child >5 yr:* IV 1 mg/min q3-5min, up to a maximum of 10 mg; repeat in 2-4 hr if necessary; *child 1 mo to 5 yr:* 0.2-0.5 mg slowly q2-5min, to a maximum of 5 mg
- *Available forms:* tabs 2, 5, 10 mg; caps time-rel 15 mg, IM/IV inj 5 mg/ml; oral solution 5 mg/5 ml, 5 mg/ml

Diphenhydramine

ALLERDRYL, BARAMINE, BAX, BENACHLOR, BENADRYL, BENAHIST, BENTRACT, COMPŌZ, DIPHENACEN, FENYLHIST, NORDRYL, ROHYORA, SPANLANIN, VAIDRENE, WEHDRYL (dye-fen-hye´-dra-meen)

Functional classification: Antihistamine
Chemical classifications: H₁-receptor antagonist, ethanolamine
FDA pregnancy category: C

Indications: Parkinsonism, EPSEs, motion sickness, allergies and allergic reactions, sedation, other nonpsychiatric uses

Contraindications: Hypersensitivity, acute asthma attacks, lower respiratory tract disease

Pharmacologic Effects: Competes with histamine for H₁-receptor sites; blocks allergic responses by blocking histamine

Pharmacokinetics: Absorbed readily in GI tract; PO peaks in 1-3 hr; duration of action 4-7 hr; IM onset ½ hr, peak 1-4 hr, duration 4-7 hr; IV onset immediate, duration 4-7 hr; metabolized in liver, excreted in urine, crosses placenta, excreted in breast milk, half-life 2-7 hr

Side Effects: *CNS:* drowsiness (usually transient), sedation, dizziness, disturbed coordination; *less common:* fatigue, confusion, restlessness, nervousness; *peripheral:* nausea and vomiting, dry mouth, blood dyscrasias, urinary retention, blurred vision, nasal stuffiness, dry throat and nose

Interactions
- *CNS depressants:* increased depression
- *Heparin:* decreased effect of heparin
- *MAOIs:* increased anticholinergic effect

Implications
Assess
- For urinary retention
- Blood studies with long-term use

Planning/Implementation
- Have patient take with meals to decrease GI upset.
- Give IV at 25 mg/min.
- Give IM in large muscle.

Teaching
- To use hard candies, gum for dry mouth
- To avoid driving
- To avoid CNS depressants (e.g., alcohol)

Evaluate
- For EPSEs: therapeutic responses
- For congestion: ability to breathe
- Insomnia: sleep
- For wheezing and chest tightness

Treatment of Overdose: Anticholinergic toxicity includes flushing, dry mouth, hyperthermia (up to 107° F); initiate gastric lavage or induced emesis; give diazepam, vasopressors, and short-acting barbiturates.

Administration
- *Parkinsonism and EPSEs: PO: adult:* 25-50 mg/day tid-qid; *child >20 lb:* 12.5-25 mg/day tid-qid or 5 mg/kg/day, not to exceed 300 mg/day; *IM or IV: adult:* 10-50 mg, 100 mg if required, maximum daily dosage is 400 mg; *child:* 5 mg/kg/day divided into 4 doses, maximum daily dosage 300 mg
- *Available forms:* caps 25, 50 mg; tabs 25, 50 mg; elixir 12.5 mg/5 ml; syr 12.5 mg/5 ml; IM, IV 10, 50 mg/ml

Disulfiram

ANTABUSE
(dye-sul´-fi-ram)

Functional classification: Alcohol deterrent
Chemical classification: Aldehyde dehydrogenase inhibitor
FDA pregnancy category: X

Indications: Treatment of chronic alcoholism

Contraindications: Hypersensitivity, alcohol intoxication, psychoses, CV disease, patients who have received paraldehyde

    Cautious use: Hypothyroidism, hepatic disease, diabetes mellitus, seizure disorders, nephritis

Pharmacologic Effects: Blocks oxidation of alcohol at acetaldehyde stage by inhibiting aldehyde dehydrogenase

Pharmacokinetics: *PO:* onset 12 hr, oxidized by liver, excreted in urine

Side Effects: *CNS:* headache, drowsiness, restlessness, dizziness, fatigue, tremors, psychosis, neuritis, sweating, convulsions, death; *peripheral:* nausea, vomiting, anorexia, severe thirst, hepatotoxicity; rash, dermatitis, urticaria; respiratory depression, hyperventilation; tachycardia, chest pain, hypotension, arrhythmia

Interactions
- *Alcohol:* violent symptoms of sweating, throbbing headache, nausea and profuse vomiting, flushed face and neck, palpitations, tightness of chest, tremor, dyspnea
- *Metronidazole, isoniazid:* psychosis
- *TCAs, diazepam, hydantoins, oral anticoagulants, paraldehyde, phenytoin, chlordiazepoxide:* increased effects of these drugs

Implications
Assess
- Liver function studies q2wk during therapy; AST, ALT, CBC, SMA-12 q3-6mo to detect any abnormality

Planning/Implementation
- If drowsiness occurs, give once per day in morning or hs.
- Give only after patient has not been drinking for >12 hr.

Teaching
- To be aware of the effect of this drug when alcohol is taken; written consent for disulfiram therapy should be obtained
- That shaving lotions, creams, cough preparations, skin products must be checked for alcohol content; even in small amount, alcohol can produce a reaction
- That tolerance does not develop when treatment is prolonged
- That reaction might occur for 14 days after last dose
- That tabs can be crushed, mixed with beverage
- To carry identification that lists disulfiram therapy and physician phone number
- To avoid driving or hazardous tasks when drowsiness occurs
- That disulfiram reaction can be fatal and occurs 15 min after drinking

Evaluate
- Mental status: ability to abstain from alcohol

---

*Infrequently used.   †Available in Canada only.

Treatment of Overdose: Give IV vitamin C, ephedrine sulfate, antihistamines, O_2.

Administration

- *Adult:* PO 250-500 mg qd for 1-2 wk, then 125-500 mg qd until desired response
- *Available forms:* tabs 250 mg

Donepezil
ARICEPT
(dah-nep'-eh-zil)

Functional classification: Drug for Alzheimer's disease

Chemical classification: Cholinesterase inhibitor

FDA pregnancy category: C

Indications: Treatment of mild to moderate dementia of the Alzheimer's type

Contraindications: Hypersensitivity to donepezil or to piperidine derivatives

Cautious use: History of ulcers, patients with history of asthma or obstructive pulmonary disease

Pharmacologic Effects: Cholinesterase inhibitor that does not cure dementia but is thought to slow degenerative processes; increases amount of acetylcholine in cortex; because only remaining cholinergic neurons are affected, this and similarly acting drugs become less effective as the disease progresses; peak response ~6 wk, then a plateau and slight decline in function, but significantly better on Alzheimer's Disease Assessment Scale-Cognitive Subscale than placebo (from manufacturer's research report)

Pharmacokinetics: Bioavailability 100%; highly bound to serum proteins (96%); half-life ~60 hr; metabolized by P-450 2D6 and 3A4

Side Effects: Does not cause liver damage as does tacrine (from manufacturer's report of research); *CNS:* potential for seizures, insomnia (6%), headache (10%), dizziness (8%), depression (3%), delusions, tremors, irritability, aggression, ataxia, increased libido; *peripheral:* bradycardia, syncopal episodes (2%); GI bleeding, diarrhea (10%); nausea (11%); vomiting (5%); potential for urinary obstruction, fatigue (5%); muscle cramps (6%); anorexia (4%); donepezil not associated with hepatotoxicity

Interactions

- *Anesthesia:* likely to exaggerate effects of succinylcholine
- *Anticholinergics:* reduced anticholinergic effect
- *Ketoconazole, quinidine:* inhibition of donepezil metabolism
- *NSAIDs:* can lead to pronounced GI irritation (e.g., GI bleeding)

- *Phenytoin, carbamazepine, phenobarbital:* potential for increasing donepezil elimination

Treatment of Overdose: Overdose can cause cholinergic crisis. Anticholinergics (e.g., atropine) may be used as an antidote.

Administration

- Usually 5-10 mg qd hs; special note: abrupt cessation might result in rapid deterioration of patient function
- *Available forms:* tabs 5, 10 mg

Doxepin HCl
ADAPIN, SINEQUAN
(dox'-e-pin)

Functional classification: Antidepressant

Chemical classifications: Tricyclic, tertiary amine

FDA pregnancy category: C

Indications: Depression, anxiety (a cream form [Zonalon] is used for pruritus)

Contraindications: Hypersensitivity to TCAs, urinary retention, narrow-angle glaucoma, prostatic hypertrophy

Cautious use: Suicidal or elderly patients, lactation, MAOI therapy, children <12 yr

Pharmacologic Effects: Blocks reuptake of norepinephrine (+) and serotonin (++) into presynaptic neurons; also thought to be r/t downregulation of beta-adrenergic receptors; also receptor antagonist for acetylcholine (+++), histamine (+++++), and alpha-1 (+++); therapeutic plasma levels 100-200 ng/ml

Pharmacokinetics: *PO:* steady state 2-8 days; metabolized by liver, excreted in kidneys, crosses placenta, protein binding (>90%), excreted in breast milk, half-life 8-24 hr

Side Effects: *CNS:* sedation (~30%), ataxia, confusion (~2%), delirium; *peripheral:* blurred vision (~10%), photophobia, increased intraocular pressure, decreased tearing; orthostatic hypotension (~10%), arrhythmias, tachycardia (~2%), palpitations; dry mouth (~30%), constipation (~10%), diarrhea; decreased sweating, urinary hesitancy (~2%)

Interactions: See Amitriptyline

Implications: See Amitriptyline

Treatment of Overdose: ECG monitoring; induce emesis, lavage, activated charcoal; administer anticonvulsant.

Administration

- *Adult:* PO 10-25 mg tid to start, may increase to 300 mg/day or may give daily dose hs; optimal dose usually 75-150 mg/day
- *Available forms:* caps 10, 25, 50, 75, 100, 150 mg; oral conc 10 mg/ml

Droperidol

INAPSINE
(droe-per´-i-dole)

Functional classification: Antipsychotic, antiemetic
Chemical classification: Butyrophenone
FDA pregnancy category: C

Psychiatric Indication: Management of delirium

Contraindications: Hypersensitivity, impaired liver and renal function
  Cautious use: Has the toxic potential of phenothiazines and the usual precautions should be observed

Pharmacologic Effects: Has pharmacologic activity similar to haloperidol and the phenothiazines

Pharmacokinetics: Onset within 3-10 min, peak effects 30 min, metabolized in liver, excreted in urine and feces with 10% unchanged

Side Effects: Adverse effects are qualitatively similar to those of haloperidol; CNS: EPSEs, restlessness, hyperactivity, anxiety, drowsiness, headaches; peripheral: mild to moderate hypotension, tachycardia, facial sweating, laryngospasm, bronchospasm

Interactions
- CNS depressants: additive effect

Administration
- Management of delirium: usual adult dose 5 mg IM
- Available forms: for injection, 2.5 mg/ml

Estazolam

PROSOM
(ess´-ta-zoe-lam)

Functional classifications: Sedative, hypnotic
Chemical classification: Benzodiazepine
Controlled substance schedule IV
FDA pregnancy category: X

Indications: Insomnia

Contraindications: Hypersensitivity, sleep apnea

Pharmacologic Effects: Believed to potentiate GABA receptors, which are inhibitory, causing CNS depression; might affect BZ_1 (sleep) receptors

Pharmacokinetics: Peak levels 2 hr, half-life 10-24 hr, protein binding 93%, <5% excreted unchanged in urine, metabolized in liver

Side Effects: CNS: somnolence (42%), asthenia (11%), hypokinesia (8%), hangover (3%), headache, nervousness, talkativeness, drowsiness, dizziness, confusion; see Diazepam for other benzodiazepine side effects; peripheral: nausea and vomiting, other GI upsets, constipation, skin eruptions, blood dyscrasias

Interactions
- Cimetidine, disulfiram, isoniazid, probenecid: increased effect of estazolam
- CNS depressants and alcohol: additive CNS depression
- Theophylline, rifampin: decreased effect of estazolam

Implications
  Assess
- BP
- Blood studies, if indicated

Planning/Implementation
- Give ½-1 hr before bedtime.
- Give with food to prevent GI upset.
- Maintain safety.

Teaching
- To avoid driving
- To avoid alcohol

Evaluate
- Therapeutic response, sleeping
- Mental status

Treatment of Overdose: No recorded deaths caused by benzodiazepine overdose alone; lavage, monitor VS, provide supportive care.

Administration
- Insomnia: adult: 1 mg hs, up to 2 mg; elderly: if healthy, 1 mg hs; if small or debilitated, 0.5 mg hs (effectiveness not clear)
- Available forms: tabs 1, 2 mg

Ethchlorvynol*

PLACIDYL
(eth-klor-vi´-nole)

Functional classifications: Sedative, hypnotic
Chemical classification: Tertiary acetylenic alcohol
Controlled substance schedule IV
FDA pregnancy category: C

Indications: Sedation, insomnia

Contraindications: Hypersensitivity, severe pain, porphyria, lactation
  Cautious use: Moderate pain

Pharmacologic Effects: Mechanism of action not known, produces CNS depression

Pharmacokinetics: Rapidly absorbed from GI tract; onset 15-30 min, peak level 2 hr, duration 5

---

hr, metabolized in liver, excreted in urine, half-life 10-20 hr for parent compound

Side Effects: *CNS:* dizziness, facial numbness, giddiness; *peripheral:* nausea and vomiting; GI upset, blood dyscrasias, blurred vision, hypotension, rash

Interactions
- *Alcohol and other CNS depressants:* additive depressive effect
- *MAOIs:* increased CNS depression
- *Oral anticoagulants:* decreased thrombin time
- *TCAs:* transient delirium

Implications
Assess
- Blood studies might be indicated

Planning/Implementation
- Give with food ½-1 hr before bedtime for sleeplessness, to decrease dizziness and giddiness; maintain patient's safety (e.g., protect from falls, keep bed rails up)

Teaching
- To avoid driving
- To avoid alcohol and other CNS depressants

Evaluate
- Decreased respiration (if <10 breaths/min, withhold drug)

Treatment of Overdose: Overdose characterized by deep coma, severe respiratory depression, hypothermia, hypotension, bradycardia; death has been reported at dosages of 6 g, but dosages as high as 50 g have been survived; lavage or other approaches to gastric evacuation should be performed immediately; provide supportive care; forced diuresis with high urinary output is helpful.

Administration
- Do not prescribe for >1 wk
- *Sedation: adult:* PO 100-200 mg bid or tid
- *Insomnia: adult:* PO 500-1000 mg ½ hr before bedtime, may repeat 200 mg, if original dose was 500-750 mg
- *Available forms:* caps 200, 500, 750 mg

Ethopropazine HCl*

PARSIDOL
(eth-oh-proe´-pa-zeen)

Functional classification: Anticholinergic
Chemical classification: Phenothiazine
FDA pregnancy category: C

Indications: Parkinsonism and EPSEs (but not frequently prescribed)

Contraindications: See Trihexyphenidyl

Pharmacologic Effects: See Trihexyphenidyl

Pharmacokinetics: See Trihexyphenidyl

Side Effects: *CNS:* see Trihexyphenidyl; *peripheral:* see Trihexyphenidyl

Interactions: See Trihexyphenidyl

Implications: See Trihexyphenidyl

Treatment of Overdose: See Trihexyphenidyl

Administration
- *Parkinsonism and EPSEs: PO adult:* begin with 50 mg qd or bid, increase gradually, if necessary; *for mild to moderate symptoms:* 100-400 mg/day; *for severe cases:* gradually increase to ≥500-600 mg/day
- *Available forms:* tabs 10, 50 mg

E

Ethosuximide

ZARONTIN
(eth-oh-sux´-i-mide)

Functional classification: Antiepileptic
Chemical classification: Succinimide
FDA pregnancy category: C

Indications: Absence seizures (petit mal)

Contraindications: Hypersensitivity to succinimide derivatives
Cautious use: Lactation, hepatic or renal disease

Pharmacologic Effects: Inhibits spike and wave formation in absence seizures by interfering with calcium conductances; does not alter sodium channel activation or increase GABA inhibition; therapeutic serum level 40-100 μg/ml

Pharmacokinetics: *PO:* peak 3-7 hr; steady state 5-10 days; metabolized by liver; excreted in urine, bile, feces; half-life 40-60 hr (adult), 30 hr (child)

Side Effects: *CNS:* Drowsiness, dizziness, fatigue, euphoria, lethargy anxiety, aggressiveness, irritability, depression, insomnia; *peripheral:* nausea, vomiting, heartburn, anorexia, diarrhea, abdominal pain, cramps, constipation, vaginal bleeding, hematuria, renal damage, urticaria, pruritic erythema, hirsutism, Stevens-Johnson syndrome, myopia, gum hypertrophy, tongue swelling, blurred vision, agranulocytosis, aplastic anemia, thrombocytopenia, leukocytosis, eosinophilia, pancytopenia (some blood dyscrasias have been fatal)

Interactions
- *Estrogens:* decreased effects of oral contraceptives
- *TCAs:* antagonist effect (imipramine, doxepin); also lower seizure threshold

Implications
Assess
- Mental status: mood, sensorium, affect
- CNS depressants: increased CNS depression

- Renal studies: urinalysis, BUN and urine creatinine levels
- Blood studies: CBC, hematocrit and hemoglobin levels
- Hepatic studies: AST, ALT, bilirubin, and creatinine levels
- Drug levels during initial treatment, therapeutic range 40-100 mg/ml

Planning/Implementation
- Have patient take with milk or food to decrease GI symptoms.
- Assist with ambulation during early part of treatment; dizziness occurs.

Teaching
- To carry identification card or MedicAlert bracelet stating drugs taken, condition, physician's name and phone number
- To avoid driving, other activities that require alertness
- To avoid alcohol ingestion, CNS depressants; increased sedation might occur
- Not to discontinue medication quickly after long-term use

Evaluate
- Therapeutic response: decreased seizure activity, document on patient's chart
- Mental status
- Allergic reaction: red raised rash, exfoliative dermatitis; if these occur, drug should be discontinued
- Blood dyscrasias: fever, sore throat, bruising, rash, jaundice
- Toxic effects: bone marrow depression, lupus have been reported

Treatment of Overdose: Lavage, activated charcoal, monitor electrolyte levels, VS.

Administration
- *Adult and child >6 yr:* PO 500 mg/day or 250 mg bid initially; may increase by 250 mg every 4-7 days, not to exceed 1.5 g/day; *child 3-6 yr:* PO 250 mg/day or 125 mg bid; may increase by 250 mg every 4-7 days, not to exceed 1.5 g/day; optimal dose 20 mg/kg/day
- *Available forms:* caps 250 mg, syr 250 mg/5 ml

Ethotoin*

PEGANONE
(eth´-oh-toyin)

Functional classification: Antiepileptic
Chemical classification: Hydantoin derivative
FDA pregnancy category: D

Indications: Generalized tonic-clonic or psychomotor seizures

Contraindications: Hypersensitivity to hydantoins, blood dyscrasias, hematologic disease, hepatic disease, lactation
　　Cautious use: Renal disorders

Pharmacologic Effects: Inhibits spread of seizure activity in motor cortex; therapeutic plasma level 15-50 mg/ml

Pharmacokinetics: Metabolized by liver, excreted in urine, half-life 3-9 hr

Side Effects: *CNS:* drowsiness, dizziness, insomnia, paresthesias, depression, suicidal tendencies, aggression, headache; *peripheral:* nausea, vomiting, constipation, anorexia, weight loss, hepatitis, jaundice, nephritis, albuminuria, rash, agranulocytosis, leukopenia, aplastic anemia

Interactions
- *Allopurinol, cimetidine, diazepam, disulfiram, alcohol (acute ingestion), phenacemide, succinimides, valproic acid:* increased effect of hydantoins
- *Barbiturates, carbamazepine, alcohol (chronic use) theophylline, antacids, dietary calcium:* decreased effects of hydantoins
- *Corticosteroids, dicumarol, digitoxin, doxycycline, haloperidol, methadone, oral contraceptives, dopamine, furosemide, levodopa:* decreased effects of these drugs
- *Phenacemide:* causes paranoid syndrome

Implications
　Assess
- Blood studies: CBC, platelets qmo until stabilized, discontinue if marked depression of blood cell count occurs

Planning/Implementation
- Describe seizures accurately.

Teaching
- To understand all aspects of drug administration (i.e., route, action, dose)
- To report side effects
- To avoid driving or operating dangerous equipment
- To practice good oral hygiene
- Not to discontinue drug abruptly
- To wear MedicAlert identification bracelet

Evaluate
- Mental status: mood, sensorium, affect, memory (long-term, short-term)
- Respiratory depression
- Blood dyscrasias: fever, sore throat, bruising, rash, jaundice

Treatment of Overdose: Mean lethal dose in adults is thought to be 2-5 g; initial symptoms are nystagmus, ataxia; death results from respiratory and circulatory depression; lavage, emesis, activated charcoal.

Administration
- *Adult:* PO 250 mg qid (1000 mg/day) or less initially, may increase over several days to 3 g/day in divided doses; *child:* PO 250 mg tid, may increase to 250 mg qid (1000 mg/day)
- *Available forms:* tabs 250, 500 mg

Flumazenil
ROMAZICON
(floo-maz´-eh-nill)

Functional classifications: Benzodiazepine receptor antagonist, antidote
Chemical classification: Imidazobenzodiazepine derivative
FDA pregnancy category: C

Indications: Complete or partial reversal of the sedative effects of benzodiazepines in cases in which general anesthesia has been induced or maintained with benzodiazepines; management of benzodiazepine overdose

Contraindications: Hypersensitivity to flumazenil or to benzodiazepines; in patients administered benzodiazepines for potentially life-threatening disorders; patients showing signs of serious cyclic antidepressant overdose
Cautious use: History of seizure; hepatic dysfunction; lactation

Pharmacologic Effects: Antagonizes the actions of benzodiazepines on the CNS and inhibits activity of GABA/benzodiazepine receptor sites

Pharmacokinetics: Initial distribution half-life 7-15 min, then a terminal half-life of 41-79 min; protein binding 50%; elimination is through the renal system and is essentially complete within 72 hr

Side Effects: *CNS:* dizziness (10%), agitation, emotional lability, confusion; *peripheral:* nausea, vomiting (11%), headache, blurred vision, paresthesia

Interactions
- *Benzodiazepines:* pharmacokinetics unaltered in presence of flumazenil
- *CNS depressants:* theoretically possible interaction

- *Food:* increased clearance of flumazenil

Implications
Assess
- Hypersensitivity to flumazenil or benzodiazepines

Planning/Implementation
- Administer by IV only.
- Ensure that emergency equipment is available.
- Secure airway during administration.
- Monitor clinical response to drug.
- Inject into running IV.

Teaching
- That flumazenil does not consistently reverse amnesia
- That although patient feels alert at time of discharge, the effects of benzodiazepines might recur
- To avoid activities requiring alertness
- To refuse alcohol and not to take nonprescription drugs for 18-24 hr after flumazenil given

Evaluate
- Hepatic status
- Emergence of withdrawal symptoms

Treatment of Overdose: No serious adverse reactions or clinically significant test abnormalities reported; most adverse responses are extensions of pharmacologic effects of the drug because it reverses a benzodiazepine

Administration
- *Benzodiazepine overdose: adult:* IV: initially 0.2 mg (2 ml) over 30 sec; if desired level of consciousness not obtained, wait 30 sec and give 0.3 mg (3 ml) over 30 sec; further doses of 0.5 mg (5 ml) can be administered over 30 sec at 1-min intervals up to a total cumulative dose of 3 mg
- *IV compatibility:* flumazenil is compatible with 5% dextrose in water, lactated Ringer's solution, and normal saline solutions; discard after 24 hr; do not remove from vial until ready for use
- *Available forms:* inj 0.1 mg/ml in 5- and 10-ml vials

Fluoxetine
PROZAC, SARAFEM
(floo-ox´-e-teen)

Functional classification: SSRI antidepressant
Chemical classification: Selective serotonin reuptake inhibitor; bicyclic
FDA pregnancy category: B

Indications: Depression, bulimia, premenstrual dysphoric disorder

Unlabeled uses: Dysthymia, atypical depression, aggression, PTSD, pervasive developmental disorder, premature ejaculation, phantom pain, fibromyalgia, enuresis (?)

Contraindications: Hypersensitivity; use with MAO inhibitors because of the possibility of causing the (sometimes fatal) serotonin syndrome
Cautious use: Anxiety, insomnia, lactation, children, elderly patients, MAOI therapy

Pharmacologic Effects: Inhibits CNS neuron uptake of serotonin; also slightly antagonizes acetylcholine (+), histamine (+), and alpha-1 (+) receptors

Pharmacokinetics: *PO:* peak 6-8 hr; 95% protein bound; metabolized in liver, excreted in urine; half-life 48-216 hr (including metabolite); metabolism involves P-450 isoenzymes; fluoxetine is a substrate of 2D6 and inhibits 2D6

Side Effects: *CNS:* anxiety (9.4%), nervousness (14.9%), insomnia (13.8%), drowsiness, headache (20.3%), tremor, dizziness, fatigue; *peripheral:* nausea (21.1%), diarrhea (12.3%), dry mouth (9.5%), anorexia (8.7%), dyspepsia, constipation, cramps, vomiting, taste changes, flatulence, sweating (8.4%), rash, pruritus, acne, alopecia, urticaria, infection (7.6%), nasal congestion, hot flashes (1.8%), palpitations, dysmenorrhea (2%), decreased libido, urinary frequency, urinary tract infection, visual changes (2.8%), ear or eye pain, photophobia, tinnitus, asthenia (4.4%), viral infection (3.4%)

Interactions
- *Diazepam:* half-life of diazepam increases
- *Highly protein-bound drugs* (i.e., digitoxin): increased side effects
- *L-tryptophan:* Agitation
- *MAOIs:* do not use; might precipitate a serotonin syndrome
- *TCAs:* toxic effects of tricyclics increased, suicidal tendencies, increase in psychiatric symptoms, depression, panic

Implications
Assess
- BP (lying, standing), pulse q4h; if systolic BP drops 20 mm Hg, withhold drug, notify physician; VS q4h in patients with CV disease
- Blood studies: CBC, leukocyte count, differential blood cell count; cardiac enzyme level when patient is receiving long-term therapy
- Hepatic studies: AST, ALT, bilirubin, and creatinine levels
- Weight: qwk, appetite might increase
- ECG: for flattening of T wave, bundle branch or AV block, arrhythmias in cardiac disease

Planning/Implementation
- If patient is constipated, urinary retention may occur; increase fluids, bulk in diet

- Do not give with MAOIs; if switching from MAOI to fluoxetine, wait at least 14 days; if switching from fluoxetine to an MAOI, wait at least 6 wk.
- Have patient take with food or milk to prevent GI symptoms.
- Empty pulvule if patient is unable to swallow medication whole.
- Give dose hs if oversedation occurs during day; may take entire dose hs; elderly patients may not tolerate once-per-day dosage.
- Have patient chew sugarless gum, suck on hard candy, and take frequent sips of water for dry mouth.
- Store at room temperature, do not freeze.
- Assist with ambulation during therapy because drowsiness, dizziness occur.
- Provide safety measures, including side rails, primarily with elderly patients.
- Check to see that PO medication is swallowed.

Teaching
- That therapeutic effect might take several days to weeks
- To use caution when driving or performing other activities requiring alertness because of drowsiness, dizziness, or blurred vision
- Not to discontinue medication suddenly after long-term use because abrupt discontinuance might cause nausea, headache, malaise
- To avoid ingesting alcohol or other CNS depressants
- To notify physician when pregnant or when planning to become pregnant or to breast-feed

Evaluate
- EPSEs, primarily in elderly; rigidity, dystonia, akathisia
- Urinary retention, constipation
- Withdrawal symptoms: headache, nausea, vomiting, muscle pain, weakness; do not usually occur unless drug is discontinued abruptly
- Alcohol consumption: if alcohol is consumed, withhold dose until morning

Treatment of Overdose: No antidotes; establish and maintain airway; ensure adequate oxygenation and ventilation; activated charcoal may be more effective than emesis or lavage.

Administration
- *Adult:* PO 20 mg qd in morning; after several weeks, if no clinical improvement noted, dose may be increased to 20 mg bid in morning, noon; not to exceed 80 mg/day
- *Available forms:* Pulvules 10, 20 mg; liquid 20 mg/5 ml

---

*Infrequently used.   †Available in Canada only.

Fluphenazine decanoate, fluphenazine enanthate, fluphenazine HCl

MODECATE DECANOATE,† PROLIXIN DECANOATE/MODITEN ENANTHATE,† PROXLIN ENANTHATE/MODITEN HCL,† PERMITIL HCL, PROLIXIN HCL†
(floo-fen´-a-zeen)

Functional classifications: Traditional antipsychotic, neuroleptic, high potency
Chemical classifications: Phenothiazine, piperazine
FDA pregnancy category: C

Indications: Psychotic disorders, schizophrenia

Contraindications: Hypersensitivity to sesame seeds or fluphenazine, liver damage, CV disease, severe hypertension or hypotension, blood dyscrasias, coma, child <12 yr, brain damage, bone marrow depression, alcohol and barbiturate withdrawal states
Cautious use: Lactation, seizure disorders, hypertension, hepatic disease, cardiac disease, extreme heat

Pharmacologic Effects: Traditional antipsychotic drugs produce a neuroleptic effect characterized by sedation, emotional quieting, psychomotor slowing, and affective indifference; exact mode of action not fully understood; blocks D_2 receptors (+++++) in the basal ganglia, hypothalamus, limbic system, brainstem, and medulla; blockade of these receptors accounts for both therapeutic and adverse responses; because of their nonselective actions, many other neurotransmitters systems are affected as well; acetylcholine (+), histamine (+++), and alpha-1 (+++); therapeutic plasma levels 0.13-2.8 ng/ml

Pharmacokinetics: *PO/IM (HCl):* onset 1 hr, peak 2-4 hr, duration 6-8 hr, half-life 13-56 hr; *decanoate:* onset 1-3 days, peak 1-2 days, duration >4 wk, half-life (single dose) 6.8-9.6 days, (multiple dose) 14.3 days; metabolized by liver, excreted in urine (metabolites) and breast milk, crosses placenta

Side Effects: *CNS:* parkinsonism, akathisias, dystonias, tardive dyskinesis, oculogyric crisis, neuroleptic malignant syndrome; *peripheral:* blurred vision (cycloplegia or paralysis of accommodation), ocular pain, photophobia, mydriasis, impaired vision; intolerance of extreme heat or cold, possible heat stroke or fatal hyperthermia; nasal congestion, wheezing, dyspnea; hypotension, especially orthostatic, leading to dizziness, syncope, tachycardia, irregular pulse, arrhythmias; dry mouth; constipation; jaundice; abdominal pain; urinary retention, urinary hesitancy, galactorrhea, gynecomastia, impaired ejaculation, amenorrhea: sedation (~2%), EPSEs (~30%), orthostasis (~2%-10%), anticholinergic (~2%), weight gain (~2%), sexual dysfunction (~2%)

Interactions: See Chlorpromazine

Implications: See Chlorpromazine

Treatment of Overdose: Lavage; if orally ingested; provide an airway; do not induce vomiting; control EPSEs and hypotension.

Administration
- *Decanoate: adult and child >12 yr:* IM or SC 12.5-25 mg q1-3wk HCl; *adult:* PO 0.5-10 mg in divided doses q6-8h, typically not to exceed 20 mg qd; *geriatric:* start with 1-2.5 mg/day, adjust according to response; IM initially 1.25 mg, then 2.5-10 mg in divided doses q6-8h
- Concentrate should not be mixed with caffeine, tannics, or pectinates
- *Available forms:* HCl tabs 1, 2.5, 5, 10 mg; elixir 2.5 mg/5 ml; concentrate 5 mg/ml; inj IM, 2.5 mg/ml; decanoate, inj SC, IM 25 mg/ml

Flurazepam

DALMANE, SOMNOL†
(flure-az´-e-pam)

Functional classifications: Sedative, hypnotic
Chemical classification: Benzodiazepine derivative
Controlled substance schedule IV
FDA pregnancy category: NR

Indications: Insomnia

Contraindications: Hypersensitivity to benzodiazepines, pregnancy, lactation, intermittent porphyria
Cautious use: Anemia, hepatic or renal disease, suicidal patients, drug abuse, elderly patients, child <15 yr, psychosis

Pharmacologic Effects: Produces CNS depression

Pharmacokinetics: PO onset 0.5-1 hr, duration 7-8 hr; active metabolite peak plasma level 1-3 hr; metabolized by liver, excreted by kidneys, crosses placenta, excreted in breast milk; half-life 3-150 hr (with metabolites)

Side Effects: *CNS:* lethargy, drowsiness, daytime sedation, dizziness, confusion, light-headedness, headache, anxiety, irritability; *peripheral:* nausea, vomiting, diarrhea, heartburn, abdominal pain, constipation, chest pain, pulse changes, palpitations

Interactions
- *Alcohol, CNS depressants:* CNS depression
- *Antacids:* decrease effects of flurazepam
- *Cimetidine, disulfiram:* prolong half-life of flurazepam

Implications
Assess
- Blood studies: hematocrit, hemoglobin levels; RBCS (if on long-term therapy regimen)
- Suicide potential: use with caution in suicidal patients

Planning/Implementation
- Have patient take ½-1 hr before bedtime for sleeplessness.
- Fast onset on empty stomach, but if GI symptoms occur, may be taken with food.
- Assist with ambulation after receiving dose.
- Provide safety measures: side rails, nightlight, call bell within easy reach.
- Check to see that PO medication has been swallowed.

Teaching
- To avoid driving or engaging in other activities requiring alertness until drug regimen is stabilized
- To avoid alcohol ingestion or CNS depressants because serious CNS depression might result
- To allow 2 nights for clinical effect
- To alternate measures to improve sleep: reading, exercise several hours before bedtime, warm bath, warm milk, television, self-hypnosis, deep breathing
- That hangover is common in elderly patients but less common than with barbiturates

Evaluate
- Therapeutic response: ability to sleep at night, decreased amount of early-morning awakening when taking drug for insomnia
- Mental status: mood, sensorium, affect, memory (long-term, short-term)
- Blood dyscrasias (rare): fever, sore throat, bruising, rash, jaundice, epistaxis
- Type of sleep problem: falling asleep, staying asleep

Treatment of Overdose:
Lavage, activated charcoal, monitor electrolyte levels, VS.

Administration
- *Adult:* PO 15-30 mg hs, may repeat dose once, if needed; *geriatric:* PO 15 mg hs, may increase, if needed
- *Available forms:* caps 15, 30 mg

Fluvoxamine maleate
LUVOX
(floo-vox′-a-meen)

Functional classification: SSRI antidepressant
Chemical classification: Selective serotonin reuptake inhibitor, monocyclic
FDA pregnancy category: C

Indications: Obsessive-compulsive disorder

Contraindications: Coadministration with terfenadine or astemizole; history of hypersensitivity to fluvoxamine
   Cautious use: Mania, hypomania, history of seizures, pregnancy, lactation

Pharmacologic Effects: Inhibits CNS neuronal uptake of serotonin (++++); has "+" antagonistic effect on acetylcholine and alpha-1 receptors

Pharmacokinetics: Peak levels 3-8 hr; half-life 15-19 hr; extensive metabolism; excreted in urine; protein binding 80%; inhibits P-450 isoenzymes 1A2, 2C19, 2D6, 3A4; is a substrate of 1A2

Side Effects: *CNS:* sexual disturbance (>30%), somnolence (22%), headache (22%), insomnia (21%), nervousness (12%), dizziness (11%); *peripheral:* nausea (40%), asthenia (14%), dry mouth (14%), diarrhea (11%), constipation (10%), dyspepsia (10%)

Interactions
- *Cigarettes:* 25% increase in fluvoxamine metabolism
- *Haloperidol:* haloperidol serum levels might double; negative and positive symptoms might increase
- *MAOIs, tryptophan:* possible enhancement of serotonin effect (serotonin syndrome), leading to fatal outcomes
- *Substrate of P-450 isoenzymes 1A2, 2C19, 2D6,3A4:* potential interactions with drugs metabolized by these isoenzymes
- *Terfenadine, astemizole:* fatal reactions might occur as a result of reduced metabolism of these drugs
- *Theophylline:* theophylline clearance decreased significantly
- *Triazolam, alprazolam, warfarin, carbamazepine, methadone, clozapine, TCAs, betablockers, diltiazem:* increased effects of these drugs

Implications
Assess
- For history of hypersensitivity to fluvoxamine; impaired hepatic or renal function; suicidal tendencies
- BP, VS

---

*Infrequently used.   †Available in Canada only.

- Urinary output, CBC
- Activation of mania

Planning/Implementation
- Maintain safety.
- Closely supervise patients at high risk for suicide because there might be a relationship between suicide and alterations in serotonin levels.

Teaching
- To be cautious about driving (although problems in this area are not established)
- To avoid alcohol
- To be cautious about the use of OTC products
- If dose >100 mg/day, divide in 2 and give larger dose hs

Evaluate
- For therapeutic effect (e.g., improvement of obsessive-compulsive disorder)
- Mental status
- Take drug hs
- Report rash, mania, seizures

Treatment of Overdose: Some fatalities occurred in conjunction with fluvoxamine overdose; treatment includes airway maintenance; close observation, including VS and ECG; activated charcoal or emesis; be aware of possibility of multiple drug overdose; no known antidote exists for fluvoxamine overdose.

Administration
- *Adult:* PO 50 mg hs to start; increase by 50 mg/day every 4-7 days until therapeutic response achieved; therapeutic dose typically 100-300 mg/day; maximum dose 300 mg/day; if dosage >100 mg/day, divide in 2 and give larger dose hs; *elderly and hepatically impaired:* give reduced dosage and titrate more slowly; *child and adolescent:* not approved for children <18 yr
- *Available forms:* tabs 25, 50, 100 mg

Gabapentin

NEURONTIN
(gab-ah-pen´-tin)

Functional classification: Antiepileptic
Chemical classification: Structurally related to GABA
FDA pregnancy category: C

Indications: Adjunctive therapy in the treatment of partial seizures with and without secondary generalization in adults with epilepsy

Contraindications: Hypersensitivity to gabapentin, lactation, children <12 yr

Pharmacologic Effects: Therapeutic actions not fully understood but thought to be caused by increasing the release of GABA from presynaptic neurons

Pharmacokinetics: Absorption is dose dependent (as dose increases, bioavailability decreases), and food does not alter absorption; half-life 5-8 hr; protein binding <3%; gabapentin is not metabolized; excreted unchanged in the urine; therapeutic serum levels >2 µg/ml

Side Effects: *CNS:* somnolence (19%), dizziness (17%), ataxia (12%); *peripheral:* fatigue (11%)

Interactions
- *Antacids:* reduced bioavailability of gabapentin by 20%
- *Cimetidine:* increased bioavailability of gabapentin
- *Oral contraceptives:* increased serum levels of oral contraceptives
- *Other antiepileptics:* gabapentin does not interact with other antiepileptics

Implications
Assess
- History of hypersensitivity to gabapentin
- Baseline physical data

Planning/Implementation
- Give with food to prevent GI distress.

Teaching
- To take gabapentin as prescribed
- That gabapentin might cause dizziness and somnolence, so care should be taken with hazardous machinery
- Not to discontinue gabapentin abruptly because of the possibility of withdrawal-precipitated seizures
- To wear MedicAlert bracelet to alert others to seizure disorder

Evaluate
- Absence of epilepsy
- Minimal side effects

Treatment of Overdose: Gabapentin seems to be a safe drug; although not necessary to this point, hemodialysis will remove gabapentin from the system.

Administration
- *Adult and child >12 yr:* PO 300 mg on day 1, 300 mg bid on day 2, and 300 mg tid on day 3; dose on day 1 should be given hs to reduce somnolence or daytime dizziness; dosage can be increased up to 1800 mg/day; effective dosage then is between 900 and 1800 mg/day in 3 divided doses; dosage spacing should not exceed 12 hr between doses
- *Available forms:* caps 100, 300, 400 mg

G

Glutethimide*

DORIDEN
(gloo-teth´-i-mide)

Functional classifications: Sedative, hypnotic
Chemical classification: Piperidine derivative
Controlled substance schedule III
FDA pregnancy category: C

Indications: Insomnia

Contraindications: Hypersensitivity, porphyria

Pharmacologic Effects: Produces CNS depression

Pharmacokinetics: Is erratically absorbed from GI tract; average half-life 10-12 hr; 50% bound to plasma proteins; conjugant excreted in urine

Side Effects: *CNS:* hangover (1.1%), drowsiness (1%); *peripheral:* skin rash (8.6%), nausea (2.7%), blood dyscrasias (rare)

Interactions
- *Alcohol and CNS depressants:* additive depressant effect
- *Oral anticoagulants:* decreased effect of anticoagulant

Implications
  Assess
- Blood studies for rare individual with blood dyscrasias

Planning/Implementation
- Give ½-1 hr before bedtime.
- Maintain safety.

Teaching
- To avoid driving and operating heavy machinery
- To avoid alcohol and other CNS depressants
- To taper drug discontinuance to prevent withdrawal syndrome

Evaluate
- Ability to sleep through night
- Mental status
- Blood dyscrasias (rare)

Treatment of Overdose: Lethal dose ranges from 10 to 20 g; a low dosage of 5 g has killed a patient, and a high dosage of 35 g has been survived; symptoms same as barbiturate intoxication; maintain airway, monitor VS, gastric lavage (induce emesis only in alert patient); lavage in all cases, regardless of elapsed time, with a 11 mixture of castor oil and water; charcoal delays absorption.

Administration
- *Insomnia: adult:* PO 250-500 mg hs, may repeat dose if >4 hr before usual awakening; not to exceed 1 g

- *Available forms:* tabs 250, 500 mg; caps 500 mg

Halazepam

PAXIPAM
(hal-az´-e-pam)

Functional classification: Antianxiety
Chemical classification: Benzodiazepine
Controlled substance schedule IV
FDA pregnancy category: D

Indications: Anxiety

Contraindications: Hypersensitivity, psychosis, narrow-angle glaucoma, child <18 yr

Pharmacologic Effects: Depresses CNS (i.e., limbic and reticular formation)

Pharmacokinetics: Speed of onset: intermediate to slow; PO peak level 1-3 hr, duration 3-6 hr, metabolized by liver, excreted by kidneys, crosses placenta and breast milk, half-life 14-100 hr (with metabolites)

Side Effects: *CNS:* see Diazepam; *peripheral:* see Diazepam

Interactions: See Diazepam

Implications: See Diazepam

Treatment of Overdose: See Diazepam

Administration
- *Adult:* PO 60-160 mg/day in divided doses; *geriatric:* PO 20 mg qd-bid
- *Available forms:* tabs 20, 40 mg

Haloperidol, haloperidol decanoate

HALDOL, HALDOL DECANOATE
(ha-loe-per´-i-dole)

Functional classifications: Traditional antipsychotic, neuroleptic, high potency
Chemical classification: Butyrophenone
FDA pregnancy category: C

Indications: Psychotic disorders, control of tics and vocal utterances in Tourette's syndrome, short-term treatment of hyperactive children with excessive motor activity, severe behavioral problems in children

Contraindications: Hypersensitivity, blood dyscrasias, coma, child <3 yr, brain damage, bone marrow depression, alcohol and barbiturate withdrawal states, parkinsonism
  Cautious use: Lactation, seizure disorders,

---

*Infrequently used.   †Available in Canada only.

hypertension, hepatic disease, cardiac disease, breast cancer

Pharmacologic Effects: Traditional antipsychotic drugs produce a neuroleptic effect characterized by sedation, emotional quieting, psychomotor slowing, and affective indifference; exact mode of action not fully understood; blocks D_2 receptors (++++) in the basal ganglia, hypothalamus, limbic system, brainstem, and medulla; blockade of these receptors accounts for both therapeutic and adverse responses; because of their nonselective actions, many other neurotransmitters systems are affected as well; ACh (+), histamine (+), and alpha-1 (+); plasma levels 5-20 ng/ml

Pharmacokinetics: *PO:* onset erratic, peak 3-5 hr, half-life 12-36 hr; *IM:* onset 15-30 min, peak 15-20 min; *IM (decanoate):* peak 4-11 days, half-life 3 wk; metabolized by liver, excreted in urine (40%) and bile (15%), crosses placenta, excreted in breast milk

Side Effects: *CNS:* parkinsonism, akathisias, dystonias, tardive dyskinesia, oculogyric crisis, NMS; *peripheral:* blurred vision (cycloplegia or paralysis of accommodation), ocular pain, photophobia, mydriasis, impaired vision; intolerance of extreme heat or cold, possible heat stroke or fatal hyperthermia; nasal congestion; wheezing, dyspnea; hypotension, especially orthostatic, leading to dizziness, syncope; tachycardia, irregular pulse, arrhythmias; dry mouth; constipation; jaundice; abdominal pain; urinary retention and hesitancy, galactorrhea, gynecomastia, impaired ejaculation, amenorrhea, sedation (~2%), EPSEs (~30%), orthostasis (~2%), anticholinergic (~2%), weight gain (~2%), sexual dysfunction (min)

Interactions

- *Alcohol and other CNS depressants* (barbiturates, antihistamines, antianxiety, or antidepressant drugs): increased CNS depression, increased risk of EPSEs
- *Amphetamines:* possible decreased antipsychotic effect
- *Antacids* (magnesium and aluminum products): possible decreased antipsychotic effect
- *Anticholinergics* (e.g., atropine, H_1-type antihistamines, antidepressants): increased risk of excessive atropine-like side effects or toxic effects
- *Benztropine:* possible decreased antipsychotic effect, increased risk of severity of peripheral anticholinergic side effects
- *Diazoxide:* possible severe hyperglycemia, prediabetic coma
- *Fluoxetine:* EPSEs
- *Fluvoxamine:* might double haloperidol serum levels, leading to increase in both negative and positive symptoms
- *Guanethidine:* poor control of hypertension by guanethidine

- *Hypoglycemia drugs* (insulin, oral hypoglycemia agents): poor diabetic control
- *Lithium:* disorientation, unconsciousness, EPSEs, and potentially neurotoxic effects
- *Meperidine, morphine:* increased risk of severe CNS depression, respiratory depression, hypotension
- *Propranolol:* increased pharmacologic effects of either drug

Implications: See Chlorpromazine

Treatment of Overdose: Lavage; if orally ingested, provide an airway; do not induce vomiting.

Administration

- *Psychosis: adult:* PO 0.5-5 mg bid or tid initially depending on severity of condition; dosage is increased to desired dosage, max 100 mg/day; *elderly:* 0.5-2.0 mg bid or tid; *chronic or resistive patients:* 3.0-5.0 mg bid or tid; IM 2-5 mg q1-8h; *child 3-12 yr:* PO/IM 0.05-0.15 mg/kg/day; *decanoate:* initial dose IM is 10-15 times the daily oral dose at 4-wk intervals; do not administer IV
- *Tourette's syndrome: adult:* PO 0.5-5 mg bid or tid, increased until desired response occurs; *child 3-12 yr:* PO 0.05-0.075 mg/kg/day (0.5-2.0 mg/day)
- *Hyperactive children: child 3-12 yr:* PO 0.05-0.075 mg/kg/day
- *Available forms:* tabs 0.5, 1, 2, 5, 10, 20 mg; conc 2 mg/ml; inj IM 5 mg/ml; decanoate IM 50, 100 mg/ml

H

Hydroxyzine*

ATARAX, QUIESS, VISTARIL/VISTARIL IM
(hye-drox´-i-zeen)

Functional classification: Antianxiety agent
Chemical classification: Piperazine
FDA pregnancy category: C

Indications: Anxiety, often used preoperatively to prevent nausea; IM form for hysterical patients

Contraindications: Hypersensitivity, early pregnancy

Pharmacologic Effects: Depresses subcortical CNS (i.e., limbic and reticular areas)

Pharmacokinetics: Rapidly absorbed from gut; clinical effect in 15-30 min; half-life 3 hr but longer in elderly patients; metabolized by liver

Side Effects: *CNS:* drowsiness (transient); rarely reported: tremor and seizures; *peripheral:* dry mouth; respiratory problems

Interactions

- *CNS depressants:* additive effect
- *Phenothiazines:* decreased antipsychotic effect

Implications

Assess
- BP

Planning/Implementation
- Give with food or milk.
- Assist with ambulation.
- Maintain safety.

Teaching
- To take hard candies and gum for dry mouth
- To avoid alcohol, CNS depressants
- To avoid driving and operating other heavy machinery

Evaluate
- Mental status

Treatment of Overdose: Oversedation most common problem; induce vomiting, gastric lavage; if hypotension occurs, give IV fluids and norepinephrine (do not use epinephrine).

Administration
- *Anxiety: adult:* PO 50-100 mg qid; *child >6 yr:* 50-100 mg/day in divided doses; *child <6 yr:* 50 mg/day in divided doses
- *Available forms:* tabs 10, 25, 50, 100 mg; caps 25, 50, 100 mg; syr 10 mg/5 ml; oral susp 25 mg/5 ml; IM inj 25, 50 mg/ml

Imipramine HCl

JANIMINE, NOVOPRAMINE,† TOFRANIL
(im-ip´-ra-meen)

Functional classification: Antidepressant
Chemical classifications: Tricyclic, tertiary amine
FDA pregnancy category: C

Indications: Depression, enuresis in children
Unlabeled use: Panic disorder

Contraindications: Hypersensitivity to TCAs, recovery phase of myocardial infarction
Cautious use: Suicidal patients, severe depression, increased intraocular pressure, narrow-angle glaucoma, urinary retention, cardiac disease, hepatic disease, hyperthyroidism, ECT, elective surgery, elderly patients, MAOI therapy, convulsive disorders, prostatic hypertrophy

Pharmacologic Effects: Blocks reuptake of norepinephrine (++) and serotonin (+++) into presynaptic neurons; also thought to be r/t downregulation of beta-adrenergic receptors; also receptor antagonist for ACh (+++), histamine (+++), and alpha-1 (+++); therapeutic plasma levels 200-350 ng/ml

Pharmacokinetics: *PO:* steady state 2-5 days, metabolized by liver, excreted by kidneys and feces, crosses placenta, excreted in breast milk, half-life 11-25 hr; desipramine is a metabolite

Side Effects: *CNS:* sedation (~10%), ataxia, confusion (~2%), delirium; *peripheral:* blurred vision (~10%), photophobia, increased intraocular pressure, decreased tearing; orthostatic hypotension (~30%), arrhythmias, tachycardia (~10%), palpitations; dry mouth (~30%); constipation (~10%), diarrhea; decreased sweating, urinary hesitancy (~10%)

Interactions: See Amitriptyline

Implications: See Amitriptyline

Treatment of Overdose: ECG monitoring; induce emesis; lavage, activated charcoal; administer anticonvulsant, if needed; treat anticholinergic effects.

Administration
- *Depression: adult:* PO/IM 75-100 mg/day in divided doses, may gradually increase to 200 mg, not to exceed 300 mg/day; may give daily dose hs; *child:* 1.5 mg/kg/day in 3 divided doses to start; may increase by 1-1.5 mg/kg/day every 3-5 days; maximum dose 5 mg/kg/day; *adolescent and geriatric:* 10 mg tid-qid, typically not necessary to exceed 100 mg/day
- *Enuresis: child 6-12 yr:* 25 mg/day 1 hr before bedtime; if no improvement in 1 wk, may increase to 50 mg/night; *adolescent:* may give up to 75 mg/night
- *Available forms:* tabs 10, 25, 50, mg; inj IM 25 mg/2 ml; Pamoate salt (slow-release capsules) 75, 100, 125, 150 mg

Lamotrigine

LAMICTAL
(la-moe´-tri-jeen)

Functional classification: Antiepileptic
Chemical classification: Phenyltriazine derivative
FDA pregnancy category: C

Indications: Adjunctive treatment for partial seizures; may have implications for more generalized seizures

Contraindications: Lactation
Cautious use: Impaired hepatic, renal, cardiac function

Pharmacologic Effects: Blocks sustained repetitive firing of neurons by prolonging the inactivation of sodium channels; therapeutic serum levels are >2 μg/ml

Pharmacokinetics: Almost completely absorbed after oral ingestion, with or without food; bioavailability 90%; moderately bound to serum proteins (55%); peak serum levels 1.5-4 hr; half-life 25 hr, but if combined with enzyme inducers (i.e., carbamazepine, phenytoin, phenobarbital) the half-life can decrease to 10 hr, and if given with

---

*Infrequently used.   †Available in Canada only.

enzyme inhibitors (e.g., valproic acid) the half-life can increase to 60 hr; protein binding 55%

Side Effects: *CNS:* dizziness (14%), diplopia (14%), somnolence (13%), headache (12%), ataxia (11%), asthenia (10%); *peripheral:* blurred vision, nausea, vomiting, rash (5%-10%); deaths have occurred r/t Stevens-Johnson syndrome; disseminated intravascular coagulation has been reported

Interactions

- *Carbamazepine, phenytoin, phenobarbital, primidone* (all are enzyme-inducing agents): decrease the half-life of lamotrigine to about 15 hr; carbamazepine serum levels are reported to increase, sometimes to toxic levels
- *Valproic acid:* increases half-life of lamotrigine to about 60 hr; valproic acid concentrations decrease by about 25%

Implications

Assess

- History of hepatic, renal, or cardiac problems
- Lactation
- Baseline physical data (e.g., VS, BP, skin, orientation)

Planning/Implementation

- Monitor renal, hepatic, and cardiac functions.
- Reevaluate if abnormal test results are found.
- Monitor drug dosage. Carefully assess when changing the dosage of another antiepileptic (because lamotrigine is an adjunctive agent).
- When discontinuing, taper drug over 2-wk period.

Teaching

- To take drug as prescribed
- Not to stop drug abruptly because of possibility of withdrawal-precipitated seizures
- To avoid driving or working with hazardous machinery because of dizziness and somnolence
- To take drug with meals if GI upset occurs
- To self-assess skin changes and to report skin yellowing, fever, sore throat, mouth sores, unusual bleeding, skin rash, bruising (see Side Effects)
- To wear MedicAlert bracelet so that others will have information about seizure disorder

Evaluate

- Seizure status
- Minimal effect of adverse reactions

Administration

- *Adults taking an enzyme-inducing antiepileptic* (carbamazepine, phenytoin, phenobarbital, primidone): 50 mg qd for 2 wk; then can increase to 50 mg bid for 2 more wk; then weekly changes of 100 mg/day up to a maintenance dosage of 150-250 mg bid; if taken with valproic acid, start with 25 mg qod then gradually increase to between 50 and 75 mg bid; not recommended for children <16 yr

Lithium carbonate

CIBALITH-S, ESKALITH, LITHANE, LITHIUM CITRATE, LITHOBID, LITHONATE, LITHONATE-S, LITHOTABS (li´-thee-um)

Functional classification: Antimanic
Chemical classification: Alkali metal ion salt
FDA pregnancy category: D

Indications: Manic-depressive illness (manic phase), prevention of bipolar manic depressive psychosis

Contraindications: Children <12 yr, hepatic or renal disease, brain trauma, lactation, schizophrenia, severe cardiac disease, severe dehydration, organic mental syndrome, sodium depletion
Cautious use: Concomitant neuroleptic therapy, elderly patients, hypothyroidism, seizure disorders, diabetes mellitus, systemic infection, urinary retention

Pharmacologic Effects: Alters sodium ion transport in nerve, muscle cells; affects norepinephrine reuptake, stabilizes calcium channels, decreases neuronal activity via second messenger systems, enhances ACh formation, and increases serotonin receptor sensitivity, all perhaps contributing to its therapeutic effect; therapeutic serum levels 0.6-1.2 mEq/L.

Pharmacokinetics: *PO:* onset rapid, peak 1-4 hr, half-life about 24 hr, depending on age; crosses blood-brain barrier, 95% excreted unchanged in urine, crosses placenta, excreted in breast milk, well absorbed by oral method; sodium loading increases lithium excretion

Side Effects: *CNS:* headache, drowsiness, dizziness, tremors, twitching, ataxia, seizure, slurred speech, restlessness, confusion, stupor, memory loss, clonic movements; *peripheral:* dry mouth, anorexia, nausea, vomiting, diarrhea, hypotension, leukocytosis, blurred vision, hypothyroidism, hyponatremia, muscle weakness

Interactions

- *Captopril, lisinopril* (ACE inhibitors): reported to produce a threefold to fourfold increase in serum lithium levels (a potentially fatal combination)
- *Carbamazepine:* neurotoxic effects
- *Haloperidol:* encephalopathy
- *Indomethacin, thiazide diuretics, NSAIDs:* increased toxic effects

L

- *Neuromuscular blocking agents, phenothiazines:* increased effects of these drugs
- *Sodium bicarbonate, acetazolamide, mannitol, aminophylline:* increased renal clearance
- *Theophylline, urinary alkalinizers:* decreased effects of lithium

Implications
Assess
- Initiate serum creatinine and thyroid function studies before starting lithium regimen
- Weigh daily, check for edema in legs, ankles, wrists; if present, report
- Sodium intake; decreased sodium intake with decreased fluid intake might lead to lithium retention; increased sodium and fluids might decrease lithium retention
- Skin turgor, at least daily
- Urine for albuminuria, glycosuria, uric acid during beginning of treatment, q2mo thereafter
- Neurologic status: gait, motor reflexes, hand tremors
- Serum lithium levels weekly initially, then obtain lithium levels 8-12 hr after previous dose (therapeutic serum level 0.6-1.2 mEq/L)

Planning/Implementation
- Have patient take with meals to prevent GI upset.
- Instruct patient to have adequate fluids (2-3 L/day) to prevent dehydration during initial treatment, 1-2 L/day during maintenance.

Teaching
- To know symptoms of minor toxic effects (vomiting, diarrhea, poor coordination, fine-motor tremors, weakness, lassitude) and major toxic effects (coarse tremors, severe thirst, tinnitus, dilute urine)
- To understand action, dosage, side effects; when to notify physician
- To monitor urine specific gravity
- That contraception is necessary because lithium might harm fetus
- Not to operate machinery until lithium serum levels are stable

Evaluate
- Reduction in manic symptoms
- Patient verbalization of understanding of side effects, symptoms of toxic effects, and need for compliance

Treatment of Overdose: Lavage, maintain airway, respiratory function; dialysis for severe intoxication.
- *Lithium levels 1.5-2 mEq/L:* diarrhea, vomiting, nausea, drowsiness, weakness
- *Lithium levels 2-3 mEq/L:* giddiness, ataxia, blurred vision, tinnitus, slurred speech, blackouts, fasciculations, incontinence
- *Lithium levels >3 mEq/L:* multiple organs and

organ systems failure, seizures, vascular collapse, coma

Administration
- *Adult:* PO 600 mg tid, maintenance 300 mg tid or qid; slow-rel tabs 450 mg bid, dosage should be individualized to maintain blood levels at 0.5-1.5 mEq/L; maintenance serum concentrations 0.6-1.2 mEq/L
- *Available forms:* caps 150, 30 0, 600 mg; tabs 300 mg; tabs slow-rel 300, 450 mg; syr 8 mEq/5 ml (as citrate)

Lorazepam
ATIVAN
(lor-a´-ze-pam)

Functional classification: Antianxiety agent
Chemical classification: Benzodiazepine
Controlled substance schedule IV
FDA pregnancy category: D

Indications: Anxiety; status epilepticus

Contraindications: Hypersensitivity to benzodiazepines, narrow-angle glaucoma, psychosis, child <18 yr (inj), child <12 yr (oral)
Cautious use: Elderly or debilitated patients, hepatic or renal disease

Pharmacologic Effects: Increases the affinity of GABA molecules for their specific receptor increasing the frequency with which chloride channels open in response to GABA; may also decrease norepinephrine and serotonin turnover rates

Pharmacokinetics: Speed of onset: intermediate PO peak 1-6 hr, duration 3-6 hr, metabolized by liver by oxidative processes, excreted by kidneys, crosses placenta, excreted in breast milk, half-life 10-20 hr

Side Effects: *CNS:* drowsiness, dizziness, confusion, headache, anxiety, tremor, stimulation, fatigue, depression, insomnia; *peripheral:* photophobia caused by mydriasis, blurred vision caused by cycloplegia; sleeplike slowing of respirations with therapeutic doses, cough; orthostatic hypotension, tachycardia, hypotension; constipation; dry mouth

Interactions: See Alprazolam

Implications: See Alprazolam

Treatment of Overdose: Lavage, VS, supportive care; few deaths, if any, reported as resulting from benzodiazepine overdose alone; deaths occur when benzodiazepines are mixed with other drugs

Administration
- *Anxiety: adult:* PO 2-6 mg/day in divided doses, not to exceed 10 mg/day; take largest dose before bedtime; *geriatric:* initially 1-2

---

mg/day in divided doses, adjust as needed or tolerated
- *Insomnia: adult:* PO 2-4 mg hs
- *Status epilepticus: adult:* IV: 4 mg administered as a 2-minute IV push; may be repeated in 5-10 min if needed; maximum dose 8 mg; *infant and child:* 0.1 mg/kg over 25 min; maximum 4 mg as a single dose
- *Available forms:* tabs 0.5, 1, 2 mg; IM/IV inj 2-4 mg/ml: must refrigerate

Loxapine succinate/ loxapine HCl

LOXAPAC,† LOXITANE, LOXITANE-C
(lox-a´-peen)

Functional classifications: Traditional antipsychotic, neuroleptic, moderate potency
Chemical classification: Dibenzoxazepine
FDA pregnancy category: C

Indications: Psychotic disorders

Contraindications: Hypersensitivity, blood dyscrasias, coma, child <16 yr, brain damage, bone marrow depression, alcohol and barbiturate withdrawal states
Cautious use: Lactation, seizure disorders, hypertension, hepatic disease, cardiac disease, glaucoma, urinary retention

Pharmacologic Effects: Traditional antipsychotic drugs produce a neuroleptic effect characterized by sedation, emotional quieting, psychomotor slowing, and affective indifference; exact mode of action not fully understood; blocks D_2 receptors (++++) in the basal ganglia, hypothalamus, limbic system, brainstem, and medulla; blockade of these receptors accounts for both therapeutic and adverse responses; because of their nonselective actions, many other neurotransmitters systems are affected as well; ACh (++), histamine (+++), and alpha-1 (++++)

Pharmacokinetics: *PO:* onset 20-30 min, peak 2-4 hr, duration 12 hr, half-life 8-30 hr; *IM:* onset 15-30 min, peak 15-20 min, duration 12 hr; metabolized by liver, excreted in urine, crosses placenta, excreted in breast milk

Side Effects: See Chlorpromazine; specific for loxapine: sedation (~30%), EPSEs (~30%), orthostasis (~10%), anticholinergic (~10%), weight gain (~2%), sexual dysfunction (~2%)

Interactions: See Chlorpromazine

Implications: See Chlorpromazine

Treatment of Overdose: Lavage, if orally ingested; provide an airway; do not induce vomiting.

Administration
- *Adult and child >15 yr:* PO 10 mg bid initially,

may be rapidly increased depending on severity of condition, maintenance 20-60 mg/day, range 20-250 mg/day; IM 12.5-50 mg q4-6h or more until desired response, then start PO form
- Mix concentrate in orange or grapefruit juice
- *Available forms:* caps 5, 10, 25, 50 mg; conc 25 mg/ml; inj IM 50 mg/ml

Maprotiline HCl

LUDIOMIL
(ma-proe´-ti-leen)

Functional classification: Antidepressant
Chemical classification: Tetracyclic
FDA pregnancy category: B

Indications: Depression, dysthymic disorder, bipolar—depressed, anxiety associated with depression

Contraindications: Hypersensitivity to TCAs, CV disease, convulsive disorders
Cautious use: Suicidal patients, severe depression, increased intraocular pressure, narrow-angle glaucoma, urinary retention, cardiac disease, hepatic disease, hypothyroidism, hyperthyroidism, ECT, elective surgery, elderly patients, lactation, child <18 yr, prostatic hypertrophy

Pharmacologic Effects: Blocks reuptake of norepinephrine (++) and serotonin (+); also r/t downregulation of beta-adrenergic receptors; also antagonizes ACh (++), histamine (++++), and alpha-1 (+++) receptors; therapeutic plasma levels 200-300 ng/ml

Pharmacokinetics: *PO:* onset 15-30 min, peak 12 hr, duration up to 3 wk, steady state 6-10 days; metabolized by liver, excreted by kidneys and feces; crosses placenta, half-life 21-25 hr

Side Effects: *CNS:* sedation (~10%), ataxia; confusion (~2%), delirium; *peripheral:* blurred vision (~10%), photophobia, increased intraocular pressure; decreased tearing; orthostatic hypotension (~2%), arrhythmias, tachycardia (~2%), palpitations; dry mouth (~30%); constipation (~10%), diarrhea; decreased sweating, urinary hesitancy (~2%); weight gain (~10%); tremor (~10%)

Interactions: See Amitriptyline

Implications: See Amitriptyline

Teaching
- That maprotiline might produce clinical effects faster than TCAs do, sometimes within 3-7 days; however, a lag time of 2-3 wk occurs in many patients

Treatment of Overdose: ECG, monitoring, induce emesis, lavage, activated charcoal, rapid digitalization for CV failure, reduce tendency for convulsions, control fever.

M

Administration

- *Adult:* PO 75 mg/day in moderate depression, may increase to 150 mg/day; not to exceed 225 mg in hospitalized patients; severely depressed patients who are hospitalized may be given 300 mg/day; *geriatric:* 50-75 mg/day
- *Available forms:* tabs 25, 50, 75 mg

Mephenytoin*

MESANTOIN
(me-fen´-i-toyn)

Functional classification: Antiepileptic
Chemical classification: Hydantoin derivative
FDA pregnancy category: C

Indications: Generalized tonic-clonic, psychomotor, focal seizures refractory to other agents

Contraindications: Hypersensitivity to hydantoins, sinus bradycardia, heart block, Adams-Stokes syndrome
   Cautious use: Alcoholism, hepatic or renal disease, blood dyscrasias, CHF, elderly patients, respiratory depression, diabetes mellitus, lactation

Pharmacologic Effects: Inhibits spread of seizure activity in motor cortex

Pharmacokinetics: *PO:* onset 30 min, duration 24-48 hr, metabolized by liver, excreted by kidneys, half-life unknown

Side Effects: See Ethotoin

Interactions: See Ethotoin

Implications: See Ethotoin

Treatment of Overdose: Mean lethal dose in adults is thought to be 2-5 g; initial symptoms are nystagmus, ataxia; death results from respiratory and circulatory depression; lavage, emesis, activated charcoal.

Administration

- *Adult:* PO 50-100 mg/day, may increase by 50-100 mg every 7 days, up to 200 mg tid (600 mg/day); *child:* usually requires 100-400 mg/day
- *Available forms:* tabs 100 mg

Mephobarbital

MEBARAL
(me-foe-bar´-bi-tal)

Functional classification: Antiepileptic (long-acting)
Chemical classification: Barbiturate
Controlled substance schedule IV
FDA pregnancy category: D

Indications: Generalized tonic-clonic, absence seizures

Contraindications: Hypersensitivity to barbiturates
   Cautious use: Hepatic or renal disease, lactation, alcoholism, drug abuse, hyperthyroidism, myasthenia gravis, myxedema, vitamin D and K deficiency

Pharmacologic Effects: Therapeutic effect caused by its ability to bind to GABA receptors (at a specific barbiturate site); barbiturates both enhance the inhibitory effects of GABA and mimic GABA, resulting in prolonged opening of the chloride

Pharmacokinetics: *PO:* onset 30-60 min, duration 10-12 hr; metabolized by liver, excreted by kidneys, half-life 34 hr (mean)

Side Effects: *CNS:* somnolence, drowsiness, lethargy, hangover headache, flushing, hallucinations, coma, dizziness; *peripheral:* nausea, vomiting; hypoventilation; bradycardia, hypotension; rash, urticaria, angioedema; local pain, swelling, necrosis, thrombophlebitis, blood dyscrasias

Interactions: See Phenobarbital

Implications: See Phenobarbital

Treatment of Overdose: 1 g can cause serious poisoning in an adult; 2-10 g can be fatal; toxic effects can be confused with drunkenness; emesis, if feasible; gastric lavage, if conscious; 30 g activated charcoal, maintain airway, good nursing care to prevent pneumonia.

Administration

- *Epilepsy: adult:* PO 400-600 mg/day or in divided doses; *child <5 yr:* 16-32 mg tid or qid; *child >5 yr:* 32-64 mg tid or qid
- *Available forms:* tabs 32, 50, 100, 250 mg

Methadone HCl

DOLOPHINE, METHADONE HCL
(meth´-a-done)

Functional classification: Narcotic analgesic
Chemical classifications: Opiate, synthetic diphenylheptane derivative
Controlled substance schedule II
FDA pregnancy category: C

Indications: Narcotic withdrawal, severe pain

Contraindications: Hypersensitivity, addiction (narcotic)
   Cautious use: Addictive personality, lactation, increased intracranial pressure, asthma, hypotension, acute abdominal condition, respiratory depression, hepatic or renal disease, child <18

---

yr, Addison's disease, prostatic hypertrophy, urethral stricture

Pharmacologic Effects: Acts on mu and kappa opiate receptors

Pharmacokinetics: *PO:* onset 30-60 min, duration 4-6 hr; peak 2-6 hr, metabolized by liver, excreted by kidneys, crosses placenta, excreted in breast milk, half-life 15-30 hr

Side Effects: *CNS:* drowsiness, dizziness, confusion, headache, sedation, euphoria; *peripheral:* nausea, vomiting, anorexia, constipation, cramps, increased urinary output, dysuria, rash, urticaria, bruising, flushing, diaphoresis, pruritus, respiratory depression, tinnitus, blurred vision, miosis, diplopia, palpitations, bradycardia, change in BP

Interactions
- *Alcohol, narcotics, sedative hypnotics, antipsychotics, skeletal muscle relaxants, rifampin, phenytoin:* increased CNS depression
- *Droperidol:* hypotension
- *Hydantoins:* increase effects of methadone
- *MAOIs:* unpredictable, have caused fatalities when used with related drugs

Implications
> *Assess*
- I&O ratio: check for decreasing output; might indicate urinary retention

Planning/Implementation
- If nausea, vomiting occurs, give with antiemetic.
- Rotate injection sites.
- Assist with ambulation.
- Provide safety measures: side rails, nightlight, call bell within easy reach.

Teaching
- To report any symptoms of CNS changes
- That dependency could result
- That withdrawal symptoms might occur (e.g., nausea, vomiting, cramps, fever, faintness, anorexia)

Evaluate
- Therapeutic response
- CNS changes: dizziness, drowsiness, hallucinations, euphoria, pupil reaction
- Respiratory dysfunction: respiratory depression; if respirations are <12 breaths/min, notify physician
- Physical dependence

Treatment of Overdose: Give naloxone 0.2-0.8 mg IV, O$_2$, IV fluids, vasopressors.

Administration
- *Pain: adult:* PO/SC/IM 2.5-10 mg q3-4h prn
- *Narcotic withdrawal: adult:* PO 10-20 mg/day but highly individualized initially, then up to ≥40-60 mg/day as patient response indicates, some patients might need as much as 100 mg/day
- *Available forms:* inj SC, IM 10 mg/ml; tabs 5,

10 mg; oral sol 5, 10 mg/5 ml, 10 mg/10 ml; dispersible tabs 40 mg, oral conc 10 mg/ml

Methamphetamine HCl
DESOXYN, DESOXYN GRADUMET
(meth-am-fet´-a-meen)

Functional classification: Cerebral stimulant
Chemical classification: Amphetamine
Controlled substance schedule II
FDA pregnancy category: C

Indications: ADHD, exogenous obesity

Contraindications: Hypersensitivity to sympathomimetic amines, hyperthyroidism, hypertension, glaucoma, severe arteriosclerosis, parkinsonism, drug abuse, anxiety, MAOI use
> *Cautious use:* Tourette's syndrome, lactation, child <3 yr

Pharmacologic Effects: Mechanism of action not clearly understood; stimulates dopamine function in the brain probably as a result of blocking of both dopamine and norepinephrine reuptake; might also promote release of dopamine into synaptic cleft; theoretically, these effects enhance inhibitory subcortical-cortical pathways, resulting in better concentration and impulse control, with a subsequent decrease in motor activity; therapeutic plasma levels 5-10 mg/dl

Pharmacokinetics: *PO:* duration 3-6 hr, metabolized by liver, excreted by kidneys, crosses blood-brain barrier, half-life 4-5 hr

Side Effects: *CNS:* hyperactivity, insomnia, restlessness, talkativeness, dizziness, headache, chills, stimulation, dysphoria, irritability, aggressiveness; *peripheral:* nausea, vomiting, anorexia, dry mouth, diarrhea, constipation, weight loss, metallic taste, cramps, erectile dysfunction, change in libido, palpitations, tachycardia, hypertension, hypotension

Interactions
- *Acetazolamide, antacids, sodium bicarbonate, ascorbic acid, ammonium chloride, phenothiazines, haloperidol:* increase half-life of amphetamine
- *Barbiturates:* decreased effects of this drug
- *Guanethidine, other antihypertensives:* decreased hypotensive effect
- *Insulin:* might alter insulin requirements
- *MAOIs or within 14 days of MAOIs:* hypertensive crisis
- *Phenothiazines:* antagonize amphetamines *Urinary acidifiers:* increase amphetamine excretion

Implications
> *Assess*
- VS, BP because this drug might reverse

M

antihypertensives; check patients with cardiac disease more often

- CBC, urinalysis; in diabetes, blood and urine glucose levels, insulin changes might need to be made because eating might decrease
- Height, growth rate in children (growth rate might be decreased)

Planning/Implementation
- Have patient take dose at least 6 hr before bedtime to prevent sleeplessness
- For obesity, only when patient is on weight-reduction program that includes dietary changes, exercise; tolerance develops, and weight loss will not occur without additional methods.
- Instruct patient to chew sugarless gum, suck on hard candies, and take frequent sips of water for dry mouth.
- If drug is for obesity, have patient take dose 30-60 min before meals.
- Dispense least amount feasible to minimize risk of overdose.
- Check to see that PO medication has been swallowed

Teaching
- To decrease caffeine consumption (coffee, tea, cola, chocolate), which might increase irritability, stimulation
- To avoid OTC preparations unless approved by physician
- To taper off drug over several weeks, or depression, increased sleeping, lethargy might occur
- To avoid alcohol ingestion
- To avoid hazardous activities until condition is stabilized on medication
- To get needed rest; patients feel more tired at end of day

Evaluate
- Mental status: mood, sensorium, affect, stimulation, insomnia; aggressiveness might occur
- Physical dependency: should not be used for extended time; dose should be discontinued gradually
- Withdrawal symptoms: headache, nausea, vomiting, muscle pain, weakness
- Drug tolerance: develops after long-term use; if tolerance develops, dosage should not be increased

Treatment of Overdose: Gastric evacuation if overdose occurred in preceding 24 hr; otherwise, acidify urine; administer fluids until urine flow is 3-6 ml/kg/hr; hemodialysis or peritoneal dialysis; antihypertensives for increased BP; ammonium chloride for increased excretion; chlorpromazine for CNS stimulation.

Administration
- *ADHD: child >6 yr:* 2.5-5 mg qd or bid, increasing by 5 mg/wk; usual effective dose 20-25 mg/day
- *Obesity: adult:* PO 5 mg 30 min ac or 10-15 mg long-acting qAM
- *Available forms:* tabs 5 mg; long-acting tabs 5, 10, 15 mg

Methohexital

BREVITAL SODIUM, BRIETAL SODIUM†
(meth-oh-hex´-i-tal)

Functional classification: General anesthetic
Chemical classification: Barbiturate
Controlled substance schedule IV
FDA pregnancy category: D

Indications: General anesthesia for ECT

Contraindications: Hypersensitivity, status asthmaticus, porphyria

Pharmacologic Effects: Ultrashortacting barbiturate depresses CNS to produce anesthesia

Pharmacokinetics: Highly lipophilic; onset rapid (unconsciousness achieved within 10-15 sec) but of brief duration (5-7 min) because of natural redistribution to adipose tissue and other less vascular sites; plasma half-life 3-8 hr

Side Effects: *CNS:* delirium, headache, prolonged somnolence and recovery; *peripheral:* circulatory depression, arrhythmias, respiratory depression, apnea, laryngospasm, bronchospasm, nausea, vomiting

Interactions
- *CNS depressants including alcohol:* additive effect
- *Furosemide:* aggravates orthostatic hypotension

Implications
Assess
- VS q3-5min until recovered from ECT

Planning/Implementation
- Have emergency drugs and resuscitation equipment available.

Evaluate
- Cardiac status
- Respirations
- Mental status

Treatment of Overdose: Usually occurs because of rapid injection, resulting in apnea and respiratory difficulties; discontinue drug, maintain airway, give oxygen prn; ventilatory assistance prn.

Administration
- *Adult:* IV 50-120 mg (5-12 ml of 1% sol); this amount provides anesthesia for 5-7 min

---

- *Available forms:* powder for IV inj; ampules 2.5, 5 g; vials 500 mg/50 ml, 2.5 g/250 ml, 5 g/500 ml

Methsuximide*

CELONTIN
(meth-sux´-i-mide)

Functional classification: Antiepileptic
Chemical classification: Succinimide
FDA pregnancy category: C

Indications: Second-choice drug for absence seizures

Contraindications: Hypersensitivity

Pharmacologic Effects: See Ethosuximide

Pharmacokinetics: Onset in 15-30 min, peak level 1-4 hr, duration of effect 3-4 hr, excreted in urine, half-life 2.6-4 hr

Side Effects: *CNS:* drowsiness, ataxia, and dizziness most common side effect; see ethosuximide for other CNS effects; *peripheral:* see Ethosuximide

Interactions: See Ethosuximide

Implications: See Ethosuximide

Treatment of Overdose: See ethosuximide

Administration
- *Adult and child:* 300 mg/day at first, increase by 300 mg/day at weekly intervals as needed; do not exceed 1200 mg/day in divided doses
- *Available forms:* caps half-strength 150 mg; caps 300 mg

Methylphenidate HCl

RITALIN, RITALIN SR
(meth-ill-fen´-i-date)

Functional classification: Cerebral stimulant
Chemical classification: Piperidine derivative
Controlled substance schedule II
FDA pregnancy category: C

Indications: ADHD, narcolepsy

Contraindications: Hypersensitivity to sympathomimetic amines, anxiety, Tourette's syndrome, history of seizures, child <6 yr (not approved)
Cautious use: Hypertension, severe depression, seizures, drug abuse, lactation, tension, agitation

Pharmacologic Effects: Although mechanism of action not clearly understood, it is known that stimulants enhance dopaminergic function in the brain; this is because of blockade of the reuptake of dopamine and norepinephrine; stimulants might also promote release of dopamine into the synaptic cleft; these effects are proposed to enhance inhibitory subcortical-cortical pathways, resulting in better communication, impulse control, and decreased motor activity

Pharmacokinetics: *PO:* onset 1/2-1 hr, duration 4-6 hr, metabolized by liver, excreted by kidneys, half-life 1-3 hr

Side Effects: *CNS:* hyperactivity, insomnia, restlessness, talkativeness, dizziness, headache, chills, stimulation, dysphoria, irritability, aggressiveness; *peripheral:* nausea, vomiting, anorexia, dry mouth, diarrhea, constipation, weight loss, metallic taste, cramps, erectile dysfunction, change in libido, palpitations, tachycardia, hypertension, hypotension

Interactions
- *Acetazolamide, antacids, sodium bicarbonate, ascorbic acid, ammonium chloride, phenothiazines, haloperidol:* increase effects of amphetamine
- *Barbiturates:* decreased effects of this drug
- *Guanethidine, other antihypertensives:* decreased effects of these drugs
- *MAOIs or within 14 days of MAOIs:* hypertensive crisis

Implications
Assess
- VS, BP
- Appetite: might be decreased
- Height, growth rate in children might be decreased

Planning/Implementation
- Instruct patient to take dose at least 6 hr before bedtime to prevent sleeplessness.
- Check to see that PO medication has been swallowed.

Teaching
- To decrease caffeine consumption (coffee, tea, cola, chocolate), which might increase irritability, stimulation
- To avoid OTC preparations unless approved by physician
- To taper off drug over several weeks, or depression, increased sleeping, lethargy might occur
- To avoid alcohol ingestion
- To avoid hazardous activities until condition is stabilized on medication
- To get needed rest; patients feel more tired at end of day

Evaluate
- Mental status: mood, sensorium, affect, stimulation, insomnia; aggressiveness might occur
- Physical dependency: should not be used for extended time; drug should be discontinued gradually
- Withdrawal symptoms: headache, nausea, vomiting, muscle pain, weakness

M

- Drug tolerance: if tolerance develops, dosage should not be increased

Treatment of Overdose: Supportive measures; protect against self-injury; evacuate gastric contents, if possible; maintain circulation; external cooling, if hyperpyrexia occurs.

Administration

- *ADHD:* not recommended for children <6 yr; *child >6 yr:* start at 2.5-10 mg bid (just before breakfast and lunch) or 0.3 mg/kg; may increase in increments of 5-10 mg every 4-6 days; doses are given 3.5-4 hours apart on a bid or tid schedule; third dose is half the others to minimize rebound effects; dosages >35 mg/day in younger children and 60 mg/day in older children are not recommended
- *Narcolepsy: adult:* PO 10 mg bid-tid, 30-45 min before meals, may increase to 40-60 mg/day
- *Available forms:* tabs 5, 10, 20 mg; tabs time-rel 20 mg

Mirtazapine

REMERON
(mir-taz´-a-peen)

Functional classification: Novel antidepressant
Chemical classification: Piperazinoazepine
FDA pregnancy category: C

Indications: Depression; might be particularly useful in patients with sleep disturbance, poor appetite, or medical illness on multiple medications (because of its low potential for drug interactions)

Unlabeled use: Can be used as an antidote for SSRI-induced sexual dysfunction

Contraindications: Hypersensitivity

Pharmacologic Effects: Apparently reduces depression by selectively antagonizing alpha-2 autoreceptors and heteroreceptors, which increases the release of norepinephrine and serotonin; also blocks $5HT_2$ and $5HT_3$ receptors, accounting for lack of sexual dysfunction and GI side effects

Pharmacokinetics: Rapidly and completely absorbed following oral administration; bioavailability 50%; peak levels 2 hr; metabolized by P-450 2C, 2D6, 1A2, 3A; does not significantly inhibit P-450 isoenzymes; half-life 35 hr; excreted in urine (75%) and feces (15%)

Side Effects: *CNS:* somnolence (54%), increased appetite (17%), dizziness (7%), headache, hypomania (~2%); *peripheral:* weight gain (12%), cholesterol increase of ≥20% (15%), dry mouth (~10%), constipation (~10%)

Interactions

- *Alcohol, diazepam:* cognitive and motor impairment increased
- *Drugs affecting hepatic metabolism:* metabolism and pharmacokinetics of mirtazepine might be affected
- *Drugs metabolized or inhibitor of CYP-450 isoenzymes:* metabolism and pharmacokinetics of mirtazepine or these drugs might be affected

Treatment of Overdose: Relatively safe in overdose; no specific antidote available, and there is limited experience with mirtazepine overdose; general measures for antidepressant overdose should be used.

Administration

- Initially 15 mg/day in single dose hs and titrated after 1-2 wk if necessary; range 15-45 mg/day
- *Available forms:* tabs 15, 30 mg

Moclobemide

MANERIX
(mo-clo´-be-mide)

Functional classification: Antidepressant; reversible inhibitor of monoamine oxidase-A (RIMA)
Chemical classification: Benzamide derivative
FDA pregnancy category: Data on safety in pregnancy is lacking

Indications: Major depression, chronic dysthymia

Unlabeled uses: Potential for use in ADHD, social phobia, memory problems as a result of cognitive disorders

Contraindications: Hypersensitivity, pheochromocytoma (?), thyrotoxicosis

Cautious use: Hypertensive patients should avoid ingesting large amounts of tyramine-rich food when combining with serotonergic drugs (because of serotonin syndrome), severe liver impairment

Pharmacologic Effects: Inhibits activity of MAO-A enzyme that metabolizes serotonin and norepinephrine; inhibition reversible within 24 hr; thought to have more rapid clinical effect than other antidepressants; antagonizes ACh (++), histamine (+), and alpha-1 (++) receptors

Pharmacokinetics: Rapidly absorbed, high first-pass metabolism; peak 0.7-3 hr, half-life 1-3 hr, protein binding 50%, about 1% of maternal dose excreted in breast milk; age does not affect pharmacokinetics; metabolized by P-450 2D6, 2C; weakly inhibits 2D6

Side Effects: Does not pose same risk for

---

hypertensive crisis as irreversible MAOIs; *CNS:* insomnia (>10%), headache (>10%), drowsiness, hypomania, disorientation; *peripheral:* dry mouth (>10%), blurred vision (>10%), nausea (>10%), orthostatic hypotension (>10%), constipation, sweating, tremor, tachycardia, arrhythmias

Interactions

- *Anticholinergics:* additive effect
- *Buspirone:* potential serotonergic reaction
- *Cimetidine:* increases moclobemide serum levels
- *Dextromethorphan* (in most cough syrups): serotonergic reaction possible
- *Food:* does not have the same food restrictions as do the irreversible MAOIs; however, still recommended that food high in tyramine be avoided
- *L-tryptophan:* potential for serotonin syndrome
- *MAO-B inhibitor* (i.e., selegiline): dietary restrictions now needed
- *Meperidine:* serotonergic reaction; do not mix these two drugs
- *Narcotics:* serotonergic reaction possible
- *SSRIs, clomipramine, nefazodone:* increase serotonergic effect
- *Sympathomimetics:* hypertension

Implications
Assess
- For sleeping difficulties; if insomnia occurs, give last dose before 5 PM

Planning/Implementation
- *Diet:* patients do not need to be on a special diet but should still not overconsume tyramine-laden foods.
- *Sleep:* if patient having difficulty sleeping, instruct to take last dose by 5 PM.

Teaching
- To take moclobemide after eating to reduce side effects
- Not to eat a large meal after taking moclobemide
- That although a special diet not necessary (as with irreversible MAOIs) should still watch amounts of tyramine-rich foods (because of headaches)
- Not to take drugs (even OTC drugs) without consulting prescriber

Treatment of Overdose: Symptoms extension of side effects: drowsiness, disorientation, stupor, hypotension, tachycardia, hyperreflexia, sweating, agitation, and hallucinations; gastric lavage, emesis, activated charcoal are appropriate measures along with supportive care and close monitoring of vital functions.

Administration
- Usually 300-600 mg/day
- *Available forms:* tabs 100, 150 mg

Modafinil
PROVIGIL
(mo-daf´-ih-nil)

Functional classification: Wakefulness promoting agent
Chemical classification: Benzhydrylsulfinylacetamide compound
FDA pregnancy category: C

Indications: Narcolepsy

Contraindications: Known hypersensitivity
Cautious use: Elderly, nursing mothers

Pharmacologic Effects: Precise mechanism of action unknown; has wake promoting actions like sympathomimetics agents such as amphetamine

Pharmacokinetics: Half-life (after ~15 doses) 15 hr, absorption is rapid (food has no effect on overall bioavailability, but absorption can be delayed), peak concentrations 2-4 hr; metabolized by P-450 3A4 and also induces its own metabolism after chronic administration; inhibits 2C19

Side Effects: (based on manufacturer research information); *CNS:* headache (50%), nervousness (8%), dizziness (4%), depression (4%), anxiety (4%), insomnia, confusion, tremor; *peripheral:* nausea (13%), rhinitis (11%), diarrhea (8%), pharyngitis (6%), dry mouth (5%), anorexia (5%), chest pain (2%), neck pain, chills, abnormal liver function

Interactions

- *Deficiency of 2D6* (~7%-10% of Caucasians) (e.g., TCAs, SSRIs): serum levels might increase for these drugs if given with modafinil
- *Drugs metabolized by 2C19* (diazepam, phenytoin, propranolol): increased levels of these drugs
- *Methylphenidate:* absorption of modafinil delayed 1 hr
- *MAOIs:* interaction studies have not been done but because of the many MAOI-drug interactions, caution should be observed.
- *Potent inducers of 3A4* (e.g., carbamazepine, phenobarbital, rifampin) *or inhibitors* (ketoconazole): could alter levels of modafinil
- *Steroidal contraceptives, cyclosporine, theophylline:* possibly reduced levels of these drugs

Implications
Assess
- For alterations in judgment, thinking, motor skills
- Baseline CV information because this drug does cause chest pain

Teaching
- That effectiveness of oral contraceptives might be reduced

M

- That elderly patients by need a reduced dosage
- To avoid OTC preparations unless approved by prescriber
- To avoid alcohol ingestion (although studies have not confirmed this to be a problem)

Evaluate
- Effectiveness in helping patient stay awake

Treatment of Overdose: No specific antidote to the toxic effects of modafinil overdose has been identified; dosages up to 4500 mg/day have been taken without life-threatening effects; nonetheless, overdosed patients should be provided supportive care (including CV monitoring), and emesis or gastric lavage should be considered; apparently neither hemodialysis nor urinary acidification/alkalinization speeds elimination.

Administration
- 200 mg/day as a single dose in the morning; 400 mg/day has been well tolerated
- *Available forms:* caps 100, 200, 400 mg

Molindone HCl

MOBAN
(moe-lin´-done)

Functional classifications: Traditional antipsychotic, neuroleptic, moderate potency
Chemical classification: Dihydroindolone
FDA pregnancy category: C

Indications: Psychotic disorders

Contraindications: Hypersensitivity, coma, child <12 yr, brain damage, bone marrow depression, alcohol and barbiturate withdrawal states
Cautious use: Lactation, hypertension, hepatic disease, cardiac disease

Pharmacologic Effects: Traditional antipsychotic drugs produce a neuroleptic effect characterized by sedation, emotional quieting, psychomotor slowing, and affective indifference; exact mode of action not fully understood; blocks D_2 receptors (++++) in the basal ganglia, hypothalamus, limbic system, brainstem, and medulla; blockade of these receptors accounts for both therapeutic and adverse responses; because of their nonselective actions, many other neurotransmitters systems are affected as well; ACh (–), histamine (+), and alpha-1 (+).

Pharmacokinetics: *PO:* onset erratic, peak 1½ hr, duration 24-36 hr; metabolized by liver, excreted in urine and feces, might cross placenta, excreted in breast milk, half-life 6.5 hr

Side Effects: See Chlorpromazine; *specific for molindone:* sedation (~30%), EPSEs (~30%), CV (minimal), anticholinergic (~10%), weight gain

(~2%), sexual dysfunction (min); menses in previously amenorrheic women

Interactions: See Chlorpromazine

Implications: See Chlorpromazine

Treatment of Overdose: If orally ingested, lavage, providing an airway; do not induce vomiting; provide symptomatic, supportive care.

Administration
- *Adult and child >12 yr:* PO 50-75 mg/day, increasing to 225 mg/day, if needed; maintenance dosage for mild condition 5-15 mg tid-qid; moderate condition 10-25 mg tid or qid; severe condition, 225 mg/day
- Concentrate mixed with orange or grapefruit juice
- *Available forms:* tabs 5, 10, 25, 50, 100 mg; conc 20 mg/ml

Naloxone HCl

NARCAN
(nal-oks´-one)

Functional classification: Narcotic antagonist
Chemical classification: Thebaine derivative
FDA pregnancy category: B

Indications: Narcotic-induced respiratory depression

Contraindications: Hypersensitivity
Cautious use: Children

Pharmacologic Effects: Competes with narcotics at opioid receptor sites

Pharmacokinetics: *PO:* onset 2 min (IV), half-life 30-81 min (this short half-life makes it impractical to use naloxone for treating opioid dependence); duration 1-4 hr; metabolized by liver, excreted by kidneys, crosses placenta

Side Effects: *CNS:* stimulation, drowsiness, nervousness; *peripheral:* hypotension, hypertension, ventricular tachycardia, hyperpnea; withdrawal symptoms (e.g., nausea, vomiting, sweating, increased blood pressure, tremulousness)

Interactions
- *Opioids:* loss of analgesia
- *Potentially cardiotoxic drugs:* hypotension, hypertension, ventricular tachycardia

Implications
Assess
- VS q3-5min

Planning/Implementation
- Remember that naloxone does not improve respiratory depression caused by nonnarcotic drugs.
- Have resuscitative equipment nearby.
- Give solutions prepared within 24 hr.

Evaluate
- Signs of withdrawal in drug-dependent individuals
- Cardiac status: tachycardia, hypertension
- Respiratory dysfunction: respiratory depression, character, rate, and rhythm; if respirations are <10 breaths/min, respiratory stimulant should be administered

Administration
- *Narcotic-induced respiratory depression: adult:* IV/SC/IM 0.4-0.8 mg; repeat q2-3min, if needed; *neonate:* 0.01 mg/kg IV, IM, SC
- *Postoperative respiratory depression: adult:* IV 0.1-0.2 mg q2-3min prn; *child:* IV/IM/SC 0.01 mg/kg q2-3min prn
- *Available forms:* inj IV, IM, SC 0.02, 0.4, 1 mg/ml

Naltrexone HCl
REVIA
(nal-trex´-one)

Functional classification: Narcotic antagonist
Chemical classification: Thebaine derivative
FDA pregnancy category: C

Indications: Treatment of alcohol dependence (reduces craving and increases abstinence); blockage of opioid analgesics, narcotic addiction; longer-acting than naloxone; prevention of readdiction

Contraindications: Patients receiving opioid analgesics; patients currently dependent on opioids; patients in acute opioid withdrawal; any individual who has failed the naloxone challenge test or who has a positive urine screen for opioids; any individual with a history of sensitivity to naltrexone; acute hepatitis or liver failure; child <18 yr
Cautious use: Anemia, hepatic or renal disease, Hodgkin's disease

Pharmacologic Effects: Opioid receptor antagonist and blocks opioid induced euphoria but does not block craving for these drugs

Pharmacokinetics: *PO:* onset 15-30 min, peak 1-2 hr, duration 4-6 hr; *REC:* onset slow, duration 4-6 hr; metabolized by liver, excreted by kidneys, crosses placenta, excreted in breast milk, half-life 4 hr for naltrexone and 13 hr for active metabolite

Side Effects: *CNS:* low energy (10%), nervousness (4%) drowsiness, dizziness (10%), confusion, convulsion, headache (7%), flushing, hallucinations, coma; *peripheral:* nausea, vomiting (>10%), diarrhea, constipation (<10%), decreased potency (<10%), rash (<10%), increased thirst (<10%), anorexia, hepatitis, urticaria, bruising, tinnitus, hearing loss, rapid pulse, pulmonary edema, wheezing, hyperpnea, hypoglycemia, hyponatremia, hypokalemia

Interactions
- *Opioids:* loss of analgesia
- *Potentially cardiotoxic drugs:* hypotension, hypertension, ventricular tachycardia

Implications
Assess
- VS q3-5min

Planning/Implementation
- Remember that naltrexone might precipitate an abstinence syndrome.

Teaching
- That naltrexone is part of the treatment plan
- To carry MedicAlert bracelet to alert health care provider
- That large doses of heroin might kill the patient

Evaluate
- Cardiac status: tachycardia, hypertension
- Respiratory dysfunction: respiratory depression, character, rate, and rhythm; if respirations are <10 breaths/min, respiratory stimulant should be administered

Treatment of Overdose: There is a lack of information concerning naltrexone overdose. Treat symptoms and possibly call poison control center for up-to-date information.

Administration
- *Alcohol treatment: adult:* PO: 50 mg once per day
- *Narcotic dependence: adult:* administer naloxone challenge first: (1) do not give until patient opioid free for 7-10 days; (2) give naloxone challenge test (see the following)
- If opioid withdrawal signs are observed, do not treat with naltrexone

Naloxone Challenge Test
- *IV challenge:* Draw 2 ampules of naloxone, 2 ml into a syringe. Inject 0.5 ml. Leave needle in vein and observe for 30 sec. If no signs of withdrawal occur, inject remaining 1.5 ml and observe for 20 min for signs and symptoms of withdrawal.
- *SC challenge:* Administer 2 ml (0.8 mg) SC, and observe the patient for signs and symptoms of withdrawal.
- *Interpretation of challenge test:* The elicitation of withdrawal signs and symptoms indicates a potential risk to the subject, and naltrexone should not be given.
- *Withdrawal signs and symptoms:* These include stuffiness or running nose, tearing, yawning, sweating, tremor, vomiting, piloerection, feeling of temperature change, joint, bone, muscle pain, abdominal cramps, skin crawling.
- *Initiation of treatment:* Give 25 mg PO, may then give another 25 mg after 1 hr if there are no withdrawal symptoms; usual maintenance dose is 50 mg in 24-hr period. A more

flexible dosing strategy might improve compliance (e.g., 100 mg qod or 150 mg every third day).

Administration
- *Available forms:* tabs 50 mg

Nefazodone HCl
SERZONE
(neh-faz´-oh-doan)

Functional classification: Novel antidepressant (unique molecular configuration)
Chemical classification: Phenylpiperazine
FDA pregnancy category: C

Indications: Depression

Contraindications: Hypersensitivity to phenylpiperazine antidepressants
    Cautious use: Patients susceptible to orthostatic hypotension; might activate mania

Pharmacologic Effects: Is a selective $5HT_2$ receptor blocker and also inhibits presynaptic reuptake of serotonin and norepinephrine; potent blocker of $5HT_{2A}$; Inhibits P-450 3A4 enzyme system; does not significantly bind to histaminergic, cholinergic, or alpha-adrenergic receptors

Pharmacokinetics: Is rapidly and completely absorbed, but food delays absorption and decrease bioavailability by 20%; is extensively metabolized in the liver; peak plasma levels occur in about an hour; half-life 2-4 hr; protein binding 99%; a substrate of the P-450 3A4 and inhibits this isoenzyme as well

Side Effects (at dosage of 300-600 mg/day):
CNS: headache (36%), somnolence (25%), dizziness (17%), insomnia (11%), light-headedness (10%), confusion (7%); *peripheral:* dry mouth (25%), nausea (22%), constipation (14%), asthenia (11%)

Interactions
- *Drugs highly bound to plasma proteins:* because nefazodone is highly bound (99%), it could displace or be displaced, causing adverse effects
- *Drugs metabolized by P-450 3A4:* increased levels of these drugs
- *MAOIs, terfenadine, astemizole:* serious interactions possible
- *Triazolam, alprazolam:* increased serum levels of these benzodiazepines

Implications
    Assess
- For history of pregnancy, CV illness, stroke, mania, hypomania, suicidal tendencies
- Establish baseline physical and psychologic status

- Signs of noncompliance (e.g., poor response to drug)

Planning/Implementation
- Monitor for drug compliance.
- Monitor for suicide because nefazodone might "energize" the patient to carry out plans to commit suicide.
- Monitor BP, particularly when patient complains of light-headedness.

Teaching
- That as with other antidepressants, several weeks might be needed for a full antidepressant response
- To adhere to drug regimen
- To avoid drugs listed in section on interactions
- To deal with dry mouth, constipation, light-headedness, headache, insomnia

Evaluate
- Verbalized decrease in subjective symptoms
- Observed decrease in objective symptoms
- Minimal to no adverse effects
- Stable VS
- Less anxiety; able to sleep, eat, and talk better

Treatment of Overdose: No serious overdoses of nefazodone have been reported.

Administration
- *Adult:* PO 50-100 mg bid for 1 wk; increase doses by 100 per day at 1-wk intervals; effective dose range typically between 300 and 500 mg/day but can reach 600 mg/day; *elderly:* PO 50 mg bid to start up to 150-300 mg/day if needed; *adolescent and child:* not recommended for this age group
- *Available forms:* tabs 50, 100, 150, 200, 250 mg

Nortriptyline HCl
AVENTYL, PAMELOR
(nor-trip´-ti-leen)

Functional classification: TCA
Chemical classification: Dibenzocycloheptene, secondary amine
FDA pregnancy category: C

Indications: Depression
    Unlabeled use: Panic disorder, adjunct to management of chronic neurogenic pain

Contraindications: Hypersensitivity to TCAs, recovery phase of myocardial infarction
    Cautious use: Convulsive disorders, prostatic hypertrophy, suicidal patients, severe depression, increased intraocular pressure, narrow-angle glaucoma, urinary retention, cardiac disease, hepatic

---

disease, hyperthyroidism, ECT, elective surgery, children

Pharmacologic Effects: Blocks reuptake of norepinephrine (+++) and serotonin (++) into presynaptic neurons, increasing action of norepinephrine and serotonin in nerve cells; also r/t downregulation of beta-adrenergic receptors; also antagonizes ACh (++), histamine (++), and alpha-1 (+++) receptors; therapeutic plasma levels 50-150 ng/ml

Pharmacokinetics: *PO:* steady state 4-19 days; metabolized by liver (a metabolite of amitriptyline), excreted by kidneys, crosses placenta, excreted in breast milk, half-life 18-44 hr, protein binding >90%

Side Effects: See Amitriptyline; *specific for nortriptyline:* dry mouth (~10%), blurred vision (~2%), constipation (~10%), sedation (~2%), orthostasis (~2%), tachycardia (~2%), sexual disturbance (~2%)

Interactions: See Amitriptyline

Implications: See Amitriptyline

Treatment of Overdose: ECG monitoring, induce emesis, lavage, activated charcoal, administer anticonvulsant, treat anticholinergic response if needed.

Administration
- *Adult:* PO 25 mg bid or qid, may increase to 200 mg/day; may give daily dose hs; *adolescent and geriatric:* 30-50 mg/day in divided doses
- *Available forms:* caps 10, 25, 50, 75 mg; sol 10 mg/5 ml

Olanzapine

ZYPREXA
(o-lan´-za-peen)

Functional classification: Atypical antipsychotic
Chemical classification: Thienobenzodiazepine
FDA pregnancy category: C

Indications: Acute and chronic psychosis, prophylaxis of schizophrenia

Contraindications: Hypersensitivity
Cautious use: Patients with signs and symptoms of hepatic dysfunction, patients receiving concomitant treatment with hepatotoxic drugs; <18 yr

Pharmacologic Effects: Blocks D_1 (+++), D_2 (+++), D_3 (+++), and D_4 (++++) receptors; also blocks histamine (++++), ACh (++++), $5HT_1$ (++++), and $5HT_2$ (++++); is a somewhat less potent blocker of alpha-1 (+++) receptors; clinical response weeks to months

Pharmacokinetics: Well absorbed (food has no effect), half-life 21-54 hr, metabolized by P-450 1A, 2D6, 2C; provides low inhibition for 1A2, 2D6, 3A4

Side Effects: Produces few EPSEs or orthostatic symptoms and only mild to moderate anticholinergic symptoms; very sedating; *CNS:* insomnia (++), sedation (++ to +++); *peripheral:* orthostatic hypotension (+), anticholinergic side effects (+), EPSEs (– to +), sexual dysfunction (+), CV effects (+), blood dyscrasias (–), weight gain (++)

Interactions
- *Carbamazepine:* decreased serum levels of olanzapine (by 50%)
- *Cigarettes:* decreased plasma level of olanzapine possible (clearance 40% higher)
- *Cimetidine:* inhibits metabolism of olanzapine
- *CNS depressants:* might increase absorption of olanzapine increasing CNS effect
- *Diazepam, alcohol:* orthostatic effect of olanzapine increased
- *Drugs that use P-450 enzyme system:* might inhibit metabolism of olanzapine
- *Fluvoxamine:* might inhibit metabolism of olanzapine
- *Levodopa:* effect of levodopa might be antagonized

Treatment of Overdose: In premarketing trials, overdosages to 300 mg caused only drowsiness and slurred speech; VS were typically stable. In acute overdose, establish airway and ensure adequate oxygenation and ventilation; no specific antidote. Gastric lavage and activated charcoal can be used to minimize absorption. Provide supportive care.

Administration
- Usually 10 mg/day; range 5-20 mg/day
- *Available forms:* tabs 5, 7.5, 10 mg

Oxazepam

SERAX
(ox-a´-ze-pam)

Functional classification: Antianxiety agent
Chemical classification: Benzodiazepine
Controlled substance schedule IV
FDA pregnancy category: D

Indications: Anxiety, alcohol withdrawal, anxiety and tension in elderly

Contraindications: Hypersensitivity to benzodiazepines, psychoses, narrow-angle glaucoma, psychosis, child <12 yr
Cautious use: Elderly or debilitated patients, hepatic or renal disease

Pharmacologic Effects: Increases affinity of GABA molecules for their specific receptor, increasing the frequency with which chloride

O

channels open in response to GABA; might also decrease norepinephrine and serotonin turnover rates

Pharmacokinetics: *Speed of onset:* intermediate to slow; *PO:* peak 2-4 hr, undergoes conjugation so a good drug for the elderly, excreted by kidneys, half-life 5-20 hr

Side Effects: *CNS:* drowsiness, dizziness, confusion, headache, anxiety, tremor, stimulation, fatigue, depression, insomnia; *peripheral:* photophobia as a result of mydriasis, blurred vision as a result of cycloplegia; sleeplike slowing of respirations with therapeutic doses, cough; orthostatic hypotension, tachycardia, hypotension; constipation; dry mouth

Interactions: See Alprazolam

Implications: See Alprazolam

Treatment of Overdose: Lavage, VS, supportive care; few deaths, if any, reported as resulting from benzodiazepine overdose alone; deaths occur when benzodiazepines are mixed with other drugs, especially alcohol.

Administration
- *Anxiety: adult:* PO 10-30 mg tid-qid (30-120 mg/day); *geriatric:* 10 mg tid, up to 15 mg tid-qid (use cautiously)
- *Alcohol withdrawal: adult:* PO 15-30 mg tid-qid
- *Available forms:* caps, 10, 15, 30 mg; tabs 15 mg

Paraldehyde

PARAL
(par-al´-de-hyde)

Functional classification: Anticonvulsant
Chemical classification: Cyclic ether
Controlled substance schedule IV
FDA pregnancy category: C

Indications: Refractory seizures, status epilepticus, alcohol withdrawal, tetanus, eclampsia, sedation

Contraindications: Hypersensitivity, gastroenteritis, asthma, hepatic disease, pulmonary disease
Cautious use: Labor, children

Pharmacologic Effects: CNS depressant; mechanism of action unknown

Pharmacokinetics: *PO:* onset 10-15 min, peak 1 hr, duration 8-12 hr; *REC:* onset slow, duration 4-6 hr; metabolized by liver, excreted by kidneys and lungs, crosses placenta, half-life 3-10 hr

Side Effects: *CNS:* stimulation, drowsiness, dizziness, confusion, convulsions, headache, flushing, hallucinations, coma; *peripheral:* foul breath, irritation, nephrosis, rash, erythema, local pain, esophagitis, yellowing of eyes

Interactions
- *Alcohol, CNS depressants, general anesthetics, disulfiram:* increased paraldehyde blood levels
- *Disulfiram:* blocks metabolism of paraldehyde; avoid use
- *Sulfonamides:* increased crystallization in kidneys

Implications
Assess
- VS q30min after parenteral route
- Hepatic studies: AST, ALT, bilirubin, and creatinine levels

Planning/Implementation
- IM injection in deep, large muscle (Z-track) mass to prevent tissue sloughing; maximum, 5 ml at one site.
- Give rectally, after diluting in cottonseed oil or olive oil, as retention enema or 200 ml NS for enema.
- Give orally with juice or milk to cover taste and smell and decrease GI symptoms (orally).
- Ventilate room.
- Use glass containers; not compatible with plastics.
- Do not use if brownish or if vinegar odor is evident.

Teaching
- That physical dependency might result when used for extended periods
- To avoid driving, other activities that require alertness
- Not to discontinue medication quickly after long-term use; taper over several weeks

Evaluate
- Mental status
- Respiratory dysfunction

Treatment of Overdose: Do not lavage; support respirations, treat acidosis.

Administration
- *Seizures: adult:* IM 5-10 ml; IV 0.2-0.4 ml/kg in NS inj; *child:* IM 0.15 ml/kg; REC 0.3 ml/kg q4-6h; IV 0.1-0.15 ml/kg ml NS inj
- For other uses, see PDR
- *Available forms:* inj IM/IV, oral and rectal liquids 1 g/ml

---

Paroxetine
PAXIL
(par-ox´-e-teen)

Functional classification: SSRI antidepressant
Chemical classification: Selective serotonin reuptake inhibitor; phenylpiperidine
Pregnancy category: B

Indications: Depression, panic disorder, obsessive-compulsive disorder, social anxiety disorder

Contraindications: Use with MAOIs; allow at least 2 wk after stopping paroxetine before starting an MAOI
Cautious use: History of seizures, history of mania or hypomania, renal or hepatic disorder; elderly, pregnancy, lactation, suicidal patients

Pharmacologic Effects: Inhibits CNS neuronal uptake of serotonin (+++++) and norepinephrine (+); also antagonizes ACh (++), histamine (+), and alpha-1 (++) receptors

Pharmacokinetics: Peak plasma level 5 hr; half-life 21 hr; protein binding 95%; steady state reached in about 10 days; elimination both renal (64%) and hepatic (36%)

Side Effects: *CNS:* somnolence (23%), headache (17%), asthenia (15%), dizziness (13%), insomnia (13%); *peripheral:* nausea (26%), dry mouth (18%), constipation (14%), sweating (11%), diarrhea (11%), ejaculatory disturbance (13%), other male genital disorders (10%)

Interactions
- *Alcohol:* although impairment has not been observed, potential for CNS depression suggests caution
- *Cimetidine:* increases concentrations of paroxetine
- *Digoxin:* decreased therapeutic effect of digoxin
- *Drugs metabolized by or that inhibit P-450 2D6 isoenzymes:* might need to reduce dosage of one or both agents
- *Highly protein-bound drugs:* might shift plasma concentrations resulting in adverse effects from either drug
- *L-tryptophan:* might cause a serotonin syndrome
- *MAOIs:* serious and sometimes fatal interaction; serotonin syndrome might result and can be fatal; wait 14 days after stopping paroxetine before initiating an MAOI; wait at least 14 days after stopping MAOI before starting paroxetine
- *Phenobarbital:* increases the half-life of paroxetine
- *Phenytoin:* half-life of both drugs reduced
- *Procyclidine, warfarin:* increased serum levels of these drugs
- *TCAs:* elevated levels of TCAs

Implications
Assess
- BP, VS
- Activation of mania
- Baseline physical data

Planning/Implementation
- Maintain safety.
- Closely supervise patients with a high risk of suicide because there might be a relationship between suicide and alterations in serotonin levels.

Teaching
- To take medication as prescribed even if feeling better before course of treatment is completed
- To be cautious about driving (although no impairment in driving ability has been recorded with use of paroxetine)
- To avoid alcohol (although no impairment resulting from this combination has been recorded)
- To be cautious about the use of OTC products
- To notify primary care provider if intending to become pregnant
- To notify primary care provider if rash develops

Evaluate
- Therapeutic effect: depression
- Mental status

Treatment of Overdose: Paroxetine is a relatively safe drug alone or in combination with other drugs or alcohol. Signs and symptoms of overdose include nausea, vomiting, drowsiness, sinus tachycardia, dilated pupils. No specific antidotes exist. Maintain airway, ensure adequate oxygenation, give activated charcoal or lavage; give emetic. Monitor VS. Dialysis and forced diuresis unlikely to help.

Administration
- *Adult:* PO 20 mg/day as 1 dose qAM; usual range 10-60 mg/day; dosage changes should occur at a minimum of 1-wk intervals; *elderly, debilitated, or hepatic or renal impairment:* PO 10 mg/day; increase may be made if indicated; maximum dosage 40 mg/day; *child and adolescent:* not approved for children
- *Available forms:* tabs 20, 30 mg

P

Pemoline
CYLERT
(pem´-oh-leen)

Functional classification: Cerebral stimulant
Chemical classification: Oxazolidine
Controlled substance schedule IV
FDA pregnancy category: B

Indications: ADHD

Contraindications: Hypersensitivity
  Cautious use: Renal disease, child <6 yr

Pharmacologic Effects: Exact mechanism not known but may work by increasing storage and synthesis of dopamine; pemoline causes less cerebral stimulation than the amphetamines or methylphenidate and is less effective; also it has a lower abuse potential

Pharmacokinetics: Well absorbed, PO peak 2-4 hr, duration 8 hr, metabolized by liver, excreted by kidneys, half-life 12 hr in adults and 7 hr in children

Side Effects: *CNS:* hyperactivity, insomnia, restlessness, dizziness, depression, headache, stimulation, irritability, aggressiveness, hallucinations, seizures; *peripheral:* nausea, anorexia, diarrhea, abdominal pain, increased liver enzyme levels, hepatitis, growth suppression in children, rashes

Interactions: None known

Implications
  Assess
- Hepatic function studies: ALT, AST, bilirubin, and creatinine levels
- Growth rate: growth retardation possible

Planning/Implementation
- Give at least 6 hr before bedtime.
- Instruct patient to chew gum, suck on hard candies, and take frequent sips of water for dry mouth.

Teaching
- To decrease caffeine consumption (coffee, tea, cola, chocolate) because caffeine might increase irritability
- To avoid OTC preparations unless approved by physician
- To taper off drug over several weeks
- To avoid alcohol ingestion
- To avoid hazardous activities until condition is stabilized on medication
- That therapeutic effect might take 3-4 wk

Evaluate
- Mental status

Treatment of Overdose: *Symptoms:* CNS overstimulation and excessive sympathomimetic effect; vomiting, agitation, tremors, twitching, convulsions; *treatment:* supportive measures, if not too severe; gastric contents might be evacuated; chlorpromazine might decrease CNS stimulation.

Administration
- *Child >6 yr:* 37.5 mg qAM, increasing by 18.75 mg/wk, not to exceed 112.5 mg/day; maintenance dose usually 37.25-75 mg/day
- *Available forms:* tabs 18.75, 37.5, 75 mg; chewable tabs 37.5 mg

Pentobarbital, pentobarbital sodium
NEMBUTAL SODIUM, NOVA-RECTAL,† PENTOGEN†
(pen-toe-bar´-bi-tal)

Functional classifications: Sedative, hypnotic
Chemical classification: Barbiturate
Controlled substance schedule II
FDA pregnancy category: D

Indications: Insomnia, sedation, emergency control of seizures, preanesthetic

Contraindications: Hypersensitivity, respiratory depression, barbiturate dependence, marked liver dysfunction, acute pain
  Cautious use: Seizure disorders, elderly patients, lactation, children

Pharmacologic Effects: Short-acting barbiturate; depresses sensory cortex to produce drowsiness, sedation, and sleep

Pharmacokinetics: *PO:* onset 10-15 min, duration 3-4 hr, half-life 15-50 hr

Side Effects: *CNS:* see Secobarbital; *peripheral:* see Secobarbital

Interactions: See Secobarbital

Implications: See Secobarbital

Treatment of Overdose: Gastric lavage, activated charcoal; warm the patient; monitor VS, I&O; hemodialysis might be effective; roll patient from side to side q30min.

Administration
- *Insomnia: adult:* PO 100 mg hs
- *Available forms:* caps 50, 100 mg; elix 18.2 mg/5 ml; rectal supp 30, 60, 120, 200 mg; IM inj, IV 50 mg/ml

---

*Infrequently used.   †Available in Canada only.

Perphenazine

**ETRAFON, PHENAZINE, TRIAVIL
(PERPHENAZINE + AMITRIPTYLINE),
TRILAFON**
(per-fen´-a-zeen)

Functional classifications: Traditional antipsychotic, neuroleptic, moderate potency
Chemical classifications: Phenothiazine, piperazine
FDA pregnancy category: C

Indications: Psychotic disorders, nausea, vomiting

Contraindications: Hypersensitivity, blood dyscrasias, coma, child <12 yr, brain damage, bone marrow depression, adynamic ileus
Cautious use: Lactation, seizure disorders, hypertension, hepatic disease, cardiac disease, glaucoma, renal impairment, ECT

Pharmacologic Effects: Traditional antipsychotic drugs produce a neuroleptic effect characterized by sedation, emotional quieting, psychomotor slowing, and affective indifference; exact mode of action not fully understood; blocks D_2 receptors (++++) in the basal ganglia, hypothalamus, limbic system, brainstem, and medulla; blockade of these receptors accounts for both therapeutic and adverse responses; because of their nonselective actions, many other neurotransmitters systems are affected as well; ACh (+), histamine (++++), and alpha-1 (+++); antiemetic effect r/t inhibition of chemoreceptor trigger zone; therapeutic plasma levels 0.8-1.2 ng/ml

Pharmacokinetics: *PO:* onset erratic, peak 2-4 hr; *IM:* onset 10 min, peak 1-2 hr, duration 6 hr, half-life 9-21 hr; metabolized by liver, excreted in urine, crosses placenta, excreted in breast milk

Side Effects: See Chlorpromazine; *specific for perphenazine:* sedation (~10%), EPSEs (~30%), orthostasis (~2%), anticholinergic (~2%), weight gain (-), sexual dysfunction (min)

Interactions: See Chlorpromazine

Implications: See Chlorpromazine

Treatment of Overdose: Lavage, if orally ingested; provide an airway; do not induce vomiting, control EPSEs and hypotension.

Administration
- *Psychiatric indications:* psychiatric use in hospitalized patients: *adult:* PO 8-16 bid-qid, gradually increased to desired dose, not to exceed 64 mg/day; IM 5 mg q6h, not to exceed 30 mg/day; *child >12 yr:* PO 8 mg in divided doses; *geriatric:* half to one third of adult dose
- *Nonhospitalized patients: adult:* PO 4-8 mg tid; IM 5 mg q6h

- Do not mix concentrate with liquids containing caffeine, tannics, or pectinates
- *Available forms:* tabs 2, 4, 8, 16; conc 16 mg/5 ml; inj IM 5 mg/ml

Phenelzine sulfate

NARDIL
(fen´-el-zeen)

Functional classifications: MAOI antidepressant
Chemical classification: Hydrazine
FDA pregnancy category: C

Indications: Depression in treatment-resistant patients, patients with mixed anxiety-depression, atypical depression
Unlabeled uses: Bulimia, cocaine deterrent

Contraindications: Hypersensitivity to MAOIs, elderly patients (>60 yr), children <16 yr, hypertension, CHF, severe hepatic disease, pheochromocytoma, severe renal disease, severe cardiac disease *Cautious use:* Suicidal patients, convulsive disorders, hyperactivity, diabetes mellitus, hypomania, agitation, hyperthyroidism

Pharmacologic Effects: Inhibits monoamine oxidase by irreversibly binding to monoamine oxidase A and B, thus increasing the concentration of endogenous epinephrine, norepinephrine, serotonin, dopamine in storage sites in CNS

Pharmacokinetics: Metabolized by liver monoamine oxidase A and monoamine oxidase B, excreted by kidneys, half-life 2-3 hr

Side Effects: *CNS:* dizziness, drowsiness, confusion, headache, anxiety, tremors, stimulation, weakness, hyperreflexia, mania, insomnia, fatigue, weight gain; *peripheral:* change in libido, constipation, dry mouth, nausea and vomiting, anorexia, diarrhea, rash, flushing, increased perspiration, jaundice, orthostatic hypotension, hypertension, arrhythmias, hypertensive crisis, blurred vision

Interactions
- *Anticholinergic drugs:* additive effect
- *Antihypertensives* (diuretics, beta-blockers, hydralazine, nitroglycerin, prazosin): hypotension
- *Buspirone:* serotonergic reaction possible
- *Drug-drug: sympathomimetics* (indirect or mixed acting): severe headache, hypertension, hyperpyrexia, and hypertensive crisis; sympathomimetic drugs include amphetamines; levodopa; tryptophan; methylphenidate; OTC compounds containing phenylpropanolamine, ephedrine, and pseudoephedrine; TCAs, other MAOIs, guanethidine, methyldopa, guanadrel, reserpine
- *Drug-food: tyramine-rich foods* (see text): hypertensive crisis

P

- *Serotonergic drugs:* potential for a serotonin syndrome

Implications
Assess
- BP (lying, standing), pulse: if systolic BP drops 20 mm Hg, withhold drug, notify physician
- Blood studies: CBC, leukocyte counts, cardiac enzyme levels (if patient is receiving long-term therapy)
- Hepatic studies: hepatotoxic effects might occur

Planning/Implementation
- Instruct patient to increase fluids, bulk in diet, if constipation, urinary retention occurs.
- Instruct patient to take dose with food or milk to prevent GI symptoms.
- Tell patient to chew sugarless gum, suck on hard candies, or take frequent sips of water for dry mouth.
- Use phentolamine for severe hypertension.
- Store in tight container in cool environment.
- Assist with ambulation during beginning of therapy because drowsiness or dizziness occurs.
- Provide safety measures, including side rails.
- Check to see that oral medication is swallowed.

Teaching
- That therapeutic effects might take 1-4 wk
- To avoid driving or other activities that require alertness
- To avoid ingesting alcohol and CNS depressants, or OTC medications for cold, weight loss, hay fever, cough
- Not to discontinue medication abruptly after long-term use
- To avoid high-tyramine foods (e.g., cheese [aged], caviar, dried fish, game meat, beer, wine, pickled products, liver, raisins, bananas, figs, avocados, meat tenderizers, chocolate, yogurt, increased caffeine, soy sauce)
- To report headache, palpitations, neck stiffness

Evaluate
- Toxic effects: increased headache, palpitations; discontinue drug immediately
- Mental status
- Urinary retention, constipation
- Withdrawal symptoms: headache, nausea, vomiting, muscle pain, weakness

Treatment of Overdose: Lavage, activated charcoal, monitor electrolyte levels, VS, treat hypotension.

Administration
- *Adult:* PO 15 mg tid, may increase to 60 mg/day, dosage should be reduced to 15 mg/day, not to exceed 90 mg/day
- *Available forms:* tabs 15 mg

Phenobarbital, phenobarbital sodium
GARDENAL, LUMINAL SODIUM, SOLFOTON
(fee-noe-bar´-bi-tal)

Functional classification: Antiepileptic (long-acting)
Chemical classification: Barbiturate
Controlled substance schedule IV
FDA pregnancy category: D

Indications: Tonic-clonic, simple partial, complex partial, status epilepticus

Contraindications: Hypersensitivity to barbiturates, porphyria, hepatic disease, respiratory disease, nephritis, diabetes mellitus, elderly, lactation, barbiturate addiction
Cautious use: Anemia, cardiac disease, children, fever, hyperthyroidism

Pharmacologic Effects: Antiepileptic effect caused by the ability to bind to GABA receptors; in fact, a specific barbiturate site on that receptor has been identified; both enhances GABA's inhibitory effects and mimics GABA, resulting in a prolonged opening of the chloride channel; therapeutic serum level 15-40 mg/ml

Pharmacokinetics: *PO:* onset 20-60 min, peak 8-12 hr, duration 10-12 hr, metabolized by liver, 25%-50% excreted unchanged by kidneys, crosses placenta, excreted in breast milk, half-life 80 hr, with a range of 53-118 hr; 40%-60% bound to plasma proteins

Side Effects: *CNS:* somnolence, drowsiness, lethargy, hangover headache, flushing, hallucinations, coma; *peripheral:* nausea, vomiting, hypoventilation, bradycardia, hypotension, rash, urticaria, angioedema, local pain, swelling, necrosis, thrombophlebitis, blood dyscrasias

Interactions
- *Acetaminophen, digitoxin, oral anticoagulants, oral contraceptives, TCAs, possibly phenytoin:* effects of these drugs are decreased by barbiturates
- *CNS depressants, other antiepileptics:* these drugs increase the effects of barbiturates (toxic effects)

Implications
Assess
- Blood studies, liver function tests during long-term therapy
- Check VS, neurologic values regularly

Planning/Implementation
- Describe seizure accurately.
- Offer consistent emotional support.
- Monitor for early signs of toxic effects (slurred speech, ataxia, respiratory and CNS depression).

Teaching
- To report any side effects or adverse reactions
- To avoid driving or operating dangerous equipment
- To change position slowly
- To take drugs as prescribed
- Not to discontinue drug abruptly
- To wear MedicAlert identification bracelet
- To consult physician before becoming pregnant

Evaluate
- Mental status
- Respiratory depression
- Blood dyscrasias: fever, sore throat, bruising, rash, jaundice

Treatment of Overdose: 1 g can cause serious poisoning in an adult; 2-10 g can be fatal; toxic effects can be confused with drunkenness. Emesis, gastric lavage, if conscious; 30 g activated charcoal, maintain airway, good nursing care to prevent pneumonia.

Administration
- *Seizures: adult:* PO 60-100 mg/day; *child:* PO 3-5 mg/kg/day in 3 divided doses; may be given as single dose hs
- *Status epilepticus: adult:* IV 15-18 mg/kg over 10-15 min not to exceed 30 mg/kg, run no faster than 50 mg/min; *child:* IV; same, run no faster than 50 mg/min
- *Available forms:* caps 16 mg; elix 15, 20 mg/5 ml; tabs 8, 16, 32, 65, 100 mg; inj 30, 60, 65, 130 mg/ml

Phensuximide*

MILONTIN
(fen-sux´-i-mide)

Functional classification: Antiepileptic
Chemical classification: Succinimide
FDA pregnancy category: D

Indications: Absence seizures (petit mal) refractory to other drugs

Contraindications: Hypersensitivity to succinimide derivatives
    Cautious use: Lactation, hepatic or renal disease

Pharmacologic Effects: Inhibits spike and wave formation in absence seizures by interfering with calcium conductances; does not alter sodium channel activation nor increase GABA inhibition

Pharmacokinetics: *PO:* peak 1-4 hr, metabolized by liver, excreted by kidneys, half-life 4 hr

Side Effects: See Ethosuximide

Interactions: See Ethosuximide

Implications: See Ethosuximide

Administration
- *Adult and child:* PO 500 mg-1 g bid or tid
- *Available forms:* caps 500 mg

Phenytoin, phenytoin sodium extended, phenytoin sodium prompt

DILANTIN, DILANTIN CAPSULES, DIPHENYLAN
(fen´-i-toy-in)

Functional classification: Anticonvulsant
Chemical classification: Hydantoin
FDA pregnancy category: D

Indications: Tonic-clonic seizures; status epilepticus, psychomotor seizures, simple partial seizures

Contraindications: Hypersensitivity, psychiatric disease, sinus bradycardia (IV use), lactation
    Cautious use: Allergies, hepatic or renal disease, hypotension, myocardial insufficiency

Pharmacologic Effects: Inhibits spread of seizure activity in motor cortex by normalizing abnormal sodium fluxes across the nerve cell membrane during or after depolarization; also decreases activity of brainstem centers responsible for the tonic phase of grand mal seizures; therapeutic serum levels 10-20 µg/ml

Pharmacokinetics: *PO:* slowly absorbed, bioavailability can vary as much as 10%-90% among different brands; peak 4-12 hr (extended), 1.5-3 hr (prompt); duration 5 hr; time to steady state 7-10 days; average half-life 22 hr but can be tripled in some people (60 hr) but dose dependent and has little clinical importance; protein binding ~90%; metabolized by liver but nonlinear, so plasma concentrations can increase significantly with small changes is dose; excreted by kidneys; *IM:* slowly absorbed (up to 5 days)

Side Effects: *CNS:* nystagmus, ataxia, drowsiness, dizziness, insomnia, paresthesias, depression, suicidal tendencies, aggression, headache; *peripheral:* nausea, vomiting, constipation, anorexia, weight loss, hepatitis, jaundice, nephritis, albuminuria, rash, gingival hyperplasia, agranulocytosis, leukopenia, aplastic anemia

P

Interactions

- *Allopurinol, alcohol (acute ingestion), amiodarone, chloramphenicol, chlordiazepoxide, cimetidine, diazepam, disulfiram, estrogens, H_2 blockers, isoniazid, phenacemide, succinimides, sulfonamides, trazodone, valproic acid, others:* increased effect of hydantoins
- *Barbiturates, carbamazepine, alcohol (chronic use) theophylline, antacids, dietary calcium, molindone:* decreased effects of hydantoins
- *Corticosteroids, dicumarol, digitoxin, doxycycline, haloperidol, methadone, oral contraceptives, dopamine, furosemide, levodopa:* decreased effects of these drugs

Implications

Assess

- Blood studies: CBC, platelet count qmo until stabilized, discontinue drug, if marked depression of the blood cell count occurs

Planning/Implementation

- Observe for gingival hyperplasia.
- Describe seizures accurately.

Teaching

- All aspects of drug administration (route, action, dose)
- To report side effects
- To avoid driving or operating dangerous equipment
- To practice good oral hygiene
- Not to discontinue abruptly
- To wear MedicAlert identification bracelet

Evaluate

- Mental status
- Respiratory depression
- Blood dyscrasias: fever, sore throat, bruising, rash, jaundice

Treatment of Overdose: Mean lethal dose in adults is thought to be 2-5 g; initial symptoms are nystagmus, ataxia; death results from respiratory and circulatory depression; lavage, emesis, activated charcoal.

Administration

- *Seizures: PO: adult:* 100-200 mg tid or qid; Dilantin Kapseals (extended form) can be given once daily; *child:* 5 mg/kg/day; *child >6 yr:* may require adult dosage.
- *Status epilepticus: IV: adult:* give a loading dose 10-15 mg/kg, rate not to exceed 50 mg/min (or, in elderly patients, 25 mg/min); initial dose should be followed by maintenance dose of 100 mg orally or IV q6-8h; *child:* 15-20 mg/kg slowly (not more than 1-3 mg/kg/min); use normal saline to avoid precipitation
- Use normal saline to avoid precipitation
- *Available forms:* susp 30, 125 mg/5 ml; tabs, chewable 50 mg; inj 50 mg/ml; caps ext-rel 30, 100 mg; caps, prompt 30, 100 mg

Pimozide

ORAP

(pi´-moe-zide)

Functional classifications: Antipsychotic, neuroleptic
Chemical classification: Diphenylbutylpiperidine
FDA pregnancy category: C

Indications: Tourette's syndrome

Contraindications: Hypersensitivity, CNS depression, coma, tics other than those of Tourette's syndrome, cardiac arrhythmias, long QT interval
    Cautious use: Child <12 yr, lactation, seizure disorders, hypertension, hepatic or renal disease, cardiac disease, hypokalemia

Pharmacologic Effects: Blocks CNS D_2 receptors

Pharmacokinetics: *PO:* peak 6-8 hr; metabolized by liver, excreted in urine, half-life 55 hr; partly metabolized by P-450 3A and 1A2 might also contribute

Side Effects: *CNS:* parkinsonism, akathisias, dystonias, tardive dyskinesia, oculogyric crisis; *peripheral:* blurred vision (cycloplegia or paralysis of accommodation), ocular pain, photophobia, mydriasis, impaired vision, intolerance of extreme heat or cold, possible heat stroke or fatal hyperthermia, nasal congestion, wheezing, dyspnea, hypotension, especially orthostatic, leading to dizziness, syncope; tachycardia, irregular pulse, arrhythmias, dry mouth, constipation, jaundice, abdominal pain; urinary frequency, galactorrhea, gynecomastia, impaired ejaculation, amenorrhea, prolonged QT interval, sudden death has occurred at doses >20 mg/day

Interactions

- *Antiarrhythmics, phenothiazines:* increased QT interval
- *Anticonvulsants:* decreased convulsive threshold
- *Increased CNS depression:* alcohol and other CNS depressants
- *Other antipsychotics:* increased EPSEs

Implications

Assess

- For prolonged QT interval
- Establish baseline VS, laboratory values to assess side effects, allergic or hypersensitivity reactions
- Physiologic and psychologic status before therapy to determine needs and evaluate progress

- For early stages of tardive dyskinesia by using abnormal involuntary movement scale
- Identify concurrent symptoms that might be aggravated by antipsychotics (e.g., glaucoma, diabetes)

Planning/Implementation
- Ensure that drug has been taken; check mouth for "cheeking."
- Keep patient quiet after injection to prevent falls associated with postural hypotension.
- For dry mouth, give chewing gum, hard candies, lip balm, monitor urinary output; check for bladder distention in inactive patients, older men, and patients receiving high dosages.
- Assist with ambulation if patient is having blurred vision; dim room lights for photosensitivity.
- Ensure safety with hypotension; instruct patient to sit on side of bed before rising, head-low position for dizziness, avoid hot showers, wear elastic stockings.
- Check BP (supine, sitting, standing) and pulse before and after each dose when possible; observe for side effects.
- Monitor body temperature for indications of NMS (e.g., muscle rigidity, fever, depressed neurologic status); ensure adequate hydration, nutrition, and ventilation.
- Protect patient from exposure to extreme heat or cold.
- Recognize impending hypersensitivity to pruritus or jaundice with hepatitis; flulike or coldlike symptoms; evidence of bleeding with blood dyscrasia.
- Observe for involuntary movements.

Teaching
- To comply with drug treatment
- To avoid activities requiring clear vision for a few weeks after treatment starts; to report eye pain immediately
- To understand the importance of exercise, fluids, and fiber in diet
- To watch for symptoms of heart failure (e.g., weight gain, dyspnea, distended neck veins, tachycardia)
- That male sexual performance failure is possible; suggest relaxed, stress-free environment
- To avoid conception; women should practice effective contraception
- To avoid exposure to sunlight; keep skin covered but with temperature-appropriate clothing
- That it is not possible to become addicted to antipsychotic drugs

Evaluate
- Whether patient follows prescribed regimen, takes medications as ordered
- Whether patient avoids injury; reports dizziness or need for assistance
- Whether patient verbalizes reduced anxiety
- Whether patient experiences minimal or no adverse responses
- Whether patient uses appropriate interventions to minimize side effects
- Whether patient achieves improved mental status

Treatment of Overdose: Lavage, if orally ingested; provide an airway; monitor ECG; do not induce vomiting; do not use epinephrine for hypotension; observe patient for at least 4 days.

Administration
- *Adult and child >12 yr:* PO 1-2 mg qd in divided doses; increase dose qod, if needed; maintenance 0.2 mg/kg/day or 10 mg/day, whichever is less; not to exceed 0.2 mg/kg/day or 10 mg/day
- *Available forms:* tabs 2 mg

Prazepam
CENTRAX
(pra´-ze-pam)

Functional classification: Antianxiety agent
Chemical classification: Benzodiazepine
Controlled substance schedule IV
FDA pregnancy category: D

P

Indications: Anxiety

Contraindications: Hypersensitivity, narrow-angle glaucoma, psychosis, children <18 yr

Pharmacologic Effects: Depresses CNS, including limbic and reticular areas, by potentiating GABA inhibitory neurotransmitters

Pharmacokinetics: *Speed of onset:* slow; *PO:* peak levels 6 hr, half-life 30-100 hr; metabolized by liver, excreted in urine

Side Effects: *CNS:* dizziness, drowsiness (main effects); see Diazepam for other side effects; *peripheral:* GI effects (dry mouth, nausea, vomiting), blurred vision, orthostatic hypotension; see Diazepam for other side effects

Interactions
- *CNS depressants, alcohol, disulfiram:* increased CNS depression
- *Valproic acid:* increased effect of prazepam

Implications
Assess
- BP

Planning/Implementation
- Give with food or milk to decrease GI upset.
- Provide gum, hard candies for dry mouth.
- Maintain safety.

Teaching
- To avoid driving
- To avoid alcohol

- To check with clinician before taking OTC drugs

Evaluate
- Mental status
- Therapeutic response: level of anxiety

Treatment of Overdose: Lavage, monitor VS, provide supportive care as indicated; there are no recorded deaths with benzodiazepines alone; death occurs when these drugs are mixed with other CNS depressants.

Administration
- *Adult:* PO 20-40 mg/day in divided doses, range 20-60 mg/day; *geriatric:* 10-15 mg/day in divided doses, can be given as single dose hs
- *Available forms:* caps 5, 10, 20 mg; tabs 10 mg

Primidone

MYSOLINE, SERTAN†
(pri´-mi-done)

Functional classification: Antiepileptic
Chemical classification: Barbiturate derivative
FDA pregnancy category: D

Indications: Generalized tonic-clonic, complex partial seizures

Contraindications: Hypersensitivity, porphyria
Cautious use: Lactation

Pharmacologic Effects: Two metabolites of primidone (phenobarbital and phenylethylmalonamide) are responsible for its antiepileptic effects; primidone raises seizure threshold; therapeutic serum level 5-12 µg/ml

Pharmacokinetics: *PO:* peak 3 hr; excreted in breast milk; half-life 3-12 hr, but active metabolites are longer (i.e., phenylethylmalonamide [PEMA] 24-48 hr; phenobarbital 53-118 hr); bioequivalence among brands not established

Side Effects: *CNS:* ataxia, vertigo, emotional disturbances, paranoid thinking, mood fluctuations, fatigue, drowsiness, nystagmus; *peripheral:* nausea, vomiting, anorexia; rash, alopecia, lupuslike syndrome, diplopia, nystagmus, erectile dysfunction, thrombocytopenia, leukopenia, megaloblastic anemia

Interactions
- *Acetazolamide:* decreased effect of primidone
- *Alcohol, heparin, carbamazepine, CNS depressants, isoniazid, phenytoin, phenobarbital:* increased levels of primidone

Implications
Assess
- Establish baseline data

Planning/Implementation
- Monitor for early signs of toxic effects.

Teaching
- All aspects of drug administration (action, route, dose)
- Not to withdraw drug quickly; withdrawal symptoms might occur
- Not to drive
- To notify physician if rash or symptoms of blood dyscrasia occur
- To wear MedicAlert identification bracelet

Evaluate
- Mental status
- Respiratory depression
- Blood dyscrasias: fever, sore throat, bruising, rash, jaundice

Administration
- *Adult and child >8 yr:* 100 mg hs for adults, 50 mg hs for children; dosage then carefully titrated over next 10 days; maintenance around 125-250 mg bid-qid; adults never given >2 g/day; *child <8 yr:* half adult dose
- *Available forms:* tabs 50, 250 mg; susp 250 mg/5 ml

Procyclidine

KEMADRIN
(proe-sye´-kli-deen)

Functional classification: Anticholinergic
Chemical classification: Synthetic tertiary amine
FDA pregnancy category: C

Indications: Parkinsonism, EPSEs

Contraindications: Hypersensitivity, narrow-angle glaucoma, duodenal obstruction, peptic ulcer, prostatic hypertrophy, myasthenia gravis, megacolon

Pharmacologic Effects: Blocks cholinergic receptors; might inhibit the reuptake and storage of dopamine

Pharmacokinetics: Peak 1.1-2 hr, half-life 11.5-12.6 hr; little pharmacokinetic information is known

Side Effects: *CNS:* Depression (19%-30%), disorientation, confusion, memory loss, hallucinations, psychoses, agitation, delusions, nervousness; *peripheral:* tachycardia, palpitations, hypotension, orthostatic hypotension, dry mouth, nausea, vomiting, constipation, paralytic ileus, blurred vision, mydriasis, diplopia, urinary retention and hesitancy, elevated temperature

Interactions
- *Amantadine:* increased anticholinergic effect
- *Digoxin:* increased digoxin serum levels

---

*Infrequently used.   †Available in Canada only.

- *Haloperidol:* worsening of schizophrenia, decreased haloperidol serum levels
- *Levodopa:* possible reduction of levodopa efficacy
- *Phenothiazines:* increased anticholinergic effect, decreased antipsychotic effect

Implications: See Benztropine

Treatment of Overdose: Emesis, lavage, activated charcoal, treat respiratory depression, hyperpyrexia.

Administration
- EPSEs: *Adult:* PO 2.5 mg tid, up to 10-20 mg/day
- *Available forms:* tabs 5mg

Promazine*

PROMANYL,† PROZINE, SPARINE
(proe´-ma-zeen)

Functional classification: Antipsychotic
Chemical classification: Aliphatic phenothiazine
FDA pregnancy category: C

Indications: Psychosis; occasionally used as antipsychotic

Contraindications: Hypersensitivity, blood dyscrasias, coma, children <12 yr, bone marrow depression; see Chlorpromazine

Pharmacologic Effects: Provides antipsychotic effect by antagonizing dopamine receptors; also antiadrenergic, anticholinergic, and antiemetic; see Chlorpromazine for more extensive explanation

Pharmacokinetics: *PO:* peak level 2-4 hr; *IM:* onset 15 min, peak level 1 hr, duration 4-6 hr; metabolized by liver, excreted in urine, crosses placenta, excreted in breast milk

Side Effects: *CNS:* see Chlorpromazine; *peripheral:* see Chlorpromazine

Interactions: See Chlorpromazine

Implications: See Chlorpromazine

Treatment of Overdose: Do not induce vomiting; lavage for oral dose; maintain airway and provide supportive care prn.

Administration
- *Psychosis: adult:* PO 10-200 mg q4-6h; range 40-1200 mg/day; however, it is recommended dose not exceed 1000 mg/day
- *Severe agitation: adult:* 50-150 mg IM; if not effective in 30 min, give additional doses up to total dose of 300 mg; *child >12 yr:* PO 10-25 mg q4-6h
- *Available forms:* tabs 25, 50, 100 mg; inj IM, IV, 25, 50 mg/ml

Propranolol HCl

INDERAL
(proe-pran´-oh-lole)

Functional classifications: Antihypertensive, antianginal
Chemical classification: Beta-adrenergic blocker
FDA pregnancy category: C

Indications: Chronic stable angina pectoris, prophylaxis of angina pain
Unapproved uses: "stage fright" (controversial), anxiety, acute panic

Contraindications: Hypersensitivity to this drug, cardiac failure, cardiogenic shock, second- or third-degree heart block, asthma, sinus bradycardia
Cautious use: Diabetes mellitus, pheochromocytoma, hypotension, renal disease, lactation, CHF, hyperthyroidism, cardiopulmonary distress, peripheral vascular disease

Pharmacologic Effects: Nonselective beta-blockers; reduces major symptoms of anxiety (e.g., tachycardia, palpitations, muscle tremors)

Pharmacokinetics: *PO:* onset 30 min, peak 1-1½ hr, duration 6 hr; *IV:* onset 2 min, peak 15 min, duration 3-6 hr; half-life 3-5 hr, metabolized by liver, crosses placenta and blood-brain barrier, excreted in breast milk

Side Effects: *CNS:* depression, hallucinations, dizziness, fatigue, lethargy, paresthesias; *peripheral:* dyspnea, respiratory dysfunction, bronchospasm; bradycardia, hypotension, CHF, palpitations, agranulocytosis, thrombocytopenia, nausea, vomiting, diarrhea, colitis, constipation, cramps, dry mouth, rash, pruritus, fever, sore throat, laryngospasm

Interactions
- *Cimetidine, morphine:* increased beta-blocking effect
- *Norepinephrine, isoproterenol, barbiturates, rifampin, dopamine:* reduced beta-blocking effects
- *Quinidine, haloperidol:* increased hypotension
- *Reserpine:* increased effects
- *Verapamil, disopyramide:* increased propranolol effect

Implications
Assess
- BP, pulse, respirations during beginning of therapy

Teaching
- That drug may be taken before stressful activity (e.g., exercise, sexual activity)

P

- To avoid hazardous activities if dizziness occurs
- To understand the importance of patient compliance with complete medical regimen
- To make position changes slowly to prevent fainting

Evaluate
- Headache, light-headedness, decreased BP; might indicate need for decreased dosage

Administration
- *Stage fright: adult:* 10 mg before appearances
- *Arrhythmia, hypertension, angina, myocardial infarction, pheochromocytoma, migraines:* see PDR
- *Available forms:* caps ext-rel 60, 80, 120, 160 mg; tabs 10, 20, 40, 60, 80, 90 mg; inj 1 mg/ml, oral sol 4, 8, 80 mg/ml

Protriptyline HCl
TRIPTIL, VIVACTIL
(proe-trip´-te-leen)

Functional classification: Antidepressant
Chemical classification: Tricyclic, secondary amine
FDA pregnancy category: C

Indications: Depression

Contraindications: Hypersensitivity to TCAs, recovery phase of myocardial infarction, patients taking cisapride, convulsive disorders, prostatic hypertrophy, MAOI therapy
  Cautious use: Suicidal patients, narrow-angle glaucoma, urinary retention, cardiac disease, hyperthyroidism, ECT, elective surgery, children

Pharmacologic Effects: Known as an "activating" antidepressant; blocks reuptake of norepinephrine (+++++) and serotonin (++) into presynaptic neuron; also antagonizes ACh (+++), histamine (+++), and alpha-1 (++) receptors; therapeutic serum levels 100-200 ng/ml

Pharmacokinetics: *PO:* onset 15-30 min, peak 24-30 hr, duration 4-6 hr; therapeutic effect 2-3 wk; metabolized by liver, excreted by kidneys, crosses placenta, half-life 67-89 hr, protein binding >90%

Side Effects: See Amitriptyline; *specific for protriptyline:* excitement (~10%), dry mouth (~10%), blurred vision (~10%), constipation (~10%), sedation (~2%), insomnia (~10%), orthostasis (~10%), ECG changes (~10%), tachycardia (~2%), sexual disturbance (~2%)

Interactions: See Amitriptyline
- *Cisapride:* cardiac interaction

Implications: See Amitriptyline

Treatment of Overdose: ECG monitoring; induce emesis, lavage, activated charcoal; administer anticonvulsant; treat anticholinergic effects if needed.

Administration
- *Adult:* PO 15-40 mg/day in divided doses, may increase to 60 mg/day; *adolescent and geriatric:* 5 mg tid, increase gradually if needed; CV monitoring necessary for elderly patient receiving dosages >20 mg/day
- *Available forms:* tabs 5, 10 mg

Quetiapine
SEROQUEL
(kwe-tye´-a-peen)

Functional classification: Atypical antipsychotic
Chemical classification: Dibenzothiazepine
FDA pregnancy category: C

Indications: Psychosis, schizophrenia

Contraindications: Hypersensitivity, <18 yr

Pharmacologic Effects: Antipsychotic effect thought to be r/t D_2 and $5HT_2$ antagonism; has greater affinity for $5HT_2$ receptors; has high affinity for alpha-1 and histamine receptors and low affinity for alpha-2 and ACh receptors

Pharmacokinetics: Rapidly absorbed, peak plasma levels 1.5 hr, protein binding 83%, highly metabolized (P-450 3A4 involved in metabolism), half-life 4-10 hr, excreted in the urine (73%) and feces (20%)

Side Effects: Has relatively good side effect profile with few anticholinergic, antiadrenergic, or histaminic side effects; *CNS:* headache (19%), somnolence (18%), dizziness (10%); *peripheral:* constipation (9%), dry mouth (7%), dyspepsia (6%), orthostasis (7%), tachycardia (7%), rash (4%)

Interactions
- *Cimetidine:* reduced clearance of quetiapine
- *Lorazepam:* reduced clearance of lorazepam
- *P-450 3A inhibitors* (e.g. ketoconazole): increased serum levels of quetiapine
- *Phenytoin:* increased clearance of quetiapine
- *Thioridazine:* increased clearance of quetiapine

Administration
- Initially 25 mg bid, dosage may be increased in increments of 25-50 mg bid-tid on 2nd or 3rd day to a target dose of 300-400 mg/day in 2 or 3 divided doses
- *Available forms:* tabs 25, 100, 200 mg

Risperidone

RISPERDAL

(ris-peer´-i-dohn)

Functional classification: Atypical antipsychotic, neuroleptic, serotonin/dopamine antagonist
Chemical classification: Benzisoxazole
FDA pregnancy category: C

Indications: Psychotic disorders, agitated aggressive behavior in dementia, Tourette's syndrome
Unlabeled uses: Antimanic, antidepressant, delusional major depression, augmentation in refractory obsessive-compulsive disorder

Contraindications: Hypersensitivity to risperidone
Cautious use: Elderly, who are susceptible to orthostatic hypotension; patients with history of CV disease because risperidone is thought to lengthen the QT interval; history of seizures

Pharmacologic effects: Mechanism of action unknown; antipsychotic effect is thought to be related to risperidone's antagonism of both D_2 (+++++) and $5HT_2$ (+++++) receptors; theoretically, by blocking D_2 receptors in the mesolimbic area, positive symptoms respond, and by blocking $5HT_2$ receptors in the cortex, negative symptoms respond; also blocks D_1 (+++), D_4 (+++++), histamine (++++), ACh (+), and alpha-1 (+++++) receptors

Pharmacokinetics: Well absorbed; extensively metabolized in the liver to a major metabolite, 9-hydroxyrisperidone, which is equipotent; is a substrate of P-450 2D6; half-life of both risperidone and its metabolite is about 20-24 hr; protein binding 90% and 77%, respectively; decreased renal clearance, and prolonged half-life in elderly

Side Effects: Does not antagonize muscarinic receptors, so it causes few anticholinergic side effects; also produces significant sedation (>30%); *CNS:* initial orthostatic hypotension (>30%) then declines; insomnia (>10%), agitation (>10%), headache (14%), anxiety (12%); EPSEs (17%) occur but less so than with most antipsychotics; *peripheral:* tachycardia (10%), anticholinergic effects (>2%), rhinitis (10%), nausea (6%), constipation (7%); photosensitivity (1%); ECG abnormalities (<2%), sexual dysfunction (>10%), weight gain (>10%)

Interactions

- *Carbamazepine:* risperidone clearance increased so decreased serum levels
- *Clozapine:* chronic combined administration might decrease risperidone clearance and increase serum levels due to competition for 2D6 isoenzymes
- *Drugs that inhibit P-450 2D6:* increased serum levels of risperidone
- *Levodopa:* risperidone might antagonize the effect of levodopa

Implications

Assess

- Establish baseline ECG, VS, laboratory values, and potential hypersensitivity to risperidone
- Physiologic and psychologic status before starting drug to evaluate progress

Planning/Intervention

- Ensure drug is taken.
- Be alert for hypotensive effect that could lead to falls.
- If orthostatic hypotension occurs, have patient sit on side of bed before rising, place head in head-low position for dizziness, avoid hot showers, wear elastic stockings.
- Check BP, using orthostatic protocols.
- Monitor temperature for potential NMS.
- Observe for involuntary movements.

Teaching

- That orthostatic hypotension is possible, especially during period of initial dose titration
- To be cautious about operation of hazardous machinery
- To notify health care provider if pregnant or intend to become pregnant; not to breastfeed while taking risperidone
- To notify care provider before taking OTC drugs (possible drug interaction)
- To avoid exposure to ultraviolet light or sunlight (photosensitivity)

Evaluate

- Decrease in positive and/or negative symptoms
- Whether patient follows prescribed regimen, takes medications as ordered
- Whether patient avoids injury; reports dizziness
- Whether patient uses appropriate interventions to minimize side effects

Treatment of Overdose: Risperidone is a relatively safe drug. In acute overdose, establish and maintain airway and provide adequate oxygenation. Gastric lavage, activated charcoal, and laxatives are all reasonable approaches. Monitor ECG. There is no specific antidote to risperidone.

Administration

- *Psychosis: adult:* PO 1 mg bid on day 1; 2 mg bid on day 2; 3 mg bid on day 3 and thereafter; further upward adjustments may be made at weekly intervals up to 16 mg/day; typical daily dose 4-6 mg/day; *elderly or debilitated patient:* start with 0.5 mg bid; increase by 0.5 mg bid; after reaching 1.5 mg bid, incremental changes should occur on

R

weekly basis; *adolescent:* not recommended for use with this age group
- When switching from another antipsychotic agent, minimize period of overlap
- *Available forms:* tabs 1, 2, 3, 4 mg; oral sol 1 mg/ml

Rivastigmine

EXELON
(ree-va-stig´-mean)

Functional classification: Drug for treatment of Alzheimer's disease
Chemical classification: Second-generation carbamate cholinesterase inhibitor
FDA pregnancy class:

Indications: Alzheimer's disease (approved April 2000)

Pharmacologic Effects: Causes pseudoreversible cholinesterase inhibition; carbamate compounds interact with the catalytic subsite of the active site of acetylcholine synthesis; forms carbamoylated complexes with cholinesterase, rendering the cholinesterase molecule unavailable for ACh reduction (this activity of rivastigmine causes it to have an anticholinesterase effect much longer than the plasma half-life would suggest); rivastigmine's mechanism is pseudoreversible; thus cessation of medication allows recovery of acetylcholinesterase function within 24 hr

Pharmacokinetics: Inhibition half-life 10 hr, plasma half-life 2 hr; metabolized during its interaction with cholinesterase without hepatic involvement (so there are no drug interactions with drugs metabolized by the P-450 system), excreted in the urine

Side Effects: Not associated with liver toxicities; hence, monitoring liver enzymes is not required; *CNS:* dizziness (14%); *peripheral:* nausea (20%), vomiting (16%)

Interactions: No drug interactions noted at this time; not metabolized by the P-450 system and hence does not interact with drugs metabolized by this system

Implications: See Tacrine for general considerations (minus liver function and multiple dosing concerns)

Treating Overdose: Because rivastigmine is new to the market, there is very limited experience with overdosage.

Administration: 6-12 mg/day

Secobarbital, secobarbital sodium

SECOGEN SODIUM,† SECONAL, SECONAL SODIUM, SERAL†
(see-koe-bar´-bi-tal)

Functional classifications: Sedative, hypnotic
Chemical classification: Barbitone
Controlled substance schedule II
FDA pregnancy category: D

Indications: Insomnia, status epilepticus, other uses

Contraindications: Hypersensitivity, respiratory depression, barbiturate dependency, liver impairment, blood dyscrasias

Pharmacologic Effects: Short-acting barbiturate, causing CNS depression in limbic and reticular areas

Pharmacokinetics: Onset 10-15 min, duration 3-4 hr, half-life 15-40 hr, metabolized by liver, excreted in urine; of barbiturates, is the most lipophilic and has highest protein binding

Side Effects: *CNS:* drowsiness, lethargy, hangover (primary side effects); see Phenobarbital for general barbiturate effects; *peripheral:* respiratory depression, laryngospasm, bronchospasm, GI upset, blood dyscrasias; see Phenobarbital

Interactions
- *CNS depressants and alcohol:* additive CNS depression
- *Doxycycline:* Decreased half-life
- *MAOIs:* CNS depression
- *Oral anticoagulants, corticosteroids:* decreased effects of these drugs

Implications
Assess
- BP; blood studies, if indicated

Planning/Implementation
- Give IM in large muscles.
- If given IV, have emergency equipment nearby.
- Give ½ hr before bedtime.
- Maintain safety.

Teaching
- To avoid driving
- To avoid alcohol
- To avoid discontinuing drug abruptly (withdrawal)

Evaluate
- Therapeutic response: sleeping
- Mental status
- Dependence?
- Toxic effects

Treatment of Overdose: Gastric lavage, charcoal to absorb drug; monitor BP, VS, I&O; warm patient; hemodialysis might be effective.

Administration
- *Insomnia: adult:* PO/IM 100-200 mg hs; *REC:* 4-5 mg/kg
- *Status epilepticus: adult and child:* IM/IV 5.5 mg/kg; repeat q3-4h; rate not to exceed 50 mg/15 sec
- *Available forms:* caps 50, 100 mg; tabs 100 mg; inj IM, IV 50 mg/ml; rec inj 50 mg/ml

Selegiline HCl

ELDEPRYL
(seh-leg´-ill-ene)

Functional classification: Antiparkinson
Chemical classification: MAOI
FDA pregnancy category: C

Indications: Parkinsonism adjunct to carbidopa/levodopa

Contraindications: Hypersensitivity

Pharmacologic Effects: Inhibits monoamine oxidase type B, increasing dopamine

Pharmacokinetics: Rapidly absorbed, peak 0.5-2 hr; 3 active metabolites, including amphetamine (half-life 18 hr) and methamphetamine (half-life 20 hr); excreted in urine

Side Effects: *CNS:* dizziness and lightheadedness (7%), Parkinson-like symptoms, confusion (3%), hallucinations (3%), dyskinesias (2%), headache (2%), anxiety; *peripheral:* nausea (10%), abdominal pain (4%), dry mouth (3%), generalized aches, diarrhea, leg and back pain, urinary retention, weight loss

Interactions
- *Meperidine:* fatalities have been reported with this combination
- *SSRIs, TCAs:* risk of serious toxicity

Implications
  Assess
- BP, respirations

Planning/Implementation
- Give with meals; limit protein taken with drug.
- Keep doses <10 mg/day because monoamine oxidase inhibition might not be selective (might also inhibit monoamine oxidase type A, which could precipitate hypertensive crisis).

Teaching
- That patient might need to reduce levodopa
- Not to exceed 10 mg/day

Evaluate
- Therapeutic response: decrease in symptoms of parkinsonism

Treatment of Overdose: *Symptoms:* If selegiline nonselectively inhibits monoamine oxidase, look for symptoms similar to those found with MAOI overdose; see Isocarboxazid.

Administration
- *Adult:* PO 5 mg at breakfast and at lunch (10 mg total); after 2-3 days, begin reducing carbidopa/levodopa by 10%-30%
- *Available forms:* tabs 5 mg

Sertraline

ZOLOFT
(ser´-tra-leen)

Functional classification: SSRI antidepressant
Chemical classification: SSRI; tetrahydronaphthyl-methylamine
FDA pregnancy category: B

Indications: Depression, panic disorders, obsessive-compulsive disorder
  Unlabeled uses: Dysthymia, atypical depression, aggression, premenstrual dysphoria, PTSD, pervasive developmental disorder, premature ejaculation

Contraindications: Hepatic dysfunction, renal impairment, lactation

Pharmacologic Effects: Inhibits CNS neuronal uptake of serotonin (++++); also inhibits dopamine reuptake (++) and blocks these receptors, ACh (++) and alpha-1 (++)

Pharmacokinetics: Peak levels 4.5-8.4 hr; half-life 26-98 hr (with metabolites); sertraline undergoes extensive first-pass metabolism; excreted in urine; protein binding 99%; inhibits P-450 2D6

Side Effects: *CNS* (from premarketing trials): headache (20%), dizziness (11%), tremor (10%), paresthesia (2%), insomnia (16%), somnolence (13%), agitation (5.6%); *peripheral* (from premarketing trials): dry mouth (16%), increased sweating (8%), palpitations (3.5%), rash (2%), diarrhea (17%), constipation (8%), dyspepsia (6%), vomiting (4%), gas (3%), anorexia (3%), abdominal pain (2.4%), sexual dysfunction (15.5%), abnormal vision (4%)

Interactions
- *Alcohol:* CNS depression
- *Anorexiants:* increased serotonin effects
- *Cimetidine:* increased plasma levels of sertraline

S

- *Diazepam:* decreased clearance of diazepam
- *Drugs highly bound to plasma proteins:* displacement of sertraline or one of these drugs could result in adverse responses
- *Grapefruit juice:* increased plasma levels of sertraline
- *MAOIs:* fatal hypertensive crises (serotonin syndrome) have resulted from combining MAOIs and SSRIs
- *Serotonergic drugs:* the serotonin syndrome can result from combining SSRIs and serotonin-enhancing agents

Implications
Assess
- BP, VS
- Hepatic studies because of sertraline's extensive liver metabolism
- Weight loss
- Activation of mania

Planning/Implementation
- Maintain safety.
- Closely supervise patients at high risk for suicide because some professionals believe that a relationship exists between suicide and alterations in serotonin levels.
- Give with food to minimize first-pass metabolism.

Teaching
- To be cautious about driving (although no impairment in driving ability has been recorded with use of sertraline)
- To avoid alcohol (although no impairment resulting from this combination has been recorded)
- To be cautious about use of OTC products
- To avoid exposure to temperature extremes because SSRIs affect temperature regulation
- To avoid grapefruit juice because it can inhibit sertraline metabolism and increase plasma levels

Evaluate
- Therapeutic effect: depression
- Mental status

Treatment of Overdose: Deaths have occurred when SSRIs, including sertraline, were combined with other serotonergic drugs. Some evidence indicates that treatment with methysergide, a serotonin antagonist, is effective. For overdose with sertraline alone, establish and maintain airway; administer oxygen prn; charcoal might inhibit absorption and might be more effective than induced vomiting.

Administration
- *Adult:* PO 50 mg initially, once daily (morning or evening); increases can be made weekly (because of long half-life); maximum dose, 200 mg/day
- *Available forms:* tabs 50, 100 mg

Sildenafil
VIAGRA
(sill-den´-a-fill)

Functional classification: Drug to treat erectile dysfunction
FDA pregnancy category: B

Indications: Impotence

Contraindications: Use of nitrates
Cautious use: Myocardial infarction, stroke, or life-threatening arrhythmia within last 6 mo, patients with resting hypotension (<90/50 mm Hg), patients with resting hypertension (>170/110 mm Hg), patients with cardiac failure or coronary artery disease, patients with retinitis pigmentosa

Pharmacologic Effects: Inhibits phosphodiesterase type 5 (PDE5), which is responsible for degradation of cGMP, causing increased levels of cGMP in the corpus cavernosum; this results in smooth muscle relaxation and increased inflow of blood to the corpus cavernosum, causing an erection (if sexually stimulated)

Pharmacokinetics: Rapidly absorbed, bioavailability 40%; protein binding 96%; metabolized by P-450 3A4 (major) and 2C9 (minor); half-life 4 hr; excreted in feces (80%) and urine (13%)

Side Effects: *CNS:* headache (16%), dizziness (2%); *peripheral:* flushing (10%), dyspepsia (7%), nasal congestion (4%), UTI (3%), abnormal vision (3%), diarrhea (2%), rash (2%); *CV:* serious CV events, including myocardial infarctions and deaths have been reported in temporal association with sildenafil; most of these events occurred during or shortly after sexual activity

Interactions
- *Cimetidine:* causes 56% increase in sildenafil serum levels
- *Drugs that inhibit P-450 3A4 (primarily) and 2C9:* increased serum levels of sildenafil
- *Nitrates:* increase hypotensive effect

Treatment of Overdose: Standard supportive measures should be adopted

Administration
- 50 mg as needed 1 hr before sexual activity; maximum 100 mg
- *Available forms:* tabs 25, 50, 100 mg

---

*Infrequently used.   †Available in Canada only.

Succinylcholine chloride

ANECTINE, ANECTINE FLO-PACK,
QUELICIN, SCALINE,† SUCOSTRIN†
(suk-sin-ill-koe´-leen)

Functional classification: Neuromuscular blocker
(depolarizing, ultrashort)
FDA pregnancy category: C

Indications: Facilitates endotracheal intubation during ECT; reduces intensity of convulsions during ECT; other indications for use with general anesthesia are given in PDR

Contraindications: Hypersensitivity, malignant hyperthermia, decreased plasma pseudocholinesterase (~4% of population), elevated CPK

Cautious use: Cardiac disease, severe burns, fractures, lactation, children <2 yr, electrolyte imbalances, dehydration, neuromuscular disease, respiratory disease, collagen diseases, glaucoma, eye surgery, penetrating eye wounds, elderly or debilitated patients

Pharmacologic Effects: Inhibits transmission of nerve impulses by binding with cholinergic receptors at motor endplate; muscle depolarizes and can be seen as fasciculations head to foot; recovery follows a reverse process

Pharmacokinetics: *IV:* onset 30-60 sec, peak 2-3 min, duration 4-6 min; *IM:* onset 1-3 min; rapidly metabolized by plasma and liver pseudocholinesterases

Side Effects: *Peripheral:* bradycardia, tachycardia, increased and decreased BP, sinus arrest, arrhythmias, prolonged apnea, bronchospasm, cyanosis, increased secretions, increased intraocular pressure, weakness, muscle pain, fasciculations, prolonged relaxation, myoglobulinemia, rash, flushing, pruritus, urticaria, malignant hyperthermia

Interactions
- *Barbiturates:* do not mix with barbiturates in solution or syringe
- *Cholinesterase inhibitors:* increases the effects of succinylcholine
- *Diazepam:* reduction of neuromuscular block
- *Narcotic analgesics:* bradycardia
- *Phenelzine, promazine, oxytocin, beta-blockers, procainamide, anticholinesterases, quinidine, local anesthetics, aminoglycosides, tetracyclines, lithium, thiazides, enflurane, isoflurane:* increased neuromuscular blockade
- *Theophylline:* arrhythmias

Implications

Assess
- For electrolyte imbalances (K, Mg); might lead to increased action of this drug
- VS until fully recovered from ECT; rate, depth, pattern of respirations, strength of hand grip

Planning/Implementation
- If communication is difficult during recovery from neuromuscular blockade, offer reassurance

Evaluate
- Therapeutic response: paralysis
- Recovery
- Prolonged apnea, allergic reactions: rash, fever, respiratory distress, pruritus; drug should be discontinued

Treatment of Overdose: Overdose can cause a prolonged apnea. Management is supportive because there is no antidote.

Administration
- *Adult:* IV 25-75 mg (average dose 0.6 mg/kg), then 2.5 mg/min prn; IM 2.5 mg/kg, not to exceed 150 mg; *child:* IV 1-2 mg/kg, IM 3-4 mg/kg, not to exceed 150 mg IM
- *Available forms:* inj IM IV 20, 50, 100 mg/ml; powder for inj 100, 500 mg/vial, 1 g/vial

Tacrine

COGNEX
(tak´-rin)

Functional classification: Drug for Alzheimer's disease
Chemical classification: Cholinesterase inhibitor; monoamine acridine
FDA pregnancy category: C

Indications: Mild to moderate dementia of the Alzheimer's type

Contraindications: Hypersensitivity to tacrine or acridine derivatives; jaundice associated with prior tacrine use; pregnancy

Cautious use: Renal or hepatic disease, bladder obstruction, GI bleeding, anesthesia

Pharmacologic Effects: Centrally acting reversible inhibitor of cholinesterase (binds with cholinesterase), which increases the amount of ACh in the cortex; might also stimulate the release of ACh; because only remaining cholinergic neurons are affected, this and similarly acting drugs become less effective as the disease progresses; might have direct effect on muscarinic and nicotinic receptors; also inhibits MAO-A; does

T

not cure dementia but is thought to slow degeneration

Pharmacokinetics: Peak level 1-2 hr; half-life 2-4 hr; protein binding 55%; metabolized in liver by CYP-450 isoenzymes; crosses placenta; might enter breast milk; excreted in urine; bioavailability is low (17%)

Side Effects: *CNS:* headache, fatigue, dizziness, confusion, ataxia, insomnia, tremor, agitation, depression, anxiety, abnormal thinking; *peripheral:* major concern is hepatotoxicity: transaminase (ALT) levels should be assessed regularly (typically every other week); other side effects: GI upset, nausea, vomiting, diarrhea, anorexia, abdominal pain, gas, constipation, URIs, UTIs, skin rash and flushing, bradycardia

Interactions
- *Anticholinergics:* decreased effect of anticholinergics
- *Cigarettes:* decreases serum levels of tacrine
- *Cimetidine:* increased effects of tacrine
- *Food:* decreased absorption of tacrine if taken with food (30%-40%)
- *Lecithin:* apparently potentiates effect of tacrine
- *Succinylcholine:* increases effect of succinylcholine
- *Theophylline:* increased effects of theophylline

Implications
Assess
- Cognitive functioning
- Baseline ALT levels

Planning/Implementation
- Administer at regular intervals between meals. If GI upset requires giving with food, then be aware dosage might need adjusting to accommodate decreased absorption.

Teaching
- To understand the importance of taking medication at regular intervals and concerns about foods decreasing absorption
- To avoid abrupt cessation because it can cause an increase in cognitive decline
- To contact physician or nurse should nausea, vomiting, diarrhea, rash, jaundice, or changes in stool color occur

Evaluate
- Monitor cognitive function

Treatment of Overdose: Overdose can cause cholinergic crisis. Anticholinergics (e.g., atropine) might be used as an antidote.

Administration
- Initially 10 mg qid for 4 wk; range typically 40-160 mg/day in 4 divided doses; usually given between meals; incremental changes

are made in conjunction with ALT monitoring
- *Available forms:* caps 10, 20, 30, 40 mg

Temazepam
RESTORIL
(te-maz´-e-pam)

Functional classifications: Sedative, hypnotic
Chemical classification: Benzodiazepine
Controlled substance schedule IV
FDA pregnancy category: X

Indications: Insomnia

Contraindications: Hypersensitivity to benzodiazepines, lactation
Cautious use: Sleep apnea, hepatic or renal disease, suicidal individuals, drug abuse, elderly patients, depression, child <18 yr

Pharmacologic Effects: Produces CNS depression

Pharmacokinetics: *PO:* onset 2-3 hr, duration 6-8 hr, half-life 10-15 hr; metabolized by liver, excreted by kidneys, crosses placenta, excreted in breast milk

Side Effects: *CNS:* euphoria, drowsiness, daytime sedation, dizziness, confusion, lightheadedness, headache, depression, irritability; *peripheral:* nausea, vomiting, diarrhea, heartburn, abdominal pain, constipation, chest pain, palpitations

Interactions
- *Alcohol, CNS depressants:* CNS depression
- *Antacids:* decrease effects of benzodiazepines
- *Cimetidine, disulfiram:* prolong half-life of benzodiazepines
- *Digoxin:* digoxin intoxication

Implications
Assess
- VS

Planning/Implementation
- For sleeplessness, instruct patient to take dose ½-1 hr before bedtime.
- If GI symptoms occur, the dose may be taken with food.
- Assist with ambulation.
- Ensure that side rails, night-light, call bell are within easy reach.
- Check to see that medication has been swallowed.

Teaching
- To avoid driving or other activities requiring alertness until drug regimen is stabilized
- To avoid ingestion of alcohol or CNS depressants
- That it might take 2 nights for benefits to be noticed

---

*Infrequently used.   †Available in Canada only.

- That hangover is common in elderly persons but less common than with barbiturates

Evaluate
- Therapeutic response: ability to sleep at night, decreased amount of early-morning awakening when taking drug for insomnia
- Mental status
- Type of sleep problem, falling asleep, staying asleep

Treatment of Overdose: Lavage; monitor electrolytes, VS; provide supportive care.

Administration
- *Adult:* PO 10-60 mg hs; *geriatric, debilitated:* 10-20 mg until individual response is determined
- *Available forms:* caps 15, 30 mg

Thioridazine HCl

MELLARIL, NOVORIDAZINE,†
THIORIDAZINE
(thye-or-rid´-a-zeen)

Functional classifications: Traditional antipsychotic, neuroleptic, low potency
Chemical classifications: Phenothiazine, piperidine
FDA pregnancy category: C

Indications: Psychotic disorders, behavioral problems in children, anxiety, major depressive disorders
Unlabeled uses: Short-term treatment of depression accompanied by anxiety; agitation, insomnia, anxiety, depressed mood in geriatric patients; children with severe behavioral problems

Contraindications: Hypersensitivity, blood dyscrasias, coma, child <2 yr, brain damage, bone marrow depression, parkinsonism
Cautious use: Lactation, seizure disorders, hypertension, hepatic disease, cardiac disease

Pharmacologic Effects: Traditional antipsychotic drugs produce a neuroleptic effect characterized by sedation, emotional quieting, psychomotor slowing, and affective indifference; exact mode of action not fully understood; blocks D_2 receptors (+++++) in the basal ganglia, hypothalamus, limbic system, brainstem, and medulla; blockade of these receptors accounts for both therapeutic and adverse responses; because of their nonselective actions, many other neurotransmitters systems are affected as well; ACh (++++), histamine (+++), and alpha-1 (++++); least antiemetic of all phenothiazines

Pharmacokinetics: *PO:* onset erratic, peak 2-4 hr; metabolized by liver, excreted in urine, crosses placenta, excreted in breast milk, half-life 9-30 hr; a substrate and inhibitor of the P-450 2D6 isoenzyme

Side Effects: See Chlorpromazine; *specific for thioridazine:* sedation (~30%), EPSEs (~2%), orthostasis (30%), anticholinergic (~30%), weight gain (~30%), sexual dysfunction (~30) (including retrograde ejaculation and priapism); also pigmentary retinopathy with thioridazine (necessitating a maximum dose of 800 mg/day)

Interactions: See Chlorpromazine
- *Antiarrhythmics:* additive cardiac depression
- *Antihistamines:* increased QT interval
- *Cimetidine:* increased plasma levels of thioridazine
- *Drugs metabolized by P-450 2D6:* inhibition of their metabolism

Implications: See Chlorpromazine

Treatment of Overdose: Lavage, provide an airway; do not induce vomiting; control EPSEs and hypotension

Administration
- *Psychosis: adult:* PO 50-100 mg tid, maximum dose 800 mg/day; dosage is gradually increased to desired response, then reduced to minimum maintenance dose
- *Depression, behavioral problems: adult:* PO 25 tid, range from 10 mg bid-qid to 50 mg tid-bid; *child 2-12 yr:* PO 0.5-3 mg/kg/day in divided doses
- Mix concentrate in distilled water or orange or grapefruit juice
- *Available forms:* tabs 10, 15, 25, 50, 100, 150, 200 mg; conc 30, 100 mg/ml; susp 25, 100 mg/5 ml

Thiothixene

NAVANE
(thye-oh-thix´-een)

Functional classifications: Antipsychotic, neuroleptic, high potency
Chemical classification: Thioxanthene
FDA pregnancy category: C

Indications: Psychotic disorders

Contraindications: Hypersensitivity, blood dyscrasias, child <12 yr, bone marrow depression
Cautious use: Lactation, seizure disorders, hypertension, hepatic disease

Pharmacologic Effects: Traditional antipsychotic drugs produce a neuroleptic effect characterized by sedation, emotional quieting, psychomotor slowing, and affective indifference; exact mode of action not fully understood; blocks D_2 receptors (++++) in the basal ganglia, hypothalamus, limbic system, brainstem, and medulla; blockade of these receptors accounts for both therapeutic and adverse responses; because of

T

their nonselective actions, many other neurotransmitters systems are affected as well; ACh (+), histamine (+++), and alpha-1 (++)

Pharmacokinetics: *PO:* onset slow, peak 2-8 hr, duration up to 12 hr; *IM:* onset 15-30 min, peak 1-6 hr, duration up to 12 hr; metabolized by liver, excreted in urine, crosses placenta, excreted in breast milk, half-life 34 hr; metabolized by P-450 1A, which is affected by cigarette smoking

Side Effects: See Chlorpromazine; *specific for thiothixene:* sedation (~10%), EPSEs (~30%), orthostasis (minimal), anticholinergic (~2%), weight gain (~10%), sexual dysfunction (min)

Interactions: See Chlorpromazine

Implications: See Chlorpromazine

Treatment of Overdose: Lavage, if orally ingested; provide an airway; do not induce vomiting.

Administration
- *Adult:* PO 2-5 mg bid-qid, depending on severity of condition; dosage gradually increased to 20-30 mg, if needed; IM 4 mg bid-qid, maximum dose is 30 mg qd; administer PO dose as soon as possible
- Mix concentrate in orange or grapefruit juice
- *Available forms:* caps 1, 2, 5, 10, 20 mg; conc 5 mg/ml; inj IM 2 mg/ml; powder for inj 5 mg/ml

Tiagabine
GABATRIL
(ti-ah-ga´-bean)

Functional classification: Antiepileptic
Chemical classification: Nipecotic acid derivative
FDA pregnancy category: C

Indications: Adjunctive treatment of partial seizures in adults and children >12

Contraindications: Hypersensitivity
Cautious use: Hepatically impaired, rash, patients taking other CNS depressants, breast-feeding

Pharmacologic Effects: Antiepileptic effect thought to be related to its ability to inhibit the reuptake of GABA into presynaptic neurons and surrounding glial cells; the net effect is greater availability of GABA for postsynaptic cells, thus prolonging the GABA-mediated inhibition

Pharmacokinetics: Rapidly and completely absorbed with a bioavailability of 90%; food slows absorption but does not alter the extent of bioavailability; peak serum levels 1-2.5 hr; probably metabolized by P-450 3A; steady state achieved in 2 days; half-life 7-9 hr but reduced with coadministration of certain drugs (see Inter-

actions); protein binding ~96%; excreted in urine (25%) and feces (63%) with 2% unchanged

Side Effects: (Based on manufacturer research report indicates) *CNS:* dizziness (27%), asthenia (20%), somnolence (18%), nervousness (10%), tremor (9%), poor concentration (6%), insomnia (6%), confusion (5%), memory problems (4%), depression (3%); *peripheral:* abdominal pain (7%), nausea (11%), diarrhea (7%), pharyngitis (7%), increased cough (4%), rash (5%)

Interactions
- *Alcohol:* at this point, studies do not indicate a potentiation of alcohol effects but because of the potential for additive CNS effects, caution should be used
- *Carbamazepine, phenytoin, phenobarbital, primidone:* tiagabine clearance increased 60%, half-life decreased to 4-7 hr
- *Valproic acid:* tiagabine causes slight decrease (10%) in valproate concentrations; valproate causes a decrease in tiagabine binding increasing free tiagabine by 40%

Treatment of Overdose: Experience with tiagabine overdose is limited. The manufacturer reports dosages as high as 800 mg ($N = 11$). These patients recovered with 1 day. The most common symptoms reported from overdose were somnolence, impaired consciousness, agitation, confusion, speech difficulty, hostility, depression, weakness, and myoclonus. There is no specific antidote for tiagabine. If indicated, tiagabine should be eliminated by emesis or gastric lavage. General supportive measures should be used. Dialysis is not likely to be effective because of tiagabine's high protein binding and its metabolism by the liver.

Administration
- *Adult:* begin at 4 mg qd and increase by 4-8 mg/wk up to 30-56 mg/day in 2-4 divided doses; *child 12-18 yr:* begin at 4 mg/day then can be increased by 4 mg/wk up to 32 mg/day in 2-4 divided doses
- *Available forms:* tabs 4, 12, 16, 20 mg

Topiramate
TOPAMAX
(toe-peer´-a-mate)

Functional classification: Antiepileptic
Chemical classification: Sulfamate-substituted monosaccharide
FDA pregnancy category: C

Indications: Adjunctive treatment of partial seizures
Unlabeled uses: Might also be effective in the treatment of partial onset seizures in children; tonic-clonic seizures, and drop attacks associated with Lennox-Gastaut syndrome; bipolar disorder

Contraindications: Hypersensitivity

Cautious use: Kidney stones, paresthesia, renal decreased renal function, patient taking a carbonic anhydrase inhibitor; safety and effectiveness in children (i.e., <18 yr) not established

Pharmacologic Effects: Mode of action not precisely known but three separate mechanisms contribute to its antiepileptic capabilities: (1) sodium channel normalization, (2) GABA potentiation, and (3) antagonism of non-NMDA glutamate receptors

Pharmacokinetics: Absorption is rapid and is not hampered by food; bioavailability 80%; peak concentrations ~2 hr; mean half-life 21 hr; steady state reached within 4 days (if patient has normal renal function); protein binding 13%-17%; 70% excreted unchanged

Side Effects: (From manufacturer's research report): *CNS:* somnolence (30%), dizziness (28%), ataxia (21%), speech problems (~17%), nystagmus (15%), memory problems (12%), tremor (~11%), nervousness (~16%), confusion (~10%), depression (8%); *peripheral:* URI (12%), nausea (~11%), dyspepsia (8%), abnormal vision (14%), psychomotor slowing (~17%), speech disorders, diplopia (14%), anorexia (5%), weight loss (7%)

Interactions: Interactions are few and typically are not severe.

- *Carbonic anhydrase inhibitors* (e.g., acetazolamide): may increase risk of kidney stones-*Digoxin:* reduced levels of digoxin
- *Oral contraceptives:* may lose their effectiveness
- *Phenytoin, carbamazepine, valproic acid:* topiramate's sera are decreased

Treatment of Overdose: If overdose is acute, the stomach should be emptied immediately by lavage or induced emesis. Activated charcoal has not been shown to absorb topiramate. Treatment should be supportive. Hemodialysis will remove topiramate.

Administration

- *Epilepsy: adult:* begin at 50 mg/day and then incrementally increase to 200 mg bid (400 mg/day)
- *Bipolar:* reported effective at dosages of 200-614 mg/day; responses at low dosages (i.e., 25 mg bid), have also been reported
- *Available forms:* sprinkle caps 15, 25 mg

Tranylcypromine sulfate
PARNATE
(tran-ill-sip´-roe-meen)

Functional classifications: MAOI antidepressant
Chemical classification: Nonhydrazine
FDA pregnancy category: C

Indications: Depression refractory to drug therapy

Contraindications: Hypersensitivity to MAOIs, elderly patients (>60 yr), children <16 yr, hypertension, CHF, severe hepatic disease, pheochromocytoma, severe renal disease, severe cardiac disease

Cautious use: Suicidal patients, convulsive disorders, schizophrenia, hyperactivity, diabetes mellitus, hypomania, agitation, hyperthyroidism

Pharmacologic Effects: Inhibits monoamine oxidase by irreversibly binding to monoamine oxidase A and B, thus increasing the concentration of endogenous epinephrine, norepinephrine, serotonin, dopamine in storage sites in CNS

Pharmacokinetics: Metabolized by liver monoamine oxidase A and monoamine oxidase B, excreted by kidneys, half-life 2-3 hr

Side Effects: *CNS:* dizziness, drowsiness, confusion, headache, anxiety, tremors, stimulation, weakness, hyperreflexia, mania, insomnia, fatigue, weight gain; *peripheral:* change in libido; constipation, dry mouth, nausea and vomiting, anorexia, diarrhea, rash, flushing, increased perspiration, jaundice, orthostatic hypotension, hypertension, arrhythmias, hypertensive crisis, blurred vision

Interactions

- *Anticholinergic drugs:* additive effect
- *Antihypertensives* (diuretics, beta-blockers, hydralazine, nitroglycerin, prazosin): hypotension
- *Buspirone:* serotonergic reaction possible
- *Drug-drug: sympathomimetics* (indirect or mixed acting): severe headache, hypertension, hyperpyrexia, and hypertensive crisis; sympathomimetic drugs include amphetamines; levodopa; tryptophan; methylphenidate; OTC compounds containing phenylpropanolamine, ephedrine, and pseudoephedrine; TCAs; other MAOIs; guanethidine; methyldopa; guanadrel; reserpine
- *Drug-food: tyramine-rich foods* (see text): hypertensive crisis
- *Serotonergic drugs:* potential for serotonin syndrome

T

Implications

Assess

- BP (lying, standing), pulse; if systolic BP drops 20 mm Hg, withhold drug, notify physician
- Blood studies: CBC, leukocyte count, cardiac enzyme levels (if patient is receiving long-term therapy)
- Hepatic studies: hepatotoxicity might occur

Planning/Implementation

- Instruct patient to increase fluids, bulk in diet if constipation, urinary retention occurs.
- Instruct patient to take dose with food or milk to prevent GI symptoms.
- Tell patient to chew gum, suck on hard candies, or take frequent sips of water for dry mouth.
- Give phentolamine for severe hypertension.
- Store drug in tight container in cool environment.
- Assist with ambulation during beginning of therapy because drowsiness or dizziness occurs.
- Maintain safety measures, including side rails.
- Check to see that PO medication is swallowed.

Teaching

- That therapeutic effects might take 2 days to 3 wk
- To avoid driving or performing other activities that require alertness
- To avoid alcohol ingestion, CNS depressants, or OTC medications for cold, weight, hay fever, cough
- Not to discontinue medication suddenly after long-term use
- To avoid high-tyramine foods: cheese (aged), caviar, dried fish, game meat, beer, wine, pickled products, liver, raisins, bananas, figs, avocados, meat tenderizers, chocolate, yogurt, increased caffeine, soy sauce
- To report headache, palpitations, neck stiffness

Evaluate

- Toxic effects: increased headache, palpitations; discontinue drug immediately
- Mental status
- Urinary retention, constipation
- Withdrawal symptoms: headache, nausea, vomiting, muscle pain, weakness

Treatment of Overdose: Lavage, activated charcoal; monitor electrolytes, VS; treat hypotension.

Administration

- *Adult:* 30 mg/day in divided doses; if no improvement after 2 wk, increase by 10 mg/day in increments of 1-3 wk, maximum dose 60 mg/day
- *Available forms:* tabs 10 mg

Trazodone HCl
DESYREL
(tray´-zoe-done)

Functional classification: Tricyclic-like antidepressant
Chemical classification: Triazolopyridine
FDA pregnancy category: C

Indications: Depression, insomnia
Unlabeled uses: Cocaine withdrawal, aggressive behavior, panic disorder

Contraindications: Hypersensitivity to trazodone, child <18 yr
Cautious use: Suicidal patients, hypotension, priapism, narrow-angle glaucoma, urinary retention, cardiac disease, hepatic disease, hyperthyroidism, ECT, elective surgery

Pharmacologic Effects: Potentiates serotonin through $5HT_2$ antagonism; selectively inhibits serotonin uptake (++) in brain; does not block ACh (−) receptors but does block histamine (++) and alpha-1 (+++) receptors; therapeutic plasma levels 800-1600 ng/ml

Pharmacokinetics: Metabolized by liver, excreted by kidneys and feces; peak 1 hr without food; half-life 4-9 hr; protein binding ~90% or greater

Side Effects: *CNS:* anger, ataxia, confusion, delirium; *peripheral:* blurred vision, photophobia, increased intraocular pressure, decreased tearing, orthostatic hypotension, arrhythmias, tachycardia, palpitations, dry mouth, constipation, diarrhea, decreased sweating, priapism

Interactions

- *CNS depressants:* additive depressant effect
- *MAOIs:* hypertensive crisis, atropine-like poisoning
- *Phenytoin:* might increase phenytoin level

Implications: See Amitriptyline

Teaching: Specific teaching for trazodone:
- To notify physician and discontinue use of the drug if prolonged, painful erection occurs
- To take dose with food

Treatment of Overdose: Deaths have occurred as a result of use of trazodone and another drug (i.e., alcohol); there is no antidote; supportive care of hypotension and excessive sedation, gastric lavage.

Administration

- *Adult:* PO 150 mg/day in divided doses, may be increased by 50 mg/day every 3-4 days, not to exceed 600 mg/day
- *Available forms:* tabs 50, 100, 150, 300 mg

---

*Infrequently used. †Available in Canada only.

Triazolam

HALCION
(trye-ay´-zoe lam)

Functional classifications: Sedative, hypnotic
Chemical classification: Benzodiazepine
Controlled substance schedule IV
FDA pregnancy category: X

Indications: Short-term treatment of insomnia

Contraindications: Pregnancy, hypersensitivity to benzodiazepines, lactation
Cautious use: Depression, hepatic or renal disease, elderly patients, drug abuse, narrow-angle glaucoma, child <18 yr

Pharmacologic Effects: Produces CNS depression

Pharmacokinetics: *PO:* onset 1-2 hr, peak 0.5-2 hr, duration 6-8 hr, metabolized by liver, excreted by kidneys, crosses placenta, excreted in breast milk, half-life 1.5-5.5 hr; metabolized by P-450 3A

Side Effects: *CNS:* anterograde amnesia, drowsiness, daytime sedation, dizziness, confusion, light-headedness, headache, irritability; *peripheral:* nausea, vomiting, diarrhea, heartburn, abdominal pain, constipation, chest pain, palpitations

Interactions
- *Alcohol, CNS depressants:* CNS depression
- *Antacids:* decrease effects of benzodiazepines
- *Antifungals* (ketoconazole, itraconazole): triazolam can reach dangerous concentrations when mixed with these drugs
- *Cimetidine, disulfiram:* prolong half-life of benzodiazepines
- *Digoxin:* digoxin intoxication
- *Drugs that inhibit P-450 3A:* increased serum levels of triazolam

Implications
Assess
- VS

Planning/Implementation
- For sleeplessness, instruct patient to take dose ½-1 hr before bedtime.
- If GI symptoms occur, tell patient that dose may be taken with food.
- Assist with ambulation.
- Ensure that side rails, night-light, call bell are within easy reach.
- Check to see that medication has been swallowed.

Teaching
- To avoid driving or other activities requiring alertness until drug is stabilized
- To avoid ingestion of alcohol or CNS depressants; serious CNS depression might result
- That it might take 2 nights to be able to sleep
- That triazolam should not be taken if a full night's rest cannot be obtained
- That hangover is common in elderly patients but less common than with barbiturates

Evaluate
- Therapeutic response: ability to sleep at night, decreased amount of early-morning awakening if taking drug for insomnia
- Mental status: mood, sensorium, affect, memory (long-term, short-term)
- Blood dyscrasias: fever, sore throat, bruising, rash, jaundice, epistaxis (rare)
- Type of sleep problem: falling asleep, staying asleep

Treatment of Overdose: Lavage; monitor electrolytes, VS; provide supportive care.

Administration
- *Adult:* PO 0.125-0.5 mg hs; *elderly patient:* PO 0.125-0.25 mg hs
- *Available forms:* tabs 0.125, 0.25 mg (prescriptions not to be written for amount exceeding 1 month's supply)

Trifluoperazine HCl

**NOVOFLURAZINE,† SOLAZINE,†
STELAZINE, TERFLUZINE,† TRIFLURIN†**
(trye-floo-oh-per´-a-zeen)

Functional classifications: Traditional antipsychotic, neuroleptic, high potency
Chemical classifications: Phenothiazine, piperazine
FDA pregnancy category: C

Indications: Psychosis, anxiety

Contraindications: Hypersensitivity, coma, child <6 yr

Pharmacologic Effects: Traditional antipsychotic drugs produce a neuroleptic effect characterized by sedation, emotional quieting, psychomotor slowing, and affective indifference; exact mode of action not fully understood; blocks D_2 receptors (++++) in the basal ganglia, hypothalamus, limbic system, brainstem, and medulla; blockade of these receptors accounts for both therapeutic and adverse responses; because of their nonselective actions, many other neurotransmitters systems are affected as well; ACh (+), histamine (++), and alpha-1 (+++)

Pharmacokinetics: *PO:* onset erratic, peak 2-4 hr, duration 4-6 hr, half-life 13 hr; *IM:* onset 15-30 min, peak 15-20 min, duration 4-6 hr; metabolized by liver, excreted in urine and feces, crosses placenta, excreted in breast milk

Side Effects: See Chlorpromazine; *specific for trifluoperazine:* sedation (~2%), EPSEs (~2%-10%), orthostasis (10%), anticholinergic (~2%), weight gain (~2%), sexual dysfunction (min)

Interactions: See Chlorpromazine

Implications: See Chlorpromazine

Treatment of Overdose: Lavage, if orally ingested; provide an airway; do not induce vomiting, control EPSEs and hypotension.

Administration

- *Psychosis: adult:* PO 2-5 mg bid, usual range 15-20 mg/day, might require ≥40 mg/day; IM 1-2 mg q4-6h; *child >6 yr:* PO 1 mg qd or bid, maximum up to 15 mg/day; IM not recommended for children, but 1 mg may be given qd or bid
- *Anxiety: adult:* PO 1-2 mg bid, not to exceed 6 mg/day; do not give for >12 wk
- *Available forms:* tabs 1, 2, 5, 10 mg; conc 10 mg/ml; inj IM 2 mg/ml

Triflupromazine*

VESPRIN
(trye-floo-proe´-ma-zeen)

Functional classification: Antipsychotic
Chemical classification: Aliphatic phenothiazine
FDA pregnancy category: C

Indications: Occasionally used for psychosis, schizophrenia

Contraindications: Hypersensitivity, children <2.5 yr

Pharmacologic Effects: See Chlorpromazine

Pharmacokinetics: *PO:* peak levels 2-4 hr, duration 4-6 hr, *IM:* onset 15-30 min, peak levels 15-20 min, duration 4-6 hr; metabolized by liver, excreted in urine and feces, crosses placenta, excreted in breast milk

Side Effects: *CNS:* EPSEs, drowsiness, seizures; *peripheral:* respiratory depression, laryngospasm, blood dyscrasias, dry mouth, GI disturbances, blurred vision, nausea and vomiting, orthostatic hypotension, tachycardia, hypertension

Interactions: See Chlorpromazine

Treatment of Overdose: See Chlorpromazine

Administration

- *Psychosis: adult:* IM 60 mg, up to 150 mg/day; *child >2½ yr:* IM 0.2-0.25 mg/kg, up to a maximum dose of 10 mg/day
- *Available forms:* inj 10, 20 mg/ml

Trihexyphenidyl

ARTANE
(tyre-hex-ee-fen´-i-dill)

Functional classification: Anticholinergic, antiparkinson
Chemical classification: Synthetic tertiary amine
FDA pregnancy category: C

Indications: Parkinsonism, EPSEs

Contraindications: Hypersensitivity, narrow-angle glaucoma, duodenal obstruction, peptic ulcer, prostatic hypertrophy, myasthenia gravis, megacolon

Pharmacologic Effects: Blocks cholinergic receptors, might inhibit the reuptake and storage of dopamine

Pharmacokinetics: Peak 1-1.3 hr, half-life 5.6-10.2 hr; little pharmacokinetic information is known

Side Effects: *CNS:* depression (19%-30%), disorientation, confusion, memory loss, hallucinations, psychoses, agitation, delusions, nervousness; *peripheral:* tachycardia, palpitations, hypotension, orthostatic hypotension, dry mouth, nausea, vomiting, constipation, paralytic ileus, blurred vision, mydriasis, diplopia, urinary retention and hesitancy, elevated temperature

Interactions

- *Amantadine:* increased anticholinergic effect
- *Digoxin:* increased digoxin serum levels
- *Haloperidol:* worsening of schizophrenia, decreased haloperidol serum levels
- *Levodopa:* possible reduction of levodopa efficacy
- *Phenothiazines:* increased anticholinergic effect, decreased antipsychotic effect

Implications
Assess
- VS, BP
- For glaucoma
- Mental status

Planning/Implementation
- Provide instructions for anticholinergic responses (i.e., dry mouth, constipation, urinary hesitancy, decreased sweating).

Teaching
- To take dose with meals
- That drug may cause drowsiness, blurred vision, dizziness; emphasize safety
- To avoid alcohol and other CNS depressants
- To notify physician should rapid or pounding heartbeat occur
- To use caution in hot weather

Evaluate
- EPSE improvement
- For adverse effects
- Mental status: confusion, delirium memory

Treatment of Overdose: Emesis, lavage, activated charcoal; treat respiratory depression, hyperpyrexia.

Administration
- *Parkinsonism: adult:* PO initially, 1-2 mg first day, increase by 2-mg increments at 3- to 5-day intervals, up to a daily dose of 5-15 mg in 3 divided doses at mealtime
- *EPSEs:* to start, 1 mg with 1 mg every few hours until symptoms controlled; maintenance or prophylactic use, 5-15 mg/day
- *Available forms:* tabs 2, 5 mg

Trimethadione*

TRIDIONE
(trye-meth-a-dye´-one)

Functional classification: Antiepileptic
Chemical classification: Oxazolidinedione
FDA pregnancy category: D

Indications: Refractory absence seizures (used only when other drugs have failed)

Contraindications: Hypersensitivity, blood dyscrasias
Cautious use: Hepatic or renal disease

Pharmacologic Effects: The exact nature of its action not known; therapeutic serum level 700 mg/ml

Pharmacokinetics: *PO:* peak 30 min-2 hr; excreted in kidneys; half-life of 12-24 hr, with a half-life of 6-13 days for the active metabolite dimethadione

Side Effects: Can be quite serious and have resulted in death; *CNS:* drowsiness, dizziness, fatigue, paresthesia, irritability, headache; *peripheral:* vaginal bleeding, albuminuria, nephrosis, abdominal pain, hepatic impairment, weight loss, nausea, vomiting, bleeding gums, abnormal liver function test, exfoliative dermatitis, systemic lupus erythematosus, lymphadenopathy, rash, alopecia, petechiae, erythema, photophobia, diplopia, epistaxis, retinal hemorrhage, hypertension, hypotension, thrombocytopenia, agranulocytosis, leukopenia, neutropenia, hemolytic anemia

Interactions: None known

Implications
Assess
- Blood studies: hematocrit, hemoglobin level, RBCs, serum folate and vitamin D values, if on long-term therapy regimen
- Hepatic studies: ALT, AST, bilirubin, and creatinine levels

- Skin; if rash occurs, withhold drug

Planning/Implementation
- Dilute oral solution with water.
- Instruct patient to take oral dose with juice or milk to cover taste and smell and to decrease GI symptoms.

Teaching
- To take with food if GI upset occurs
- To carry MedicAlert identification bracelet
- To notify physician if visual disturbances, sore throat, etc., occur
- To avoid driving and other activities that require alertness
- Not to discontinue medication abruptly after long-term use because convulsions might result

Evaluate
- Mental status
- Renal and hematologic problems

Treatment of Overdose: Symptoms include nausea, drowsiness, dizziness, ataxia, visual disturbances; coma in cases of massive overdose. Emesis, lavage; provide supportive care.

Administration
- *Adult:* PO 300 mg tid (900 mg/day), may increase by 300 mg/wk, not to exceed 600 mg qid (2400 mg/day); *child:* 300-900 mg/day in 3 or 4 equally divided doses
- *Available forms:* caps 300 mg; chew tabs 150 mg; oral sol 40 mg/ml

Trimipramine maleate

SURMONTIL
(tri-mip´-ra-meen)

Functional classification: Antidepressant
Chemical classification: Tricyclic, tertiary amine
FDA pregnancy category: C

Indications: Depression

Contraindications: Hypersensitivity to TCAs, recovery phase of myocardial infarction, convulsive disorders, prostatic hypertrophy, children
Cautious use: Suicidal patients, severe depression, increased intraocular pressure, narrow-angle glaucoma, urinary retention, cardiac disease, hepatic disease, hyperthyroidism, ECT, elective surgery, MAOI therapy

Pharmacologic Effects: Inhibits serotonin (+) and norepinephrine (+) uptake; also blocks ACh (+), histamine (+++++), and alpha-1 (+++) receptors; it is sedating with moderate anticholinergic effects; therapeutic plasma level 180 ng/ml

Pharmacokinetics: Metabolized by liver (P-450 2D6), excreted by kidneys, steady state 2-6 days; half-life 7-30 hr

T

Side Effects: See Amitriptyline; *specific for trimipramine:* dry mouth (~10%), blurred vision (~2%), constipation (~10%), sedation (~30%), orthostasis (~10%), tachycardia (~2%), sexual disturbance (-), weight gain (~10%), tremor (~10%)

Interactions: See Amitriptyline
- *Drugs metabolized by P-450 2D6:* increased serum levels of trimipramine

Implications: See Amitriptyline

Treatment of Overdose: ECG monitoring; induce emesis; lavage, activated charcoal; administer anticonvulsant; treat anticholinergic effects if needed.

Administration
- *Adult:* PO 75 mg/day in divided doses, may be increased to 300 mg/day; *adolescent and geriatric:* 50 mg/day to start, gradually increase to 100 mg/day
- *Available forms:* caps 25, 50, 100 mg

Valproates

- **DIVALPROEX SODIUM**
(dye-val-proe´-ex)
Depakote
- **VALPROATE SODIUM**
(val-proe´-ate)
Depacon
- **VALPROIC ACID**
(val-proe´-ik)
Depakene

Functional classification: Anticonvulsant
Chemical classification: Carboxylic acid derivative
FDA pregnancy category: D

Indications: Drug of choice for tonic-clonic and absence seizures; complex partial seizures, myoclonic seizures; bipolar disorders

Contraindications: Hypersensitivity to valproic acid; hepatic disease or significant hepatic dysfunction; teratogenic birth defects have been reported with valproic acid
Cautious use: Children with metabolic disorders, lactation, children <2 yr

Pharmacologic Effects: Apparently inhibits the spread of abnormal discharges through the brain by one or more of four hypothesized mechanisms: (1) increase of GABA by decreasing its metabolism or reducing its uptake, (2) an increased postsynaptic response to GABA, (3) an increase in the resting membrane potential r/t sodium channel regulation, and (4) by suppressing calcium influx through specific calcium channels; therapeutic serum levels 50-100 mg/ml

Pharmacokinetics: *PO:* rapidly absorbed, peak

levels 1-4 hr, time to steady state 2-4 days, half-life 6-16 hr, children with immature livers and older patients with cirrhosis or acute hepatitis have prolonged half lives (67 and 25 hours, respectively); serum protein binding (90%-95%)

Side Effects: Serious side effects not common; *CNS:* sedation but usually dissipates; *peripheral:* nausea; vomiting; indigestion; other GI symptoms; emotional upset; minor elevation in SGOT and LDH; severe hepatotoxicity might occur and has been linked to some fatalities; blood dyscrasias; rash

Interactions
- *Alcohol and other CNS depressants:* CNS depression
- *Anticonvulsants:* might increase serum levels of phenobarbital; clonazepam toxicity might be increased; phenytoin causes two opposite interactions: increase in serum phenytoin and decrease in serum phenytoin levels
- *Aspirin, warfarin:* prolonged bleeding time
- *Carbamazepine, phenytoin:* decreased valproic acid sera levels
- *Chlorpromazine, aspirin:* increased valproic acid half-life
- *Felbamate:* increase in mean valproic acid peak concentration
- *Rifampin:* increased oral clearance of valproic acid

Implications
Assess
- Blood studies, hepatic studies

Planning/Implementation
- Serious side effects are uncommon.
- Do not dilute elixir with carbonated beverage.

Teaching
- To take dose with food for GI upset
- To swallow tabs and caps whole to avoid irritation
- To take hs to avoid drowsiness during day
- That valproic acid alters blood and urine volume in diabetes
- To wear MedicAlert identification bracelet

Evaluate
- Efficacy of treatment

Treatment of Overdose: *Symptoms:* coma and death have occurred; however, more typical symptoms of overdose include motor restlessness, visual hallucinations; provide supportive care, paying close attention to adequate urinary output. Because the fraction of the drug not bound to serum proteins is high in overdose, hemodialysis might be helpful. Naloxone has been reported to reverse the CNS depression associated with valproic acid overdose.

Administration
- *Seizure control: adult and child:* PO 15 mg/kg/day; increase at weekly intervals by

5-10 mg/kg/day until seizures are controlled or as side effects dictate up to a maintenance dose of 20-60 mg/kg/day in divided doses

- *Bipolar disorder—manic phase: adult:* PO: start with 750 mg/day in divided doses; increase daily dose by 250 mg every 2-3 days to achieve lowest therapeutic dose that produces the desired clinical effect or the desired serum concentrations; maximum recommended dose 60 mg/kg/day; *child and adolescent:* use of valproic acid in patients <18 yr not established
- *Available forms: valproic acid:* caps 250 mg; syr 250 mg/5 ml; *valproate sodium–valproic acid:* tabs 125, 250, 500 mg

Venlafaxine

EFFEXOR
(ven-lah-facks´-in)

Functional classification: Novel antidepressant, selective serotonin norepinephrine reuptake inhibitor (SNRI)

Chemical classification: Phenethylamine

FDA pregnancy category: C

Indications: Depression, generalized anxiety disorder

Contraindications: Hypersensitivity to venlafaxine, pregnancy, lactation, use of MAOIs

Pharmacologic Effects: Inhibits norepinephrine (++) and serotonin uptake (+++); lacks affinity for histamine, ACh, or alpha-1 receptors

Pharmacokinetics: Well absorbed (98%) and extensively metabolized; undergoes significant first-pass metabolism but has a shorter half-life (5-11 hr) and lower protein binding (23%) than most antidepressants; is metabolized to an active metabolite, *O*-desmethylvenlafaxine, which has similar biochemical properties; venlafaxine's half-life is 5 hr; the active metabolite is 11 hr; protein binding 23%; steady state achieved in 3-4 days; excreted in urine; not a potent inhibitor of P-450 isoenzymes but is metabolized by P-450 2D6

Side Effects: *CNS:* headache (25%), somnolence (23%), dizziness (19%), insomnia (18%), nervousness (13%); *peripheral:* nausea (37%), dry mouth (22%), constipation (15%), asthenia (12%), sweating (12%), abnormal ejaculation/orgasm (12%), anorexia (11%), weight loss, hypertension (2%-5%) at high dosages (>225 mg/day)

Interactions
- *Cimetidine:* inhibits first-pass metabolism of venlafaxine
- *Drugs that inhibit cytochrome P-450 IID6:* potential for interaction

- *MAOIs:* risk of a serotonin syndrome, which can be fatal
- *Selegiline:* serotonergic reaction possible

Implications
Assess
- Use of MAOIs
- BP, VS, weight
- Baseline physical data
- Hepatic studies because of venlafaxine's extensive liver metabolism
- Activation of mania

Planning/Implementation
- Maintain safety.
- Administer with food to decrease GI upset.
- If discontinuing venlafaxine, do so gradually.
- If switching to MAOI, wait 7 days after stopping venlafaxine; if switching from MAOI to venlafaxine, wait at least 14 days before starting venlafaxine.

Teaching
- To take dose with food to prevent GI upset.
- To understand side effects that can occur and appropriate interventions to minimize them
- To avoid alcohol while taking venlafaxine
- To report rash, hives, swelling, sore throat, etc., indicative of allergic reaction
- To report pregnancy, intent to become pregnant, or lactation
- To report use of OTCs
- To avoid operating hazardous machinery

Evaluate
- Depression
- Mental status
- Minimal side effects
- Weight loss

Treatment of Overdose: Few overdoses have been reported, no fatalities have been reported, and symptoms, if any, are ill defined. Treatment of overdose includes maintenance of an airway, oxygenation, monitoring of VS, and supportive care. Consider use of charcoal, emetic, or lavage. Dialysis or forced diuresis seems to hold little promise of benefit for the patient. No specific antidotes are known.

Administration
- *Adult:* PO: starting dose is 75 mg/day in 2 or 3 divided doses taken with food; dosage may be increased to 150-225 mg/day in increments of 75 mg/day every 4 or more days; severely depressed patients might respond to a higher dosage up to 375-450 mg/day in 3 divided doses; *hepatic impairment:* reduce adult dose by 50%; *geriatric:* no dosage adjustment required; *child and adolescent:* not approved for use in children <18 yr
- *Available forms:* tabs 25, 37.5, 50, 75, 100 mg

V

Vigabatrin

SABRIL
(vi-gab´-a-trin)

Functional classification: Antiepileptic
Chemical classification: Structural analog of GABA
FDA pregnancy category:

Indications: Partial epilepsy, infantile spasms

Contraindications: Hypersensitivity
Cautious use: Renal disease

Pharmacologic Effects: Vigabatrin's antiepileptic effect is caused by its ability to irreversibly inhibit GABA-transaminase; this effectively increases brain GABA levels and decreases GABA-transaminase

Pharmacokinetics: Rapidly absorbed with or without food; bioavailability high; is not bound to plasma proteins; half-life 5-8 hr but half-life can be extended; is completely excreted by the kidneys unchanged; half-life is extended in elderly

Side Effects: *CNS:* drowsiness (13%-40%), fatigue, headache, depression (~12%), psychosis, irritability, severe behavior disturbance (3.4% adults, 6% children), visual field defects; *peripheral:* weight gain, GI complaints

Interactions: Because vigabatrin is not metabolized by the P-450 enzyme system, few drug-drug interactions have been reported; only known interaction is with phenytoin in which there is 15%-30% reduction in phenytoin serum levels

Implications: Withdrawal from vigabatrin should be gradual and should follow the administration titration schedule noted next; abrupt cessation can produce seizure exacerbation or status epilepticus

Treatment of Overdose: An encephalopathy might occur with vigabatrin overdose.

Administration

- *Adult*s: initially 0.5-1 g/day and then titrate upward at that dose on a weekly basis until reaching 2-3 g/day; can be increased to 4 g/day in some patients
- *Available forms:* tabs 500 mg

Zaleplon

SONATA
(zae-la´-plon)

Functional classification: Sedative and hypnotic

Chemical classification: Pyrazolapyrimidine derivative
FDA pregnancy category: C

Indications: Short-term treatment of insomnia

Contraindications: None known
Cautious use: Some abuse potential, elderly, COPD, child <18 yr, hepatic impairment

Pharmacologic Effects: Interacts with GABA receptor chloride channel complex at the benzodiazepine site (BZ-1)

Pharmacokinetics: Extensively metabolized primarily by aldehyde oxidase (major) and by P-450 3A4 isoenzymes; is more rapidly metabolized and excreted than is zolpidem; rapid onset of action; not highly protein bound; half-life 1 hr

Side Effects: >1% of patients report the following side effects: *CNS:* headache (28%), asthenia (5%), dizziness (7%), somnolence (5%), amnesia, anxiety (2%); *peripheral:* nausea (7%), dyspepsia (4%), abdominal pain (5%), myalgia (7%), dysmenorrhea (2%), ocular pain, fever, malaise, anorexia, tremor (2%)

Interactions

- *Cimetine:* increases half-life of zaleplon
- *CNS depressants:* additive effect
- *CYP-450 3A4 inducers* (carbamazepine, phenytoin, rifampin, phenobarbital): decreased sera levels of zaleplon
- *CYP-450 3A4 inhibitors:* no likely interaction

Implications
Assess
- Baseline physical data
- BP, US
- History of hypersensitivity
- History of heatic or renal disorder

Planning/Implementation
- Assist with ambulation.
- Carefully observe patients with history of addiction.
- Ensure side rails, night-light, and call bell are within reach.

Teaching
- To take immediately before bedtime and get at least 4 hr sleep
- Not to take with a high-fat meal
- To take as prescribed
- To use caution if driving or operating hazardous machinery
- To report to clinician any adverse effects
- To report to clinician if taking a new medication or an OTC drug
- That women should notify prescriber if planning on becoming pregnant

Treatment of Overdose: There is limited information at this time about zaleplon overdose. Symptoms are expected to be exaggerations of pharmacologic effects. Mild cases will no doubt manifest as drowsiness, mental confusion, and lethargy. More severe cases will present as ataxia, hypotonia, hypotension, respiratory, depression, and rarely coma. Treatment is supportive along with gastric lavage when appropriate.

Administration
- *Adult:* 5-10 mg hs
- *Available forms:* caps 5, 10 mg

Ziprasidone
ZELDOX (NOT APPROVED AT THIS WRITING)
(zee-praz´-uh-dohn)

Functional classification: Atypical antipsychotic
Chemical classification: Benzisothiazolyl piperazine
FDA pregnancy category: Pregnancy information not available at this time

Indications: Psychoses

Contraindications: Hypersensitivity

Pharmacologic Effects: Has a higher affinity and antagonism for $5HT_{2A}$ and moderate for D_2; also an agonist for the $5HT_{1A}$ receptor and blocks the reuptake of norepinephrine; these mechanisms suggest a potential for both positive and negative schizophrenia and a potential for relieving anxiety and depression that is often associated with schizophrenia; has low modest affinity for D_1, muscarinic, and alpha-2 receptors

Pharmacokinetics: Is about 5 times more potent than chlorpromazine, peak plasma concentrations occur within 4 hr; baseline bioavailability is 30% but increases to 60% if taken with food; protein binding 98%-99%; metabolized by P-450 3A4 to nonactive metabolites; half-life 5-10 hr; ziprasidone does not inhibit the P-450 system

Side Effects: Ziprasidone, in early reports, is thought to produce few EPSEs, anticholinergic, antiadrenergic, or antihistaminic side effects; also these reports suggest less weight gain than the other atypical agents cause; most common side effects reported are as follows: *CNS:* headache, somnolence, dizziness; *peripheral:* nausea, dyspepsia, weakness, nasal discharge, orthostatic hypotension, tachycardia

Treatment of Overdose: There is little experience with ziprasidone overdose at this time.

Administration: In some studies, ziprasidone has been successfully dosed at 80 and 160 mg/day in divided doses

Zolpidem
AMBIEN
(zol´-pih-dem)

Functional classification: Sedative, hypnotic (nonbarbiturate)
Chemical classification: Imidazopyridine
Controlled substance schedule IV
FDA pregnancy category: B

Indications: Short-term treatment of insomnia

Contraindications: Hypersensitivity to zolpidem *Cautious use:* Acute intermittent porphyria, impaired hepatic or renal function; susceptibility to respiratory problems; depression; history of drug dependence

Pharmacologic Effects: Modulation of GABA receptor chloride channels might be responsible for several therapeutic effects, including sedation

Pharmacokinetics: Onset 0.5-1 hr; rapid absorption from GI tract; half-life 2.6 hr; protein binding 92%; half-life and bioavailability increased in elderly and patients with hepatic function impairment; zolpidem converted to inactive metabolites and excreted in urine

Side Effects: *CNS:* headache (19%); drowsiness (8%); dizziness (5%); *peripheral:* myalgia (7%); nausea (6%); dyspepsia (5%)

Interactions
- *Food:* peak concentrations are decreased, and time to concentration is prolonged

Implications
Assess
- Baseline physical data
- BP, VS
- History of hypersensitivity
- History of hepatic or renal disorders

Planning/Implementation
- Carefully observe patients known to be suicidal.
- Taper drug slowly if discontinuance is warranted.
- Assist with ambulation.
- Ensure that side rails, night-light, call bell are within reach.

Teaching
- To avoid alcohol and other CNS depressants
- That drug might cause drowsiness; to use caution in operating hazardous machinery

Evaluate
- Therapeutic response: ability to sleep at night, decreased amount of early-morning awakening
- Mental status

- Type of sleep problem: falling asleep or staying asleep

Treatment of Overdose: With zolpidem alone, symptoms range from somnolence to light coma; recovery has been reported when 400 mg have been taken, which is 40 times the recommended dose; when mixed with CNS depressant agents, fatalities have occurred; supportive care is required, with immediate lavage; monitor hypotension and CNS depression; withhold sedating drugs, even if CNS excitement occurs; flumazenil might be useful; dialysis will probably not be very useful.

Administration

- *Adult:* PO: usual dose 5-10 mg immediately before bedtime; maximum dose 10 mg; *elderly or debilitated patient:* PO: initially 5 mg immediately before bedtime; *child and adolescent:* not approved for children <18 yr
- *Available forms:* tabs 5, 10 mg

INDEX

Page numbers in italics indicate illustra-
tions; *t* indicates tables. Drug names
appear in bold.